Periodontics

The Complete Summary

Library of Congress Cataloging-in-Publication Data

Names: Suárez López del Amo, Fernando, editor.
Title: Periodontics: The Complete Summary / edited by Fernando Suárez López del Amo.
Description: Batavia, IL : Quintessence Publishing Co, Inc, [2021] | Includes bibliographical references and index. | Summary: "Textbook covers a broad range of topics to prepare aspiring periodontists for exams as well as dental practice, including vocab words, tables, diagrams, and illustrations for additional context"-- Provided by publisher.
Identifiers: LCCN 2020007624 (print) | LCCN 2020007625 (ebook) | ISBN 9780867159608 (softcover) | ISBN 9781647240301 (ebook) | ISBN 9781647240318 (ebook)
Subjects: MESH: Periodontal Diseases | Periodontium | Periodontics--methods | Study Guide
Classification: LCC RK450.P4 (print) | LCC RK450.P4 (ebook) | NLM WU 18.2 | DDC 617.6/32--dc23
LC record available at https://lccn.loc.gov/2020007624
LC ebook record available at https://lccn.loc.gov/2020007625

QUINTESSENCE PUBLISHING USA

Quintessence Publishing Co, Inc
411 N Raddant Road
Batavia, IL 60510
www.quintpub.com

5 4 3 2 1

Editor: Marieke Zaffron
Design: Sue Zubek
Production: Sarah Minor

Printed in the USA

PERIODONTICS
The Complete Summary

Edited by

Fernando Suárez López del Amo, DDS, MS

Private Practice
Tacoma, Washington

QUINTESSENCE PUBLISHING

Berlin | Chicago | Tokyo
Barcelona | London | Milan | Mexico City | Moscow | Paris | Prague | Seoul | Warsaw
Beijing | Istanbul | Sao Paulo | Zagreb

CONTENTS

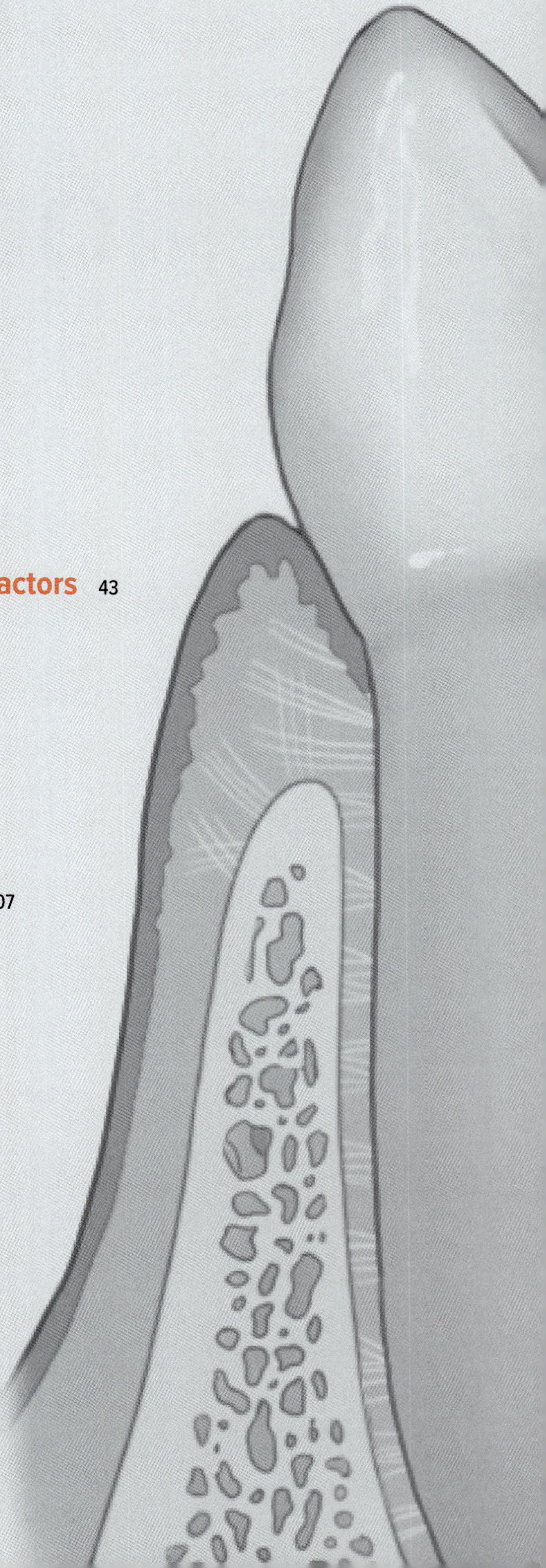

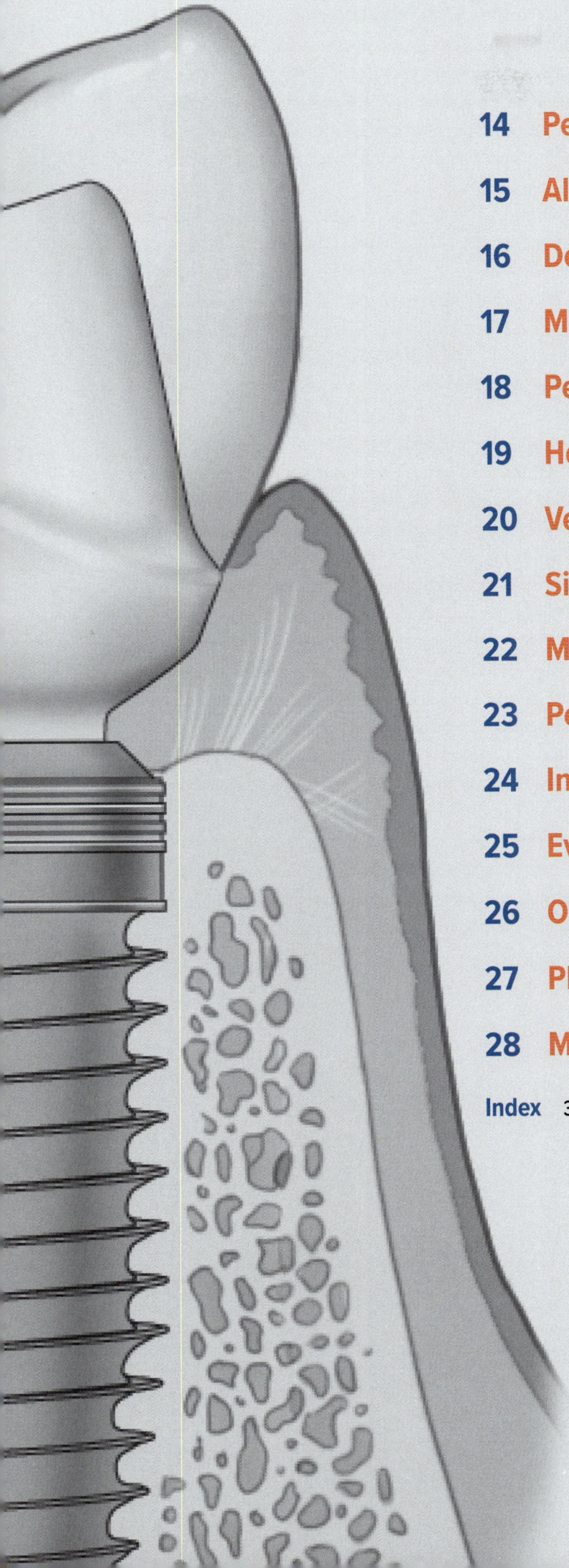

FOREWORD

In this day and age, an overwhelming influx of information is flooding the scientific literature. Separating wheat from chaff can be an arduous and demanding task for any oral health care professional, expert or novice, when reviewing the best available evidence in the fields of periodontics and oral implantology. A well-curated and comprehensive compilation of essential knowledge can be an invaluable compass to navigate what may seem to be an insurmountable ocean of data and concepts.

That is why I enthusiastically applaud Dr Fernando Suárez López del Amo for his vision and dedication in leading the efforts that have culminated in making this book, *Periodontics: The Complete Summary*, a reality. Knowing Fernando for more than a decade now, I have truly enjoyed witnessing his development and inexorable growth in becoming an excellent clinician, outstanding scholar, and tremendously effective teacher. It is rare for an individual of such virtues to also seek to engage and elevate the profession by generating quality didactic materials. This textbook is a clear representation of Fernando's commitment.

Spanning from the anatomy of periodontal and peri-implant structures to the management of medical emergencies, this book contains a cleverly weaved sequence of meticulously selected topics covering the most relevant literature pertaining to the diagnosis, prevention, and treatment of common periodontal and peri-implant diseases and conditions. Readers will notice that a great deal of attention was paid to scrupulously select and present pertinent information stemming both from classic and contemporary literature sources, providing it in a succinct and understandable manner. Although this book is primarily geared to serve as a guide for students throughout their formal training and in their preparation for standardized exams, more experienced professionals will also find it an excellent reference or "refresher" resource.

While Fernando is responsible for its genesis, organization, and successful completion, it must be acknowledged that this book is also the result of a collective endeavor carried out by a marvelous bunch of young and emerging clinicians, researchers, and educators from different geographic locations across the globe. It is exciting to see such a talented group coming together to generate an up-to-date and valuable compendium of foundational knowledge germane to periodontics and oral implantology. Congratulations to all of them for this superb contribution!

With my best wishes,

Gustavo Avila-Ortiz, DDS, MS, PhD
Professor and Chair
Department of Periodontics
College of Dentistry
University of Iowa
Iowa City, Iowa

PREFACE

The fields of periodontics and oral implantology have greatly advanced and evolved over the last decades. Numerous investigations and developments have redefined the instruments, materials, and techniques used in daily practice, and we, the scientists and clinicians, should always be at the forefront of this continuous evolution. However, while remaining up to date is imperative to provide the best possible patient care, it is of utmost importance to acknowledge and understand the scientific discoveries and investigations previously performed. It is critical to appreciate the lessons learned decades ago to continue with the progression of the periodontal and dental implant fields. For this reason, I decided to embark on this project, and along with the outstanding contribution of a talented group of friends and colleagues, we have created this summary aimed at describing the underlying scientific basis and rationale for the numerous challenges and decisions that periodontists face in clinical practice. Special attention was given to provide the fundamental classic literature as well as newer and more current evidence.

The information presented in this book is a comprehensive review of the most essential knowledge pertaining to the different aspects of periodontics and oral implantology. From anatomy to medical emergencies, the 28 chapters summarize topics related to diagnosis, nonsurgical and surgical therapy, guided tissue regeneration, dental implants, and oral pathology. Students in the dental and periodontal fields will find this book of utmost value during their training. Nevertheless, this book was also conceived with the objective of being a source of information and consultation guide for more senior professionals, including investigators and clinicians.

ACKNOWLEDGMENTS

First, I would like to thank my parents, Antonio and Mónica, for their unconditional love, endless support, and encouragement. For showing me that with passion and sacrifice, everything is possible. I also want to thank Morgan for her love, patience, and support throughout these years from when the idea of creating the book first originated until the final chapter was proofread. I would most like to thank my mentors in Spain and at the University of Michigan, who instilled in me the love for this profession. I have been tremendously fortunate to have mentors throughout my career who have not only taught me dentistry and periodontics, but also served as inspiration and role models. Last but not least, I deeply thank all the authors and coauthors that have collaborated on this project. Their hard work and dedication have made the completion of this book possible. I also want to thank the staff of Quintessence Publishing and particularly Bryn Grisham, as well as Marieke Zaffron for her excellent work editing this book.

CONTRIBUTORS

Aeshah Alkanderi, BMedSc, BDM, MS
Periodontist
Department of Periodontics
Jaber Al Ahmad Al Sabah Dental Specialty Center
Shuhada, Kuwait

Farah Asa'ad, BDS, MSc, PhD
Postdoctoral Researcher
Department of Biomaterials
Institute of Clinical Sciences
Sahlgrenska Academy
University of Gothenburg
Gothenburg, Sweden

Federico Ausenda, DDS, MS
Visiting Assistant Professor
Department of Periodontology
School of Dental Medicine
Tufts University
Boston, Massachusetts

Clinical Instructor
Department of Biomedical, Surgical, and Dental Sciences
University of Milan

Private Practice
Milan, Italy

Lucía Barallat, DDS, MS, PhD
Associate Professor
Department of Periodontology
The University Dental Clinic
International University of Catalonia

Private Practice Limited to Periodontology and Implant Dentistry
Barcelona, Spain

Alvaro Blasi, DDS, CDT
Adjunct Assistant Professor
Department of Restorative Sciences
Dental College of Georgia
Augusta University
Augusta, Georgia

Private Practice
Barcelona, Spain

Gonzalo Blasi, DDS, MS
Dean's Faculty
Division of Periodontics
School of Dentistry
University of Maryland
Baltimore, Maryland

Associate Faculty
Department of Periodontics
The University Dental Clinic
International University of Catalonia

Private Practice
Barcelona, Spain

Ignacio Blasi, DDS, MS, PhD
Dean's Faculty
Division of Orthodontics
School of Dentistry
University of Maryland
Baltimore, Maryland

Private Practice
Fairfax, Virginia

Private Practice
Barcelona, Spain

Miguel Romero Bustillos, DDS, PhD
Resident
Iowa Institute for Oral Health Research
Department of Periodontics
College of Dentistry and Dental Clinics
University of Iowa
Iowa City, Iowa

Carlos Parra Carrasquer, DDS
Clinical Assistant Professor
Assistant Program Director
Department of Periodontics
Texas A&M University College of Dentistry
Dallas, Texas

Emilio Couso-Queiruga, DDS, MS
Resident
Department of Periodontics
College of Dentistry and Dental Clinics
University of Iowa
Iowa City, Iowa

Anusha Reddy Etikala, BDS, MS
Private Practice Limited to Periodontics and Implant Dentistry
Seattle, Washington

Basel Elnayef, DDS, MS, PhD
Assistant Professor
Department of Oral and Maxillofacial Surgery
The University Dental Clinic
International University of Catalonia

Private Practice
Barcelona, Spain

Carlos Garaicoa-Pazmiño, DDS, MS
Associate Professor
Department of Periodontology
School of Dentistry
Oregon Health & Science University
Portland, Oregon

Alexandra Plonka Hosking, DDS, MS
Adjunct Clinical Lecturer in Dentistry
Department of Periodontics and Oral Medicine
School of Dentistry
University of Michigan
Ann Arbor, Michigan

Private Practice Limited to Periodontics and Implantology
Grosse Pointe Woods, Michigan

Theodoros Katsaros, DDS, MSD
Clinical Assistant Professor
Graduate Program Director
Department of Periodontics
College of Dentistry and Dental Clinics
University of Iowa
Iowa City, Iowa

Arash Khojasteh, DDS, MS, PhD
Chairman and Program Director
Department of Tissue Engineering and Applied Cell Sciences
Associate Professor
Department of Oral and Maxillofacial Surgery
Shahid Beheshti University of Medical Sciences
Tehran, Iran

Vahid Khoshkam, DDS, MS
Private Practice Limited to Periodontics and Implantology
El Paso, Texas

Private Practice Limited to Periodontics and Implantology
Karaj, Iran

Guo-Hao Lin, DDS, MS
Health Sciences Assistant Clinical Professor
Department of Orofacial Sciences
School of Dentistry
University of California, San Francisco
San Francisco, California

Manoela Domingues Martins, DDS, PhD
Associate Professor
Department of Oral Pathology
School of Dentistry
Federal University of Rio Grande do Sul
Porto Alegre, Brazil

Alberto Monje, DDS, MS, PhD
Assistant Lecturer
Department of Periodontology
The University Dental Clinic
International University of Catalonia
Barcelona, Spain

Adjunct Clinical Assistant Professor
Department of Periodontology
School of Dentistry
University of Michigan
Ann Arbor, Michigan

Private Practice
Badajoz, Spain

Jose Nart, DDS, PhD
Professor
Chairman and Program Director
Department of Periodontology
The University Dental Clinic
International University of Catalonia
Barcelona, Spain

Vice President
Spanish Society of Periodontics and Osseointegration

Andrea Ravidà, DDS, MS
Resident
Department of Periodontics and Oral Medicine
School of Dentistry
University of Michigan
Ann Arbor, Michigan

Juan C. Rodríguez, DDS, MS
Private Practice
East Lansing, Michigan

Adjunct Clinical Assistant Professor
Department of Periodontics and Oral Medicine
School of Dentistry
University of Michigan
Ann Arbor, Michigan

Rachel Sheridan Sinacola, DDS, MS
Private Practice
Grand Rapids, Michigan

Adjunct Clinical Lecturer in Dentistry
Department of Periodontics and Oral Medicine
School of Dentistry
University of Michigan
Ann Arbor, Michigan

Fernando Suárez López del Amo, DDS, MS
Private Practice
Tacoma, Washington

Mustafa Tattan, BDS
Resident
Department of Periodontics
College of Dentistry and Dental Clinics
University of Iowa
Iowa City, Iowa

Lorenzo Tavelli, DDS, MS
Adjunct Clinical Assistant Professor and Research Fellow
Department of Periodontics and Oral Medicine
School of Dentistry
University of Michigan
Ann Arbor, Michigan

Vivian Petersen Wagner, DDS, PhD
Postdoctoral Researcher
Department of Oral Diagnosis
Piracicaba School of Dentistry
University of Campinas
Campinas, Brazil

Shan-Huey Yu, DDS, MS
Clinical Assistant Professor
Department of Periodontics and Oral Medicine
School of Dentistry
University of Michigan
Ann Arbor, Michigan

1

ANATOMY

Miguel Romero Bustillos, DDS, PhD

The **periodontium** comprises the supporting structures of the dentition. It is composed of four main elements: gingiva, cementum, periodontal ligament (PDL), and bone. Understanding this dynamic network of tissues is pivotal for the proper performance of the many procedures related to periodontal therapy. This chapter describes the different structures of the periodontium from microscopic and macroscopic points of view.

The **attachment apparatus**, also known as *periodontal attachment*, is an aggregate of tissues with the main function of anchoring teeth to the alveolus. It consists of cementum, alveolar bone, PDL, and gingiva. Several terms are highly relevant with this regard and are described by the American Academy of Periodontology (AAP) *Glossary of Periodontal Terms* (see sidebar).[1]

Periodontium: Attachment Apparatus

PERIODONTAL LIGAMENT

The **PDL** is a specialized connective tissue located between the bony walls of the dental socket and the dental root. It surrounds the majority of the dental root and attaches the teeth to the alveolar bone. In the most coronal portion, the PDL is continued with the lamina propria of the gingiva. Characterized by its hourglass shape, this specialized connective tissue narrows at the middle part, with an average width ranging from 0.2 to 0.4 mm.[3] The PDL space decreases with age and increases under excessive load.

Origin

The PDL develops in a cell population from the dental follicle. As the crown approaches the oral mucosa, fibroblasts produce collagen fibrils without organized orientation. Later, prior to tooth eruption, the fibroblasts adopt an oblique orientation adjacent to the cementum. Finally, after this fibroblast arrangement, fibers with organized orientation are developed at the cementum surface as well as at the alveolar bone proper. These fibers will continue elongating until they reach each other at the middle portion of the

DEFINITIONS AND TERMINOLOGY

Alveolar bone proper: Compact bone that composes the alveolus (tooth socket). Also known as the *lamina dura* or *cribriform plate*, the fibers of the periodontal ligament insert into it.

Alveolar process: The compact and cancellous bony structure that surrounds and supports the teeth.

Attached gingiva: The portion of the gingiva that is firm, dense, stippled, and tightly bound to the underlying periosteum, tooth, and bone.

Attachment apparatus: The cementum, periodontal ligament, and alveolar bone.

Biologic width: The dimension of soft tissue composed of a connective tissue and epithelial attachment extending from the crest of bone to the most apical extent of the pocket or sulcus. This term was recently redefined as "supracrestal tissue attachment."[2]

Bundle bone: A type of alveolar bone, so-called because of the "bundle" pattern caused by the continuation of the principal (Sharpey) fibers into it.

Fibroblast: The predominant connective tissue cell; a flattened, irregularly branched cell with a large oval nucleus that is responsible in part for the production and remodeling of the extracellular matrix.

TABLE 1-1 Principal periodontal ligament fibers[4,5]

	Location	Origin	Insertion	Orientation	Function
Alveolar crest fibers	Between CEJ and alveolar bone crest	Cementum	Alveolar crest	Mostly bucco-lingual but also mesiodistal	Prevent extrusion of the teeth and resist lateral tooth movements
Horizontal fibers	Directly apical to the crest	Cementum	Alveolar bone proper	Horizontal across the PDL	Prevent lateral tooth movement
Oblique fibers	Middle two-thirds of the PDL	Cementum	Alveolar bone proper	Oblique in a coronal direction	Resist apically directed chewing forces
Apical fibers	Apical portion of the PDL	Apical portion of cementum	Apical portion of alveolar bone proper	Irregular fashion in horizontal or vertical dimension	Resist forces of luxation
Interradicular fibers	Furcation region	Interradicular cementum	Interradicular coronal portion of alveolar bone proper	Vertical and horizontal	Resist tooth tipping, torquing, and luxation
Transalveolar fibers	Primarily crestal region	Cementum	Cementum of adjacent tooth	Horizontal	Provide support and stability, prevent tooth movement

CEJ, cementoenamel junction.

Free gingiva: The part of the gingiva that surrounds the tooth and is not directly attached to the tooth surface.

Gingival groove: A shallow, V-shaped groove that is closely associated with the apical extent of free gingiva and runs parallel to the margin of the gingiva. The frequency of its occurrence varies widely.

Gingival papilla: The portion of the gingiva that occupies the interproximal spaces. The interdental extension of the gingiva.

Hertwig epithelial root sheath (HERS): An extension of the enamel organ (cervical loop) Determines the shape of the roots and initiates dentin formation during tooth development. Its remnants persist as epithelial rests of Malassez in the periodontal ligament.

PDL. The orientation of the fibers will be determined by the location within the PDL (Table 1-1).[4,5]

Composition

The PDL is formed by different cell types. The fibroblasts are the most abundant as they are responsible for the metabolism of the extracellular components. Within this heterogeneous population of fibroblasts within the PDL, osteoblast-like fibroblasts are also present, and these are rich in alkaline phosphatase.[6,7] In addition, the PDL contains stem cells, epithelial cell rests of Malassez, cells from the blood vessels, and cells associated with the immune and nervous systems.

The extracellular matrix of the PDL consists of collagenous and noncollagenous proteins. Collagen type I is the most abundant, and it is also the primary constituent of the Sharpey fibers, together with collagen II, V, VI, XII, and XIV.[8] Other noncollagenous proteins present in the PDL are tenascin, fibronectin, vitronectin, elastin, and glycoproteins. In addition, hyaluronate, heparan sulfate, chondroitin sulfate, and dermatan sulfate are the glycosaminoglycans identified in the PDL. Dermatan sulfate is the principal glycosaminoglycan, while versican and decorin are the main proteoglycans.[8,9]

ALVEOLAR BONE

One of the two mineralized tissues that comprises the attachment apparatus is the alveolar bone. Just like any other type of bone in the human body, it is composed of a mineralized matrix and a nonmineralized connective tissue. Within the mineralized tissues, calcium is the most prevalent mineral in the form of hydroxyapatite. The alveolar bone, also known as **alveolar process**, consists of spongy bone, cortical plates, and the **alveolar bone proper** (Table 1-2). The crest of the alveolar bone refers to the most coronal portion of it, and its distance from the cementoenamel junction (CEJ) in a healthy periodontium is within the range of 1 to 3 mm.

The alveolar bone is created following an intramembranous ossification with ectomesenchymal cells from the dental follicle intervening in the developmental process. The presence of teeth is essential for the development of the alveolar bone. As such, in absence of a PDL, the alveolar bone proper will not develop.[5]

The alveolar bone houses the teeth, providing protection and support and allowing proper functioning during mastication, absorbing and distributing the occlusal forces. The primary function of the alveolar bone is to provide a structure where the Sharpey fibers of the PDL anchor to keep the tooth in position and function.

The chemical composition of alveolar bone is 65% hydroxyapatite and 35% organic material such as collagen and noncollagenous proteins (eg, osteocalcin, bone sialoprotein, phosphoprotein, osteonectin, and bone morphogenetic proteins).

Microscopically, two different types of mature bone can be observed based on the organization: *(1)* the lamellar bone, containing osteons which consist of a blood vessel surrounded by concentric lamellae, and *(2)* the **bundle bone** where PDL fibers (Sharpey fibers) anchor. In the bundle bone, lamellae can be found parallel to adjacent marrow spaces, and the disposition is parallel to the tooth surface.

CEMENTUM

Cementum is the second mineralized tissue of the attachment apparatus. It is an avascular mineralized connective tissue that surrounds the dentin at the level of the dental root. Its primary function is to allow for the anchorage of Sharpey fibers that will keep the tooth in the alveolus as well as to adapt and protect during tooth wear and movement. The thickness of cementum increases with age. Also, apical portions of the dental root present with thicker cementum than the coronal counterparts.[5] The CEJ is the anatomical area where the crown meets the root. Schroeder and Scherle[10] described three types of relationships between cementum and enamel: edge to edge; cementum covering the enamel; or a gap between both structures where dentin is exposed. The most prevalent interrelation is cementum covering the enamel, followed by edge to edge and gap.[11]

Based on the presence of cementocytes embedded in its extracellular matrix, the cementum can be classified as cellular or acellular. In addition,

Lamina propria: In the mucous membrane, the connective tissue coat just beneath the epithelium and basement membrane. In skin, this layer is known as the *dermis*.

Mucogingival junction: The junction of the gingiva and the alveolar mucosa.

Osseointegration: A direct contact, at the light microscopic level, between living bone tissue and an implant.

Periodontal ligament (PDL): A specialized fibrous connective tissue that surrounds and attaches roots of teeth to the alveolar bone. Also known as the *periodontal membrane*.

Periodontium: The tissues that invest and support the teeth, including the gingiva, alveolar mucosa, cementum, periodontal ligament, and alveolar supporting bone. Also known as the *supporting structure of the tooth*.

Rete pegs: Ridge-like projections of epithelium into the underlying stroma of connective tissue that normally occur in the mucous membrane and dermal tissue subject to functional stimulation.

TABLE 1-2 Features of alveolar bone

	Location	Thickness	Composition	Characteristics
Alveolar bone proper	Wall of the socket	0.1 to 0.4 mm	Lamellated and bundle bone	• Perforated, carrying interalveolar nerves and blood vessels. • Radiographically identified as cribriform plate or lamina dura.
Spongy bone	Between alveolar bone proper and cortical plates	More volume present in maxilla at interdental and interradicular septa. Very limited in buccal sites followed by lingual and palate sites.	Trabeculae surrounded by marrow that contains adipocytes and pluripotent stem cells	• Highly vascularized. The amount and organization will determine the classification. • Regular or irregular orientation of trabeculae can be identified based on the location.
Cortical plates	Outline the alveolar process	Variable from posterior to anterior sites. Buccal thinner than lingual.	Osteons and interstitial lamellae	• Poor intrinsic vascularization. Highly remodeled in the most coronal portion after tooth extraction.

TABLE 1-3 Features of the different types of cementum

	Location	Thickness	Contain cells	Intrinsic collagen fibers	Extrinsic collagen fibers	Developed by
Acellular afibrillar cementum	Coronal part, covering enamel surface. One of the components of acellular extrinsic fiber cementum.	1 to 15 μm	No	No	No	Cementoblasts
Acellular extrinsic fiber cementum	Cervical third of the root	30 to 230 μm	No	No	Yes (composed of bundles of Sharpey fibers)	Cementoblasts and fibroblasts
Cellular mixed stratified cementum	Apical third of the root and furcation. Tip of the apex.	100 to 1,000 μm	Yes	Yes	Yes (composed of bundles of Sharpey fibers)	Cementoblasts and fibroblasts
Cellular intrinsic fiber cementum	Filling resorption lacunae of the root	Varies	Yes	Yes	No	Cementoblasts

the fibers that form the cementum will contribute to the classification of the different types[5] (Table 1-3).

As in the formation of the PDL, cementum starts developing in a prefunctional stage prior to the eruption of the tooth. After the crown is formed, the cells of the inner and outer enamel epithelium that constitute the cervical loop will proliferate deeper into the ectomesenchyme driving the development of the dental root. This structure is known as the **Hertwig epithelial root sheath (HERS)**. The most apical portion of the HERS, which encloses the dental papilla, is known as the *epithelial diaphragm*. Cells from the HERS induce the differentiation of the dental papilla cells in a coronoapical direction to become odontoblasts that will form the dentin of the root. The number and morphology of the dental roots will be determined by the disposition of the HERS. The cementum, the mineral portion of the root facing the PDL, is formed by cementoblasts that are believed to originate from the ectomesenchymal cells of the dental follicle after the disintegration of the HERS. Cells from the HERS produce different proteins and mediators to induce the differentiation of the dental follicle cells into cementoblasts. Fibroblasts in the area produce bundles of collagen fibrils that form fringe fibers, and these are anchored to the tooth by the deposition of a mineral matrix by cementoblasts.

When the tooth is near to entering its functional stage, a shift in the formation of cementum can be seen from acellular extrinsic fibrillar cementum to mixed stratified cementum. The rate of growth of cementum is 1.5 to 3 μm per year.[12]

Even though the previously described formation of cementum is the most accepted theory, an alternative hypothesis has been proposed. This theory suggests an enhanced role of the HERS in the formation of cementum through the differentiation of HERS cells to become cementoblasts.[13]

The chemical composition of cementum is similar to bone with approximately one-third organic material, one-third mineral phase, and one-third water. The primary inorganic structure of cementum is also hydroxyapatite crystals. The organic material is composed of collagen, glycoproteins, and proteoglycans (Box 1-1).

BOX 1-1 Organic chemical composition of cementum

Collagenous proteins	Collagen I (90%) Collagen III (5%)
Noncollagenous proteins	Glycoproteins Glycolipids Proteoglycans Enamel-related proteins

GINGIVA

The oral mucosa is composed of the mucosal tissues that cover the mouth, and it can be classified as masticatory mucosa (gingiva and hard palate), lining mucosa (alveolar mucosa, floor of the month, and internal surface of lips), and specialized mucosa (tongue). The lining or alveolar mucosa extends inside the cheeks, floor of the mouth, as well as soft palate, and it is characterized by the presence of a basal layer (which is positive to the expression of keratin 5, 14, and 19), an intermediate layer, and a superficial layer expressing keratin 13 and 4.[14]

The gingiva (masticatory mucosa) is composed of **free gingiva** and **attached gingiva**, and it is characterized by the presence of keratin in the most superficial layer. Histologically, four layers of cells have been described (Fig 1-1):

1. Stratum basale, which is characterized by the expression of keratin 5 and 14
2. Stratum spinous, named due to the spinous morphology of the cells in this layer
3. Stratum granulosum, characterized by the presence of round cytoplasmic granules
4. Stratum corneum with cornified cells

Gingiva has different names and presents with slight morphologic differences depending on the tissue that it covers (ie, free gingiva or attached gingiva; Fig 1-2).

Free gingiva

Free gingiva is the portion of the gingival epithelium that extends from the free gingival margin to the gingival groove (see Fig 1-2). The **gingival groove** is defined as the "shallow linear depression on the gingiva surface that demarcates the free gingiva and the attached gingiva."[1] The free gingiva covers the teeth at the vestibular and lingual sites following the contour of the tooth and the dental papilla. In normal conditions, the free gingiva presents as a coral pink color. The location of the gingival groove is determined by the position of the CEJ, and it is present in 4% to 54% of teeth with differences based on tooth type.[15,16]

Attached gingiva

Attached to the tooth and/or alveolar bone, the attached gingiva is delimited by the gingival groove at the coronal end and the mucogingival junction at the apical end. In healthy conditions, it also presents with a coral pink color. A morphologic characteristic of the attached gingiva is the stippling or orange peel appearance. The stippling corresponds to small epithelial ridges and is developed in areas of high keratinization. When the attached gingiva is inflamed, it loses the superficial stippling, and the color turns to a darker red.[15,17,18]

The **mucogingival junction**, which is the interphase between the attached gingiva and the oral mucosa, is located between 3 to 5 mm apical to the alveolar crest, and it has been shown to be stable over the years in reference to the base of the mandible or floor of the nose. Consequently, an increase in attached gingiva with age has been associated with the continuous eruption of the dentition.[19,20] The dimensions of the attached gingiva have been investigated in classic studies by Bowers[21] and Voigt

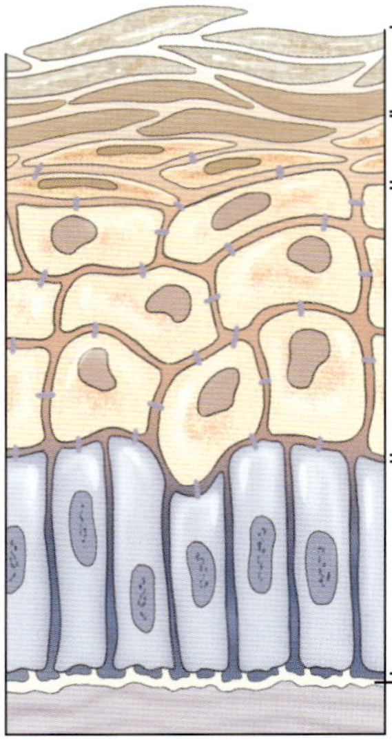

Fig 1-1 Layers of keratinized gingiva.

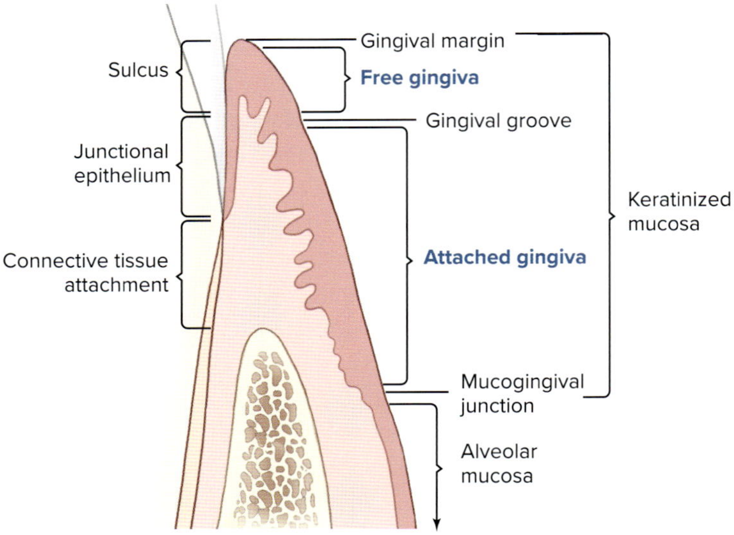

Fig 1-2 The gingiva.

et al.[22] In the maxilla, the sites with the greatest width of attached gingiva are the central and lateral incisors. There is a decrease in canines and first premolars, and a slight increase over the second premolar and molar locations. In the mandible, the incisors also present with the greatest amount of attached gingiva with a sharp decrease around the canines and first premolars. At the second premolar site, the attached gingiva increases, and a decrease at the mandibular molar area is also observed. On the lingual aspect, the molar area presents with the greatest attached gingiva followed by premolars, incisors, and canines.

Based on the location and microscopic appearance, the gingival epithelium can be classified into three types: oral, sulcular, and junctional epithelium.

Oral epithelium

The oral epithelium is a keratinized stratified squamous epithelium that extends from the mucogingival junction to the free gingival margin. In some areas of the most superficial layer, the stratum corneum, the cells maintain their nuclei and are considered parakeratinized. If no nuclei are present in the stratum corneum, this epithelium is considered orthokeratinized. In addition to the keratinocytes, other cells can be found in the oral epithelium, such as melanocytes, which give pigmentation to the epithelium; Langerhans cells, which play a role in the immune response; and Merkel cells, which are important for sensory function.

Sulcular epithelium

This is the epithelial tissue located in the sulcus, and it extends from the free gingival margin to the most coronal portion of the junctional epithelium. It is a nonkeratinized stratified squamous epithelium.

Junctional epithelium

The junctional epithelium extends apically from the base of the gingival sulcus following the tooth structure, and it is a nondifferentiated stratified squamous epithelium.[23] In healthy situations with no history of periodontal disease or gingival deformities, the deepest portion of the junctional epithelium is located around the CEJ. It has a triangular shape with the base at the bottom of the sulcus and a vertex located apically. The base of the junctional epithelium has a layer 20 to 30 cells thick, which decreases in number to become a bilayer at the level of the CEJ.[24] The junctional epithelium is attached to the tooth surface through hemidesmosomes, while the connections in between the epithelial cells are established by desmosomes, adherents, gaps, and tight junctions.[25]

The gingival epithelial tissue lies over connective tissue establishing finger-type indentations of epithelial tissue

TABLE 1-4 Main connective tissue fibers[5,28]

	Subclassification	Origin	Direction
Dentogingival fibers	Subgroup A	Cementum	Free gingiva
	Subgroup B	Cementum	Attached gingiva
	Subgroup C	Sweep down and across the crest	NA
Alveologingival fibers	NA	Periosteum	Free gingiva and attached gingiva
Circular fibers	NA	Encircle each tooth within the connective tissue	
Dentoperiosteal fibers	NA	Cementum apical to the dento-gingival fibers	Crest of the alveolar bone. Some fibers may insert into muscles of the vestibule.
Transseptal fibers	NA	Cementum	Cementum of adjacent tooth

NA, not applicable.

termed *ridges*. This connective tissue subjacent to the epithelium of the attached gingiva is known as **lamina propria**. The lamina propria is a highly vascularized tissue with two known portions: the papillary layer, which is the most superficial, and the reticular layer. In the papillary layer, the interphase between the connective tissue of the lamina propria and the epithelium follow a wavy morphology with projections of connective tissue called *papillae* and epithelial ridges known as **rete pegs**. The interface between the sulcular epithelium, the junctional epithelium, and the connective tissue is characterized by the absence of rete pegs. The lamina propria consists of 57% to 60% connective tissue fibers/fibrous proteins, 5% to 8% cells, and 35% other components such as blood vessels, nerves, and ground substance of the intercellular matrix.[5,26]

The main cell type in the lamina propria is the **fibroblast**, which is the main cell responsible for the formation and remodeling of the connective tissue. The main fibers of the lamina propria are comprised by collagen type I, III, IV, and V, with minor presence of elastic fibers and oxytalan fibers. The fibers in the gingiva follow a specific orientation and are classified into different bundles. The main connective tissue fibers are dentogingival, alveologingival, circular, dentoperiosteal, and transseptal (Table 1-4 and Figs 1-3 and 1-4).[5,27,28] In addition, secondary connective tissue fibers are periosteogingival, interpapillary, transgingival, intercircular, semicircular, and intergingival.[29] The main as well as the secondary fibers are part of the connective tissue attachment.

The interface between the connective tissue and the epithelium is a specialized form of extracellular matrix named the *basement membrane* or *basal membrane*. The basal membrane consists of a highly crosslinked matrix of collagen and glycoproteins such as laminin, perlecan, and entactin, and it is composed of several layers. Under electron microscopy, three components can be differentiated: the lamina lucida, the lamina densa, and the lamina reticularis.[27]

The interdental gingiva or papilla refers to the soft tissue that occupies the space between the teeth and consists of an epithelium with a subjacent dense connective tissue. The shape of this interdental gingiva is determined by the morphology of the teeth and the CEJ. In anterior sites, it presents with a pyramidal shape, whereas in posterior sites, it presents with a concave shape. The epithelium that covers this concave portion is known as the *col epithelium*.[28,30]

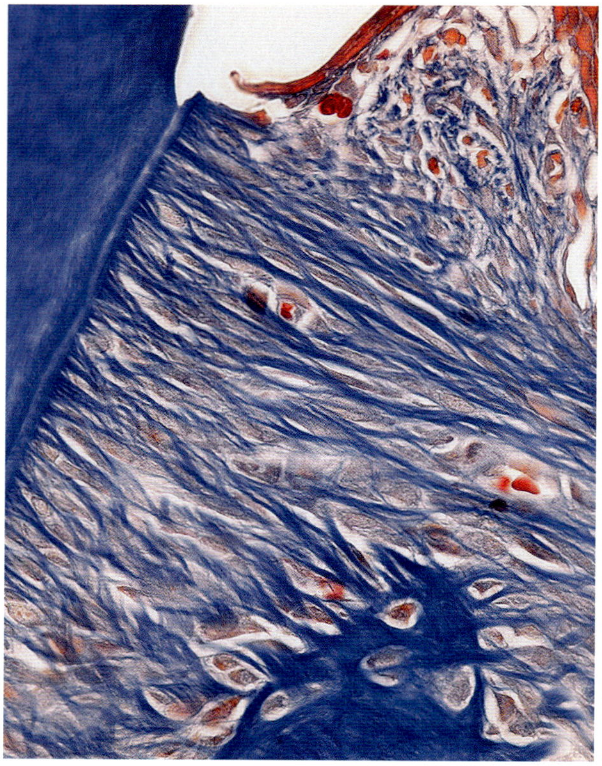

Fig 1-3 Dentogingival fibers in a mouse model (100× magnification).

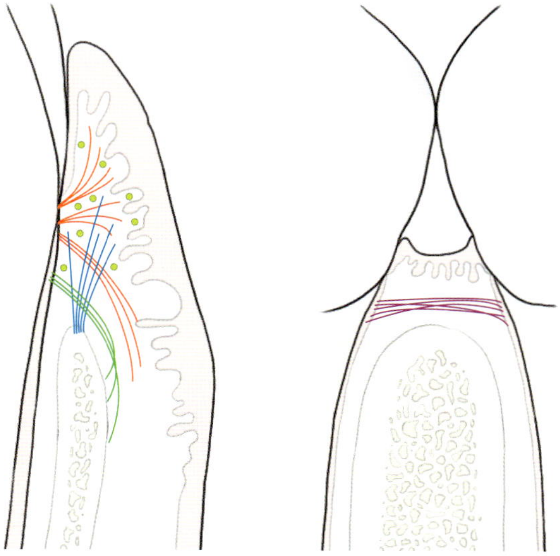

Fig 1-4 Gingival fibers.

TABLE 1-5 Classic studies on the dimensions of supracrestal tissue attachment and sulcus

	Sulcular epithelium (mm)	Junctional epithelium (mm)	Connective tissue (mm)
Gargiulo et al[32]	0.69	0.97	1.07
Vacek et al[33]	1.34	1.14	0.77

SUPRACRESTAL TISSUE ATTACHMENT

The junctional epithelium and connective tissue attachment together are known as the *supracrestal attached tissues* (formerly referred to as **biologic width**).[2,31] The dimensions of these structures were investigated by Gargiulo et al[32] and Vacek et al[33] in human cadavers reporting an average distance of 2.04 mm and 1.91 mm, respectively (Table 1-5).

A meta-analysis by Schmidt et al[34] in 2013 concluded that the biologic width ranges from 2.15 mm to 2.30 mm, with posterior teeth having longer junctional epithelium and the dimension of connective tissue attachment being larger in buccal and lingual surfaces compared with interproximal sites.[34]

Peri-Implant Attachment Apparatus

The replacement and restoration of the missing dentition by means of dental implants has become a routine procedure in daily practice. As such, a plethora of systems with different macro- and microstructures are available on the market. However, independently of the design, the proper functioning of dental implants is primarily based on the process of **osseointegration**. This phenomenon is defined as the direct contact between the surface of a loaded implant and vital bone.

Considerable differences exist between the structures giving support to dental implants and natural dentition, the most important being the lack of PDL for osseointegrated implants. However, at the most coronal portion, some similarities can be found. Similar to the supracrestal attached tissues in the natural dentition, implants also present in their most coronal portion with a sulcus epithelium, junctional epithelium, and connective tissue.[35] In 1991 in an animal model, Berglundh et al[35] described the differences in the arrangement of collagenous fibers in the connective tissue between teeth and implants. Essentially, while the collagenous fibers run perpendicular to the axis of the tooth, they run parallel to the surface of an implant. The composition of the connective tissue also seems to differ between implants and teeth. As such, more collagen and fewer cells have been found around dental implants in comparison with teeth.[35] Moon et al[36] also described that although generally a reduced number of cells have been found in the peri-implant tissue, a cell-rich zone is present in the connective tissue adjacent to the implant-abutment surface with high concentration of fibroblasts.

The absence of PDL space around dental implants also determines the lack of vascularization from this structure. Consequently, the blood vessels that irrigate the peri-implant mucosa are terminal branches from the periosteum. On the other hand, both natural dentition and dental implants present with a vascular plexus adjacent to the junctional epithelium.[37]

References

1. American Academy of Periodontology. Glossary of Periodontal Terms. American Academy of Periodontology, 2001.
2. Jepsen S, Caton JG, Albandar JM, et al. Periodontal manifestations of systemic diseases and developmental and acquired conditions: Consensus report of workgroup 3 of the 2017 World Workshop on the Classification of Periodontal and Peri-Implant Diseases and Conditions. J Periodontol 2018;89(suppl 1):S237–S248.
3. Nanci A, Bosshardt DD. Structure of periodontal tissues in health and disease. Periodontol 2000 2006;40:11–28.
4. Sicher H. The principal fibers of the periodontal membrane. Bur 1954;55:2–6.
5. Schroeder HE. Handbook of Microscopic Anatomy. Vol 5: The Periodontium. Berlin: Springer-Verlag, 1986.
6. Cho MI, Garant PR. Development and general structure of the periodontium. Periodontol 2000 2000;24:9–27.
7. Goseki T, Shimizu N, Iwasawa T, Takiguchi H, Abiko Y. Effects of in vitro cellular aging on alkaline phosphatase, cathepsin activities and collagen secretion of human periodontal ligament derived cells. Mech Ageing Dev 1996;91:171–183.
8. Narayanan AS, Page RC. Connective tissues of the periodontium: A summary of current work. Coll Relat Res 1983;3:33–64.
9. Bartold PM. Connective tissues of the periodontium. Research and clinical implications. Aust Dent J 1991;36:255–268.
10. Schroeder HE, Scherle WF. Cemento-enamel junction: Revisited. J Periodontal Res 1988;23:53–59.
11. Neuvald L, Consolaro A. Cementoenamel junction: Microscopic analysis and external cervical resorption. J Endod 2000;26:503–508.
12. Bosshardt DD, Selvig KA. Dental cementum: The dynamic tissue covering of the root. Periodontol 2000 1997;13:41–75.
13. Foster BL, Popowics TE, Fong HK, Somerman MJ. Advances in defining regulators of cementum development and periodontal regeneration. Curr Top Devl Biol 2007;78:47–126.
14. Presland RB, Dale BA. Epithelial structural proteins of the skin and oral cavity: Function in health and disease. Crit Rev Oral Biol Med 2000;11:383–408.
15. Ainamo J, Löe H. Anatomical characteristics of gingiva. A clinical and microscopic study of the free and attached gingiva. J Periodontol 1966;37:5–13.
16. Shirmohammadi A, Faramarzie M, Lafzi A. A clinical evaluation of anatomic features of gingiva in dental students in Tabriz, Iran. J Dent Res Dent Clin Dent Prospects 2008;2:90–94.
17. Orban B. Clinical and histologic study of the surface characteristics of the gingiva. Oral Surg Oral Med Oral Pathol 1948;1:827–841.
18. Kyllar M, Witter K, Tichy F. Gingival stippling in dogs: Clinical and structural characteristics. Res Vet Sci 2010;88:195–202.
19. Ainamo A. Influence of age on the location of the maxillary mucogingival junction. J Periodontol Res 1978;13:189–193.
20. Ainamo A. Optimal reference line for determination of the location of the maxillary mucogingival junction in the orthopantomogram. Proc Finn Dent Soc 1977;73:70–75.
21. Bowers GM. A study of the width of the attached gingiva. J Periodontol 1963;34:201–209.
22. Voigt JP, Goran ML, Flesher RM. The width of lingual mandibular attached gingiva. J Periodontol 1978;49:77–80.
23. Hormia M, Owaribe K, Virtanen I. The dento-epithelial junction: Cell adhesion by type I hemidesmosomes in the absence of a true basal lamina. J Periodontol 2001;72:788–797.

24. Bartold PM, Walsh LJ, Narayanan AS. Molecular and cell biology of the gingiva. Periodontol 2000 2000;24:28–55.
25. Shimono M, Sugira K, Yamamura T. Intercellular junctions of normal human gingival epithelium. A study using freeze-fracture. Bull Tokyo Dent Coll 1981;22:223–236.
26. Lang NP, Lindhe J. Clinical Periodontology and Implant Dentistry, ed 6. Ames, IA: Wiley Blackwell, 2015.
27. Kobayashi K, Rose GG, Mahan CJ. Ultrastructure of the dento-epithelial junction. J Periodontal Res 1976;11:313–330.
28. Schroeder HE, Listgarten MA. The gingival tissues: The architecture of periodontal protection. Periodontol 2000 1997;13:91–120.
29. Page RC, Ammons WF, Schectman LR, Dillingham LA. Collagen fibre bundles of the normal marginal gingiva in the marmoset. Arch Oral Biol 1974;19:1039–1043.
30. Cohen B. Pathology of the interdental tissues. Dent Pract 1959;9:167–173.
31. Cohen DW. Pathogenesis of Periodontal Disease and Its Treatment. Washington, DC: Walter Reed Army Medical Center, 1962.
32. Gargiulo AW, Wentz FM, Orban B. Dimensions and relations of the dentogingival junction in humans. J Periodontol 1961;32:261–267.
33. Vacek JS, Gher ME, Assad DA, Richardson AC, Giambarresi LI. The dimensions of the human dentogingival junction. Int J Periodontics Restorative Dent 1994;14:154–165.
34. Schmidt JC, Sahrmann P, Weiger R, Schmidlin PR, Walter C. Biologic width dimensions: A systematic review. J Clin Periodontol 2013;40:493–504.
35. Berglundh T, Lindhe J, Ericsson I, Marinello CP, Liljenberg B, Thomsen P. The soft tissue barrier at implants and teeth. Clin Oral Implants Res 1991;2:81–90.
36. Moon IS, Berglundh T, Abrahamsson I, Linder E, Lindhe J. The barrier between the keratinized mucosa and the dental implant. An experimental study in the dog. J Clin Periodontol 1999;26:658–663.
37. Berglundh T, Lindhe J, Jonsson K, Ericsson I. The topography of the vascular systems in the periodontal and peri-implant tissues in the dog. J Clin Periodontol 1994;21:189–193.

2

EXAMINATION AND DIAGNOSIS

Shan-Huey Yu, DDS, MS

A thorough and comprehensive clinical and radiographic examination is the critical first step for establishing a proper periodontal diagnosis before a treatment plan can be developed. The objective of this chapter is to review the main components of a periodontal examination and interpretation of these parameters to aid in developing a periodontal diagnosis. The second part of this chapter is an overview of the different classifications for periodontal diseases and conditions that have been proposed and developed over the years.

Clinical Examination

To determine a proper periodontal diagnosis, clinicians should perform a periodontal examination that includes but is not limited to the following parameters[2,3]:

- Probing depth (PD)
- Gingival recession
- Clinical attachment level (CAL)
- Width of keratinized gingiva (KG) and attached gingiva (AG)
- Signs of gingival inflammation (ie, bleeding on probing [BOP], suppuration, gingival color and texture)
- Tooth mobility
- Degree of furcation involvement
- Extent, distribution, and pattern of radiographic bone loss
- Patient's medical and dental history[3]

PROBING DEPTH

The measurement of PDs is considered to be one of the most important parameters of the periodontal examination because it provides an overall assessment of the periodontal pockets, which are usually considered as a critical sign for the establishment of a diagnosis. In addition, pockets

DEFINITIONS AND TERMINOLOGY

Clinical attachment level: The distance from the cementoenamel junction (CEJ) to the tip of a periodontal probe during periodontal diagnostic probing. The health of the attachment apparatus can affect the measurement.[1]

Furcation: The anatomical area of a multirooted tooth where the roots diverge.[1]

Furcation involvement: Pathologic resorption of bone within a furcation. The degree of interradicular bony destruction of a multirooted tooth. It is characterized by factors such as root trunk length, root concavities, and the extent of root separation.[2]

Recession: The migration of the marginal soft tissue to a point apical to the CEJ of a tooth or the platform of a dental implant.[1]

BOX 2-1 Common types of periodontal probes

Williams probe

- The graduations on this probe are 1-, 2-, 3-, 5-, 7-, 8-, 9-, and 10-mm. The 4- and 6-mm markings are absent to improve visibility and avoid confusion in reading the markings.

Merritt B probe

- The graduations and markings on this probe are the same as Williams probe.

Goldman-Fox probe

- This probe has a flattened tip. The graduations and markings on this probe are the same as Williams probe; however, the flat tip end might preclude easy access into tight or narrow pockets.

UNC 15 probe

- The graduations on this probe are 1-, 2-, 3-, 4-, 5-, 6-, 7-, 8-, 9-, 10-, 11-, 12-, 13-, 14-, and 15-mm. This probe is color-coded at every millimeter demarcation, and it is suitable for deeper pockets (ie, > 10 mm).

Marquis color-coded probe

- The graduations on this probe are 3-, 6-, 9-, and 12-mm. Color markings are darker at 3–6 mm and 9–12 mm. The main disadvantage of this probe is its accuracy; the measurements are usually estimated between color markings.

Michigan O probe

- The graduations on this probe are 3-, 6-, and 8-mm and are color-coded. This probe might not be suitable for deeper pockets (ie, > 8 mm), and the measurements are also estimated between color markings.

CPITN probe

- The graduations on this probe are 3.5-, 5.5-, 8.5-, and 11.5-mm. Markings are a darker color at 3.5–5.5 mm and 8.5–11.5 mm. This probe is particularly useful for screening and monitoring patients or for epidemiologic research.

UNC, University of North Carolina; CPITN, community periodontal index of treatment needs.

are also the major habitats for periodontal pathogens.[3] Currently, the most widely used instrument to obtain PDs in clinical practice is the conventional or manual probe. In 1936, periodontist Charles H. M. Williams created the first periodontal probe, and his invention—the Williams periodontal probe—has been the prototype or benchmark for all manual probes.[4] Different types of conventional periodontal probes have been developed over the years and utilized for different indications. Box 2-1 summarizes the common types of conventional probes used in the clinic and their characteristics and indications.[4]

Conventional probes are easily operated and inexpensive; therefore, these are the most commonly used probe system in dental clinics. However, conventional probes also present with several disadvantages[4]:

- The pressure applied cannot be standardized.
- Assistants are often needed to transfer measurements to a periodontal chart.
- Operator variability and errors can affect the readings of the markings.

In order to overcome these disadvantages of conventional probes, new generations of probes have been developed. These include but are not limited to the following[4]:

- *Constant-pressure probes:* Designed to be pressure sensitive, therefore allowing for standardization of the force applied during PD measurements.
- *Computer-assisted/automated probes:* This generation of probes was developed based on constant-pressure probes. Added features include automated detection of the measurement and computer-assisted data capture into a storage system. This minimizes possible errors from probe reading and data recording.
- *3D probes:* This instrument aims to develop a method to record the PD in a serial matter instead of linear measurements.
- *Noninvasive probes:* Probing into periodontal pockets can often be uncomfortable and/or painful to patients. This probe system is still under development, and it aims to identify the periodontal pocket and attachment level without the need to physically penetrate the tissues.

The usage of these newer probe systems is still very limited due to various considerations such as cost (more expensive), less tactile sensitivity, and less accessibility for most dentists. To date, the conventional periodontal probe is still the most popular system that is used in dental offices when a periodontal examination is performed.[4]

It is very important to bear in mind that, when measuring PDs with a conventional probe, there are a number of factors that can affect these measurements and their accuracy. The variables are summarized in Table 2-1.[5–14]

TABLE 2-1 Variables affecting probing measurements

Reproducibility	Operators' experience and skills would affect the inter- and intraexaminer reproducibility.	
Probing force	Probing force affects how deep the periodontal probes penetrate into the pocket and the connective tissue; greater probing force usually results in deeper PDs.[5] It has been recommended that 30 g (0.3 N) of probing force be used during periodontal examination to allow the probe tip to remain within the junctional epithelium.[6,7] Probing forces up to 50 g (0.5 N) would penetrate deeper, and the probe tip could reach closer to the alveolar bone.[6,7]	
Probe angulation	Mean PDs could be 1 mm greater with midproximal compared to line-angle measurements.[8]	
Gingiva inflammation	Periodontal probes tend to penetrate deeper into the gingival tissue when inflammation is present[9–14]:	
	Healthy dentition	Apical one-third of junctional epithelium
	Gingivitis	Apical one-third of junctional epithelium
	Periodontitis	Coronal one-third of connective tissue
	Posttreatment periodontitis	Apical one-third of junctional epithelium
Site and local anatomy	Crown contours, defective restorations and margins, tipped or rotated teeth, osseous ledges, and subgingival calculus can all affect probing accuracy.	
Type of probe	Different types of conventional probes, pressure-sensitive probes, and computer-assisted data recording probes could yield different measurements.	
Natural dentition versus dental implants	Probing at an implant site usually results in deeper depths compared with probing at a natural tooth[9–14]:	
	Healthy implant	Apical one-third of junctional epithelium to coronal one-third of connective tissue
	Peri-implant mucositis	Apical two-thirds of connective tissue
	Peri-implantitis	Apical one-third of connective tissue and close proximity to bone
	Posttreatment peri-implantitis	Apical two-thirds of connective tissue

It is also of relevance to differentiate between the terms "pocket depth" and "probing depth." The measurement obtained with a probe into the gingiva includes not only the depth of the gingival sulcus or periodontal pocket, but also an additional distance that represents varying degrees of adjacent tissue penetration.[15] Therefore, the objective when a periodontal probe is inserted into the space between the tooth and the gingiva is to measure the probing depth instead of the anatomical structure of the pocket depth, which can only be accomplished histologically.[2] Listgarten also emphasized the use of the correct terminology "probing depth" when describing periodontal probing in the literature.[15]

CLINICAL ATTACHMENT LEVEL

The definition of CAL is the distance from the cementoenamel junction (CEJ) to the tip of a periodontal probe during diagnostic periodontal probing.[1] The amount of gingival recession is needed to calculate the CAL. Recession by definition is the migration of the gingiva to a point apical to the CEJ,[1] and it is often described as the distance between CEJ and the free gingival margin. Recession can be recorded as a positive (+) or negative (–) measurement. Recession is recorded as "+" when CEJ is visible and the free gingival margin is below the CEJ. However, when there is gingival enlargement, recession is recorded as a negative "–" measurement (Fig 2-1). CAL can then be

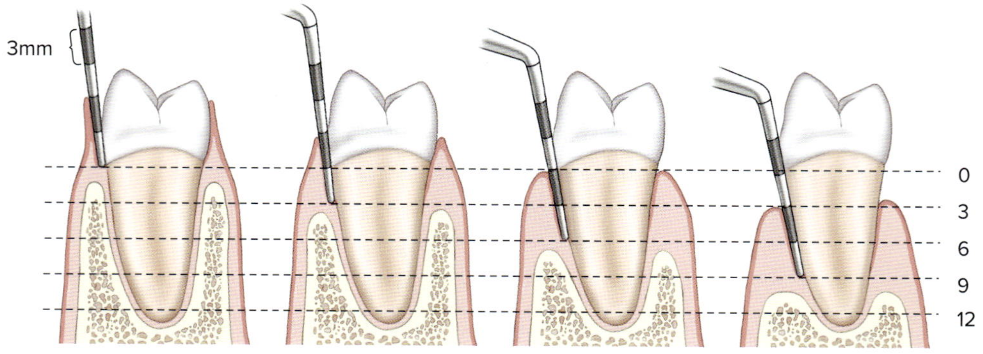

Fig 2-1 Representation of different situations with 6 mm PD and different attachment levels. Rec, recession.

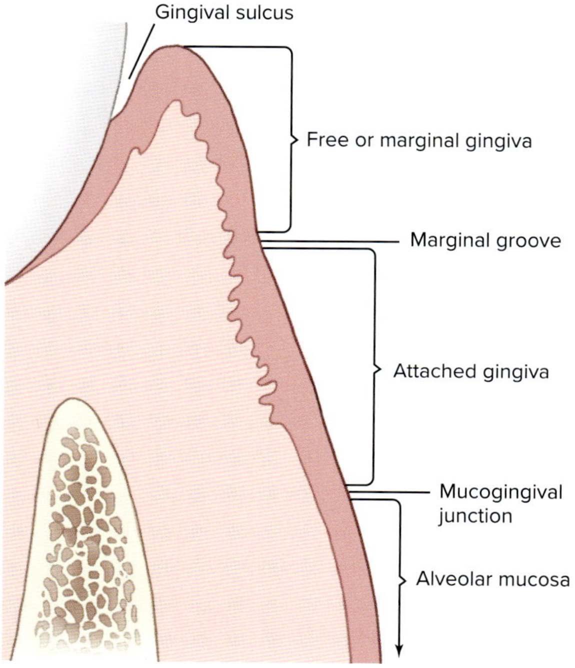

Fig 2-2 Gingival landmarks.

calculated by adding PD and recession (making sure to include "+" or "–"). In Fig 2-1, all four case scenarios measured 6 mm PD; however, when recession is taken into account to determine the CAL, it is clear that the degree of periodontal destruction of these four cases is very different. Therefore, compared with PD, the level of CAL can provide a better overall estimate of the periodontium, and it usually correlates better with radiographic bone loss.[3]

ATTACHED GINGIVA AND KERATINIZED GINGIVA

The amount of AG and the width of KG are also important clinical parameters to record during a comprehensive periodontal evaluation. AG extends from the free gingival marginal groove to the mucogingival junction (MGJ), and it is the portion of the gingiva bonded to the tooth and the alveolar bone through gingival fibers[1] (Fig 2-2). On the other hand, KG includes free (marginal) gingiva and the AG. Around teeth, healthy and uninflamed gingival tissue usually encompass a band of AG, which is crucial to defend against pathogens.[2]

Lang and Löe performed a clinical study evaluating the inflammation status by examining gingival exudate of teeth with or without 2 mm of KG.[16] The results from this investigation indicated that most teeth with < 2 mm of KG presented with clinical inflammation and varying amounts of exudate while surfaces with ≥ 2 mm of KG were healthy, and most of these surfaces showed no exudate.[16] Therefore, it was concluded that 2 mm of KG and 1 mm of AG are needed to maintain periodontal stability.[16] Nevertheless, evidence from another study demonstrated that when good plaque control is achieved through adequate home care, the presence of AG/KG is not an essential prerequisite for the maintenance of periodontal health and attachment.[17] Overall, it is generally accepted that the presence of a collar of KG and AG is beneficial for the long-term stability of the periodontium, and even more important when oral hygiene is not optimal. The MGJ and the width of KG can be determined using the methods demonstrated in Fig 2-3 and Box 2-2.[2,16]

BLEEDING ON PROBING

BOP is another important parameter to record during periodontal examination, and it indicates evidence of gingival inflammation. A prospective study by Lang and colleagues evaluated the prognostic value of sites with BOP and the risk for periodontal breakdown of at least 2 mm of attachment loss during periodontal maintenance therapy.[18] The results showed that only a 30% probability of future attachment loss may be predicted for sites repeatedly positive for BOP (Table 2-2).[18] Further calculations confirmed that frequent BOP for prediction of future attachment loss yields a specificity of 88%, and the continuous absence of BOP has a positive predictive value of 98%.[19] Therefore, it is of paramount importance to understand that BOP alone does not represent a good positive predictor for disease progression[7]; instead, studies have shown that absence of BOP is a more reliable parameter to indicate periodontal stability.[19] BOP is also sensitive to the forces applied with the probe[2,19]; therefore, Lang et al suggested a probing force of 25 g (0.25 N) when recording BOP, as heavier pressures (> 25 g) might traumatize the gingival tissue and provoke bleeding.[19] In conclusion, the presence of BOP has low sensitivity and high specificity with respect to the development of additional attachment loss. For clinicians to monitor patients' periodontal stability over time in daily practice, the absence of BOP at 25 g is a reliable indicator for periodontal stability with a negative predictive value of 98%.[7,18,19]

FURCATION INVOLVEMENT

The furcation is the anatomical area of a multirooted tooth from where the roots diverge and form bifurcation (two-rooted tooth) or trifurcation (three-rooted tooth).[2] *Furcation involvement* or *furcation invasion* describes the pathologic resorption of bone within a furcation area[1,2,20] (Fig 2-4). The Nabers furcation probe is widely used and suited for detection and examination of furcation involvement.[2,20] The extent and configuration of furcation involvement can be characterized by anatomical factors including but not limited to presence of cervical enamel projections, enamel pearls, root trunk distance, tooth surface concavities, and the extent of root separation. The following summarizes the furcation entrances of multirooted teeth to aid in detection of furcation involvement[20]:

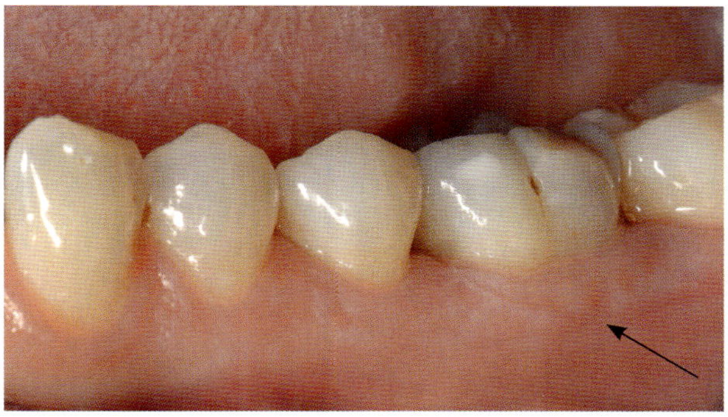

Fig 2-3 Visual examination of the MGJ. The *arrow* indicates the junction between the KG and the mucosa. KG presents as a coral pink color, while mucosa is redder.

BOX 2-2 Methods to determine the location of MGJ and the width of KG[3,16]

Visual

- Examine for color difference. AG/KG of healthy gingiva usually presents a coral pink coloration, while mucosa is darker and redder (see Fig 2-3).

Schiller's iodine test

- Oral mucosa can be stained with an iodine solution because of the glycogen distribution, while KG is iodine-negative.[16]

Roll technique

- Oral mucosa is movable while AG/KG is bonded to tooth surface and bone. A clear demarcation (MGJ) would appear when rolling from movable mucosa to AG/KG.

TABLE 2-2 Positive predictive values for loss of attachment of ≥ 2 mm in 2 years in sites that bled on probing 0, 1, 2, 3, or 4 times out of 4 maintenance visits[18]

BOP incidence	Sites with loss of attachment > 2 mm
4/4	30%
3/4	14%
2/4	6%
1/4	3%
0/4	1.5%

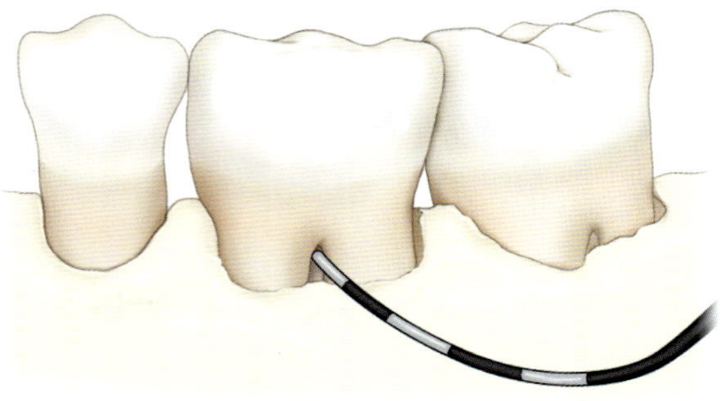

Fig 2-4 Furcation entrance on a mandibular first molar.

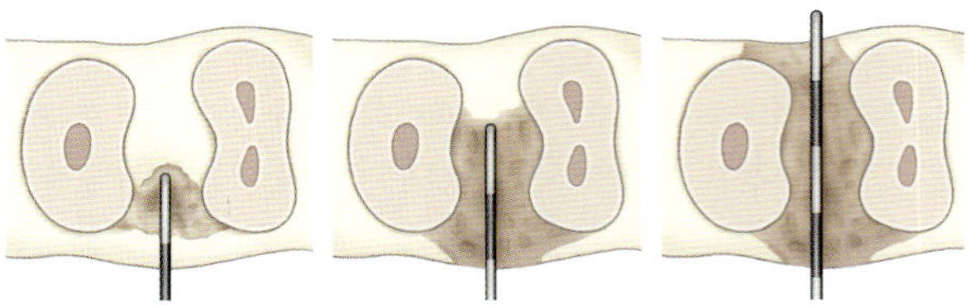

Fig 2-5 Different degrees of furcation involvement.

- Maxillary premolar:
  - Furcation involvement can be detected from the mesial or distal surface; the entrance is located at the apical third of the root and/or approximately 8 mm below the CEJ.
- Maxillary molars:
  - Buccal entrance: Centered mesiodistally.
  - Mesial entrance: Two-thirds of the buccolingual width toward the palatal aspect, easier to approach from mesiopalatal aspect.
  - Distal entrance: Furcation entrance is centered buccolingually and can be examined from either the buccal or palatal aspect.
- Mandibular molars:
  - Buccal entrance: Centered mesiodistally at the buccal surface.
  - Lingual entrance: Centered mesiodistally at the lingual surface.

The amount of furcation involvement of a multirooted tooth can be registered depending on the horizontal and vertical amount of bony destruction into the furcation area.[20–22] Many systems have been proposed for classifying furcation involvement.[2] Hamp's classification is one of the most commonly used for furcation destruction.[22] A brief review of three systems is presented in the following sections.[2,20–23]

Horizontal destruction

Glickman (1958) divided furcation involvement into 4 grades[21]:

- *Grade I:* Pocket formation into the flute but intact interradicular bone. Incipient lesion.
- *Grade II:* Loss of interradicular bone and pocket formation of varying depths into the furcation area but not completely through to the opposite side of the tooth.
- *Grade III:* Through-and-through lesion.
- *Grade IV:* Same as Grade III with through-and-through lesion with gingival recession, rendering the furcation area clearly visible on clinical examination.

Hamp et al (1975) proposed three levels of furcation involvement[22] (Fig 2-5):

- *Degree I:* Horizontal loss of periodontal tissue support < 3 mm.
- *Degree II:* Horizontal loss > 3 mm, but not passing the total width of the furcation.
- *Degree III:* Horizontal through-and-through destruction.

Vertical destruction

Tarnow and Fletcher (1985) proposed the following classification based on the vertical bone loss around furcations. It is encouraged to supplement each category of horizontal destruction with a subclass based on the vertical bone resorption.[23]

- *Subclass A:* 0 to 3 mm probeable depth.
- *Subclass B:* 4 to 6 mm probeable depth.
- *Subclass C:* ≥ 7 mm probeable depth.

MOBILITY

The definition of *tooth mobility* is the movement of a tooth in its socket resulting from an applied force.[1] Increase in tooth mobility is often a sign of periodontal breakdown and/or presence of excessive occlusal forces.[1] Tooth mobility is detected by using the ends of two instruments (eg, mirror handle) on either side of the tooth and alternately applying forces.[2] The most commonly used clinical index for tooth mobility is the Miller Index; using this index, mobility can be scored as the following[2,24]:

- *Class 0:* Normal (physiologic) movement when force is applied. It has been defined as movement up to 0.2 mm horizontally and 0.02 mm axially.
- *Class I:* First distinguishable sign of movement greater than "normal" or "physiologic."
- *Class II:* Movement of the crown up to 1 mm in any direction (buccolingual or mesiodistal).
- *Class III:* Movement of the crown more than 1 mm in any direction (buccolingual or mesiodistal) and/or vertical depression (apicocoronal) or rotation of the crown in its socket.

Radiographic Interpretation

Clinical periodontal examination provides information with regard to PDs, recession defects, AG/KG, and more; however, it cannot reveal the status of the alveolar bone. The alveolar bone is another critical aspect to take into consideration to accurately diagnose different periodontal diseases and conditions.[2] Dental radiographs are the most commonly used noninvasive method of examining alveolar bone levels. Other valuable information that can be obtained through radiographic examination includes subgingival calculus deposition, root length and form, crown-to-root ratio, presence of periapical lesions, periodontal ligament space, root proximity, and the destruction of alveolar bone.[2,7]

Clinicians should keep in mind the following limitations of conventional dental radiography when interpreting radiographs during the examination phase[3,7,25]:

- Radiographs do not show periodontal pockets.[25]
- Radiographs cannot distinguish between posttreatment periodontitis and active periodontitis.[25]
- Radiographs do not show buccal and lingual aspects of tooth and alveolar bone.[25]
- Radiographs cannot detect tooth mobility.[25]
- Radiographs can provide evidence of past destruction to the periodontium, but they cannot identify sites with active or ongoing periodontal inflammation.[7]
- Clinical attachment loss always precedes visual radiographic changes by approximately 6 to 8 months, and clinical attachment variations are greater than radiographic changes.[26]
- Radiographic changes are detectable by simple visual inspection when approximately 30% to 50% of the bone mineral has been lost.[27]

The presence or absence of the crestal lamina dura is another common interpretation of radiographs for diagnosing periodontitis. Rams et al[28] observed that the presence of intact crestal lamina dura is positively correlated to periodontal stability over a 2-year follow up period. However, no significant relationship could be found between future periodontal breakdown and lack of crestal lamina dura.[28] A recent publication by Rams et al also reported similar findings and concluded that patients with angular bony morphology and PD greater than 5 mm poses a significant risk of periodontitis progression after treatment. However, if intact crestal lamina dura is present, despite the bony morphology, clinical stability for at least 24 months can be anticipated.[29] Also, molar furcation involvement can sometimes be observed on radiographs. Hardekopf et al were the first to describe the radiographic features of maxillary molars with furcation destruction: a triangular radiographic shadow, commonly known as "furcation arrow," can be noted over the mesial and distal proximal areas of maxillary molars.[30] The clinical reliability of the presence of furcation arrow can be subjective and also greatly dependent on the degree of destruction. For instance, when furcation arrows are present on radiographs, these can only predict actual furcation invasion 70% of the time. On the other hand, when there is true furcation involvement, a furcation arrow is seen in less than 40% of the sites.[31] It has been reported that the presence of furcation arrow for diagnosing furcation involvement on maxillary molars has a low sensitivity (38.7%) and high specificity (92.2%).[31] When mandibular molars suffer from furcation involvement, radiolucency can be noted at the area where roots start to separate.

In recent years, the utilization of CBCT has been rapidly increasing in popularity. CBCT has become an integral tool for researchers and clinicians, mostly applied to the implant field. As such, the use of CBCT imaging for the diagnosis of periodontitis has also been studied. However, in 2017, the American Academy of Periodontology reported that even though its use may be beneficial in selective cases, there is limited evidence to support the use of CBCT for the different types of bony defects, and there are no guidelines for its application to periodontal treatment planning.[32]

BOX 2-3 Classification proposed in 1989 World Workshop in Clinical Periodontics[37]

- I. Adult periodontitis (> 35 y)
- II. Early-onset periodontitis (≤ 35 y)
  - A. Prepubertal periodontitis (< 13 y)
    1. Generalized
    2. Localized
  - B. Juvenile periodontitis (13 to 26 y)
    1. Generalized
    2. Localized
  - C. Rapid progressive periodontitis (25 to 35 y)
- III. Periodontitis associated with systemic diseases
- IV. Necrotizing ulcerative periodontitis
- V. Refractory periodontitis

Advanced and Emerging Examination

Periodontitis is a multifactorial disease involving the combination of dysbiosis of oral bacteria and an overreacted immune response from the host.[33] One of the disadvantages of the clinical periodontal evaluation is that these examinations only record destruction that has already occurred, such as the bone loss pattern and periodontal pockets. Therefore, patients would greatly benefit from techniques that detect the development of periodontal inflammation before tissue breakdown occurs and prevent further complications such as bone loss, tooth mobility, and ultimately tooth loss. The major rationale to develop advanced methods for examination is to detect disease activity at a subclinical level in order to provide early diagnosis and create a treatment plan tailored to each individual.[34]

Researchers and scientists have been investigating possible periodontitis-related biomarkers that could be used to distinguish between healthy and diseased patients.[34] These biomarkers can be collected from saliva, which can demonstrate overall periodontal health at a subject level, or gingival crevicular fluid, which is site specific.[34] For instance, proportions of specific periodontal pathogens, pro- and anti-inflammatory cytokines, and tissue-degradation products have all been studied to differentiate between healthy and periodontitis subjects. Among all biomarkers, interleukin-1 (IL-1) is one of the most notable proinflammatory cytokines that has been extensively studied in the periodontal field.[34,35] Periodontal pathogens that have been extensively studied and proved to be closely linked to the development of periodontitis include *Porphyromonas gingivalis*, *Treponema denticola*, *Tannerella forsythia*, *Aggregatibacter actinomycetemcomitans*, *Fusobacterium nucleatum*, and more.[2,36] Research in the field of advanced examination and biomarkers is still ongoing, and the results have indicated a promising future for early detection of periodontitis. However, these examinations are still not routinely utilized, due at least in part to the additional costs and disassociation to treatment options (ie, the test results would not alter the treatment plan).[34]

Classifications of Periodontal Diseases and Conditions

Classification systems are essential to properly study the diagnosis, etiology, pathogenesis, and treatment of the different diseases. As such, the field of periodontology has witnessed the creation and continued update of different classification systems since the early 1940s. The first World Workshop in Periodontics[37] was held in Ann Arbor, Michigan, on June 6 to 9, 1966, and the most recent World Workshop took place in Chicago on November 9 to 11, 2017, with the related publications released in June 2018.[38] Understanding the development and the variations among the different classifications is critical for comprehending the literature published in different eras.

1989 WORLD WORKSHOP IN CLINICAL PERIODONTICS

One of the first major and comprehensive classifications of periodontitis emerged from the World Workshop in 1989.[37] On this date, the World Workshop in Clinical Periodontics gathered scientists and researchers to develop a classification for periodontal diseases. There were essentially five different classifications, which are listed in Box 2-3.[37]

Under the 1989 classification system, age of onset and distribution of lesions were taken into consideration for classifying adult periodontitis and early onset periodontitis as well as the subforms of early-onset periodontitis that included prepubertal periodontitis (generalized/localized), juvenile periodontitis (generalized/ localized), and rapidly progressive periodontitis.[37]

1999 INTERNATIONAL WORKSHOP FOR A CLASSIFICATION OF PERIODONTAL DISEASES AND CONDITIONS

The 1989 classification raised problems in several areas[39]:

- Considerable overlap in disease categories
- Absence of a gingival disease component
- Inappropriate emphasis on age of onset of disease and rates of progression
- Inadequate or unclear classification criteria

Therefore, the next landmark classification was the 1999 International Workshop for a Classification of Periodontal Diseases and Conditions, which addressed some of the problems in the previous classification. The major changes in the classification system for periodontal diseases included (Box 2-4)[39]:

- Addition of a section on gingival diseases
- Replacement of "Adult periodontitis" with "Chronic periodontitis"
- Replacement of "Early-onset periodontitis" with "Aggressive periodontitis"
- Elimination of a separate disease category for Refractory periodontitis
- Clarification of the designation "Periodontitis as a manifestation of systemic diseases"
- Replacement of "Necrotizing ulcerative periodontitis" with "Necrotizing periodontal diseases"
- Addition of "Periodontal abscesses" category
- Addition of "Periodontic-endodontic lesions" category
- Addition of "Developmental or acquired deformities and conditions" category

2017 WORLD WORKSHOP ON THE CLASSIFICATION OF PERIODONTAL AND PERI-IMPLANT DISEASES AND CONDITIONS

In order to update the 1999 classification of periodontal diseases and conditions,[39] an organizing committee from the American Academy of Periodontology (AAP) and the European Federation of Periodontology (EFP) commissioned the world workshop that was held in Chicago on November 9 to 11, 2017.[38] The world workshop included expert participants in the field of periodontology and implant dentistry from around the world. The scope of the 2017 world workshop was to align and update the classification scheme to the current understanding of periodontal and peri-implant diseases and conditions. Therefore, in addition to updating the 1999 classification of periodontal diseases and conditions, this was also the first world consensus to develop a classification scheme for peri-implant diseases and conditions.[38]

A brief classification scheme for the 2017 world workshop is presented in Box 2-5,[38] and major changes to the 1999 classification include the following[40]:

- The 2017 workshop characterized periodontal health and gingival inflammation in a reduced periodontium after completion of successful treatment of a patient with periodontitis.
- The workshop agreed that, consistent with current knowledge on pathophysiology, three forms of periodontitis can be identified:
  - Necrotizing periodontitis
  - Periodontitis as a manifestation of systemic disease
  - Periodontitis
- The forms of the disease previously recognized as "chronic" or "aggressive" are now grouped under a single category, "periodontitis."
- A new classification framework for periodontitis was established and further characterized based on a multidimensional staging and grading system that can be adapted over time as new evidence emerges.
  - Goals of staging a periodontitis patient[40]:
    - Classify severity and extent of an individual based on currently measurable extent of destroyed and damaged tissue attributable to periodontitis.
    - Assess specific factors that may determine complexity of controlling current disease and managing long-term function and esthetics of the patient's dentition.
  - Goals of grading a periodontitis patient[40]:
    - Estimate future risk of periodontitis progression and responsiveness to standard therapeutic principles, to guide intensity of therapy and monitoring.
    - Estimate potential health impact of periodontitis on systemic disease and the reverse, to guide systemic monitoring and cotherapy with medical colleagues.
- A new classification scheme for dental implants was developed by the workshop, including the following: peri-implant health, peri-implant mucositis, peri-implantitis, and peri-implant soft and hard tissue deficiencies.

BOX 2-4 Summary of 1999 International Workshop for a Classification of Periodontal Diseases and Conditions[39]

I. Gingival diseases
  A. Dental plaque–induced gingival diseases
    1. Gingivitis associated with dental plaque only
    2. Gingival diseases modified by systemic factors
    3. Gingival diseases modified by medications
    4. Gingival diseases modified by malnutrition
  B. Non-plaque-induced gingival lesions
    1. Gingival diseases of specific bacterial origin
    2. Gingival diseases of viral origin
    3. Gingival diseases of fungal origin
    4. Gingival lesions of genetic origin
    5. Gingival manifestations of systemic conditions
    6. Traumatic lesions (factitious, iatrogenic, accidental)
    7. Foreign body reactions
    8. Not otherwise specified (NOS)
II. Chronic periodontitis
  A. Localized (≤ 30% of sites involved)
  B. Generalized (> 30% of sites involved)
III. Aggressive periodontitis
  A. Localized (≤ 30% of sites involved)
  B. Generalized (> 30% of sites involved)
IV. Periodontitis as a manifestation of systemic diseases
  A. Associated with hematologic disorders
    1. Acquired neutropenia
    2. Leukemias
    3. Other
  B. Associated with genetic disorders
    1. Familial and cyclic neutropenia
    2. Down syndrome
    3. Leukocyte adhesion deficiency syndromes
    4. Papillon–Lefèvre syndrome
    5. Chediak-Higashi syndrome
    6. Histiocytosis syndromes
    7. Glycogen storage disease
    8. Infantile genetic agranulocytosis
    9. Cohen syndrome
    10. Ehlers-Danlos syndrome (Types IV and VIII)
    11. Hypophosphatasia
    12. Other
  C. Not otherwise specified (NOS)
  D. Necrotizing ulcerative periodontitis (NUP)
V. Necrotizing periodontal diseases
  A. Necrotizing ulcerative gingivitis (NUG)
  B. Necrotizing ulcerative periodontitis (NUP)
VI. Abscesses of the periodontium
  A. Gingival abscess
  B. Periodontal abscess
  C. Pericoronal abscess
VII. Periodontitis associated with endodontic lesions
  A. Combined periodontic-endodontic lesions
VIII. Developmental or acquired deformities and conditions
  A. Localized tooth-related factors that modify or predispose to plaque-induced gingival diseases/periodontitis
    1. Tooth anatomical factors
    2. Dental restorations/appliances
    3. Root fractures
    4. Cervical root resorption and cemental tears
  B. Mucogingival deformities and conditions around teeth
    1. Gingival/soft tissue recession
    2. Lack of keratinized gingiva
    3. Decreased vestibular depth
    4. Aberrant frenum/muscle position
    5. Gingival excess
  C. Mucogingival deformities and conditions on edentulous ridges
    1. Vertical and/or horizontal ridge deficiency
    2. Lack of gingiva/keratinized tissue
    3. Gingival/soft tissue enlargement
    4. Aberrant frenum/muscle position
    5. Decreased vestibular depth
    6. Abnormal color
  D. Occlusal trauma
    1. Primary occlusal trauma
    2. Secondary occlusal trauma

BOX 2-5 2017 World Workshop on the Classification of Periodontal and Peri-implant Diseases and Conditions[38]

- I. Periodontal health, gingival diseases/conditions
  - A. Periodontal health and gingival health
    - 1. Clinical gingival health on an intact periodontium
    - 2. Clinical gingival health on a reduced periodontium
      - i. Stable periodontitis patient
      - ii. Non-periodontitis patient
  - B. Gingivitis: Dental biofilm–induced
    - 1. Associated with dental biofilm alone
    - 2. Meditated by systemic or local risk factors
    - 3. Drug-influenced gingival enlargement
  - C. Gingival diseases: Non-dental-biofilm-induced
    - 1. Genetic/developmental disorders
    - 2. Specific infections
    - 3. Inflammatory and immune conditions
    - 4. Reactive processes
    - 5. Neoplasms
    - 6. Endocrine, nutritional, and metabolic diseases
    - 7. Traumatic lesions
    - 8. Gingiva pigmentation
- II. Forms of periodontitis
  - A. Necrotizing periodontal diseases
    - 1. Necrotizing gingivitis
    - 2. Necrotizing periodontitis
    - 3. Necrotizing stomatitis
  - B. Periodontitis as manifestation of systemic diseases
  - C. Periodontitis
    - 1. Stages: Based on severity and complexity of management
      - i. Stage I: Initial periodontitis
      - ii. Stage II: Moderate periodontitis
      - iii. Stage III: Severe periodontitis with potential for additional tooth loss
      - iv. Stage IV: Severe periodontitis with potential for loss of the dentition
    - 2. Extent and distribution: Localized (< 30% teeth); generalized (≥ 30% teeth); molar-incisor distribution
    - 3. Grades: Evidence of risk of rapid progression, anticipated treatment
      - i. Grade A: Slow rate of progression
      - ii. Grade B: Moderate rate of progression
      - iii. Grade C: Rapid rate of progression
- III. Periodontal manifestation of systemic diseases and developmental and acquired conditions
  - A. Systemic diseases or conditions affecting the periodontal supporting tissues
  - B. Other periodontal conditions
    - 1. Periodontal abscesses
    - 2. Endodontic-periodontic lesions
  - C. Mucogingival deformities and conditions around teeth
    - 1. Gingival biotype
    - 2. Gingival/soft tissue recession
    - 3. Lack of gingiva
    - 4. Decreased vestibular depth
    - 5. Aberrant frenum/muscle position
    - 6. Gingival excess
    - 7. Abnormal color
    - 8. Condition of the exposed root surface
  - D. Traumatic occlusal forces
    - 1. Primary occlusal trauma
    - 2. Secondary occlusal trauma
    - 3. Orthodontic forces
  - E. Prosthesis- and tooth-related factors that modify or predispose to plaque-induced gingival diseases/periodontitis
    - 1. Localized tooth-related factors
    - 2. Localized dental prosthesis–related factors
- IV. Peri-implant diseases and conditions
  - A. Peri-implant health
  - B. Peri-implant mucositis
  - C. Peri-implantitis
  - D. Peri-implant soft and hard tissue deficiencies

Conclusion

The diagnosis represents the first stage and one of the most critical phases in the sequence of treatment for periodontal patients. An appropriate and accurate diagnosis is essential for continuing with the next phases of treatment (establishing an etiology, prognosis, treatment plan, etc). Without a proper diagnosis, the treatment plan may be incomplete or even harmful to the patient. Consequently, it is of paramount importance to understand and properly utilize the multitude of tools pertaining to the acquisition of data for the creation of a diagnosis. Last, while some of these parameters may be of greater diagnostic value than others, the diagnosis should be formed based on the information obtained from all these different tools and methods of examination, including both clinical and radiographic evidence. Relying on a single parameter can also result in incomplete or inadequate diagnosis.

References

1. American Academy of Periodontology. Glossary of Periodontal Terms. American Academy of Periodontology, 2001.
2. Research, Science and Therapy Committee. Position Paper: Diagnosis of Periodontal Diseases. J Periodontol 2003;74:1237–1247.
3. The American Academy of Periodontology. Periodontal literature review: The Next Generation. A Review of Periodontal Literature from 1996 – 2010. Retrieved 24 October 2019 from https://www.perio.org/plr.
4. Ramachandra SS, Mehta DS, Sandesh N, Baliga V, Amarnath J. Periodontal probing systems: A review of available equipment. Compend Contin Educ Dent 2011;32:71–77.
5. Van der Velden U, de Vries JH. The influence of probing force on the reproducibility of pocket depth measurements. J Clin Periodontol 1980;7:414–420.
6. Kalkwarf KI, Kaldahl WD, Patil KD. Comparison of manual and pressure-controlled periodontal probing. J Periodontol 1986;57:467–471.
7. Armitage GC. Periodontal diseases: Diagnosis. Ann Periodontol 1996;1:37–215.
8. Persson GR. Effects of line-angle versus midproximal periodontal probing measurements on prevalence estimates of periodontal disease. J Periodontal Res 1991;26:527–529.
9. Armitage GC, Svanberg GK, Löe H. Microscopic evaluation of clinical measurements of connective tissue attachment levels. J Clin Periodontol 1977;4:173–190.
10. Schou S, Holmstrup P, Stoltze K, Hjørting-Hansen E, Fiehn NE, Skovgaard LT. Probing around implants and teeth with healthy or inflamed peri-implant mucosa/gingiva. A histologic comparison in cynomolgus monkeys *(Macaca fascicularis)*. Clin Oral Implants Res 2002;13:113–126.
11. Abrahamsson, I, Soldini C. Probe penetration in periodontal and peri-implant tissues. An experimental study in the beagle dog. Clin Oral Implants Res 2006;17:601–605.
12. Magnusson I, Listgarten MA. Histological evaluation of probing depth following periodontal treatment. J Clin Periodontol 1980;7:26–31.
13. Fowler C, Garrett S, Crigger M, Egelberg J. Histologic probe position in treated and untreated human periodontal tissues. J Clin Periodontol 1982;9:373–385.
14. Lang NP, Wetzel AC, Stich H, Caffesse RG. Histologic probe penetration in healthy and inflamed peri-implant tissues. Clin Oral Implants Res 1994;5:191–201.
15. Listgarten MA. Re: Periodontal terminology. J Periodontol 1993;64:918.
16. Lang NP, Löe H. The relationship between the width of keratinized gingiva and gingival health. J Periodontol 1972;43:623–627.
17. Kennedy JE, Bird WC, Palcanis KG, Dorfman HS. A longitudinal evaluation of varying widths of attached gingiva. J Clin Periodontol 1985;12:667–675.
18. Lang NP, Joss A, Orsanic T, Gusberti FA, Siegrist BE. Bleeding on probing. A predictor for the progression of periodontal disease? J Clin Periodontol 1986;13:590–596.
19. Lang NP, Joss A, Tonetti MS. Monitoring diseases during supportive periodontal treatment by bleeding on probing. Periodontol 2000 1996;12:44–48.
20. Harpenau LA. Furcation involvement. In: Harpenau LA, Kao RT, Lundergan WP, Sanz M. Hall's Critical Decisions in Periodontology and Dental Implantology, ed 5. Shelton, CT: People's Medical Publishing House–USA, 2013:26–27.
21. Glickman I. Clinical Periodontology: Prevention, Diagnosis, and Treatment of Periodontal Disease in the Practice of General Dentistry, ed 4. Philadelphia: Saunders, 1972:242–245.
22. Hamp SE, Nyman S, Lindhe J. Periodontal treatment of multirooted teeth. Results after 5 years. J Clin Periodontol 1975;2:126–135.
23. Tarnow D, Fletcher P. Classification of the vertical component of furcation involvement. J Periodontol 1985;55:283–284.
24. Miller SC. Textbook of Periodontia. Philadelphia: Blakiston McGraw-Hill, 1938.
25. Prichard JF. Interpretation of radiographs in periodontics. Int J Periodontics Restorative Dent 1983;3:8–39.
26. Goodson JM, Haffajee AD, Socransky SS. The relationship between attachment level loss and alveolar bone loss. J Clin Periodontol 1984;11:348–359.
27. Ortman LF, McHenry K, Hausmann E. Relationship between alveolar bone measured by 125I absorptiometry with analysis of standardized radiographs: 2. Bjorn technique. J Periodontol 1982;53:311–314.
28. Rams TE, Listgarten MA, Slots J. Utility of radiographic crestal lamina dura for predicting periodontitis disease-activity. J Clin Periodontol 1994;21:571–576.
29. Rams TE, Listgarten MA, Slots J. Radiographic alveolar bone morphology and progressive periodontitis. J Periodontol 2018;89:424–430.
30. Hardekopf JD, Dunlap RM, Ahl DR, Pelleu GB Jr. The "furcation arrow." A reliable radiographic image? J Periodontol 1987;58:258–261.
31. Deas DE, Moritz AJ, Mealey BL, McDonnell HT, Powell CA. Clinical reliability of the "furcation arrow" as a diagnostic marker. J Periodontol 2006;77:1436–1441.
32. Kim DM, Bassir SH. When is cone-beam computed tomography imaging appropriate for diagnostic inquiry in the management of inflammatory periodontitis? An American Academy of Periodontology best evidence review. J Periodontol 2017;88:978–998.
33. Page RC, Kornman KS. The pathogenesis of human periodontitis: An introduction. Periodontol 2000 1997;14:9–11.

34. Korte DL, Kinney J. Personalized medicine: An update of salivary biomarkers for periodontal diseases. Periodontol 2000 2016;70:26–37.
35. Kornman KS, Crane A, Wang HY, et al. The interleukin-1 genotype as a severity factor in adult periodontal disease. J Clin Periodontol 1997;24:72–77.
36. Socransky SS, Haffajee AD, Cugini MA, Smith C, Kent RL, Jr. Microbial complexes in subgingival plaque. J Clin Periodontol 1998;25:134–144.
37. The American Academy of Periodontology. Proceedings of the World Workshop in Clinical Periodontics. Chicago: The American Academy of Periodontology 1989:I/23–I/24.
38. Caton JG, Armitage G, Berglundh T, et al. A new classification scheme for periodontal and peri-implant diseases and conditions: Introduction and key changes from the 1999 classification. J Periodontol 2018;89(suppl 1):S1–S8.
39. Armitage GC. Development of a classification system for periodontal diseases and conditions. Ann Periodontol 1999;4:1–6.
40. Tonetti MS, Greenwell H, Kornman KS. Staging and grading of periodontitis: Framework and proposal of a new classification and case definition. J Periodontol 2018;89(suppl 1):S159–S172.

3

GINGIVITIS AND PERIODONTITIS

Carlos Parra Carrasquer, DDS
Fernando Suárez López del Amo, DDS, MS

DEFINITIONS AND TERMINOLOGY

Aggressive periodontitis: A diverse group of highly destructive forms of periodontitis affecting primarily young individuals, including conditions formerly classified as "early-onset periodontitis" and "rapidly progressing periodontitis."[1]

Chronic periodontitis: Forms of destructive periodontal disease that are generally characterized by slow progression.[1]

Epidemiology: The study of the distribution of disease or a physiologic condition in human populations and of the factors that influence this distribution.[2]

Gingivitis: Site-specific inflammatory condition initiated by dental biofilm accumulation and characterized by gingival redness and edema and the absence of periodontal attachment loss.[3]

Incidence: The frequency in which some event, such as a disease or trait, appears in a particular population or area.

Necrotizing ulcerative gingivitis: An infection characterized by gingival necrosis presenting as "punched out" papillae, with gingival bleeding and pain. Halitosis and pseudomembrane formation may be secondary diagnostic features. Fusiform bacteria, *Prevotella*

Periodontal diseases are the result of a complex interaction between bacterial plaque, the host's immune response, and modifying factors that may impact the course of the disease. Periodontitis in particular represents a chronic inflammatory disease typically resulting in the apical migration of the junctional epithelium along with destruction of connective tissue attachment and alveolar bone. While microbial plaque and its byproducts are the main etiologic factors initiating the disease, it is the host's response to bacterial challenge that accounts for most of the periodontal destruction. Modifying factors such as diabetes, smoking, obesity, and genetic predisposition, among others, may exacerbate the progression of periodontal disease. Also, many of the features of periodontal disease are derived from the unique anatomy of the periodontium, in which a hard nonshedding structure (ie, a tooth) is partially embedded within the maxillary and mandibular processes.

This chapter focuses on the **epidemiology**, etiology, and pathogenesis, as well as the characteristics of the different forms of periodontal disease. It is important to mention that, while acknowledging the latest classification in periodontal diseases and conditions from the 2017 World Workshop (see chapter 2), several terms pertinent to previous classifications, including **chronic periodontitis** and **aggressive periodontitis**, have been used for clarification purposes.

Epidemiology

Epidemiologic studies must be conducted in humans, comprising a control or comparison group, and should consider all clinically relevant endpoints. These studies must provide data on the **prevalence** of periodontal diseases in different populations, as well as the severity of the cases. Additionally, the studies should clarify aspects of the etiology and risk factors and should provide information regarding the effectiveness of preventive and therapeutic measures on the population. Information on epidemiologic studies is gathered by clinical and radiographic assessment of the periodontal status. On the other hand, an *index* is a numeric value that is often used to describe the relative status of the population on a scale with definite upper and lower limits.[6] Since the 1950s, different clinical, laboratory, and radiologic recording systems and indices have been used to measure the prevalence, extent, and severity of periodontal diseases at individual and population levels. Indices require validity, reliability, clarity, simplicity, objectivity, quantifiability, sensitivity, and acceptability by both the examiner and the subject.[7–9] Some of the most commonly used in periodontology indices are shown in Box 3-1.[10–17]

PREVALENCE

One of the major challenges in assessing the prevalence of periodontal diseases relies on the great heterogeneity of indices used, the variations within population, the measurement errors, and the subjectivity of the examiners. However, recent epidemiologic studies have attempted to identify and overcome these issues.

Periodontitis

Between 2009 and 2014, the National Health and Nutrition Examination Survey (NHANES) conducted a survey on the prevalence of periodontitis among adults in the United States.[18] The findings were as follows:

- 42.2% of adults 30 years or older have periodontitis
  - 7.8% have severe periodontitis
  - 34.4% have mild or moderate periodontitis
- 59.8% of adults 65 years or older have periodontitis

Gingivitis

It is estimated that more than 82% of adolescents in the United States have signs of gingival bleeding and therefore **gingivitis**.[19] Additionally, more than 75% of the adults in the United States have signs of gingivitis.[20] Consequently, gingivitis is prevalent at all ages and is considered the most common form of periodontal disease.[21–23]

BOX 3-1 Commonly employed indices in periodontics[10–17]

Assessment of periodontal inflammation
- Gingival Index[10]
- Gingival Bleeding Index[11]

Assessment of plaque
- Plaque Index[12]
- Hygiene Analysis Index[13]

Assessment of loss of periodontal support
- Russell's Periodontal Index[14]
- Periodontal Disease Index[15]

Radiographic assessment of radiographic bone loss
- Schei's ruler[16]
- Percent of bone loss

Assessment of periodontal treatment needs
- Community Periodontal Index of Treatment Needs[17]

intermedia, and spirochetes have been associated with the lesion. Predisposing factors may include stress, poor diet, smoking, and HIV infection.[4]

Necrotizing ulcerative periodontitis: An infection characterized by necrosis of gingival tissues, periodontal ligament, and alveolar bone. These lesions are most commonly observed in individuals with systemic conditions, including but not limited to HIV infection, malnutrition, and immunosuppression.[4]

Periodontal health: State free of inflammatory periodontal disease.[5]

Periodontitis: Chronic multifactorial inflammatory disease associated with dysbiotic plaque biofilms and characterized by progressive destruction of the tooth-supporting apparatus.[1]

Prevalence: The proportion of a population that has a specific characteristic at a given time.

Aggressive periodontitis

It is estimated that the prevalence of aggressive periodontitis among US schoolchildren is around 0.4% for 13- to 15-year-olds and 0.8% for 16- to 19-year-olds.[24] Löe and Brown[25] in 1991 as well as Albandar et al[24] in 1997 found that the prevalence of aggressive periodontitis is highest among African Americans (2.64% and 2.6%), followed by Hispanic Americans (1.08% and 0.5%), whereas White Americans had the lowest prevalence (0.17% and 0.06%). In most populations, the prevalence of aggressive periodontitis is similar in males and females.[26]

Tooth loss

The main reason for tooth extraction in the ages up to 40 to 45 years is dental caries. On the other hand, periodontal disease is the major cause of tooth loss in older adults. In fact, extractions for periodontal reasons increase with age and account for over two-thirds of all extractions in adults over 50 years of age.[27] Second molars and mandibular incisors are the teeth most frequently extracted for periodontal reasons.[28]

Dental Biofilm

The human oral microbiome is an exceptional habitat for many different species of bacteria. Data from molecular and culture studies with the support of the United States National Institute of Health and the Human Microbiome Project have shown that approximately 700 distinct bacterial phyla may be able to live in the oral cavity.[29] Nevertheless, not all of them will be present simultaneously in a particular individual. It has been estimated that an individual subject may harbor about 100 to 200 taxa in the mouth.[30] In addition, some species are site specific, while other species are subject specific.[31]

Oral bacteria will produce various polysaccharides and glycoproteins that have the ability to adhere to other suspended or planktonic microorganisms (coaggregation) or to other already-adhering microorganisms or surfaces (coadhesion). Additionally, salivary glycoproteins and antibodies will form the acquired pellicle on the tooth surface, which facilitates bacterial adhesion.

In 1998, Socransky et al[32] were able to use the checkerboard DNA-DNA hybridization technique to identify different groups of bacteria that often exist together in subgingival plaque. Five bacterial clusters were identified and classified into different colors: red, orange, purple, yellow, and green (Fig 3-1).[32] Additionally, a relationship between those bacterial clusters was identified, categorizing them in different stages and severity of periodontal disease. Actinomyces (purple complex), Streptococcus (yellow complex), and Capnocytophaga (green complex) species are considered early colonizers because these will be the first microorganisms colonizing the tooth surface. Usually the early or primary colonizers are facultative anaerobic gram-positive cocci. Later, secondary colonizers like *Fusobacterium nucleatum* or *Prevotella intermedia* (orange complex) will interact with the early colonizers, and the shift to gram-negative anaerobic bacterial flora will begin. Finally, the late colonizers, red complex bacteria such as *Porphyromonas gingivalis*, *Treponema denticola*, or *Tannerella forsythia*, will coaggregate with the secondary colonizers, resulting in a more pathogenic microbiota (Fig 3-2).[33,34]

These bacteria associations are regulated by *quorum sensing*, which is the ability to detect and respond to cell density and thereby coordinate cell behavior. As such, bacteria secrete and detect autoinducer molecules, which accumulate in a cell density–dependent manner and regulate the expression of specific genes.[35] A major advantage for bacteria grouped in the biofilm is the protection it provides against environmental factors such as host-defense mechanisms and toxic substances in the environment, such as antimicrobials. Along with providing protection, biofilms also facilitate the uptake of nutrients and water, as well as the removal of metabolic waste products.[36] As a result, it has been estimated that organisms in biofilms could be up to 1,000 times more resistant to antibiotics as compared with their planktonic state.[37]

Dental calculus usually represents mineralized bacterial plaque. Supragingival calculus will be located coronal to the gingival margin and is usually whitish to dark yellow or brown, hard, with a claylike consistency and easily detachable from the tooth surface. Its rate of formation will depend on the bacterial plaque present and on the quality and quantity of the secretions of the salivary glands. Subgingival calculus is located apical to the gingival margin, so it is not visible on routine clinical examination. Occasionally, subgingival calculus may be visible in dental radiographs. Both sub- and supragingival calculus provide perfect environments for bacterial adhesion, growth, and maturation, as well as increase the surface for bacterial colonization. It is important to mention that sterilized[38] or disinfected[39] calculus does not trigger a marked inflammatory reaction, but the bacterial plaque attached to it will. For this, calculus is considered

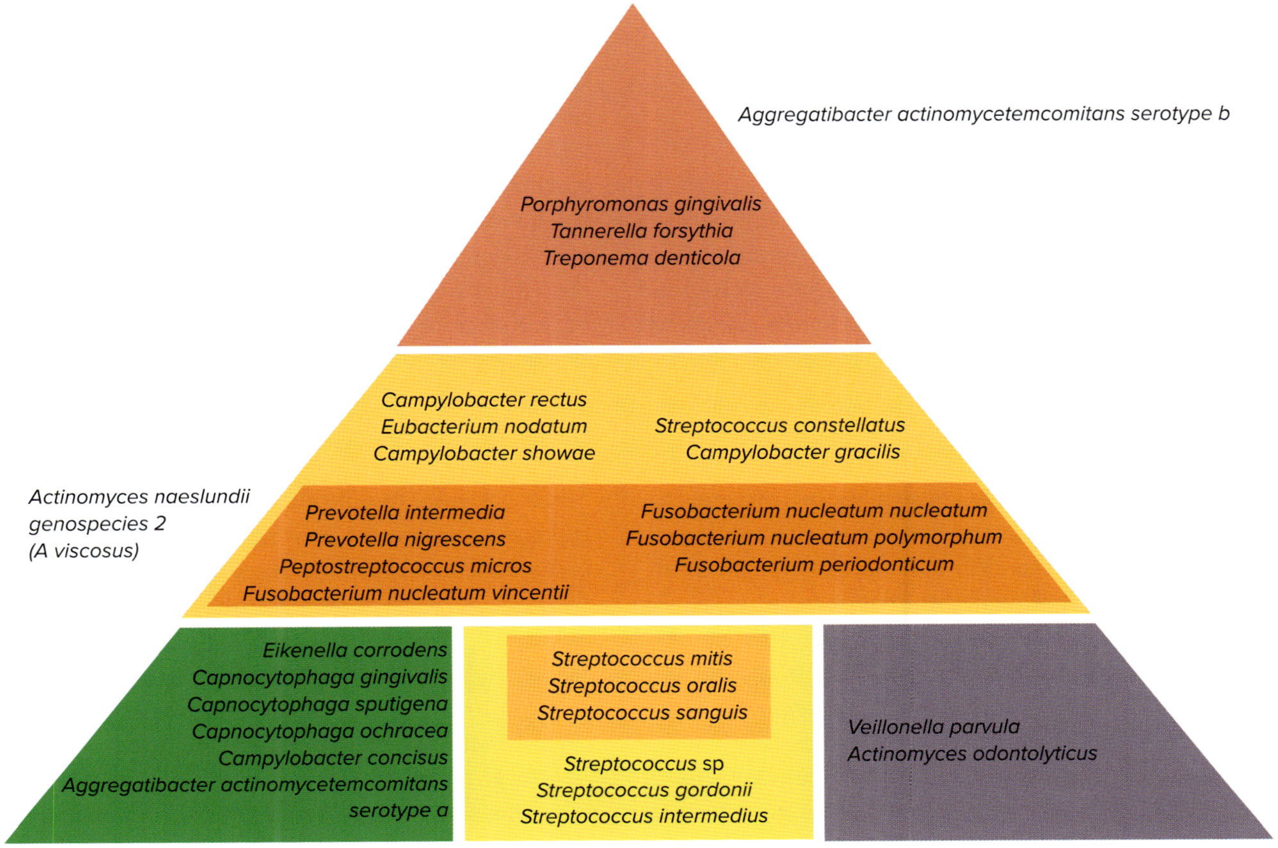

Fig 3-1 Microbial complexes. (Adapted from Socransky et al.[32])

Fig 3-2 Spatiotemporal model of oral bacteria colonizing a tooth surface. Early colonizers will attach to specific receptors on molecules of the acquired pellicle. Coadhesion of secondary colonizers, and specifically of *F nucleatum*, will play a role of "bridging" species from early and late colonizers because it has the ability to coaggregate with multiple bacteria. (Adapted with permission from Düzgünes.[34])

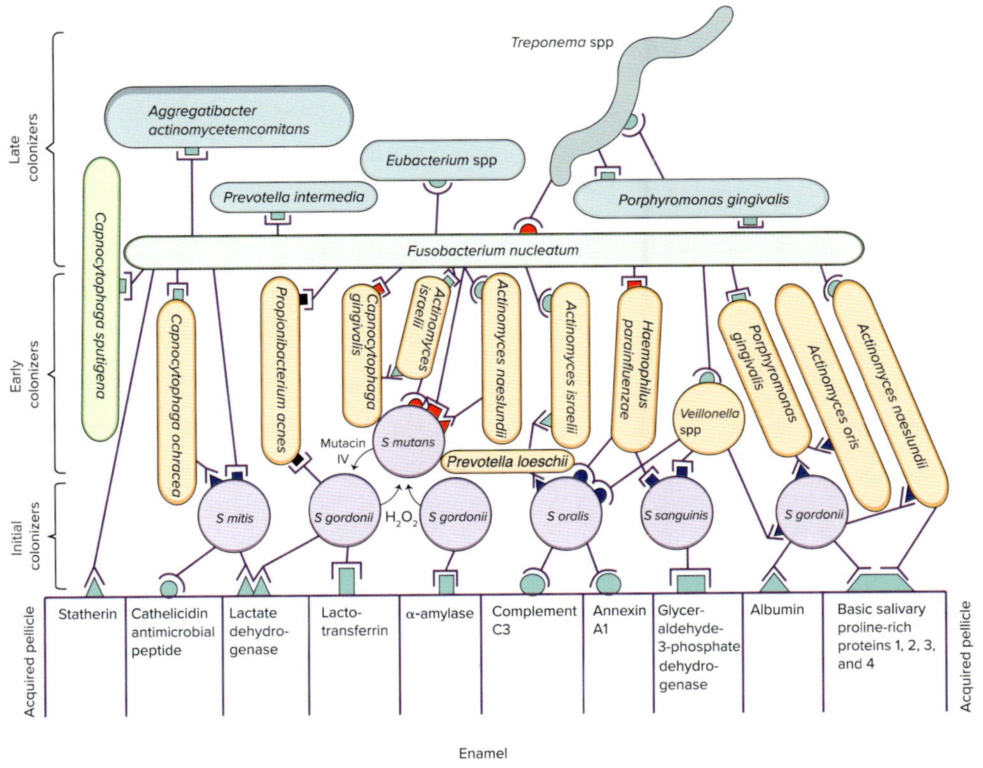

a secondary factor for periodontal disease, as it provides an ideal surface topography for plaque accumulation.

Theories of Pathogenesis

Different theories have emerged throughout the years trying to relate dental plaque and the transition from health to disease. Most of the theories have evolved and adapted based on the microbial and host response knowledge at the time.

NONSPECIFIC PLAQUE THEORY

Initially, the most common hypothesis was that periodontal infections were caused by a nonspecific overgrowth of bacteria.[40–42] Regardless of the specific types of microorganisms present, the most important factor was the increased amount of bacterial load in the periodontal tissues. Based on this hypothesis, the host would have a defined threshold, and periodontal disease would develop if that threshold became surpassed by increased amounts of bacteria, bacterial byproducts, and virulence factors.[43] This theory supports the notion that the most effective method to prevent and arrest disease progression is by the mechanical removal of plaque.

SPECIFIC PLAQUE THEORY

In 1976, Walter J. Loesche[41] described the specific plaque hypothesis, postulating that dental caries was a bacteria-specific infection, particularly originated by *Streptococcus mutans*, and that acute **necrotizing ulcerative gingivitis** was caused by specific intermediate-sized spirochetes, as well as *Bacteroides melaninogenicus* (known today as *Prevotella melaninogenica*).

The specific plaque hypothesis was further developed in the 1970s and 1980s, when more advanced culture and bacterial identification techniques were developed.[44,45] Key periodontal pathogens related to severe and aggressive periodontal diseases were identified, such as *Aggregatibacter actinomycetemcomitans*, *P gingivalis*, *T forsythia*, or *T denticola*.[32,46,47] In light of the increased microbiologic understanding, it became evident that periodontal destruction was not only influenced by quantity, but also by the qualitative composition of bacterial plaque.[41]

ECOLOGICAL PLAQUE HYPOTHESIS

In 1994, Marsh[48] described the ecological plaque hypothesis, which encompasses the previous plaque theories relating bacterial plaque and the host response. Thus, specific bacteria as well as the total amount of bacterial plaque contribute to the development and progression of periodontal disease. Changes in the environment (eg, ecological stress) increase the competitiveness of putative pathogens at the expense of species associated with oral health, resulting in an upregulation of the expression of virulence factors. Therefore, there is a link between local environmental conditions and the activity and composition of the biofilm.[49]

In conclusion, the different dental plaque and bacteria hypotheses are dynamic theories that continue to evolve as new evidence and pathogenic mechanisms are unveiled.

Gingivitis

Plaque-induced or dental biofilm–induced gingivitis refers to an inflammatory response of the gingival tissues occurring secondary to bacterial plaque accumulation around the gingival margin.[40,50] In order to understand the initiation and progression of this inflammatory condition, Löe et al[40] performed an experimental gingivitis study. For this investigation, patients with healthy gingiva were asked to withdraw from all oral hygiene methods until the inflammatory changes were observed. Gingivitis developed within 10 days for three subjects, while for the remaining nine subjects it took between 15 and 21 days. Once these inflammatory changes were observed, patients were instructed to resume oral hygiene methods, and gingival health was regained within a week, also reestablishing the original bacterial flora. While simple in design, this study proved several concepts: *(1)* the bacterial plaque is the etiology of the disease, *(2)* the differences in the response suggest different progressions models and susceptibility of patients, and *(3)* gingivitis is reversible.[40]

In addition, bacteriologic changes were also evaluated. Healthy gingiva presented with small groups of bacteria mainly composed of gram-positive cocci and short rods. The initial stages of plaque accumulation (ie, 1 to 2 days) yielded an increase in rods and cocci followed by an accumulation of filamentous forms and fusobacteria (2 to 4 days) accompanied by further leukocyte accumulation. During the last phase, the predominant bacterial flora was characterized by *Vibrio* spp and spirochetes with still a large number of cocci, rods, and filamentous organisms as well as a heavy leukocyte accumulation. One year later, the same group performed a follow-up investigation demonstrating the increase in complexity of the microbial flora when gingivitis was established.[51] During the next decades, several other investigations focused on the progression and the different stages of gingivitis.[52–54] It is important to mention the methodologic differences among these studies. Page and Schroeder[52] reviewed the progression of gingivitis based on animal and human studies. Seymour et al[54] carried out experimental gingivitis in dental students. Last, Kornman et al[53] reviewed the relationship between bacterial challenge and host immunity during the progression of gingivitis.

Clinical signs and symptoms of plaque-induced gingivitis include edema, bleeding, erythema, tenderness, gingival enlargement, and halitosis.[55,56] In addition, the severity of these symptoms can vary among individuals and can be influenced by a variety of anatomical and restorative factors.[57,58] While gingivitis does not directly cause tooth loss, the prevention and early treatment of this condition represents a key component of the prevention of periodontitis.[59]

Dental plaque–induced gingivitis can also be associated with dental biofilm alone, or on the other hand, it can be potentially modified or mediated by a variety of local and systemic factors including sex steroid hormones, hyperglycemia, leukemia, smoking, malnutrition, certain subgingival restorations, and hyposalivation.[50] Moreover, drug-influenced gingival enlargements can also occur secondary to antiepileptic drugs, certain calcium channel blockers, immunoregulators, and high-dose oral contraceptives.[50] It is important to bear in mind that while bacteria are necessary to develop gingivitis in conjunction with these medications, not all patients taking these drugs will experience gingival enlargement.

Non-Plaque-Induced Gingival Diseases

While dental biofilm–induced gingivitis is the most common form of periodontal disease, several other non-plaque-induced gingival diseases are described. Based on the 2017 World Workshop, these non-plaque-induced gingival diseases include[60]:

- Genetic/developmental disorders
- Specific infections
- Inflammatory and immune conditions
- Reactive processes
- Neoplasms
- Endocrine, nutritional, and metabolic diseases
- Traumatic lesions
- Gingival pigmentation

Chronic Periodontitis

Based on the 2017 World Workshop on the classification of periodontal and peri-implant diseases and conditions, three forms of periodontitis are recognized: necrotizing periodontitis; periodontitis (formerly known as *chronic* and *aggressive periodontitis*); and periodontitis as a manifestation of systemic diseases.[61] However, for the purpose of this chapter, both chronic and aggressive periodontitis are discussed separately.

Periodontitis was recently defined by the 2017 World Workshop as a "chronic multifactorial inflammatory disease associated with dysbiotic plaque biofilms and characterized by progressive destruction of the tooth-supporting apparatus."[1] The main features of this disease include the presence of periodontal pockets, gingival bleeding, clinical attachment loss, and alveolar bone loss (Fig 3-3). If left untreated, periodontitis could lead to tooth mobility and ultimately tooth loss. In addition, chronic periodontitis is influenced by a great variety of local and systemic factors that can significantly exacerbate disease progression. These factors are discussed in the following chapters.

As mentioned previously, periodontitis is caused by an exaggerated inflammatory response from the host caused by a dysbiosis. This process is the result of a transition from the symbiotic microbial and immune state of a healthy individual (or nonprogressive gingivitis) to an abnormal and exacerbated host response accompanied by a dysbiotic microbiome.[62] It is important to mention that while gingivitis may or may not advance to periodontitis, attachment loss and the development of periodontitis are always preceded by gingival inflammation.[63] Consequently, many authors have studied the changes and progression from gingivitis to periodontitis. In 1985, Listgarten et al[64] longitudinally followed 61 adults with varying degrees of gingivitis. Results from this investigation revealed that only 1 out of 1,000 tooth surfaces increased in probing depths by 3 mm or more from baseline regardless of the protocol for recall maintenance intervals. Therefore, the authors concluded that despite the high prevalence of

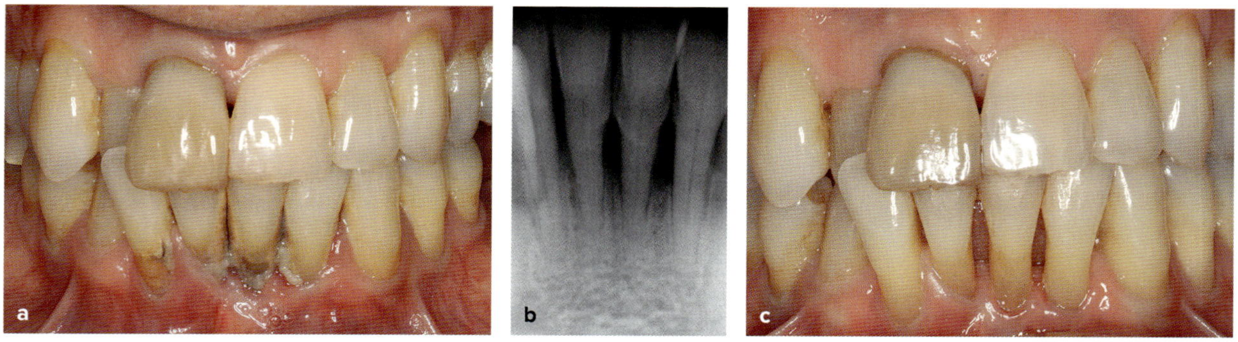

Fig 3-3 Periodontitis (formerly referred to as *chronic periodontitis*.) *(a)* Initial presentation of maxillary and mandibular anterior dentition prior to nonsurgical therapy. *(b)* Radiographic evaluation prior to nonsurgical therapy. *(c)* Reevaluation 3 months after nonsurgical therapy.

gingivitis, most individuals were relatively resistant to periodontitis. Subsequently, other investigations aimed at studying disease development, disease progression, and several other parameters related to periodontitis, such as attachment loss or changes in bone level.

Löe et al[65,66] conducted a series of landmark investigations aimed at studying the natural development and progression of periodontal disease. One of the first investigations was published by this group in 1978 and compared two populations with different geographic, cultural, socioeconomic, and educational differences. Both groups were chosen due to the extreme differences with regard to health care systems and dental care. The study population from Oslo, Norway, had access to programs for dental care while the population from Sri Lanka never had access to any programs for prevention or treatment of dental-related diseases and did not perform toothbrushing. Results from this investigation demonstrated the variability with regard to disease progression between both populations, concluding also that without proper dental care, the periodontal lesions continue progressing at a relatively even pace.[65] Years later in 1986, after following a group of 480 male Sri Lankan tea workers for 15 years, Löe et al[66] described three subpopulations presenting with *(1)* rapid progression, *(2)* moderate progression, and *(3)* no progression of periodontal disease (Table 3-1). Results from this investigation demonstrated that disease progression varies between individuals, at different ages, as well as within the same individual dentition. Also, the authors explained that although disease progresses steadily over time, there may be discrete episodes with more rapid or slower destruction. In agreement with these results, a recent systematic review by Needleman et al[67] concluded that mean attachment level change differs significantly within and between populations.

MODELS OF DISEASE PROGRESSION

The patterns of disease progression have been extensively studied, aiming at evaluating how loss of attachment occurs over time. In 1982, Goodson et al[68] described the progression of attachment level in 22 untreated patients performing measurements every month for 1 year. Results from this investigation demonstrated that the majority of the sites experienced no significant changes (82.8%), followed by 11.5% of the sites that became significantly shallower and 5.7% of sites that became significantly deeper. Within the group that suffered increase in probing depths, approximately half experienced progressive deepening and the other half presented with periods of exacerbation and spontaneous remission/recovery.[68] In 1984, Socransky et al[69] reviewed the available evidence and described three models of disease progression: continuous, random burst, and asynchronous multiple burst.[68] In 1991, Jeffcoat and Reddy[70] revisited this topic following patients with periodontitis for 6 months. In this investigation, three models were described as *(1)* linear or continuous (76% of sites), *(2)* burst (12% of sites), and *(3)* exacerbations and remission (12% of sites).[70]

TABLE 3-1 Characteristics of the groups described by Löe et al[66] in 1986

		No progression	Moderate progression	Rapid progression
Individuals		~ 11%	~ 81%	~ 8%
Annual rate of destruction (mm)		0.05–0.09	0.05–0.5	0.1–1.0
Mean attachment loss (mm)	15 years	NA	0.35	0.64
	25 years	NA	1.8	4.3
	30–40 years	< 1	~ 4	~ 11.2
	45 years	NA	~ 7	~ 13
Tooth loss (teeth)	15 years	0	NA	NA
	25 years	0	NA	5.9
	30–40 years	0	3–4	9–20
	45 years	0	7	All

NA, not available.

Aggressive Periodontitis

The term *aggressive periodontitis* has been through many modifications since 1923 when Gottlieb defined it as "diffuse alveolar atrophy."[71] Over the course of the 20th century, this inflammatory disease often changed in terminology, being referred to as *periodontosis*, *juvenile periodontitis*, and *early-onset periodontitis*, among others. Later, in 1999, the American Academy of Periodontology proposed the term *aggressive periodontitis* to refer to the highly destructive forms of periodontitis.[72] This rapidly progressing type of periodontal disease has been studied for decades as a separate entity from chronic periodontitis due to its aggressive nature, familial tendencies, the location of the lesions, and the relative low or inconsistent levels of biofilm (and secondary etiologic factors) compared with the severity of periodontal tissue destruction[73,74] (Fig 3-4). Other features recognized by the 1999 consensus report included patients that are otherwise healthy, rapid attachment loss and bone destruction that may be self-arresting, and phagocyte abnormalities.[73]

Nevertheless, chronic and aggressive periodontitis share many similarities, and the latest classification from the 2017 World Workshop on the classification of periodontal and peri-implant diseases and conditions refuted the presence of enough evidence to support the distinction between aggressive and chronic periodontitis as two separate diseases. This recent report emphasized the phenotypic differences between both entities, and more specifically, between chronic and localized aggressive periodontitis (including age of onset, location of initial lesions, and rate of progression). However, it also reiterated that both represent inflammatory diseases responding to biofilm accumulation, and it is premature to describe pathophysiologic differences until further data in larger and more controlled studies is available. In addition, both chronic and localized aggressive periodontitis have a common end result.[62] Hence, it was concluded that while there are significant variations with regard to clinical presentations, the currently available evidence does not support the distinction between chronic and aggressive periodontitis as two separate diseases.[1]

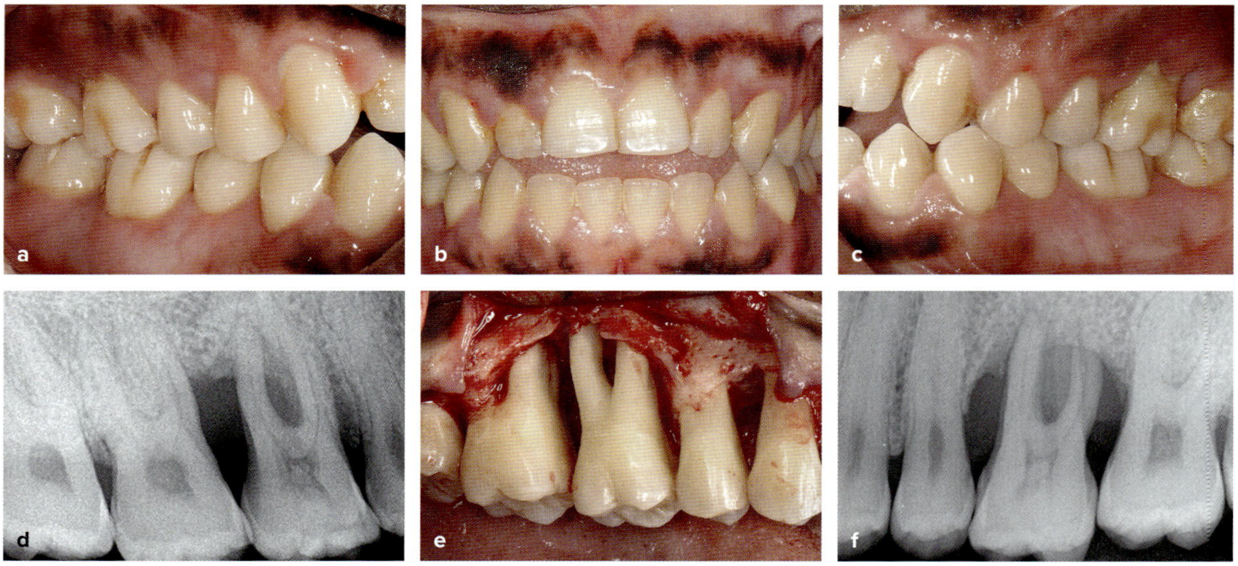

Fig 3-4 *(a to f)* Periodontitis (formerly referred to as *aggressive periodontitis*).

Periodontitis as a Manifestation of Systemic Diseases

Several systemic diseases and conditions can affect the periodontium and cause its destruction. Most of these disorders or conditions are secondary to innate mechanisms, although some are acquired through lifestyles or environmental factors. The periodontal effects of these systemic diseases and conditions are mainly through their influence on the immune and inflammatory responses. In addition, these can affect the periodontium by either influencing the course of periodontitis or by affecting the supporting tissues independently of plaque-induced inflammation.[75] Albandar et al[75] classified those diseases and conditions into three main categories. The first includes systemic disorders with a major impact on the loss of periodontal tissue by influencing periodontal inflammation. These disorders include genetic disorders (eg, Down syndrome), acquired immunodeficiency diseases (eg, HIV infection), and inflammatory diseases (eg, arthritis). The second category describes systemic disorders that influence the pathogenesis of periodontal diseases contributing to periodontal tissue loss (eg, smoking, depression). Last, the third category describes disorders that can cause destruction of the periodontal attachment independent of plaque-induced periodontitis (eg, neoplasms).[75]

Most of these conditions are determined by the genotype of the host, and they may be modified by environmental and behavioral factors. In addition, periodontitis and certain systemic disorders may share similar genetic and/or environmental risk factors. Consequently, loss of periodontal attachment is a common manifestation of several systemic disorders, which could have an important therapeutic and diagnostic value.

Necrotizing Periodontal Diseases

Necrotizing periodontal diseases belong to a group of acute lesions occurring in the periodontium and can be divided into necrotizing gingivitis (formerly referred to as *necrotizing ulcerative gingivitis*) and necrotizing periodontitis (formerly referred to as **necrotizing ulcerative periodontitis**).[76] Currently available evidence suggests that given the similar etiology, clinical features, and treatment, these entities may represent different stages of the same disease and may even progress to more severe forms such as necrotizing stomatitis and noma.[76]

Necrotizing periodontal diseases are associated with impairment in the host immune response and typically present with three clinical features: papilla necrosis, pain, and bleeding. Other signs and symptoms may include halitosis, pseudomembranes, regional lymphadenopathy, fever, sialorrhea, and rapid bone loss in cases of necrotizing periodontitis. Necrotizing stomatitis is a more severe inflammatory condition that courses with soft tissue necrosis beyond the gingiva, osteitis, and bone sequestrum.[1]

Similar to other forms of periodontitis, the etiology of necrotizing periodontal diseases is a bacterial infection; however, several other predisposing factors and immune-related conditions play a role in the pathogenesis.[76]

References

1. Papapanou PN, Sanz M, Buduneli N, et al. Periodontitis: Consensus report of workgroup 2 of the 2017 World Workshop on the Classification of Periodontal and Peri-Implant Diseases and Conditions. J Periodontol 2018;89(suppl 1):S173–S182.
2. Lilienfeld DE. Definitions of epidemiology. Am J Epidemiol 1978;107:87–90.
3. Trombelli L, Farina R, Silva CO, Tatakis DN. Plaque-induced gingivitis: Case definition and diagnostic considerations. J Periodontol 2018;89(suppl 1):S46–S73.
4. American Academy of Periodontology. Glossary of Periodontal Terms. American Academy of Periodontology, 2001.
5. Lang NP, Bartold PM. Periodontal health. J Periodontol 2018;89(suppl 1):S9–S16.
6. Russell AL. Epidemiology and the rational base of dental public health and dental practice. In: Young WO (ed). The Dentist, His Practice, and His Community, ed 2. Philadelphia: Saunders, 1969.
7. Beltrán-Aguilar ED, Eke PI, Thornton-Evans G, Petersen PE. Recording and surveillance systems for periodontal diseases. Periodontology 2000 2012;60:40–53.
8. Beltrán-Aguilar ED, Malvitz DM, Lockwood SA, Rozier RG, Tomar SL. Oral health surveillance: Past, present, and future challenges. J Public Health Dent 2003;63:141–149.
9. Burt BA, Eklund SA. The methods of oral epidemiology. In: Burt BA, Eklund SA (eds). Dentistry, Dental Practice, and the Community, ed 4. Philadelphia: Saunders, 1992.
10. Löe H, Silness J. Periodontal disease in pregnancy. I. Prevalence and severity. Acta Odontol Scand 1963;21:533–551.
11. Ainamo J, Bay I. Problems and proposals for recording gingivitis and plaque. Int Dent J 1975;25:229–235.
12. Silness J, Löe H. Periodontal disease in pregnancy. II. Correlation between oral hygiene and periodontal condtion. Acta Odontol Scand 1964;22:121–135.
13. O'Leary TJ, Drake RB, Naylor JE. The plaque control record. J Periodontol 1972;43:38.
14. Russell AL. A system of classification and scoring for prevalence surveys of periodontal disease. J Dent Res 1956;35:350–359.
15. Ramfjord SP. Indices for prevalence and incidence of periodontal disease. J Periodontol 1959;30:51–59.
16. Schei O, Waerhaug J, Lovdal A, Arno A. Alveolar bone loss as related to oral hygiene and age. J Periodontol 1959;30:7–16.
17. Ainamo J, Barmes D, Beagrie G, Cutress T, Martin J, Sardo-Infirri J. Development of the World Health Organization (WHO) community periodontal index of treatment needs (CPITN). Int Dent J 1982;32:281–291.
18. Eke PI, Thornton-Evans GO, Wei L, Borgnakke WS, Dye BA, Genco RJ. Periodontitis in US Adults: National Health and Nutrition Examination Survey 2009–2014. J Am Dent Assoc 2018;149:576–588.
19. Albandar JM, Brown LJ, Brunelle JA, Löe H. Gingival state and dental calculus in early-onset periodontitis. J Periodontol 1996;67:953–959.
20. Kingman A, Albandar JM. Methodological aspects of epidemiological studies of periodontal diseases. Periodontology 2000 2002;29:11–30.
21. White DA, Tsakos G, Pitts NB, et al. Adult Dental Health Survey 2009: Common oral health conditions and their impact on the population. Br Dent J 2012;213:567–572.
22. Dye BA. Global periodontal disease epidemiology. Periodontol 2000 2012;58:10–25.
23. Stamm JW. Epidemiology of gingivitis. J Clin Periodontol 1986;13:360–366.
24. Albandar JM, Brown LJ, Löe H. Clinical features of early-onset periodontitis. J Am Dent Assoc 1997;128:1393–1399.
25. Löe H, Brown LJ. Early onset periodontitis in the United States of America. J Periodontol 1991;62:608–616.
26. Susin C, Haas AN, Albandar JM. Epidemiology and demographics of aggressive periodontitis. Periodontol 2000 2014;65:27–45.
27. Oliver RC, Brown LJ. Periodontal diseases and tooth loss. Periodontology 2000 1993;2:117–127.
28. Ong G. Periodontal disease and tooth loss. Int Dent J 1998;48:233–238.
29. Verma D, Garg PK, Dubey AK. Insights into the human oral microbiome. Arch Microbiol 2018;200:525–540.
30. Siqueira JF Jr, Rôças IN. The oral microbiota in health and disease: An overview of molecular findings. Methods Mol Biol 2017;1537:127–138.
31. Aas JA, Paster BJ, Stokes LN, Olsen I, Dewhirst FE. Defining the normal bacterial flora of the oral cavity. J Clin Microbiol 2005; 43:5721–5732.
32. Socransky SS, Haffajee AD, Cugini MA, Smith C, Kent RL Jr. Microbial complexes in subgingival plaque. J Clin Periodontol 1998;25:134–144.
33. Kolenbrander PE, Palmer RJ Jr, Periasamy S, Jakubovics NS. Oral multispecies biofilm development and the key role of cell-cell distance. Nat Rev Microbiol 2010;8:471–480.
34. Düzgünes N. Medical Microbiology and Immunology for Dentistry. Chicago: Quintessence, 2016.
35. Nadell CD, Xavier JB, Levin SA, Foster KR. The evolution of quorum sensing in bacterial biofilms. PLoS Biol 2008;6:e14.
36. Socransky SS, Haffajee AD. Dental biofilms: Difficult therapeutic targets. Periodontol 2000 2002;28:12–55.
37. Rasmussen TB, Givskov M. Quorum-sensing inhibitors as anti-pathogenic drugs. Int J Med Microbiol 2006;296:149–161.
38. Allen DL, Kerr DA. Tissue response in the guinea pig to sterile and non-sterile calculus. J Periodontol 1965;36:121–126.
39. Listgarten MA, Ellegaard B. Electron microscopic evidence of a cellular attachment between junctional epithelium and dental calculus. J Periodontal Res 1973;8:143–150.
40. Löe H, Theilade E, Jensen SB. Experimental gingivitis in man. J Periodontol 1965;36:177–187.
41. Loesche WJ. Chemotherapy of dental plaque infections. Oral Sci Rev 1976;9:65–107.

42. Miller WD. The Micro-Organisms of the Human Mouth. Philadelphia: SS White Dental MFG, 1890.
43. Theilade E. The non-specific theory in microbial etiology of inflammatory periodontal diseases. J Clin Periodontol 1986;13:905–911.
44. Listgarten MA. Structure of the microbial flora associated with periodontal health and disease in man. A light and electron microscopic study. J Periodontol 1976;47:1–18.
45. Socransky SS, Haffajee AD. The bacterial etiology of destructive periodontal disease: Current concepts. J Periodontol 1992;63:322–331.
46. Slots J. Subgingival microflora and periodontal disease. J Clin Periodontol 1979;6:351–382.
47. Tanner AC, Izard J. *Tannerella forsythia*, a periodontal pathogen entering the genomic era. Periodontol 2000 2006;42:88–113.
48. Marsh PD. Microbial ecology of dental plaque and its significance in health and disease. Adv Dent Res 1994;8:263–271.
49. Marsh PD, Moter A, Devine DA. Dental plaque biofilms: Communities, conflict and control. Periodontol 2000 2011;55:16–35.
50. Murakami S, Mealey BL, Mariotti A, Chapple ILC. Dental plaque-induced gingival conditions. J Periodontol 2018;89(suppl 1):S17–S27.
51. Theilade E, Wright WH, Jensen SB, Löe H. Experimental gingivitis in man. II. A longitudinal clinical and bacteriological investigation. J Periodontal Res 1966;1:1–13.
52. Page RC, Schroeder HE. Pathogenesis of inflammatory periodontal disease. A summary of current work. Lab Invest 1976;34:235–249.
53. Kornman KS, Page RC, Tonetti MS. The host response to the microbial challenge in periodontitis: Assembling the players. Periodontol 2000 1997;14:33–53.
54. Seymour GJ, Powell RN, Aitken JF. Experimental gingivitis in humans. A clinical and histologic investigation. J Periodontol 1983;54:522–528.
55. Suzuki JB. Diagnosis and classification of the periodontal diseases. Dent Clin North Am 1988;32:195–216.
56. Quirynen M, Dadamio J, Van den Velde S, et al. Characteristics of 2,000 patients who visited a halitosis clinic. J Clin Periodontol 2009;36:970–975.
57. Blieden TM. Tooth-related issues. Ann Periodontol 1999;4:91–97.
58. Trombelli L, Scapoli C, Orlandini E, Tosi M, Bottega S, Tatakis DN. Modulation of clinical expression of plaque-induced gingivitis. III. Response of "high responders" and "low responders" to therapy. J Clin Periodontol 2004;31:253–259.
59. Tonetti MS, Chapple IL, Jepsen S, Sanz M. Primary and secondary prevention of periodontal and peri-implant diseases: Introduction to, and objectives of the 11th European Workshop on Periodontology consensus conference. J Clin Periodontol 2015;42(suppl 16):S1–S4.
60. Holmstrup P, Plemons J, Meyle J. Non-plaque-induced gingival diseases. J Periodontol 2018;89(suppl 1):S28–S45.
61. Caton JG, Armitage G, Berglundh T, et al. A new classification scheme for periodontal and peri-implant diseases and conditions: Introduction and key changes from the 1999 classification. J Periodontol 2018;89(suppl 1):S1–S8.
62. Fine DH, Patil AG, Loos BG. Classification and diagnosis of aggressive periodontitis. J Periodontol 2018;89(suppl 1):S103–S119.
63. Kinane DF, Attström R, European Workshop in Periodontology group B. Advances in the pathogenesis of periodontitis. Group B consensus report of the fifth European Workshop in Periodontology. J Clin Periodontol 2005;32(suppl 6):130–131.
64. Listgarten MA, Schifter CC, Laster L. 3-year longitudinal study of the periodontal status of an adult population with gingivitis. J Clin Periodontol 1985;12:225–238.
65. Löe H, Anerud A, Boysen H, Smith M. The natural history of periodontal disease in man. The rate of periodontal destruction before 40 years of age. J Periodontol 1978;49:607–620.
66. Löe H, Anerud A, Boysen H, Morrison E. Natural history of periodontal disease in man. Rapid, moderate and no loss of attachment in Sri Lankan laborers 14 to 46 years of age. J Clin Periodontol 1986;13:431–445.
67. Needleman I, Garcia R, Gkranias N, et al. Mean annual attachment, bone level, and tooth loss: A systematic review. J Periodontol 2018;89(suppl 1):S120–S139.
68. Goodson JM, Tanner AC, Haffajee AD, Sornberger GC, Socransky SS. Patterns of progression and regression of advanced destructive periodontal disease. J Clin Periodontol 1982;9:472–481.
69. Socransky SS, Haffajee AD, Goodson JM, Lindhe J. New concepts of destructive periodontal disease. J Clin Periodontol 1984;11:21–32.
70. Jeffcoat MK, Reddy MS. Progression of probing attachment loss in adult periodontitis. J Periodontol 1991;62:185–189.
71. Gottlieb B. Weitere Beiträge zur Kenntnis des Alveolarschwundes und dessen Wiedergutmachung durch Zementwachstum. Z Stomatol 1923:195–201.
72. Armitage GC. Development of a classification system for periodontal diseases and conditions. Ann Periodontol 1999;4:1–6.
73. American Academy of Periodontology Task Force Report on the Update to the 1999 Classification of Periodontal Diseases and Conditions. J Periodontol 2015;86:835–838.
74. Listgarten MA. Structure of surface coatings on teeth. A review. J Periodontol 1976;47:139–147.
75. Albandar JM, Susin C, Hughes FJ. Manifestations of systemic diseases and conditions that affect the periodontal attachment apparatus: Case definitions and diagnostic considerations. J Periodontol 2018;89(suppl 1):S183–S203.
76. Herrera D, Retamal-Valdes B, Alonso B, Feres M. Acute periodontal lesions (periodontal abscesses and necrotizing periodontal diseases) and endo-periodontal lesions. J Periodontol 2018;89(suppl 1):S85–S102.

4

RISKS

Theodoros Katsaros, DDS, MSD

Risk assessment is an essential component of periodontal patient management due to a number of local and systemic factors that can potentially affect the manifestation and progression of the disease. Accounting for these factors is an important step toward the delivery of optimal periodontal care.[1] In this chapter, the main risk factors, risk determinants, risk indicators, and risk markers are reviewed. The association between them and the onset and progression of periodontal disease is discussed, as well as the impact on treatment outcomes. It should be highlighted that this chapter is based on the current knowledge, and if new evidence emerges in the future, some of these factors may be classified under a different category.

Box 4-1 lists examples of **risk factors**, **risk determinants**, **risk indicators**, and **risk markers** or **predictors** for periodontal disease.

BOX 4-1 Classification of the main risk factors, risk determinants, risk indicators, and risk markers for periodontal disease

Risk factors	Risk determinants	Risk indicators	Risk markers
• Smoking • Diabetes • Pathogenic bacteria	• Genetics • Age • Sex • Race	• Obesity • Osteoporosis • Stress • Alcohol use • Rheumatoid arthritis	• Bleeding on probing • Probing depth • Furcation involvement

DEFINITIONS AND TERMINOLOGY

Risk determinant: A risk factor that cannot be modified (eg, genetic factors, sex, age).[2]

Risk factor: Environmental, behavioral, or biologic factors that increase the likelihood of developing the disease; identified through longitudinal studies and confirmed to be present before the onset of the disease (eg, smoking, diabetes, pathogenic bacteria).

Risk indicator: A putative risk factor that is correctly identified through cross-sectional study designs.

Risk marker or risk predictor: Characteristics or factors that have the ability to predict individuals at high risk for disease, but are not part of the causal chain.[3]

Risk Factors

SMOKING

Smoking is a well-documented risk factor for periodontal disease. The effects of smoking on the periodontal status can be classified as local and systemic.

Local effects

At the local level, smokers demonstrate increased supragingival[4] as well as subgingival calculus formation.[5] Additionally, the presence of nicotine has an effect on gingival fibroblasts, demonstrating an increase in gingival mediated collagen degradation. This action is mediated through the activation of matrix metalloproteinases (MMPs) and redistribution of the tissue inhibitors of metalloproteinases (TIMPs) to the cell membrane. Interestingly, this action is enhanced by the presence of *Porphyromonas gingivalis*.[6] With regard to the often observed fibrotic clinical appearance of the gingival tissues in smokers, in vitro investigations have demonstrated a possible explanation by the increase in the production of CCN2/CTGF (connective tissue growth factor) protein and consequently Type I collagen production.[7] The vasoconstriction and fibrosis on the gingival tissues often result in decreased bleeding on probing (BOP) even in the presence of bacterial plaque and calculus.[8]

Smokers also present with increased radiographic bone loss compared with nonsmokers, and there is a dose-dependent relationship: The odds of heavy smokers having severe bone loss are higher (odds ratio [OR] 7.28) compared with light smokers (OR 3.25).[9] These detrimental effects are also observed in populations that maintain good levels of oral hygiene. Cross-sectional studies demonstrated that smokers had significantly reduced bone levels compared with nonsmokers, with the observed amount of bone loss occurring in a shorter time frame in smokers.[10] Similar conclusions were obtained when evaluating the bone levels of a different population (Swedish hygienists) through the assessment of bitewing radiographs. Smokers had the highest amount of radiographic bone loss compared with nonsmokers or former smokers.[11]

0Van Winkelhoff et al[12] investigated the prevalence and levels of periodontal pathogens in both smokers and nonsmokers who were treated for periodontal disease as well as untreated populations. A higher prevalence of periodontal pathogens was noted in treated and untreated smokers in comparison with the respective nonsmoking populations. Based on these findings, the authors suggested integrating the use of systemic antibiotics in patients who do not exhibit a favorable response to initial treatment.[12] Haffajee and Socransky[13] performed a similar study, implementing DNA-DNA hybridization. Subjects were divided based on two criteria: *(1)* according to their smoking habits in current smokers, former smokers, and nonsmokers; *(2)* according to their periodontal status in periodontally healthy, well-maintained, and periodontitis patients. Current smokers had larger proportions of sites colonized by periodontal pathogens.[13] Zambon et al[14] came to similar conclusions after conducting a large cross-sectional study using immunofluorescence. *Tannerella forsythia* and *Aggregatibacter actinomycemetcomitans* were more likely to be identified in the subgingival microflora of smokers. Furthermore, there was a dose-dependent relationship between the risk of *T forsythia* infection and the number of pack-years.[14]

Systemic effects

Systemically, smoking can affect multiple components and mechanisms of the human immune response and subsequently the host response to periodontal pathogens. Smokers have been found to have a higher receptor activator of nuclear factor-κB ligand/osteoprotegerin (RANKL/OPG) ratio, which could partially explain the increased bone loss observed in smoking populations. This alteration in RANKL and OPG is observed not only in saliva[15] but also in serum.[16] Neutrophils constitute the first line of defense toward bacteria that accumulate in the gingival sulcus. Their function can be altered as a result of tobacco use.[17] In later disease stages, antibody production also takes place. During that period, reduced levels of serum immunoglobulin G 2 (IgG2) are identified.[18]

Treatment outcomes

In the classic longitudinal studies performed at the University of Nebraska, periodontal patients were enrolled in a maintenance program and followed up for 6 years after receiving active treatment. Smokers demonstrated poorer response to surgical and nonsurgical treatment, having lower probing depth (PD) reduction and clinical attachment level (CAL) gain.[19] When furcation sites were analyzed separately, smokers had 0.5 mm less CAL gain and 0.6 mm less PD reduction compared with nonsmokers.[19] A noteworthy observation from a different publication by the same group is that smokers exhibited a similar percentage of sites with BOP as nonsmokers.[20] Other studies reported smokers having higher percentages of

BOX 4-2 Link between smoking and periodontal status

Local effects	Systemic effects	Effects on treatment: Nonsurgical	Effects on treatment: Surgical	Effects on treatment: Maintenance
↑ Calculus formation	↑ RANKL/OPG	↓ PD reduction and CAL gain after SRP	↓ PD reduction and CAL gain	↑ Tooth loss
↑ Vasoconstriction	Altered neutrophil function	↓ PD reduction and CAL gain after SRP and local delivery of antibiotics	↓ CAL gain after GTR	↓ Periodontal stability
↑ Fibrosis	↓ Serum IgG2 levels			
↑ Radiographic bone loss				
↑ Periodontal pathogens				
↓ BOP				

GTR, guided tissue regeneration; SRP, scaling and root planing.

sites with BOP than nonsmokers with similar levels of oral hygiene.[21] The inferior response of smokers to nonsurgical periodontal treatment is also observed in cases where local delivery of antibiotics is used as an adjunct to scaling and root planing.[22]

As mentioned previously, smoking negatively affects the response to surgical as well as nonsurgical periodontal treatment.[19,22,23] Guided tissue regeneration is negatively affected as well. Clinical studies performed in private practices in Italy concluded that smokers had approximately 3 mm less CAL gain 12 months postoperatively (2.1 ± 1.2 mm) compared with nonsmokers (5.2 ± 1.9 mm).[24] When followed up for an extended period of 5 years, stable treatment outcomes were associated with patients who were not smokers, who maintained adequate oral hygiene, and who complied with supportive periodontal treatment.[25] Similarly, soft tissue grafting procedures are negatively influenced by smoking habits.[26]

It should be noted that despite the fact that the treatment response following smoking cessation is comparable with nonsmokers, this does not reverse the detrimental effects of smoking that have already manifested.[21,27] Tomar and Asma[28] analyzed the data from the Third National Health and Nutrition Examination Survey (NHANES III). The sample consisted of more than 13,000 adults, and it was estimated that it is four times more likely for current smokers to have periodontitis compared with individuals who never smoked. When former smokers were analyzed separately, the ones who had quit smoking in the previous 2 years were more likely to be diagnosed with periodontitis, and this likelihood decreased gradually. Former smokers who quit smoking for at least 11 years were as likely to have periodontitis as those who had never smoked. According to this study, almost three-fourths of periodontitis cases in the United States (74.8%) are attributed to smoking.[28]

Ultimately, smoking increases the likelihood of tooth loss. McGuire and Nunn[29] discussed the prognosis and prediction of tooth loss and followed up with periodontal maintenance patients for 14 years. They estimated the risk for tooth loss to be increased by 2.9 times for heavy smokers (Box 4-2).

DIABETES MELLITUS

According to the Centers for Disease Control and Prevention (CDC), an estimated 9.4% (30.3 million) of the U.S. population are diabetics, and almost 24% of this population (7.2 million) are undiagnosed.[30] The American Diabetes Association classifies diabetes based on its pathophysiology into the following categories:

- Type 1 (5% of diabetics): Caused by autoimmune destruction of the pancreatic β-cells. This results in inability of the pancreas to produce insulin.
- Type 2 (90%–95% of diabetics): Characterized by insulin resistance, eventually leading to loss of β-cell insulin secretion.
- Gestational (2%–10% of pregnancies): Onset usually during the second or third trimester of pregnancy.

BOX 4-3 Link between diabetes and periodontal status

Local effects	Systemic effects	Treatment outcomes
↑ BOP	↑ RANKL/OPG	Uncontrolled diabetics have poorer response to periodontal treatment, whereas well-controlled diabetics have responses similar to nondiabetics
Similar periodontal microbiota as nondiabetics	↑ Reactive oxygen species	Nonsurgical periodontal treatment can result in HbA1c level reduction (more significant in Type 2 diabetics)
	AGE–RAGE interaction that alters cell function	The average reduction in HbA1c is 0.3%–0.4% from the baseline value
	Similar IgG levels	

These individuals are more likely to develop Type 2 diabetes later in life.

- Other: Examples include diseases of the exocrine pancreas, and drug- or chemical-induced syndromes.

Diabetes is considered another major risk factor for periodontal disease. The mechanisms that link diabetes to periodontal disease have been described as associated with the interaction of the advanced glycation end products (AGEs) with their receptor (RAGE). This interaction alters cell function, increases levels of reactive oxygen species, and increases the RANKL/OPG, therefore altering bone homeostasis and eventually leading to increased tissue destruction.[31]

Local effects

The composition of periodontal microbiota does not appear to be influenced by diabetes, according to the majority of the existing literature.[31] Diabetics exhibit increased BOP, and this tendency increases as the level of diabetic control decreases.[32] In a longitudinal study in Pima Indians, more than 2,200 subjects were enrolled and followed up for 2.5 years. The incidence of periodontitis was 2.6 times higher in diabetics compared with nondiabetics.[33] Similar findings were reported from an epidemiologic study of the same population, with diabetes increasing the risk for periodontal disease by three times.[34]

Treatment outcomes

On the other hand, prediabetics or well-controlled diabetics are not at additional risk for periodontal disease.[35] The level of glycemic control has an impact on the outcome of the treatment. A favorable response is observed in well-controlled diabetics, similar to nondiabetic controls.[36]

The immunologic response of diabetics to bacterial plaque is similar to nondiabetics in terms of IgG levels, although differences can be observed in regard to the levels of E-selectin, vascular cell adhesion molecule-1 (VCAM-1), adiponectin, and plasminogen activator inhibitor-1.[37]

With regard to the effect of periodontal treatment on diabetic control, nonsurgical periodontal therapy can reduce the hemoglobin A1c (HbA1c) levels. However, this reduction may be considered insignificant, and it is not stable over time. The magnitude of the reduction is higher in Type 2 diabetics compared with Type 1 and when antibiotics were prescribed as an adjunct to nonsurgical treatment. Although the reduction of HbA1c following periodontal treatment reported from several studies can vary, based on the current evidence, it is anticipated to correspond to 0.3% to 0.4% less than the original value[38,39] (Box 4-3).

PATHOGENIC BACTERIA

Groups of bacteria with specific characteristics have been shown to be implicated as primary etiologic factors in the pathogenesis of periodontal diseases. The classic 1998 study by Socransky et al,[40] among others, investigated this association and identified specific bacterial complexes to be associated with increased PDs.

The qualitative and quantitative differences in the microflora of periodontitis and nonperiodontitis patients was also evidenced in a study by Listgarten and Hellden[41] in 1978. A significant increase in motile rods and a decrease in coccoid cells was observed in diseased sites (PD > 5 mm) compared with healthy sites.[41] See chapter 3 for further considerations.

Risk Determinants

GENETICS

The degree that periodontitis is influenced by genetics has been investigated in a number of studies. The role of genetics appears to be more significant in specific categories of periodontitis with rapid progression (previously known as *aggressive periodontitis*). The mode of transmission, however, remains unclear. The majority of the studies point toward autosomal dominant mode,[42] while others report X-linked or autosomal recessive.[43]

For the majority of the rest of the phenotypic expressions of periodontitis (chronic periodontitis), evidence from cross-sectional studies in twins suggest that genetics (heritability) are responsible for up to 50% of the manifestation of the disease.[44] Furthermore, a specific genotype of interleukin 1 β (IL-1β) has been shown to be associated with increased disease severity[45,46] and a 2.7-fold increase in risk of tooth loss.[29]

AGE

There have been studies connecting age with higher percentages of bone and attachment loss.[9,47] It is debatable, however, if the increased attachment loss observed with aging is representative of increased susceptibility to periodontal disease. Studies in different populations (Japanese and Swedish) concluded that periodontal stability can be observed over time.[48] In fact, recent evidence from epidemiologic studies supports the idea that the observed increase in clinical attachment loss is a result of changes accumulating over the years, rather than the result of periodontitis. These changes in CALs are mainly attributed to recession because PDs remain relatively stable over time.[49]

SEX

Males have been identified as being in higher risk for attachment and bone loss (OR 1.36 and 1.29, respectively), in cross-sectional[9] as well as longitudinal studies.[50] The clinical signs of gingival inflammation may be more severe in females during periods associated with hormonal changes, such as pregnancy or menstrual cycles.[51,52]

RACE

National Health and Nutrition Examination Survey (NHANES) data from the 2009–2010 period indicate that periodontitis is more prevalent among Mexican Americans, followed by non-Hispanic Black individuals, while non-Hispanic White individuals had the lowest prevalence among the three groups.[47] Furthermore, disease entities that were classified as "aggressive periodontitis" according to the 1999 classification of periodontal diseases were found to be more prevalent among African-American and Hispanic children and adolescents (OR 15.1 and 2.4, respectively).[53]

Risk Indicators

OBESITY

Adipose tissue secretes a number of proinflammatory cytokines and acute phase proteins, which can potentially affect the progression of periodontitis (among other possible mechanisms).[54] Young females who are overweight or obese also have increased risk of being diagnosed with periodontitis. The same population, however, did not demonstrate altered bacterial plaque composition compared with nonobese individuals, with the exception of increased levels of *T forsythia*.[55] Gorman et al[56] examined male subjects over a period of more than 25 years. The participants in this study who showed increase in waist circumference–to-height ratio and were obese were more likely to demonstrate signs of periodontal disease progression.[56]

OSTEOPOROSIS

Cross-sectional data suggest that there is an association in postmenopausal women between alveolar bone loss and osteopenia (T score between −2.5 and −1.0) as well as osteoporosis (T score < -2.5). This association is stronger in those 70 years old and above with worsening T scores. This subset of the population was 2.5 to 4.6 times more likely to present with loss of alveolar bone compared with subjects with normal bone scores.[57] A similar association was found between CALs and T scores, especially in women without subgingival calculus.[58]

STRESS

Genco et al[59] evaluated the association between periodontal disease and stress, distress, and inadequate coping behaviors. Analysis of questionnaires completed by more than 1,400 participants indicated that there was an association between bone loss and financial strain. This association, however, was altered depending on the approach the subjects demonstrated when coping with stress (emotional-based or problem-based).[59] The mechanisms behind these associations are not fully understood. Behavioral changes as a result of stress as well as alterations in host's immune function have been reported as possible mechanisms.[60]

ALCOHOL

A NHANES study indicated that there appears to be a dose-dependent relationship between alcohol consumption and prevalence of periodontal disease. As the number of drinks per week increases from 5 to more than 20, the odds ratio also increases from 1.22 to 1.67.[61] A smaller cross-sectional study reported similar conclusions, as alcohol dependence exhibited a linear relationship with CALs and PD.[62]

RHEUMATOID ARTHRITIS

Although there is only a low level of evidence, findings from a systematic review on the association between rheumatoid arthritis (RA) and periodontal disease indicate that patients with RA present with greater clinical attachment loss and increased tooth loss compared with individuals without RA. In the majority of cases, periodontitis precedes the manifestation of RA, but due to the quality of the existing studies, causality cannot be supported at this time.[63]

OTHER

Background characteristics, such as behavioral changes, socioeconomic status, and education level are frequently important when evaluating the associations between specific risk predictors and periodontal disease.

Risk Markers

BLEEDING ON PROBING

BOP has been thoroughly investigated in a number of longitudinal studies of periodontitis patients enrolled in maintenance programs. The high negative predictive value of this index makes it valuable in identifying the absence of clinical inflammation with high accuracy.[64] However, the presence of BOP does not necessarily indicate disease progression. Consequently, BOP presents with high specificity but low sensitivity. As demonstrated by Lang et al[65] in 1986 over a period of four consecutive maintenance appointments, a specific site may present with BOP in every maintenance visit, but there is still a 70% chance that this site will not lose attachment.

PROBING DEPTH

Another retrospective study evaluating patients in periodontal maintenance (for more than 11 years on average) showed that PDs of 5 mm and above following active periodontal therapy indicate increased risk for tooth loss. More specifically, the ORs of teeth with a deepest PD of 5, 6, or 7 mm to be extracted during the periodontal maintenance phase were 7.7, 11, and 64.2.[66]

FURCATION INVOLVEMENT

Several longitudinal studies in patients undergoing supportive periodontal treatment have demonstrated the association between furcation involvement and tooth loss. See chapter 5 for further considerations.

CRESTAL LAMINA DURA

A 3-year study by Rams et al[67] concluded that the presence of radiographic crestal lamina dura is positively associated with clinically stable periodontal status in interproximal sites. On the other hand, the absence of crestal lamina dura cannot be used as a predictor for periodontal disease recurrence due to its low positive predictive value.[67] Greenstein et al[68] performed a cross-sectional study to investigate the potential relationship between the crestal lamina dura and clinical signs of inflammation, PD, BOP, and attachment loss. No association could be established based on the study findings.[68]

References

1. Lang NP, Tonetti MS. Periodontal risk assessment (PRA) for patients in supportive periodontal therapy (SPT). Oral Health Prev Dent 2003;1:7–16.
2. American Academy of Periodontology. Glossary of Periodontal Terms. American Academy of Periodontology, 2001.
3. Page RC, Beck JD. Risk assessment for periodontal diseases. Int Dent J 1997;47:61–87.
4. Bergström J. Tobacco smoking and supragingival dental calculus. J Clin Periodontol 1999;26:541–547.
5. Bergström J. Tobacco smoking and subgingival dental calculus. J Clin Periodontol 2005;32:81–88.
6. Zhou J, Olson BL, Windsor LJ. Nicotine increases the collagen-degrading ability of human gingival fibroblasts. J Periodontal Res 2007;42:228–235.
7. Takeuchi H, Kubota S, Murakashi E, et al. Nicotine-induced CCN2: From smoking to periodontal fibrosis. J Dent Res 2010;89:34–39.
8. Preber H, Bergström J. Occurrence of gingival bleeding in smoker and non-smoker patients. Acta Odontol Scand 1985;43:315–320.
9. Grossi SG, Genco RJ, Machtei EE, et al. Assessment of risk for periodontal disease. II. Risk indicators for alveolar bone loss. J Periodontol 1995;66:23–29.
10. Bergström J, Eliasson S. Cigarette smoking and alveolar bone height in subjects with a high standard of oral hygiene. J Clin Periodontol 1987;14:466–469.
11. Bergström J, Eliasson S, Preber H. Cigarette smoking and periodontal bone loss. J Periodontol 1991;62:242–246.
12. van Winkelhoff AJ, Bosch-Tijhof CJ, Winkel EG, van der Reijden WA. Smoking affects the subgingival microflora in periodontitis. J Periodontol 2001;72:666–671.
13. Haffajee AD, Socransky SS. Relationship of cigarette smoking to the subgingival microbiota. J Clin Periodontol 2001;28:377–388.
14. Zambon JJ, Grossi SG, Machtei EE, Ho AW, Dunford R, Genco RJ. Cigarette smoking increases the risk for subgingival infection with periodontal pathogens. J Periodontol 1996;67(10 suppl):1050–1054.
15. Buduneli N, Biyikoğlu B, Sherrabeh S, Lappin DF. Saliva concentrations of RANKL and osteoprotegerin in smoker versus non-smoker chronic periodontitis patients. J Clin Periodontol 2008;35:846–852.
16. Lappin DF, Sherrabeh S, Jenkins WM, Macpherson LM. Effect of smoking on serum RANKL and OPG in sex, age and clinically matched supportive-therapy periodontitis patients. J Clin Periodontol 2007;34:271–277.
17. Pauletto NC, Liede K, Nieminen A, Larjava H, Uitto VJ. Effect of cigarette smoking on oral elastase activity in adult periodontitis patients. J Periodontol 2000;71:58–62.
18. Fredriksson MI, Figueredo CM, Gustafsson A, Bergström KG, Asman BE. Effect of periodontitis and smoking on blood leukocytes and acute-phase proteins. J Periodontol 1999;70:1355–1360.
19. Ah MK, Johnson GK, Kaldahl WB, Patil KD, Kalkwarf KL. The effect of smoking on the response to periodontal therapy. J Clin Periodontol 1994;21:91–97.
20. Kaldahl WB, Johnson GK, Patil KD, Kalkwarf KL. Levels of cigarette consumption and response to periodontal therapy. J Periodontol 1996;67:675–681.
21. Grossi SG, Zambon J, Machtei EE, et al. Effects of smoking and smoking cessation on healing after mechanical periodontal therapy. J Am Dent Assoc 1997;128:599–607.
22. Kinane DF, Radvar M. The effect of smoking on mechanical and antimicrobial periodontal therapy. J Periodontol 1997;68:467–472.
23. Preber H, Bergström J. Effect of cigarette smoking on periodontal healing following surgical therapy. J Clin Periodontol 1990;17:324–328.
24. Tonetti MS, Pini-Prato G, Cortellini P. Effect of cigarette smoking on periodontal healing following GTR in infrabony defects. A preliminary retrospective study. J Clin Periodontol 1995;22:229–234.
25. Cortellini P, Paolo G, Prato P, Tonetti MS. Long-term stability of clinical attachment following guided tissue regeneration and conventional therapy. J Clin Periodontol 1996;23:106–111.
26. Chambrone L, Chambrone D, Pustiglioni FE, Chambrone LA, Lima LA. The influence of tobacco smoking on the outcomes achieved by root-coverage procedures: A systematic review. J Am Dent Assoc 2009;140:294–306.
27. Haffajee AD, Cugini MA, Dibart S, Smith C, Kent RL Jr, Socransky SS. The effect of SRP on the clinical and microbiological parameters of periodontal diseases. J Clin Periodontol 1997;24:324–334.
28. Tomar SL, Asma S. Smoking-attributable periodontitis in the United States: Findings from NHANES III. National Health and Nutrition Examination Survey. J Periodontol 2000;71:743–751.
29. McGuire MK, Nunn ME. Prognosis versus actual outcome. IV. The effectiveness of clinical parameters and IL-1 genotype in accurately predicting prognoses and tooth survival. J Periodontol 1999;70:49–56.
30. Centers for Disease Control and Prevention. National Diabetes Statistics Report, 2017. https://www.cdc.gov/features/diabetes-statistic-report/index.html. Accessed 25 October 2019.
31. Taylor JJ, Preshaw PM, Lalla E. A review of the evidence for pathogenic mechanisms that may link periodontitis and diabetes. J Periodontol 2013;84(4 suppl):S113–S134.
32. Ervasti T, Knuuttila M, Pohjamo L, Haukipuro K. Relation between control of diabetes and gingival bleeding. J Periodontol 1985;56:154–157.
33. Nelson RG, Shlossman M, Budding LM, et al. Periodontal disease and NIDDM in Pima Indians. Diabetes Care 1990;13:836–840.
34. Emrich LJ, Shlossman M, Genco RJ. Periodontal disease in non-insulin-dependent diabetes mellitus. J Periodontol 1991;62:123–131.
35. Kowall B, Holtfreter B, Völzke H, et al. Pre-diabetes and well-controlled diabetes are not associated with periodontal disease: The SHIP Trend Study. J Clin Periodontol 2015;42:422–430.
36. Christgau M, Palitzsch KD, Schmalz G, Kreiner U, Frenzel S. Healing response to non-surgical periodontal therapy in patients with diabetes mellitus: Clinical, microbiological, and immunologic results. J Clin Periodontol 1998;25:112–124.
37. Lalla E, Kaplan S, Chang SM, et al. Periodontal infection profiles in type 1 diabetes. J Clin Periodontol 2006;33:855–862.
38. Janket SJ, Wightman A, Baird AE, Van Dyke TE, Jones JA. Does periodontal treatment improve glycemic control in diabetic patients? A meta-analysis of intervention studies. J Dent Res 2005;84:1154–1159.
39. Kiran M, Arpak N, Unsal E, Erdoğan MF. The effect of improved periodontal health on metabolic control in type 2 diabetes mellitus. J Clin Periodontol 2005;32:266–272.
40. Socransky SS, Haffajee AD, Cugini MA, Smith C, Kent RL Jr. Microbial complexes in subgingival plaque. J Clin Periodontol 1998;25:134–144.

41. Listgarten MA, Helldén L. Relative distribution of bacteria at clinically healthy and periodontally diseased sites in humans. J Clin Periodontol 1978;5:115–132.
42. Marazita ML, Burmeister JA, Gunsolley JC, Koertge TE, Lake K, Schenkein HA. Evidence for autosomal dominant inheritance and race-specific heterogeneity in early-onset periodontitis. J Periodontol 1994;65:623–630.
43. Melvin WL, Sandifer JB, Gray JL. The prevalence and sex ratio of juvenile periodontitis in a young racially mixed population. J Periodontol 1991;62:330–334.
44. Michalowicz BS, Diehl SR, Gunsolley JC, et al. Evidence of a substantial genetic basis for risk of adult periodontitis. J Periodontol 2000;71:1699–1707.
45. Papapanou PN, Neiderud AM, Sandros J, Dahlén G. Interleukin-1 gene polymorphism and periodontal status. A case-control study. J Clin Periodontol 2001;28:389–396.
46. Kornman KS, Crane A, Wang HY, di Giovine FS, Newman MG, Pirk FW, et al. The interleukin-1 genotype as a severity factor in adult periodontal disease. J Clin Periodontol 1997;24:72–77.
47. Eke PI, Dye BA, Wei L, et al. Prevalence of periodontitis in adults in the United States: 2009 and 2010. J Dent Res 2012;91:914–920.
48. Papapanou PN, Lindhe J. Preservation of probing attachment and alveolar bone levels in 2 random population samples. J Clin Periodontol 1992;19:583–588.
49. Billings M, Holtfreter B, Papapanou PN, Mitnik GL, Kocher T, Dye BA. Age-dependent distribution of periodontitis in two countries: Findings from NHANES 2009 to 2014 and SHIP-TREND 2008 to 2012. J Periodontol 2018;89(suppl 1):S140–S158.
50. Van der Velden U, Abbas F, Armand S, et al. Java project on periodontal diseases. The natural development of periodontitis: Risk factors, risk predictors and risk determinants. J Clin Periodontol 2006;33:540–548.
51. Adriaens LM, Alessandri R, Spörri S, Lang NP, Persson GR. Does pregnancy have an impact on the subgingival microbiota? J Periodontol 2009;80:72–81.
52. Mascarenhas P, Gapski R, Al-Shammari K, Wang HL. Influence of sex hormones on the periodontium. J Clin Periodontol 2003;30:671–681.
53. Löe H, Brown LJ. Early onset periodontitis in the United States of America. J Periodontol 1991;62:608–616.
54. Suvan J, D'Aiuto F, Moles DR, Petrie A, Donos N. Association between overweight/obesity and periodontitis in adults. A systematic review. Obes Rev 2011;12:e381–e404.
55. Haffajee AD, Socransky SS. Relation of body mass index, periodontitis and *Tannerella forsythia*. J Clin Periodontol 2009;36:89–99.
56. Gorman A, Kaye EK, Apovian C, Fung TT, Nunn M, Garcia RI. Overweight and obesity predict time to periodontal disease progression in men. J Clin Periodontol 2012;39:107–114.
57. Wactawski-Wende J, Hausmann E, Hovey K, Trevisan M, Grossi S, Genco RJ. The association between osteoporosis and alveolar crestal height in postmenopausal women. J Periodontol 2005;76(suppl 11S):2116–2124.
58. Brennan RM, Genco RJ, Hovey KM, Trevisan M, Wactawski-Wende J. Clinical attachment loss, systemic bone density, and subgingival calculus in postmenopausal women. J Periodontol 2007;78:2104–2111.
59. Genco RJ, Ho AW, Grossi SG, Dunford RG, Tedesco LA. Relationship of stress, distress and inadequate coping behaviors to periodontal disease. J Periodontol 1999;70:711–723.
60. da Silva AM, Newman HN, Oakley DA. Psychosocial factors in inflammatory periodontal diseases. A review. J Clin Periodontol 1995;22:516–526.
61. Tezal M, Grossi SG, Ho AW, Genco RJ. Alcohol consumption and periodontal disease. The Third National Health and Nutrition Examination Survey. J Clin Periodontol 2004;31:484–488.
62. Amaral Cda S, Luiz RR, Leão AT. The relationship between alcohol dependence and periodontal disease. J Periodontol 2008;79:993–998.
63. Kaur S, Bright R, Proudman SM, Bartold PM. Does periodontal treatment influence clinical and biochemical measures for rheumatoid arthritis? A systematic review and meta-analysis. Semin Arthritis Rheum 2014;44:113–122.
64. Lang NP, Adler R, Joss A, Nyman S. Absence of bleeding on probing. An indicator of periodontal stability. J Clin Periodontol 1990;17:714–721.
65. Lang NP, Joss A, Orsanic T, Gusberti FA, Siegrist BE. Bleeding on probing. A predictor for the progression of periodontal disease? J Clin Periodontol 1986;13:590–596.
66. Matuliene G, Pjetursson BE, Salvi GE, et al. Influence of residual pockets on progression of periodontitis and tooth loss: Results after 11 years of maintenance. J Clin Periodontol 2008;35:685–695.
67. Rams TE, Listgarten MA, Slots J. Utility of radiographic crestal lamina dura for predicting periodontitis disease-activity. J Clin Periodontol 1994;21:571–576.
68. Greenstein G, Polson A, Iker H, Meitner S. Associations between crestal lamina dura and periodontal status. J Periodontol 1981;52:362–366.

5

LOCAL ANATOMICAL AND CONTRIBUTING FACTORS

Carlos Garaicoa-Pazmiño, DDS, MS
Vahid Khoshkam, DDS, MS

The anatomy of the dentition differs significantly based on multiple factors, including but not limited to tooth type, number of roots, location of the **furcation entrance**, **root trunk** length, total root length, and root divergence/convergence. In addition, different local characteristics may alter or influence these anatomical variations. A comprehensive understanding of the tooth morphology and tooth-related factors that may influence or predispose periodontal breakdown is paramount for an accurate diagnosis and treatment plan. This chapter includes a comprehensive description of the evidence on the role of these factors in periodontal diseases.

Biofilm and Calculus

Biofilm formation is a progressive and dynamic process that facilitates bacterial attachment to tooth structures through van der Waals forces, glycocalyx, and lectin-like receptors within a salivary pellicle and negative surface charges mediated by teichoic acid of gram-positive bacteria.[14–16] The shift from gram-positive to gram-negative bacteria occurs as subgingival **plaque** develops and is influenced by biofilm thickness and gingival crevicular fluid. The process of mineralization of biofilm into dental **calculus** has been suggested by Genco et al[16] to undergo four theoretical processes: booster mechanism, epitaxic concept, inhibition theory, and transformation theory.

The inorganic and organic composition of dental calculus have been extensively explored.[17–28] Major inorganic components of dental calculus are calcium, phosphorus, carbonate, sodium, magnesium, potassium, and trace elements such as fluoride and zinc.[16] Moreover, four major crystalline forms can be noted within mature calculus, including hydroxyapatite, octacalcium phosphate (OCP), whitlockite (WHT), and brushite.[18,20,22] On the other hand, proteins (50%–60%), carbohydrates (12%–20%), and lipids (10%–15%) represent about 15% to 20% of the dry weight of mature supragingival plaque.[29] Major differences in the characteristics of dental calculus exist depending on the location. Table 5-1 summarizes the characteristics of both **supragingival** and **subgingival calculus**.[30]

DEFINITIONS AND TERMINOLOGY

Biofilm: A multispecies community of microorganisms that adhere to each other and a surface and are encased in an extracellular matrix. The extracellular matrix is a complex polymeric substance that protects the microorganisms from environmental stresses. Bacteria living in a biofilm have a different physiology from free-living bacteria and are more difficult to eradicate with antibiotics. Dental plaque is the prototypical example of a biofilm.[1]

Calculus: A hard concretion that forms on teeth or dental prostheses through calcification of microbial plaque.[1]

- **Subgingival calculus:** Calculus formed apical to the gingival margin, often brown or black, hard and tenacious. Also known as *seruminal calculus*.[1]
- **Supragingival calculus:** Calculus formed coronal to the gingival margin, usually formed more recently than subgingival calculus. Also known as *salivary calculus*.[1]

Cemental tears: A specific type of root surface fracture and characterized by the detachment of a cemental fragment.[2]

Cementicles: Calcified spherical bodies (0.2 to 0.3 mm) composed of cementum lying free within the periodontal ligament, attached to the cementum, or embedded within it.[1,3–6]

TABLE 5-1 Characteristics of supragingival and subgingival calculus*

	Supragingival	Subgingival
Location	Coronal to gingival margin	Apical to gingival margin
Color	Yellow/white	Brown/black
Distribution	Adjacent to salivary duct openings	Randomly around the oral cavity
Composition	Low concentration of Ca, Mg, F, Sr, and Zn High concentration of carbonate and Mn	High concentration of Ca, Mg, and F Lower concentration of carbonate More irregular distribution of F
Mineral content and source	Average of 37% from saliva by volume	Average of 58% from gingival crevicular fluid by volume
Crystal type	Mostly OCP and hydroxyapatite	Mostly WHT
Formation	Heterogenous nucleation and crystal growth More variable calcification	Heterogenous nucleation and crystal growth More homogenous calcification
Microorganisms	More filamentous, faster growing	Less filamentous, slower growing
Morphology	Heterogenous with small needle-shaped (100 nm), large-ribbon-like and bundle/rosettes (1–50 nm) crystals	Several crystal types (< 50 nm): spiny, crusty, nodular, ledge/ring, individual islands, smooth veneers and finger/fern-like
Pathogenic potential	Little evidence	Associated with periodontal disease

*Adapted and modified from Roberts-Harry and Clerehugh.[30]

Ca, calcium; Mg, magnesium; F, fluoride; Sr, strontium; Zn, zinc; Mn, manganese; Na, sodium.

Crowding: Discrepancy between tooth sizes and arch length and/or tooth positioning that results in malalignment and abnormal contact relationships between teeth.[1]

Enamel pearl: A focal mass of enamel that has formed apical to the cementoenamel junction (CEJ) and is typically located in the areas between the roots of molars.[1]

Enamel projection: An apical extension of enamel, usually toward a furcation.[1] May prevent true attachment of periodontal ligament fibers upon the root surface.[7]

Exostosis: A benign bone growth projection outward from the surface of a bone.[1] →

MECHANISM OF CALCULUS ATTACHMENT

In 1953, Zander explored the mechanisms of calculus attachment upon 50 freshly extracted teeth.[31] Four main types of attachment were identified: *(1)* secondary cuticle, *(2)* direct attachment into irregularities of cementum, *(3)* penetration into cementum, and *(4)* mechanical retention in areas of resorption. In addition, various forms of combinations were also described (Box 5-1).[31] Types II (20%) and III (10%) were noted as the most frequent modalities of calculus attachment, and the cementoenamel junction (CEJ) was the favored site for calculus formation.[31]

Following Zander's findings, multiple authors questioned specific types of calculus attachment and attempted to employ more sophisticated technology to test his conclusions.[19,32–40] Notably, Canis et al rejected the possibility that microorganisms can penetrate the cementum surface and considered this phenomenon as an artifact due to superimposition of a detached cementum onto the tooth structure during sample preparation.[41] These findings were confirmed using light microscopy, scanning electron microscopy (SEM), and transmission electron microscopy (TEM).

BOX 5-1 Mode of calculus attachment to cementum[31]

Type I	Secondary cuticle
Type II	Direct attachment into irregularities of cementum
Type III	Penetration into cementum
Type IV	Mechanical retention in areas of resorption
Type V	Combination of Types III and IV
Type VI	Combination of Types II, III, and IV
Type VII	Combination of Types I, II, III, and IV
Type VIII	Combination of Types I and II
Type IX	Combination of Types II and III
Type X	Combination of Types II and IV

BOX 5-2 Grading system for cervical enamel projections by Masters and Hoskins[7]

Grade I	A distinct change in CEJ attitude with enamel projecting toward the bifurcation.
Grade II	Enamel projection approaching the furcation but not actually making contact with it.
Grade III	Enamel projection extending into the furcation proper.

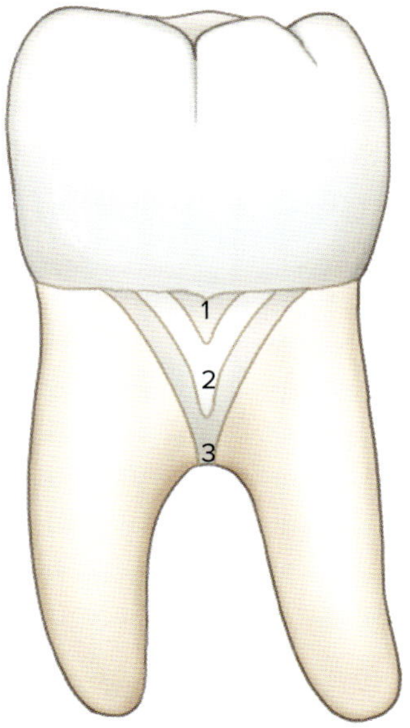

Fig 5-1 Classification of cervical enamel projections.

Developmental Deformities

ENAMEL PROJECTIONS

Defined as an apical extension of enamel usually toward a **furcation**,[1] **enamel projections** (also known as *cervical enamel projections* [CEPs]) are common anatomical variations where a definitive projection of enamel extends into the furcation area, preventing true attachment of periodontal ligament (PDL) fibers upon the root surface[7] (Fig 5-1).

Early observations in dental anatomy described how the enamel dips into the furcation area of multirooted teeth in a tongue-like fashion.[42–48] A landmark article by Masters and Hoskins examined extracted teeth with CEPs and suggested a grading system to determine the severity of these projections (Box 5-2).[7] The authors reported the prevalence of CEPs in mandibular and maxillary molars as 28.6% and 17%, respectively. In addition, clinical observations revealed that 90% of isolated **furcation involvements** were associated with CEPs and mainly affected buccal furcation entrances.[7]

A myriad of studies continued exploring the prevalence, incidence, and association between CEPs and furcation involvement (Table 5-2).[7,49–55] Variations within these investigations might arise from differences in tooth type, reason for tooth extraction (eg, caries, severe periodontitis, endodontic failure), and patient population. With the exception of Leib et al,[50] most studies confirmed a positive correlation between CEPs and furcation defects. Notably, Hou and Tsai reported a high prevalence (63.2%) of furcation defects associated with CEPs and intermediate bifurcational ridges (IBRs) affecting primarily mandibular molars.[55]

Furcation: Anatomical area of a multirooted tooth where the roots diverge.[1]

Furcation arrow: A radiographic shadow associated with a proximal furcation.[8]

Furcation entrance: Transitional area between the undivided and the divided part of the root.[9]

Furcation fornix: Roof of the furcation.[9]

Furcation involvement (invasion): Pathologic resorption of bone within the furcation. The extension of periodontitis or pulpitis into a trifurcation area.[1]

Impacted tooth (impaction): An unerupted or partially erupted tooth so positioned that complete eruption is unlikely.[1]

Intermediate bifurcational ridge (IBR): A distinct ridge running across the bifurcation in a mesiodistal direction.[10]

Overhang: Excess of dental restorative material extending beyond cavity margins.[1]

TABLE 5-2 Prevalence of enamel projections

Authors	Material and methods	Main findings
Masters and Hoskins[7]	• Extracted teeth • Population not specified	• Prevalence: – Mandibular molars: 28.6% – Maxillary molars: 17% • 90% of isolated furcation involvements were associated with CEP
Grewe et al[49]	• Extracted teeth • Population not specified	• Prevalence: – Mandibular: 25.2% – Maxillary: 15.8% • Frequency (in order): – Mandibular second molars – Maxillary second molars – Mandibular first molars – Mandibular third molars – Maxillary third molars – Maxillary first molars
Leib et al[50]	• Extracted teeth • Population not specified	• Prevalence: – Mandibular molars: 25.4% – Maxillary molars: 21.9% • Not associated with furcation defects.
Bissada and Abdelmalek[51]	• Egyptian skulls	• Incidence: – Overall: 8.6% • Frequency (in order): – Mandibular second molars – Maxillary second molars – Mandibular first molars – Mandibular third molars – Maxillary third molars – Maxillary first molars
Tsatsas et al[52]	• Extracted teeth • Population not specified	• Prevalence: – Overall: 29.9%
Swan and Hurt[53]	• East Indian skulls	• Prevalence: – Overall: 32.6% – Mandibular molars: 33.7% – Maxillary molars: 31.4% • Frequency (in order): – Mandibular second molars – Maxillary second molars – Maxillary third molars – Mandibular first molars – Mandibular third molars – Maxillary first molars
Hou and Tsai[54]	• Surgical access • Population: Taiwanese	• Prevalence: – Overall: 45.2% • Frequency (in order): – Mandibular first molars – Maxillary first molars – Mandibular second molars – Maxillary second molars
Hou and Tsai[55]	• Hopeless teeth with Class III FI • Population: Taiwanese	• Prevalence: – FI with CEPs and IBR: 63.2% – FI with CEPs alone: 21.8% – FI with IBR alone: 2.3%

FI, furcation involvement; IBR, intermediate bifurcational ridge.

TABLE 5-3 Classification of enamel pearls[61]

Enamel pearls	Extradental	Solitary	• Enamel nodules in periodontium • Enamel-cementum nodules in periodontium
		Adherent	• True enamel pearl • Enamel-dentine pearl • Enamel-dentine-pulp pearl
	Intradental	• Coronal • Cervical • Radicular	

ENAMEL PEARLS

An **enamel pearl** is defined as a focal mass of enamel that has formed apical to the CEJ and is typically located in the area between the roots of molars.[1] Historically, enamel pearls have also been referred to as *droplets*, *nodules*, *globules*, *knots*, and *exostoses*, based on their surface morphology.[46,56] Interestingly, some authors referred to them as *enamelomas* as an early inaccurate delineation of an odontogenic tumor.[57,58] These enamel anomalies are described as spheroid masses with a mean diameter of 0.96 mm and a prevalence of 4.6%. They are generally located at the coronal third of the root with a mean distance of 2.8 mm from the CEJ.[59] Moskow and Canut performed a literature review and reported an incidence rate ranging from 1.1% to 9.7% (mean: 2.69%) and a predilection for maxillary third and second molars.[60] Furthermore, Cavanha introduced a classification based on macroscopic and microscopic observations based on the number, location, and composition of the enamel pearls (Table 5-3).[61]

The formation of extradental enamel pearls is attributed to activity of the Hertwig epithelial root sheath (HERS) that failed to detach from the dental surface after root formation.[62] Interestingly, Slavkin et al developed a model to explore the HERS differentiation as well as root, cementum, and bone formation.[63] They noted deposits that resembled enamel pearls during the differentiation, disintegration, and detachment of the HERS. Conversely, others speculated that enamel pearl formation occurs at the early stages of tooth development because they have been associated with dentin and pulp.[64] In fact, this theory could explain the formation of intradental enamel pearls resulting from focal ameloblastic activity of invaginated cells or entrapped enamel epithelium from the cervical loop during root formation within newly forming dentin.[65] Nevertheless, the process of formation of enamel pearls at some locations remains to be further elucidated.[60]

Palatal groove: A developmental, anomalous groove usually found on the palatal aspect of maxillary central and lateral incisors.[1]

Plunger cusp: An active passage of food into the embrasure area during function.[11]

Plaque: An organized mass, consisting mainly of microorganisms embedded in a matrix of glycopolymers, that adheres to teeth, prostheses, and oral surfaces and is found in the gingival crevice and periodontal pockets. Other components include an organic, polysaccharide-protein matrix consisting of bacterial by-products such as enzymes, food debris, desquamated cells, and inorganic components such as calcium and phosphate.[1]

Root complex: Portion of a tooth apical to the CEJ.[9]

Root concavity: Developmental depressions as cratered, valley-like shapes in the root surface.[12]

Root cone: Divided region of the root complex.[9]

Root proximity: Closeness of roots of adjacent teeth typically associated with inadequate interdental tissue.[1]

Root surface area: Area available for periodontal attachment.[13]

Root trunk: Undivided region of the root between the CEJ and furcation.[9]

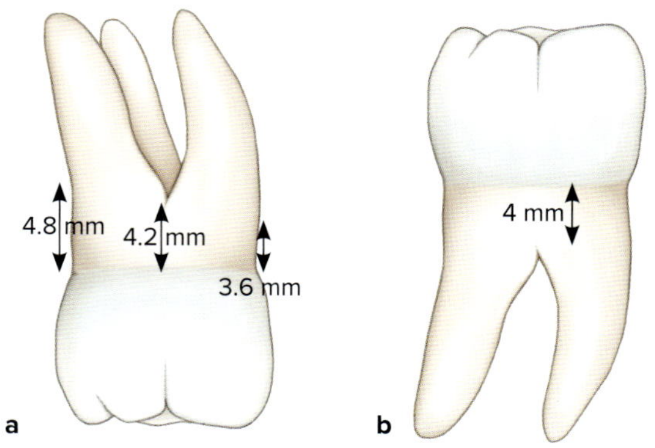

Fig 5-2 Location of furcation entrance of maxillary *(a)* and mandibular *(b)* first molars.

TABLE 5-4 Location of furcation entrance with respect to the CEJ

Tooth type	Authors	Distance from CEJ to furcation entrance (mm)
Maxillary first molars	Gher and Dunlap[68]	• Mesial: 3.6 • Buccal: 4.2 • Distal: 4.8
	Kerns et al[71]	• Mesial: 4.73 • Buccal: 4.11 • Distal: 4.66
Maxillary second molars	Kerns et al[71]	• Mesial: 6.40 • Buccal: 4.29 • Distal: 4.83
Mandibular first molars	Dunlap and Gher[69]	• Buccal/lingual: 4
	Mandelaris et al[72]	• Buccal: 3.19 • Lingual: 4.08
	Kerns et al[71]	• Buccal: 3.27 • Lingual: 4.28
	Wheeler[73]	• Buccal: 3 • Lingual: 4
Mandibular second molars	Mandelaris et al[72]	• Buccal: 3.09 • Lingual: 4.27
	Kerns[71]	• Buccal: 3.28 • Lingual: 3.83
Maxillary first premolars	Gher and Vernino[70]	• 6
	Booker and Loughlin[74]	• 7.9
	Joseph et al[75]	• Range of 7.6–7.9

Furcations

FURCATION MORPHOLOGY

The furcation morphology has been a subject of interest for multitude of investigations, including research evaluating the effectiveness of mechanical instrumentation.[66,67] Bower noted that 81% of the furcations had a diameter less than 1 mm, while 58% were less than 0.75 mm in diameter.[66] At the time, such findings were clinically relevant because the diameter of tested curettes (ie, Gracey, Columbia, and McCall) had a blade face width ranging between 0.75 and 1.1 mm, resulting in limitations for mechanical instrumentation. Similarly, Chiu et al reported that 49% of furcation entrance dimensions were equal to or less than 0.75 mm, which reinforced the need to use narrow instruments and ultrasonic devices with narrow tips for the management of furcation defects.[67]

LOCATION OF FURCATION ENTRANCE

Gher and Dunlap performed a series of studies to determine variations in the root anatomy.[13,68,69] One study reported that the mean distance from the CEJ to the furcation entrance for maxillary first molars was 3.6 mm, 4.2 mm, and 4.8 mm for mesial, buccal, and distal furcations, respectively[68] (Fig 5-2). In a similar study using mandibular first molars, the mean distance was 4 mm for both buccal and lingual furcation entrances.[69] Ultimately, the furcation anatomy of maxillary first premolars was explored, and authors reported a mean distance of 6 mm from the CEJ[70] (Table 5-4).[68–75]

CLASSIFICATION OF FURCATION DEFECTS

Classification systems for furcations were developed to help determine the extension of the defect, tooth prognosis, and treatment approaches. These classifications were mostly developed with the use of a Nabers probe. Both horizontal and vertical components represent the primary endpoints of these classification systems.[1,76–94] Table 5-5 summarizes some of the most commonly employed classifications.[1,76,83,84,87,90]

FURCATION ARROW

Early experimental studies evaluated the potential of radiographs to detect periodontal bony defects using

TABLE 5-5 Classification systems for furcation defects

Authors	Criteria
Glickman[76]	• Pattern of destruction: Horizontal and vertical component. • Grade I: Furcation area without gross or radiographic evidence of loss of alveolar bone loss (*incipient defect*). • Grade II: Bone loss in one or more aspects of the furcation area, but a portion of the alveolar bone and periodontal membrane remains intact (also known as *cul-de-sac lesion*). • Grade III: Alveolar bone destruction permits the complete passage of a probe through the furcation. Entrance might be occluded by gingival tissues (*through-and-through defect*). • Grade IV: Alveolar bone destruction creates an open area through which a probe can be passed without difficulty. The entrance is exposed and clearly visible to clinical examination.
Hamp et al,[83] Lindhe and Nyman[87]	• Pattern of destruction: Horizontal component. • Degree I: Horizontal loss of periodontal support less than 3 mm. • Degree II: Horizontal loss of periodontal support exceeding 3 mm, but not encompassing the total width of the furcation. • Degree III: Horizontal "through-and-through" destruction of the periodontal tissue in the furcation.
Nyman and Lindhe[84]	• Pattern of destruction: Horizontal component. • Class I: Horizontal loss of periodontal support not exceeding one-third of the width of the tooth. • Class II: Horizontal loss of periodontal support exceeding one-third of the width of the tooth, but not encompassing the total width of the furcation. • Class III: Horizontal "through-and-through" destruction of the periodontal tissue in the furcation.
Tarnow and Fletcher[90]	• Pattern of destruction: Vertical component. • Subclass of Lindhe and Nyman[87] classification. • Subclass A: 0–3 mm probable depth from the roof of the furcation. • Subclass B: 4–6 mm probable depth from the roof of the furcation. • Subclass C: 7 mm or greater probable depth from the roof of the furcation.
American Academy of Periodontology *Glossary of Periodontal Terms*[1]	• Pattern of destruction: Horizontal component. • Class I: Incipient loss of bone limited to the furcation flute that does not extend horizontally. • Class II: A variable degree of bone loss in a furcation, but not extending completely through the furcation. • Class III: Bone loss extending completely through the furcation.

TABLE 5-6 Average root surface area (mm^2) covered by cementum*

Tooth type	Jepsen[105] (1963)	Watt et al[104] (1958)	Hillam[106] (1973)	Müller[107] (1958)
Maxillary				
Central incisor	204 ± 31	204	177	250–330
Lateral incisor	179 ± 25	177	182	180–260
Canine	273 ± 44	266	233	250–600
First premolar	234 ± 34	220	204	180–380
Second premolar	220 ± 39	217	187	180–380
First molar	433 ± 41	455	363	700–1,000
Second molar	431 ± 62	417		600–900
Mandibular				
Central incisor	154 ± 26	162	158	180–260
Lateral incisor	168 ± 22	175	166	180–260
Canine	268 ± 42	172	227	250–600
First premolar	180 ± 27	197	207	180–380
Second premolar	207 ± 27	204	207	180–380
First molar	431 ± 60	450	358	550–850
Second molar	426 ± 70	400		500–780

*Adapted from Schroeder.[108]

human cadaver skulls.[95–102] Prichard was the first to describe a "subtle shadow" in radiographs pointing toward the opening of the mesial furcation of maxillary first molars.[99] Then, Hardekopf et al coined the term **furcation arrow** and defined it as a radiographic shadow associated with a proximal furcation involvement.[8] Using skulls with furcation-involved molars, authors reported a significant association of Degree II and III furcation defects with the presence of furcation arrows in both mesial and distal furcation entrances when compared to noninvolved molars. For Degree I defects and noninvolved furcations, the incidence of furcation arrows was low and insignificant. Nonetheless, it was concluded that the absence of a furcation arrow does not necessarily mean an absence of a furcation involvement.[8]

Overall, the usefulness of the furcation arrow as a diagnostic marker is limited. When detected on radiographs, these can predict furcation involvements only in 70% of cases; yet, furcation arrows were also seen in less than 40% of sites with truly present furcation involvement. Consequently, the furcation arrow has a sensitivity of 38.7%, a specificity of 92.2%, a positive predictive value of 71.7%, and a negative predictive value of 74.6%.[100]

Currently, a combination of both clinical and conventional radiographic assessments remains as the gold standard approach for detecting furcation defects. Limited evidence supports the use of CBCT for periodontal disease diagnosis.[101–103]

Root Morphology

ROOT SURFACE AREA

Root surface area has been extensively explored in the literature (Table 5-6).[104–108] While initially investigated as an important factor to aid clinicians in decision making for root resection therapy,[13] the calculation of this area is also helpful to determine the extent of disease progression

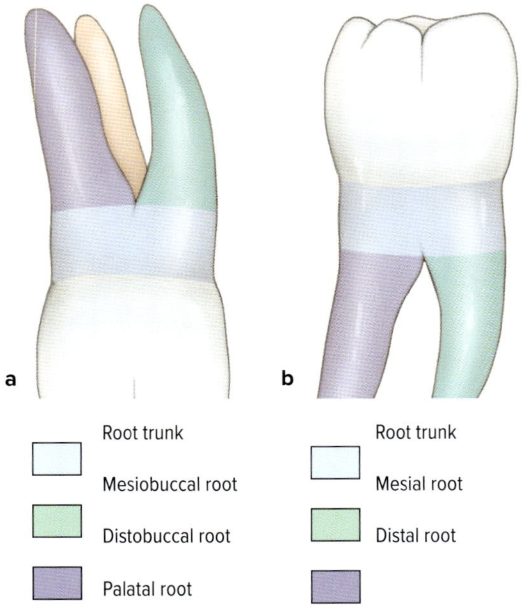

Fig 5-3 Percentage of root surface area of maxillary *(a)* and mandibular *(b)* first molars.

BOX 5-3 Percentage of root surface area in the root complex

Maxillary first molars (Hermann et al[13])		Mandibular first molars (Gher and Dunlap[68])	
Root trunk	32%	Mesial root	37%
Mesiobuccal root	25%	Distal root	32.4%
Palatal root	24%	Root trunk	30.5%
Distobuccal root	19%		

and to assist in the selection between regenerative or resective approaches.

Hermann et al[13] reported a total surface area for the maxillary first molar of 476.43 mm^2. Interestingly, the authors went further to investigate the percentage of root surface area occupied by root trunk (32%), palatal (24%), mesiobuccal (25%), and distobuccal (19%) roots (Fig 5-3a). Later, similar studies were conducted around mandibular first molars.[69,109] Dunlap and Gher reported a total surface area of 436.8 mm^2, and the percentage of root surface area for the root trunk, distal, and mesial root were 30.5%, 32.4%, and 37%, respectively[69] (Fig 5-3b). Box 5-3 includes a summary for the percentages of root surface area for each region in the **root complex**.[13,68]

ROOT CONCAVITIES

Root concavities are common features of the root configuration and act as predisposing sites for periodontal breakdown.[70] Additionally, the presence of these developmental depressions will impair mechanical instrumentation during nonsurgical and surgical therapy, especially for multirooted teeth.

Fox and Bosworth conducted a morphologic assessment to determine the presence of proximal concavities on extracted teeth among all tooth types.[110] The authors concluded that nearly every tooth has concavities at or within 5 mm apical to its CEJ.[110] For multirooted teeth specifically, Booker and Loughlin reported mesial concavity depths of 0.35 mm and 0.44 mm associated with single-rooted and two-rooted maxillary first premolars, respectively.[74] Generally, these depressions tend to be deeper on the mesial aspects and middle third of the root surface.[75] Conversely, Gher and Vernino reported a prevalence of 78% of concavities around maxillary premolars being not clinically relevant until 50% of interproximal bone loss had occurred.[70]

Bower also extensively explored the concavity depth and incidence around maxillary and mandibular first molars.[111] Within the maxillary first molar, concavities are more likely found on mesiobuccal (94%) than distobuccal (31%) or palatal (17%) root surfaces. A higher incidence was also noted among mandibular first molars on both mesial (100%) and distal (99%) root surfaces (Table 5-7).[74,111]

TABLE 5-7 Prevalence and root concavity depth around maxillary and mandibular molars[74,111]

Tooth type	Root	Prevalence	Concavity depth (mean)	Range of depth
Maxillary first premolar	Single-rooted	100%	0.35 mm	0.03–1.09 mm
	Two-rooted	100%	0.44 mm	0.13–3.03 mm
Maxillary first molar	Mesiobuccal	94%	0.3 mm	0.1–0.7 mm
	Distobuccal	31%	0.1 mm	0.1–0.2 mm
	Palatal	17%	0.1 mm	0.1–0.2 mm
Mandibular first molar	Mesial	100%	0.7 mm	0.3–1.3 mm
	Distal	99%	0.5 mm	0–1 mm

TABLE 5-8 Histologic features based on IRD[120]

Interradicular distance	Histologic features
≥ 0.5 mm	Cancellous bone, lamina dura, and PDL
< 0.5 mm	Lamina dura and PDL
< 0.3 mm	Only PDL

Root Proximity

DEFINITION AND CHARACTERISTICS

Root proximity has been defined as interradicular distances (IRDs) of less than or equal to 0.8 mm or less than 1 mm presenting as a risk marker for periodontal disease.[112–119] In a classic study, Heins and Wieder examined the nature of IRD spaces using human histology and reported a distance ranging from 0.2 to 4.5 mm between second premolars, first molars, and second molars.[120] Interestingly, sites exceeding 0.5 mm (89.6%) of IRD showed signs of cancellous bone flanked by lamina dura. When this distance is less than 0.5 mm, a fused lamina dura was observed with no signs of cancellous bone in between. Ultimately, sites with less than 0.3 mm of IRD were connected only by the PDL (Table 5-8).[120]

Vermylen et al reported a 15.3% prevalence of root proximity among 5,122 interproximal sites from 197 patients.[113] It is important to note that 68% of sites were located affecting primarily maxillary molars as well as central and lateral mandibular incisors.[113] In a case control study, root proximity was encountered more often at the coronal and middle thirds of the root.[115] Moreover, sites with bilateral root proximity had 3.6 times greater risk of developing periodontitis. Similarly, Kim et al examined 473 patients with a mean follow-up time of 23 years to evaluate the association between root proximity and the risk for alveolar bone loss.[119] The mean IRD and alveolar bone loss was 1.0 mm and 0.61 mm, respectively. Sites with less than 0.6 mm of IRD presented an increased risk for alveolar bone loss than those with 0.8 mm or more, especially in mandibular anterior teeth.

Similarly, a higher risk for occurrence of intrabony defects has been associated with IRD between 2.1 to 4.1 mm.[121] Trossello and Gianelly reported more bone loss at sites with less than 1 mm of root proximity (13.4%) and in patients who had received orthodontic treatment.[112] On the other hand, Årtun et al examined 400 patients who completed orthodontic treatment with at least a 16-year follow-up. Among them, 25 patients (6%) with root proximity had no significant differences regarding inflammation, attachment level, and bone level in comparison with neighboring control sites.[122]

TABLE 5-9 Classification for root proximity by Vermylen et al[113]

Location	A	Apical third of the root
	B	Intervening (middle) third of the root
	C	Coronal third of the root
Severity	1	> 0.5 and ≤ 0.8 mm. A small amount of cancellous bone is present between the adjacent roots.
	2	> 0.3 and ≤ 0.5 mm. Only cortical and connective tissue attachment is present between the adjacent roots.
	3	≤ 0.3 mm. Only connective tissue attachment is present between the adjacent roots.

CLASSIFICATION FOR ROOT PROXIMITY

Vermylen et al proposed a classification system for root proximity to indicate location (apical, middle, and coronal third) and severity based on modification of the ruler used by Schei et al[123] and findings from Heins and Wieder[120] as depicted in Table 5-9.[113]

Root Surface Anomalies

INTERMEDIATE BIFURCATIONAL RIDGE

Intermediate bifurcational ridge (IBR) is defined as a distinct ridge running across the bifurcation in a mesiodistal direction.[10] It originates from the mesial surface of the distal root at about 2 mm from the height of the furcation area and ends high up on the distal surface of the mesial root by merging within the root concavity.[10] Histologic evaluation of IBRs has shown that these developmental anomalies are formed mostly by dentin but also contained cementum.[10]

Everett et al reported that among 328 extracted mandibular first molars, the prevalence of IBRs was 73%.[10] This finding was confirmed by two other studies that revealed a presence of IBRs in 70% and 76.8% of extracted first molars.[68,124] Moreover, Hou and Tsai found that IBRs are highly associated with CEPs (63.2%) and Class III furcations (25.3%).[55]

Grading system

Hou and Tsai introduced a grading system for IBRs using an electronic digital caliper to calculate dimensions as less than 1 × 1 mm, between 1 × 1 mm and 2 × 2 mm, and 2 × 2 mm or greater as Grades I, II, and III, respectively.[55] It is important to bear in mind that when IBRs are present in furcation defects, these may predispose to further attachment loss by hindering the patient's plaque control and the clinician's ability for proper mechanical instrumentation during active and/or supportive therapy.

PALATORADICULAR GROOVES

The **palatal groove** is a developmental, anomalous groove usually found on the palatal aspect of maxillary central and lateral incisors. It is also known as *palatogingival groove* or *palatoradicular groove*.[1] These structures are considered a funnel-like anomaly predisposing to the accumulation of biofilm and calculus formation.[125–132] The prevalence of this condition ranges from 1.9% to 18%, affecting primarily maxillary lateral incisors and central incisors with a possible predilection for individuals of Asian descent (Table 5-10).[70,127,128,131,133–135]

Embryologically, these anomalies arise as a mild form of invagination from the folding of the enamel epithelium and are closely related to dens in dente.[133] As a result, a clinically detectable hollow groove can be observed proceeding apically for a variable distance along the length of the root. Hou and Tsai noted an increased predilection of these grooves for midpalatal areas (42.5%) when compared with mesial (27.4%) and distal (30.1%) surfaces.[134] Moreover, it has been reported that 58% of the grooves extended more than 5 mm from the CEJ,[127] whereas 8.6% can reach the root apex.[135] Radiographically, these might be detected as radiolucent, parapulpal lines representing a radicular extension of the palatal groove.[126,130]

TABLE 5-10 Prevalence of palatoradicular grooves

Authors	Population	Affected teeth	Prevalence
Everett and Kramer[133]	American	Lateral incisors	1.9%
Gher and Vernino[70]	American	Lateral incisors	3%
Withers[131]	American	Lateral and central incisors	Overall: 2.33% Bilateral: 0.75% Lateral incisors: 4.4% Central incisors: 0.28%
Kogon[127]	Canadian	Lateral and central incisors	4.6%
Bačić et al[128]	Croatian	Lateral and central incisors	1.01%
Hou and Tsai[134]	Taiwanese	Lateral and central incisors	18.06%
Albaricci et al[135]	Brazilian	Lateral and central incisors	Overall: 9.3% Lateral incisors: 11.1% Central incisors: 7%

Localized forms of periodontitis have also been associated with the presence of palatoradicular grooves.[128,130–132] Teeth with palatoradicular grooves revealed worse periodontal health as evidenced by higher gingival index, plaque index, and periodontal disease index scores when compared to teeth without grooves.[131] Similarly, Bačić et al reported significantly greater probing depths (mean: 8.8 mm) at sites with palatoradicular grooves among periodontal patients.[128] Hou and Tsai also noted deeper pocket depths when palatoradicular grooves were present.[134]

ACCESSORY CANALS

Accessory root canals are considered a lateral branch of the main root canal most often found in the apical half of the roots and in furcation areas.[1] The formation of these accessory root canals has been labeled as lines of weakness and attributed to a defect in the HERS during the development of the root at the site of a larger vessel.[136,137] The size of the foramina of these canals might range between 4 and 250 μm, and the canals are more numerous and larger in diameter among maxillary molars than mandibular molars.[138] Early studies reported the presence of an accessory apical artery entering the tooth via the periodontal ligament.[139] Kramer demonstrated large blood vessels within the furcation region running through the radicular dentin to supply one root canal vascular system.[140] At times, these vessels appeared to contribute more to the root canal vascular supply than those entering the apical foramen.[140]

The terminology used to describe root canal ramifications is diverse. De Deus identified different types of root canals based on their location (eg, apex, body, and coronal third) as *accessory*, *secondary*, and *lateral* canals.[141] Some authors have referred to them as *furcation canals* when they are exclusively located at the furcation region.[142,143]

Vertucci and Williams reported a 46% prevalence of accessory canals in a study of 100 mandibular molars.[143] The authors also established an association between their occurrence and the site of origin (pulp chamber or root surface) and the possibility to have multiple accessory canals. Conversely, Kirkham found that 23% of the teeth had accessory canals and reported an association with periodontal defects in 2% of the cases.[144] In a similar manner, Gutmann reported a prevalence of 28.4% of accessory canals at furcation regions from maxillary and mandibular molars.[142] Finally, De Deus used a sample of 1,140 teeth and reported an overall (27.4%) and a site-specific prevalence (apex: 17%; body: 8.8%; and base: 1.6% of the root)[141] (Fig 5-4).

Overall, a large variation (17% to 92.5%) for the prevalence of accessory canals has been observed. This wide range can potentially be attributed to multiple factors.[124,141–149] It is important to bear in mind that these canals are encased by dentin, and a calcification process might cause the number of canals to diminish with age.[150] Also, subtle differences can be associated with the tooth type,[143,145,146] the reason for extraction (eg, caries, periodontal disease, endodontic failure), deposition of cementum,[147] and processing methods (eg, drying, vulcanizing).[151]

Classification

A classification system to describe the site of origin and course of accessory canals within the furcation was proposed by Yoshida et al[152] and modified by Paras et al[153] as Type A (true), Type B (blind), Type C (looping), and Type D (enclosed) canals. Zuza et al labeled Type D canals as *sealed canals*.[146]

ENDODONTIC-PERIODONTAL RELATIONSHIP

Over the past century, the pulpal-periodontal relationship has been a topic of controversy and extensively studied. From a periodontal perspective, it has been suggested that the cumulative effect of biofilm-induced pocket formation might cause pulp inflammation via exposed accessory canals.[147,154,155] Nonetheless, a complete disintegration of the pulp may occur only when all main apical foramina are challenged by bacterial biofilm.[156]

Conversely, Mazur and Massler demonstrated that the pulp condition could vary from almost normal to advanced degeneration despite the presence of periodontal disease.[157] Their findings suggest that the periodontal status does not exert any great influence on the pulp and addressed possible systemic factors as the cause for pulp degeneration.

On the other hand, advanced stages of pulpitis can cause periodontal breakdown.[158–161] As such, endodontic treatment often leads to healing of untreated periodontal lesions in the presence of a endodontic-periodontal defect and supports the idea that accessory canals may act as a passageway for endodontic irritants.[158,162,163]

CEMENTICLES

Cementicles are defined as calcified spherical bodies (0.2 to 0.3 mm) composed of cementum lying free within the periodontal ligament, attached to the cementum, or embedded within it.[1,3–6] It has been suggested that their formation is influenced by epithelial rest cells of HERS and only present on a tooth surface covered with cementum.[3,5] True cementicles consists of a collagenous matrix intermixed with a noncollagenous ground substance.[6]

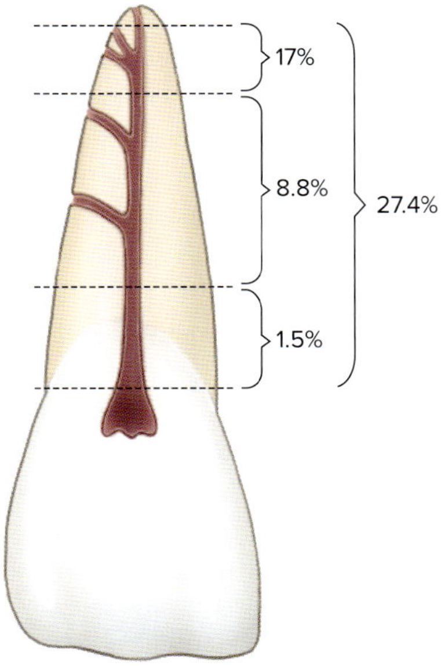

Fig 5-4 Prevalence of accessory canals.

Cementicles may enlarge by deposits of calcium salts from the connective tissue. These salts fuse with adjacent free cementicles and become embedded in the root surface during cementum deposition.[164,165] According to Holton et al, cementicles are often observed in canines and molars with an overall prevalence of 34%.[166]

The presence of cementicles has not been correlated with the pathogenesis of periodontal disease; however, root surfaces with cementicles might hinder mechanical instrumentation.

CEMENTAL TEARS

Cemental tears are defined as a specific type of root surface fracture and characterized by the detachment of a cemental fragment.[2] Cemental tears are a rare condition able to induce periodontal attachment loss[167–176] and periapical tissue destruction.[177–179] Partial or complete separations can occur along the dentin-cement junction or following cementum incremental lines from both exposed and unexposed root surfaces leading to cemental tears.[39,180,181]

The occurrence of these cemental defects remains unclear due to its rarity. Retrospective data from a multicenter study in Taiwan reported that cemental tears are more likely to occur in mandibular and maxillary incisors (76.1%), among men (77.5%), and in patients older than

TABLE 5-11 Prevalence of palatal exostosis

Authors	Prevalence
Larato[191]	• Overall: 30% • Population: Mexican
Nery et al[193]	• Overall: 40.5% • Population: European, Oceanic-Asiatic, African, and Mexican-Peruvian
Sonnier et al[192]	• Overall: 56% • Population: Caucasian and African American

60 years (73.2%).[177] A predisposition for these tears in a Hindu population has also been reported.[180,182]

Müller and Zander hypothesized that the occurrence of cementum defects could be associated with the quality of cementum rather than differences in rate, speed, or lack of cementum deposition.[182] Conversely, Moskow noted that these defects were located mostly at the coronal third of the cementum, serving as susceptible sites for calculus formation.[39] Interestingly, he pointed out that cemental tears could be the result of inadvertent root gouging during mechanical instrumentation. Additionally, observations from Leknes et al noted that cemental tears can occur away from the gingival sulcus, suggesting that these fractures can elicit a rapid periodontal breakdown in noninfected environments.[167] Hence, cemental tears can often be associated with traumatic occlusion or traumatic events.[2,167,181,183–188]

Cemental tears are detectable clinically via very localized deep pocketing and radiographically (about 50% of the cases) with a localized radiolucency surrounding a "prickle-like body."[170,177,185] Further analysis showed that teeth with cemental tears were more likely to develop an abscess and be associated with pockets greater than 6 mm, a positive vitality test, healthy opposing teeth, and moderate to severe attrition.[177]

If properly diagnosed, teeth with cemental tears can be satisfactorily treated. Treatment includes removal of the cemental tear, root debridement, pocket reduction, and/or regenerative procedures with or without endodontic therapy.[189] A recent study showed that most of the teeth with cemental tears could be treated via surgical or nonsurgical treatments; however, teeth with cemental tears in the apical third had a worse prognosis.[190]

Palatal Exostosis (Tubercles)

Exostoses are defined as benign bone growth projections outward from the surface of a bone.[1] Palatal exostoses are bony protuberances that can cause surface irregularities, leading to periodontal pockets in the area of maxillary molars. Larato proposed a classification based on their anatomical appearance as Type A (small nodule), Type B (large nodule), Type C (sharp ridge), Type D (spike-like projections), and Type E (combinations of types A to D).[191]

Several studies using human skull specimens have reported a diverse prevalence of palatal exostosis ranging between 30% and 56% (Table 5-11).[191–193] These subtle differences might be influenced by ethnic background and/or age.[192,193] Most of the palatal exostoses (62%) are commonly found in the maxillary third molar area and directly lateral to and at a mean of 11.4 mm from the greater palatine foramen.[192] The removal of these bony protuberances is often indicated to ensure proper flap adaptation during resective procedures. These can also serve as a potential source of autogenous bone for regenerative procedures.[192]

Dental Materials and Tooth Position–Related Factors

IMPACT OF DENTAL MATERIALS

The periodontium can be affected by the different types and surface characteristics (eg, surface free energy and roughness) of dental materials.[194–197] In a comparative study by Chan and Weber,[198] 150 crowns (50 porcelain crowns with aluminum-oxide framework, 68 porcelain-fused-to-metal

[PFM] restorations, 13 cast gold crowns, 19 acrylic resin veneer crowns) and 242 intact natural teeth serving as controls were compared in terms of plaque retention using Löe and Silness[199] plaque index scores in a crown-to-quadrant ratio. Results showed that crowns with an aluminum-oxide base had minor plaque retention (32%), whereas PFM crowns (90%), natural teeth (110%), cast gold restorations (148%), and acrylic resin veneer crowns (152%) had substantially more plaque retention. Other material surfaces, like lithium disilicate and zirconia, have shown a superior resistance to surface roughness changes after instrumentation with stainless steel curettes, yet zirconia revealed a greater bacterial adhesion compared with gold alloy and lithium disilicate.[200]

Despite differences in plaque retention and quality of the marginal fit, galvanic-ceramic crowns demonstrated significantly less clinical and inflammatory responses than metallic-ceramic crowns by means of plaque index, gingival index, gingival crevicular fluid flow rate, and levels of immunoglobulin G.[201] Nonetheless, these responses might differ when ceramic or metal restorations are compared with resin-bonded restorations. A study by van Dijken and Sjöström tested the effects of glass ionomer cement and composite filling materials for Class V subgingival cervical lesions and demonstrated that these materials present with no differences over time in term of the amount of plaque and degree of gingivitis when compared with enamel.[202] Konradsson et al noted a similar inflammatory biomarker response (interleukin [IL] 1α, IL-1β, and IL-1 receptor antagonist) with different materials when compared with enamel.[203]

It has been proposed that a maximum roughness threshold of Ra less than 0.2 μm be recommended to reduce plaque accumulation.[204] Moreover, periodontal therapy might have an impact in roughness changes, resulting in increased plaque accumulation. These changes are also dependent on each dental material and treatment modality.[205] An in vitro study using gold alloy specimens showed that pre- and posttreatment Ra values significantly increased after instrumentation with stainless steel curettes and prophylactic cups.[200] Interestingly, stainless steel curettes increase roughness levels nearly 13 times greater than prophylactic cups.

Proceedings from the 2017 World Workshop on the classification of Periodontal and Peri-implant Diseases and Conditions concluded that dental materials act similar to enamel as plaque retentive factors to initiate gingivitis.[197]

LOCATION OF THE RESTORATIVE MARGIN

The relationship between gingival health and the margin of the restoration has also been researched.[206–208] Newcomb showed in 51 subjects that the more apical the margin of the restoration, the more gingival inflammation was present according to a gingival index.[209] Four groups were classified depending on the distance of the crown margin to the base of the crevice (CM-BC) and found that margins as close as 0.75 mm or less can induce gingival inflammation.

A human histologic study[210] showed that restorations placed below the gingival margin were likely to accumulate plaque subgingivally, even when routine oral hygiene was performed. It was also noted that individual sites can re-form plaque as soon as 6 weeks on subgingival restorations, while others can be free of plaque for as long as 2 years.

A 26-year longitudinal study examined the long-term effects of restorations with supra- and subgingival margins on periodontal health.[211] It was concluded that subgingival margins exert a detrimental effect to gingival and periodontal health. Additionally, a "burn-out" effect was suggested as loss of attachment in teeth with subgingival margins was clinically detectable 1 to 3 years after the placement of the restoration.

SUBGINGIVAL PLAQUE AND DENTAL RESTORATIONS

The clinical and microbiologic effects of subgingival restorations have also been investigated. Lang et al found that placement of restorations with **overhanging** margins resulted in changes in subgingival microflora.[196] Also, increased proportions of gram-negative anaerobic bacteria, black-pigmented *Bacteroides*, and an increase in anaerobe:facultative ratio were noted. These changes may potentially initiate periodontal disease associated with iatrogenic factors. Similarly, the quality of plaque subjacent to bridge pontics from inflamed sites seems to harbor a higher proportion of periodontopathic bacteria (eg, *Porphyromonas gingivalis*, *Prevotella intermedia*, and *Tannerrella forsythia*) when compared with healthy sites.[212]

STATUS OF THE RESTORATIVE MARGIN

The proper contour and adaptation of the restorative margins may also influence the presence of other factors

TABLE 5-12 Prevalence of overhanging restorations

Authors	Prevalence
Gilmore and Sheiman[216]	32%
Jeffcoat and Howell[217]	71%
Pack et al[218]	56%

TABLE 5-13 Classification of overhangs by Jeffcoat and Howell[217]

Size	Percentage of interproximal space occupied by overhang
Small	< 20%
Medium	20%–50%
Large	> 50%

such as overhangs, open contacts, food retention/impaction, recurrent caries, and plaque retention—and thus play a role in periodontal breakdown.[213,214] In this sense, Chan and Weber assessed crown margins and classified them into three groups based on the transition of the probe against the margin.[198] The classification proposed included grade I, grade II, and grade III for margins with a smooth transition from restoration to tooth substance, margins with a slight irregularity, and gross imperfections of the crown margin, respectively.

OVERHANGING RESTORATIONS

An overhanging restoration that occupies the interproximal space might be conducive to periodontal breakdown and alveolar bone destruction.[215,216] Studies reporting the prevalence of overhangs are included in Table 5-12.[216–218]

The classic study by Jeffcoat and Howell randomly selected 100 periodontal patients to assess the effect of amalgam overhangs on the alveolar bone height and classified their size into small (< 20%), medium (20%–50%), and large (> 50%) based on the interproximal space occupied by the overhang[217] (Table 5-13). The authors showed that only medium and large overhanging restorations revealed significant bone loss when compared with control teeth.

Pack et al evaluated 2,117 restored surfaces and reported that most of the overhangs were associated with pockets greater than 3 mm (64.3%) and bleeding on probing (32%).[218] Also, Jansson et al concluded that sites with overhangs were associated with deeper probing depths, radiographic bone loss, and worsened parameters among susceptible periodontal patients.[219]

Removal of overhangs in combination with plaque elimination results in significant reduction of gingival inflammation,[220–222] and it is recommended during the initial phase of periodontal therapy.[223]

OPEN INTERPROXIMAL CONTACTS

The link between open contacts and periodontal breakdown has been a topic of debate. Open contacts can be measured by the visual assessment[224] or through the resistance of dental floss within the interproximal embrasure.[225] Jernberg et al used a constructed gauge consisting of calibrated metal strips 0.1 mm thick.[224] Interestingly, O'Leary et al chose a more practical assessment by using dental floss between the interproximal embrasure and classified into them tight (definitive resistance to floss), loose (minimal resistant to floss), or open contacts (no resistance to floss).[225]

Despite the inability of early studies to find a direct correlation between open contacts and periodontal destruction,[226–228] one classic study found that open contacts were directly related to food impaction, which in turn was significantly related to increased probing depths.[229] However, there was no significant relationship between contact type and periodontal pocket depth. It should be noted that the subjects in that study had 80% of sites with moderate to severe gingival inflammation, indicating poor oral hygiene. This finding was confirmed in a cross-sectional study in a group of 104 subjects with 75% of anterior open contacts, demonstrating that food impaction was more frequent in open contacts (18.3%) than closed contacts (2.9%).[224]

As a consequence of open contacts, **plunger cusps** may actively pass food into the embrasure area, causing food impaction.[11] Hence, more plaque accumulation is expected when plunger cusps are present, and thus adequate and frequent plaque removal is paramount to maintain periodontal integrity within embrasure areas.[230] It is also important to bear in mind that teeth requiring extraction with adjacent open contacts had significantly more attachment loss than sites with closed contacts.[231]

MARGINAL RIDGE DISCREPANCIES

The importance of marginal ridge relationships relies on this factor being investigated as a predisposing factor for food impaction,[232] attachment loss, and deeper probing depths.[233] It is believed that interproximal wedging of food by a "plunger cusp" could be prevented if the integrity of proximal contacts and contour of marginal ridges are well maintained.[11] A study by Kepic and O'Leary evaluated marginal ridge discrepancies in posterior teeth among 100 patients. The authors found a low correlation between marginal ridge discrepancies and periodontal parameters (probing depths, attachment loss, plaque/calculus accumulation, and gingival status).[234] As such, it was suggested that the presence and extent of plaque and calculus deposits are more important in determining periodontal health than uneven marginal ridge discrepancies.

TOOTH POSITION–RELATED CONDITIONS

Tooth **crowding**, crossbite, extreme overjet/overbite, and malposition are very common forms of malocclusion[235,236] and often associated with worsened periodontal conditions.[237–239] Studies evaluating the prevalence of crowding and periodontal diseases had reported values ranging between 58% and 95%, and their presence is seemingly influenced by age.[240–243]

Different definitions and grading scores have been proposed to assess crowding for periodontal purposes.[226,244,245] Van Kirk developed a scoring index to examine malalignment.[244] Score 0 was given to an ideal alignment with no deviation from the ideal arch line projected through contact areas. Minor and major malalignment conditions were also assessed by the degree of rotation and displacement. Score 1 includes situations where rotation is less then 45 degrees and malalignment less 1.5 mm. Score 2 includes situations of rotation exceeding 45 degrees and displacement equal to or more than 1.5 mm.

To date, it remains controversial whether tooth position–related factors exert a significant impact on the periodontium using oral hygiene as a confounding factor.[226,246–255] Early studies showed a correlation between crowding and increased loss of clinical attachment, plaque accumulation, and gingival inflammation.[241,256–258] On the other hand, other studies reported that crowding has no effect on periodontal health.[226,235,240,259–261]

Results from a cross-sectional study among 154 army recruits concluded that tooth malposition does not enhance periodontal breakdown; however, it decreases the ability for optimal oral hygiene habits.[242] Ultimately, Ingervall et al demonstrated that crowding did not favor plaque accumulation or extent of gingival inflammation in an experimental gingivitis model.[245]

Because tooth crowding is not a causal agent for the initiation of periodontal disease, it must be considered in conjunction with biofilm as a contributing factor for periodontal breakdown.[262] Hence, individuals with poor plaque control and crowding might be more susceptible to attachment loss.

IMPACTED THIRD MOLARS

Generally, third molar sites are prone to plaque accumulation due to the difficulty of proper access for oral hygiene. Also, **impaction** of these teeth might create vertical defects on the distal surfaces of second molars.

In a retrospective study, Kugelberg showed a significant correlation between bone healing of third molar extraction sites and patient age.[263] Residual probing depths greater than 7 mm and intrabony defects exceeding 4 mm in depth were evaluated in the distal surfaces of second molars after extraction of impacted mandibular third molars. Curiously, a significant improvement of the intrabony defect depth was noted among individuals under 25 years old (Table 5-14).[263]

Later, Kugelberg et al confirmed their previous findings in a prospective study and provided evidence that periodontal healing after third molar extraction is impaired in patients over 30 years.[264] One year postoperatively, 14% of patients aged 20 years or younger had residual intrabony defects of 4 mm or greater, while 47% of the patients aged 30 years or older had intrabony defects 4 mm or greater following removal of the impacted third molars. Thus, early removal of the impacted third molars with severe angulation and close positional relationship adjacent to the second molars will benefit the periodontal health.[264]

RETENTION OF HOPELESS TEETH

Several studies have investigated the potential detrimental effects of retention of a hopeless tooth. In a retrospective study with a 4-year observation period, Machtei et al defined teeth as *hopeless* when Class III furcation involvement or more than 50% alveolar bone loss was present.[265] It was later demonstrated that in the absence of periodontal therapy, an annual bone loss at dentition adjacent to hopeless teeth was 10 times greater (3.12% vs 0.23%)

TABLE 5-14 Incidence of residual intrabony defects after third molar extraction[263]

	≤ 25 years		≥ 26 years	
	Intrabony defect (> 4 mm)	PD ≥ 7 mm	Intrabony defect (> 4 mm)	PD ≥ 7 mm
2 years after extraction	16.7%	29.2%	40.7%	55.6%
4 years after extraction	4.2%	25.0%	44.4%	51.9%

PD, probing depth.

BOX 5-4 Effect of retained hopeless teeth upon the adjacent periodontium

- Negative effect (absence of periodontal therapy)
  - Machtei et al[265]
- No effect (with periodontal therapy)
  - DeVore et al[266]
  - Wojcik et al[267]
  - Machtei and Hirsch[268]

than the teeth adjacent to the healed sockets of extracted hopeless teeth. Conversely, DeVore et al and Wojcik et al presented data of 17 hopeless teeth with a mean follow-up of 3.41 years[266] and 8.4 years,[267] suggesting that retention of hopeless teeth has no effect on the proximal periodontium prior to and following periodontal therapy.

Overall, these studies demonstrated that the effect of the retention of hopeless teeth on adjacent dentition is diminished as long as active and supportive periodontal therapy is provided. Hence, Machtei revisited his previous findings and concluded that the long-term preservation of these teeth following periodontal surgery is feasible with no detrimental effects on the adjacent proximal teeth[268] (Box 5-4).[265–268]

References

1. American Academy of Periodontology. Glossary of Periodontal Terms. American Academy of Periodontology, 2001.
2. Xie C, Wang L, Yang P, Ge S. Cemental tears: A report of four cases and literature review. Oral Health Prev Dent 2017;15:337–345.
3. Mikola OJ, Bauer WH. Cementicles and fragments of cementum in the periodontal membrane. Oral Surg Oral Med Oral Pathol 1949;2:1063–1074.
4. Moskow BS. Origin, histogenesis and fate of calcified bodies in the periodontal ligament. J Periodontol 1971;42:131–143.
5. Kalnins V. Origin of enamel drops and cementicles in the teeth of rodents. J Dent Res 1952;31:582–590.
6. Bosshardt DD, Nanci A. Immunocytochemical characterization of ectopic enamel deposits and cementicles in human teeth. Eur J Oral Sci 2003;111:51–59.
7. Masters DH, Hoskins SW Jr. Projection of cervical enamel into molar furcations. J Periodontol 1964;35:49–53.
8. Hardekopf JD, Dunlap RM, Ahl DR, Pelleu GB, Jr. The "furcation arrow." A reliable radiographic image? J Periodontol 1987;58:258–261.
9. Carnevale G, Pontoriero R, Lindhe J. Treatment of furcation-involved teeth. In: Lang NP, Lindhe J. Clinical Periodontology and Implant Dentistry. Chichester: John Wiley & Sons, 2015.
10. Everett FG, Jump EB, Holder TD, Williams GC. The intermediate bifurcational ridge: A study of the morphology of the bifurcation of the lower first molar. J Dent Res 1958;37:162–169.
11. Hirschfeld I. Food impaction. J Am Dent Assoc 1930;17:1504–1528.
12. Hodges K. Concepts in nonsurgical periodontal therapy. Clifton Park: Delmar, 1998.
13. Hermann DW, Gher ME Jr, Dunlap RM, Pelleu GB Jr. The potential attachment area of the maxillary first molar. J Periodontol 1983;54:431–434.
14. van Houte J. Colonization mechanisms involved in the development of the oral flora. In: Gengo RJ, Mergenhagen SE. Host-parasite interactions in periodontal disease: Proceedings of a symposium held at Buffalo, New York, 4-6 May, 1981. Washington: American Society of Microbiology, 1982.
15. van Houte J. Bacterial adherence and dental plaque formation. Infection 1982;10:252–260.
16. Genco RJ, Goldman HM, Cohen DW. Contemporary Periodontics. St Louis: Mosby, 1990.
17. Jensen AT, Danø M. Crystallography of dental calculus and the precipitation of certain calcium phosphates. J Dent Res 1954;33:741–750.
18. Jensen AT, Hansen KG. Tetracalcium hydrogen triphosphate trihydrate, a constituent of dental calculus. Experientia 1957;13:311.

19. Forsberg A, Lagergren C. Dental calculus. A biophysical study. Oral Surg Oral Med Oral Pathol 1960;13:1051–1060.
20. Grøn P, Van Campen GJ. Mineral composition of human dental calculus. Helv Odontol Acta 1967;11:71–74.
21. Grøn P, Van Campen GJ, Lindstrom I. Human dental calculus. Inorganic chemical and crystallographic composition. Arch Oral Biol 1967;12:829–837.
22. Le Geros RZ. Variations in the crystalline components of human dental calculus. I. Crystallographic and spectroscopic methods of analysis. J Dent Res 1974;53:45–50.
23. LeGeros RZ, Shannon IL. The crystalline components of dental calculi: Human vs dog. J Dent Res 1979;58:2371–2377.
24. Schroeder HE, Bambauer HU. Stages of calcium phosphate crystallisation during calculus formation. Arch Oral Biol 1966;11:1–14.
25. Kaufman HW, Kleinberg I. X-ray diffraction examination of calcium phosphate in dental plaque. Calcif Tissue Res 1973;11:97-104.
26. Kani T, Kani M, Moriwaki Y, Doi Y. Microbeam x-ray diffraction analysis of dental calculus. J Dent Res 1983;62:92–95.
27. Friskopp J, Isacsson G. A quantitative microradiographic study of mineral content of supragingival and subgingival dental calculus. Scand J Dent Res 1984;92:25–32.
28. Friskopp J. Ultrastructure of nondecalcified supragingival and subgingival calculus. J Periodontol 1983;54:542–550.
29. Etiology and contributing factors. In: American Academy of Periodontology. Periodontal Literature Reviews: A summary of current knowledge. Chicago: American Academy of Periodontology, 1996. https://www.perio.org/sites/default/files/files/PDFs/Postdoc%20Education/1996_Periodontal_LitRev.pdf. Accessed 28 October 2019.
30. Roberts-Harry EA, Clerehugh V. Subgingival calculus: Where are we now? A comparative review. J Dent 2000;28:93–102.
31. Zander HA. The attachment of calculus to root surfaces. J Periodontol 1953;24:16–19.
32. Shroff FR. An observation on the attachment of calculus. Oral Surg Oral Med Oral Pathol 1955;8:154–160.
33. Kopczyk RA, Conroy CW. The attachment of calculus to root planed surfaces. Periodontics 1968;6:78–83.
34. Mandel ID, Levy BM. Studies on salivary calculus. I. Histochemical and chemical investigations of supra- and subgingival calculus. Oral Surg Oral Med Oral Pathol 1957;10:874–884.
35. Voreadis EG, Zander HA. Cuticular calculus attachment. Oral Surg Oral Med Oral Pathol 1958;11:1120–1125.
36. Selvig KA. Attachment of plaque and calculus to tooth surfaces. J Periodontal Res 1970;5:8–18.
37. Jones SJ. Morphology of calculus formation on the human tooth surface. Proc R Soc Med 1972;65:903–905.
38. Benson LA. The surface of cementum. J Periodontol 1959;30:126–132.
39. Moskow BS. Calculus attachment in cemental separations. J Periodontol 1969;40:125–130.
40. Sottosanti JS, Garrett JS. A rationale for root preparation: A scanning electron microscopic study of diseased cementum [abstract]. In: Abstracts of Presentations at the September, 1975 Meeting of the Academy of Periodontology. J Periodontol 1975;46:628–632.
41. Canis MF, Kramer GM, Pameijer CM. Calculus attachment. Review of the literature and new findings. J Periodontol 1979;50:406–415.
42. Bresica NJ. Applied Dental Anatomy. St Louis: Mosby, 1961.
43. Churchill HR. Human Odontography and Histology. Philadephia: Lea and Febiger, 1932.
44. Sicher H. Oral Anatomy. St Louis: Mosby, 1960.
45. Atkinson SR. Changing dynamics of the growing face. Am J Orthod 1949;35:815–836.
46. Linderer J, Linderer CJ. Handbuch der zahnheilkunde, vol 2. Berlin: Schlesinger, 1842.
47. Suzuki T. The enamel in the interradicular space portion of human multirooted teeth [in Japanese]. Kokubyogakkai Zasshi 1958;25:273–280.
48. Owens R. Odontography; or, a treatise of the comparative anatomy of the teeth, vol 2. London: Hyppolyte Bailliere, 1840.
49. Grewe JM, Meskin LH, Miller T. Cervical enamel projections: Prevalence, location, and extent; with associated periodontal implications. J Periodontol 1965;36:460–465.
50. Leib AM, Berdon JK, Sabes WR. Furcation involvements correlated with enamel projections from the cementoenamel junction. J Periodontol 1967;38:330–334.
51. Bissada NF, Abdelmalek RG. Incidence of cervical enamel projections and its relationship to furcation involvement in Egyptian skulls. J Periodontol 1973;44:583–585.
52. Tsatsas B, Mandi F, Kerani S. Cervical enamel projections in the molar teeth. J Periodontol 1973;44:312–314.
53. Swan RH, Hurt WC. Cervical enamel projections as an etiologic factor in furcation involvement. J Am Dent Assoc 1976;93:342–345.
54. Hou GL, Tsai CC. Relationship between periodontal furcation involvement and molar cervical enamel projections. J Periodontol 1987;58:715–721.
55. Hou GL, Tsai CC. Cervical enamel projection and intermediate bifurcational ridge correlated with molar furcation involvements. J Periodontol 1997;68:687–693.
56. Salter SJA. Dental pathology and surgery. New York: William Wood, 1875.
57. Schaffer WG. A Textbook of Oral Pathology. Philadelphia: Saunders, 1958.
58. Thoma KH, Goldman HM. Oral Pathology. St Louis: Mosby, 1960.
59. Risnes S. The prevalence, location, and size of enamel pearls on human molars. Scand J Dent Res 1974;82:403–412.
60. Moskow BS, Canut PM. Studies on root enamel (2). Enamel pearls. A review of their morphology, localization, nomenclature, occurrence, classification, histogenesis and incidence. J Clin Periodontol 1990;17:275–281.
61. Cavanha AO. Enamel pearls. Oral Surg Oral Med Oral Pathol 1965;19:373–382.
62. Pindborg JJ. Pathology of the dental hard tissues. Copenhagen: Munskgaard, 1970.
63. Slavkin HC, Bringas P Jr, Bessem C, et al. Hertwig's epithelial root sheath differentiation and initial cementum and bone formation during long-term organ culture of mouse mandibular first molars using serumless, chemically-defined medium. J Periodontal Res 1989;24:28–40.
64. Malassez L, Gallipe V. Notes on "enamel pearls." Abstract. Dent Cosmos 1908;49:1286.
65. Kaugars GE. Internal enamel pearls: Report of case. J Am Dent Assoc 1983;107:941–943.
66. Bower RC. Furcation morphology relative to periodontal treatment. Furcation entrance architecture. J Periodontol 1979;50:23–27.
67. Chiu BM, Zee KY, Corbet EF, Holmgren CJ. Periodontal implications of furcation entrance dimensions in Chinese first permanent molars. J Periodontol 1991;62:308–311.
68. Gher MW Jr, Dunlap RW. Linear variation of the root surface area of the maxillary first molar. J Periodontol 1985;56:39–43.
69. Dunlap RM, Gher ME. Root surface measurements of the mandibular first molar. J Periodontol 1985;56:234–238.
70. Gher ME, Vernino AR. Root morphology: Clinical significance in pathogenesis and treatment of periodontal disease. J Am Dent Assoc 1980;101:627–633.

71. Kerns DG, Greenwell H, Wittwer JW, Drisko C, Williams JN, Kerns LL. Root trunk dimensions of 5 different tooth types. Int J Periodontics Restorative Dent 1999;19:82–91.
72. Mandelaris GA, Wang HL, MacNeil RL. A morphometric analysis of the furcation region of mandibular molars. Compend Contin Educ Dent 1998;19:113–116.
73. Wheeler RC. Textbook of Dental Anatomy and Physiology, ed 4. Philadelphia: Saunders, 1965.
74. Booker BW, 3rd, Loughlin DM. A morphologic study of the mesial root surface of the adolescent maxillary first bicuspid. J Periodontol 1985;56:666–670.
75. Joseph I, Varma BR, Bhat KM. Clinical significance of furcation anatomy of the maxillary first premolar: A biometric study on extracted teeth. J Periodontol 1996;67:386–389.
76. Glickman I. Clinical Periodontology: The Periodontium in Health and Disease; Recognition, Diagnosis and Treatment of Periodontal Disease in the Practice of General Dentistry. Philadelphia: Saunders, 1953.
77. Goldman HM, Cohen DW. Periodontal Therapy, ed 6. St Louis: Mosby, 1980.
78. Heins PJ, Canter SR. The furca involvement: A classification of bony deformities. Periodontics 1968;6:84–86.
79. Easley JR, Drennan GA. Morphological classification of the furca. J Can Dent Assoc (Tor) 1969;35:104–107.
80. Eskow RN, Kapin SH. Furcation invasions: Correlating a classification system with therapeutic considerations. Part I. Examination, diagnosis, and classification. Compend Contin Educ Dent 1984;5:479–483.
81. Staffileno HJ. Surgical management of the furca invasion. Dent Clin North Am 1969;13:103–119.
82. Basaraba N. Furcation invasions. In: Yuodelis RA, Page RC, Schlunger S. Periodontal Disease. Basic Phenomena, Clinical Management, and Occlusal and Restorative Interrelationships. Philadelphia: Lea & Febiger, 1977.
83. Hamp SE, Nyman S, Lindhe J. Periodontal treatment of multirooted teeth. Results after 5 years. J Clin Periodontol 1975;2:126–135.
84. Nyman S, Lindhe J. Examination of patients with periodontal disease. In: Lindhe J. Textbook of Clinical Periodontology. Copenhagen: Munsksgaard, 1983.
85. Rosenberg MM. Management of osseous defects. In: Clark JW. Clinical Dentistry. Volume 3: Periodontal and Oral Surgery. Philadelphia: Harper & Row, 1979.
86. Ramfjord SP, Ash MM. Periodontology and Periodontics. Philadelphia: Saunders, 1979.
87. Lindhe J, Nyman S. The effect of plaque control and surgical pocket elimination on the establishment and maintenance of periodontal health. A longitudinal study of periodontal therapy in cases of advanced disease. J Clin Periodontol 1975;2:67–79.
88. Ricchetti PA. A furcation classification based on pulp chamber-furcation relationships and vertical radiographic bone loss. Int J Periodontics Restorative Dent 1982;2:50–59.
89. Tal H, Lemmer J. Furcal defects in dry mandibles. Part II: Severity of furcal defects. J Periodontol 1982;53:364–367.
90. Tarnow D, Fletcher P. Classification of the vertical component of furcation involvement. J Periodontol 1985;55:283–284.
91. Walter C, Kaner D, Berndt DC, Weiger R, Zitzmann NU. Three-dimensional imaging as a pre-operative tool in decision making for furcation surgery. J Clin Periodontol 2009;36:250–257.
92. Pilloni A, Rojas MA. Furcation involvement classification: A comprehensive review and a new system proposal. Dent J (Basel) 2018;23:6.
93. Hou GL, Chen YM, Tsai CC, Weisgold AS. A new classification of molar furcation involvement based on the root trunk and horizontal and vertical bone loss. Int J Periodontics Restorative Dent 1998;18:257–265.
94. Grant DA, Stern IB, Everett FG. Periodontics in the Tradition of Orban and Gottlieb, ed 5. St Louis: Mosby, 1979.
95. Bender IB, Seltzer S. Roentgenographic and direct observation of experimental lesions in bone: II. J Am Dent Assoc 1961;62:708–716.
96. Bender IB, Seltzer S. Roentgenographic and direct observation of experimental lesions in bone: I. J Am Dent Assoc 1961;62:152–160.
97. Goldman HM, Stallard RE. Limitations of the radiograph in the diagnosis of osseous defects in periodontal disease. J Periodontol 1973;44:626–628.
98. Rees TD, Biggs NL, Collings CK. Radiographic interpretation of periodontal osseous lesions. Oral Surg Oral Med Oral Pathol 1971;32:141–153.
99. Prichard JF. Advanced Periodontal Disease: Surgical and Prosthetic Management. Philadelphia: Saunders, 1972.
100. Deas DE, Moritz AJ, Mealey BL, McDonnell HT, Powell CA. Clinical reliability of the "furcation arrow" as a diagnostic marker. J Periodontol 2006;77:1436–1441.
101. Qiao J, Wang S, Duan J, et al. The accuracy of cone-beam computed tomography in assessing maxillary molar furcation involvement. J Clin Periodontol 2014;41:269–274.
102. Kim DM, Bassir SH. When is cone-beam computed tomography imaging appropriate for diagnostic inquiry in the management of inflammatory periodontitis? An American Academy of Periodontology best evidence review. J Periodontol 2017;88:978–998.
103. Walter C, Weiger R, Zitzmann NU. Accuracy of three-dimensional imaging in assessing maxillary molar furcation involvement. J Clin Periodontol 2010;37:436–441.
104. Watt DM, MacGregor AR, Geddes M, Cockburn A, Boyd JL. A preliminary investigation of the support of partial dentures and its relationship to vertical loads. Dent Pract 1958;9:2–15.
105. Jepsen A. Root surface measurement and a method for x-ray determination of root surface area. Acta Odontol Scand 1963;21:35–46.
106. Hillam DG. Stresses in the periodontal ligament. J Periodontal Res 1973;8:51–56.
107. Müller JJ. Die Wurzeloberfläche menschlicher Zähne und ihre Bedeutung für Ersatzkonstruktionen im Belastungsbereich des normalen und pathologischen Parodontiums. Schweiz Mschr Zahnheilk 1958;69:193-199.
108. Schroeder HE. The Periodontium. Berlin: Springer, 1986.
109. Anderson RW, McGarrah HE, Lamb RD, Eick JD. Root surface measurements of mandibular molars using stereophotogrammetry. J Am Dent Assoc 1983;107:613–615.
110. Fox SC, Bosworth BL. A morphological survey of proximal root concavities: A consideration in periodontal therapy. J Am Dent Assoc 1987;114:811–814.
111. Bower RC. Furcation morphology relative to periodontal treatment. Furcation root surface anatomy. J Periodontol 1979;50:366–374.
112. Trossello VK, Gianelly AA. Orthodontic treatment and periodontal status. J Periodontol 1979;50:665–671.
113. Vermylen K, De Quincey GN, van 't Hof MA, Wolffe GN, Renggli HH. Classification, reproducibility and prevalence of root proximity in periodontal patients. J Clin Periodontol 2005;32:254–259.

114. Vermylen K, De Quincey GN, Wolffe GN, van 't Hof MA, Renggli HH. Root proximity as a risk marker for periodontal disease: A case-control study. J Clin Periodontol 2005;32:260–265.
115. Klassman B, Zucker HW. Treatment of a periodontal defect resulting from improper tooth alignment and local factors. J Periodontol 1969;40:401–403.
116. Kramer GM. A consideration of root proximity. Int J Periodontics Restorative Dent 1987;7:8–33.
117. Nevins M. Interproximal periodontal disease: The embrasure as an etiologic factor. Int J Periodontics Restorative Dent 1982;2:8–27.
118. Kessler M. Interrelationships between orthodontics and periodontics. Am J Orthod 1976;70:154–172.
119. Kim T, Miyamoto T, Nunn ME, Garcia RI, Dietrich T. Root proximity as a risk factor for progression of alveolar bone loss: The Veterans Affairs Dental Longitudinal Study. J Periodontol 2008;79:654–659.
120. Heins PJ, Wieder SM. A histologic study of the width and nature of inter-radicular spaces in human adult pre-molars and molars. J Dent Res 1986;65:948–951.
121. Tal H. Relationship between the interproximal distance of roots and the prevalence of intrabony pockets. J Periodontol 1984;55:604–607.
122. Årtun J, Osterberg SK, Kokich VG. Long-term effect of thin interdental alveolar bone on periodontal health after orthodontic treatment. J Periodontol 1986;57:341–346.
123. Schei O, Waerhaug J, Lovdal A, Arno A. Alveolar bone loss as related to oral hygiene and age. J Periodontol 1959;30:7–16.
124. Burch JG, Hulen S. A study of the presence of accessory foramina and the topography of molar furcations. Oral Surg Oral Med Oral Pathol 1974;38:451–455.
125. Prichard J. Advanced Periodontal Disease: Surgical and Prosthetic Management. Philadelphia: Saunders, 1965.
126. Lee KW, Lee EC, Poon KY. Palato-gingival grooves in maxillary incisors. A possible predisposing factor to localised periodontal disease. Br Dent J 1968;124:14–18.
127. Kogon SL. The prevalence, location and conformation of palato-radicular grooves in maxillary incisors. J Periodontol 1986;57:231–234.
128. Bačić M, Karakas Z, Kaić Z, Sutalo J. The association between palatal grooves in upper incisors and periodontal complications. J Periodontol 1990;61:197–199.
129. Leknes KN, Lie T, Selvig KA. Root grooves: A risk factor in periodontal attachment loss. J Periodontol 1994;65:859–863.
130. Simon JH, Glick DH, Frank AL. Predictable endodontic and periodontic failures as a result of radicular anomalies. Oral Surg Oral Med Oral Pathol 1971;31:823–826.
131. Withers JA, Brunsvold MA, Killoy WJ, Rahe AJ. The relationship of palato-gingival grooves to localized periodontal disease. J Periodontol 1981;52:41–44.
132. August DS. The radicular lingual groove: An overlooked differential diagnosis. J Am Dent Assoc 1978;96:1037–1039.
133. Everett FG, Kramer GM. The disto-lingual groove in the maxillary lateral incisor; a periodontal hazard. J Periodontol 1972;43:352–361.
134. Hou GL, Tsai CC. Relationship between palato-radicular grooves and localized periodontitis. J Clin Periodontol 1993;20:678–682.
135. Albaricci MF, de Toledo BE, Zuza EP, Gomes DA, Rosetti EP. Prevalence and features of palato-radicular grooves: An in-vitro study. J Int Acad Periodontol 2008;10:2–5.
136. Addison WHF, Appleton JLT. Root development and the light it throws on certain peculiarities of the roots and root-canals. J Dent Res 1928;8:403.
137. Sicher H. Orban's Oral Histology and Embryology, ed 5. St Louis: Mosby, 1962.
138. Koenigs JF, Brilliant JD, Foreman DW. Preliminary scanning electron microscope investigations of accessory foramina in the furcation areas of human molar teeth. Oral Surg Oral Med Oral Pathol 1974;38:773–782.
139. Saunders RL. X-ray microscopy of human dental pulp vessels. Nature 1957;180:1353–1354.
140. Kramer IR. The vascular architecture of the human dental pulp. Arch Oral Biol 1960;2:177–189.
141. De Deus QD. Frequency, location, and direction of the lateral, secondary, and accessory canals. J Endod 1975;1:361–366.
142. Gutmann JL. Prevalence, location, and patency of accessory canals in the furcation region of permanent molars. J Periodontol 1978;49:21–26.
143. Vertucci FJ, Williams RG. Furcation canals in the human mandibular first molar. Oral Surg Oral Med Oral Pathol 1974;38:308–314.
144. Kirkham DB. The location and incidence of accessory pulpal canals in periodontal pockets. J Am Dent Assoc 1975;91:353–356.
145. Hess W. The Anatomy of the Root Canals of the Teeth of the Permanent Dentition. New York: William, Wood & Co, 1925.
146. Zuza EP, Toledo BE, Hetem S, Spolidório LC, Mendes AJ, Rosetti EP. Prevalence of different types of accessory canals in the furcation area of third molars. J Periodontol 2006;77:1755–1761.
147. Rubach WC, Mitchell DF. Periodontal disease, accessory canals and pulp pathosis. J Periodontol 1965;36:34–38.
148. Lowman JV, Burke RS, Pelleu GB. Patent accessory canals: Incidence in molar furcation region. Oral Surg Oral Med Oral Pathol 1973;36:580–584.
149. Pineda F, Kuttler Y. Mesiodistal and buccolingual roentgenographic investigation of 7,275 root canals. Oral Surg Oral Med Oral Pathol 1972;33:101–110.
150. Ogilvie AL, Ingle JI. An Atlas of Pulpar and Periapical Biology. Philadelphia: Lea & Febiger, 1965.
151. Green D. Morphology of the pulp cavity of the permanent teeth. Oral Surg Oral Med Oral Pathol 1955;8:743–759.
152. Yoshida H, Yakushiji M, Sugihara A, Tanaka K, Taguchi M. Accessory canals at floor of the pulp chamber of primary molars [in Japanese]. Shikwa Gakuho 1975;75:580–585.
153. Paras LG, Rapp R, Piesco NP, Zeichner SJ, Zullo TG. An investigation of accessory canals in furcation areas of human primary molars: Part 2. Latex perfusion studies of the internal and external furcation areas to demonstrate accessory canals. J Clin Pediatr Dent 1993;17:71–77.
154. Seltzer S, Bender IB, Ziontz M. The interrelationship of pulp and periodontal disease. Oral Surg Oral Med Oral Pathol 1963;16:1474–1490.
155. Bender IB, Seltzer S. The effect of periodontal disease on the pulp. Oral Surg Oral Med Oral Pathol 1972;33:458–474.
156. Langeland K, Rodrigues H, Dowden W. Periodontal disease, bacteria, and pulpal histopathology. Oral Surg Oral Med Oral Pathol 1974;37:257–270.
157. Mazur B, Massler M. Influence of periodontal disease on the dental pulp. Oral Surg Oral Med Oral Pathol 1964;17:592–603.
158. Simring M, Goldberg M. The pulpal pocket approach: Retrograde periodontitis. J Periodontol 1964;35:22–48.
159. Seltzer S, Bender IB, Nazimov H, Sinai I. Pulpitis-induced interradicular periodontal changes in experimental animals. J Periodontol 1967;38:124–129.
160. Winter GB. Changes in periodontal membrane and bone following experimental pulpal injury in deciduous molar teeth in kittens. Arch Oral Biol 1965;10:279–289.

161. Barkhordar RA, Stewart GG. The potential of periodontal pocket formation associated with untreated accessory root canals. Oral Surg Oral Med Oral Pathol 1990;70:769–772.
162. Hiatt WH. Regeneration of the periodontium after endodontic therapy and flap operation. Oral Surg Oral Med Oral Pathol 1959;12:1471–1477.
163. Rossman SR, Kaplowitz B, Baldinger SR. Therapy of the endodontically and periodontally involved tooth: Report of a case. Oral Surg Oral Med Oral Pathol 1960;13:361–367.
164. Provenza DV. Oral Histology: Inheritance and Development. Philadelphia: Lippincott, 1964.
165. Shafer WG, Hine MK, Levy BM. A Textbook of Oral Pathology. Philadelphia: Saunders, 1974.
166. Holton WL, Hancock EB, Pelleu GB, Jr. Prevalence and distribution of attached cementicles on human root surfaces. J Periodontol 1986;57:321–324.
167. Leknes KN, Lie T, Selvig KA. Cemental tear: A risk factor in periodontal attachment loss. J Periodontol 1996;67:583–588.
168. Leknes KN. The influence of anatomic and iatrogenic root surface characteristics on bacterial colonization and periodontal destruction: A review. J Periodontol 1997;68:507–516.
169. Lyons CT, Peacock ME, Cuenin MF, Swiec GD, Dickey DJ. Severe localized periodontal destruction associated with cervical cemental separation. Gen Dent 2005;53:212–214.
170. Chou J, Rawal YB, O'Neil JR, Tatakis DN. Cementodentinal tear: A case report with 7-year follow-up. J Periodontol 2004;75:1708–1713.
171. Lin HJ, Chan CP, Wu CT, Jeng JH. Cemental tear on a mandibular second molar: A case report. Odontology 2010;98:173–176.
172. Brunsvold MA, Lasho DJ. Cemental tears related to severe localized periodontal disease. Pract Periodontics Aesthet Dent 2000;12:536–540.
173. Marquam BJ. Atypical localized deep pocket due to a cemental tear: Case report. J Contemp Dent Pract 2003;4:52–64.
174. Schmidlin PR. Regenerative treatment of a cemental tear using enamel matrix derivatives: A ten-year follow-up. Open Dent J 2012;6:148–152.
175. Tulkki MJ, Baisden MK, McClanahan SB. Cemental tear: A case report of a rare root fracture. J Endod 2006;32:1005–1007.
176. Blum G, Bouquot J, Dorn S. Oral and maxillofacial pathology case of the month. Cemental tear and chronic periodontitis. Tex Dent J 2013;130:534–538.
177. Lin HJ, Chan CP, Yang CY, et al. Cemental tear: Clinical characteristics and its predisposing factors. J Endod 2011;37:611–618.
178. Lin HJ, Chang SH, Chang MC, et al. Clinical fracture site, morphologic and histopathologic characteristics of cemental tear: Role in endodontic lesions. J Endod 2012;38:1058–1062.
179. Tai TF, Chiang CP, Lin CP, Lin CC, Jeng JH. Persistent endodontic lesion due to complex cementodentinal tears in a maxillary central incisor: A case report. Oral Surg Oral Med Oral Pathol Oral Radiol Endod 2007;103:e55–e60.
180. Harvey BL, Zander HA. Root surface resorption of periodontally diseased teeth. Oral Surg Oral Med Oral Pathol 1959;12:1439–1443.
181. Haney JM, Leknes KN, Lie T, Selvig KA, Wikesjö UM. Cemental tear related to rapid periodontal breakdown: A case report. J Periodontol 1992;63:220–224.
182. Müller G, Zander HA. Cementum of periodontally diseased teeth from India. J Dent Res 1960;39:385–390.
183. Harrel SK, Wright JM. Treatment of periodontal destruction associated with a cemental tear using minimally invasive surgery. J Periodontol 2000;71:1761–1766.
184. Camargo PM, Pirih FQ, Wolinsky LE, Lekovic V, Kamrath H, White SN. Clinical repair of an osseous defect associated with a cemental tear: A case report. Int J Periodontics Restorative Dent 2003;23:79–85.
185. Ishikawa I, Oda S, Hayashi J, Arakawa S. Cervical cemental tears in older patients with adult periodontitis. Case reports. J Periodontol 1996;67:15–20.
186. Stewart ML, McClanahan SB. Cemental tear: A case report. Int Endod J 2006;39:81–86.
187. Watanabe C, Watanabe Y, Miyauchi M, Fujita M, Watanabe Y. Multiple cemental tears. Oral Surg Oral Med Oral Pathol Oral Radiol 2012;114:365–372.
188. Müller HP. Cemental tear treated with guided tissue regeneration: A case report 3 years after initial treatment. Quintessence Int 1999;30:111–115.
189. Jeng PY, Luzi AL, Pitarch RM, Chang MC, Wu YH, Jeng JH. Cemental tear: To know what we have neglected in dental practice. J Formos Med Assoc 2018;117:261–267.
190. Lin HJ, Chang MC, Chang SH, et al. Treatment outcome of the teeth with cemental tears. J Endod 2014;40:1315–1320.
191. Larato DC. Palatal exostoses of the posterior maxillary alveolar process. J Periodontol 1972;43:486–489.
192. Sonnier KE, Horning GM, Cohen ME. Palatal tubercles, palatal tori, and mandibular tori: Prevalence and anatomical features in a U.S. population. J Periodontol 1999;70:329–336.
193. Nery EB, Corn H, Eisenstein IL. Palatal exostosis in the molar region. J Periodontol 1977;48:663–666.
194. Willershausen B, Köttgen C, Ernst CP. The influence of restorative materials on marginal gingiva. Eur J Med Res 2001;6:433–439.
195. Ababnaeh KT, Al-Omari M, Alawneh TN. The effect of dental restoration type and material on periodontal health. Oral Health Prev Dent 2011;9:395–403.
196. Lang NP, Kiel RA, Anderhalden K. Clinical and microbiological effects of subgingival restorations with overhanging or clinically perfect margins. J Clin Periodontol 1983;10:563–578.
197. Ercoli C, Caton JG. Dental prostheses and tooth-related factors. J Clin Periodontol 2018;89(suppl 1):S223–S236.
198. Chan C, Weber H. Plaque retention on teeth restored with full-ceramic crowns: A comparative study. J Prosthet Dent 1986;56:666–671.
199. Löe H, Silness J. Periodontal disease in pregnancy. I. Prevalence and severity. Acta Odontol Scand 1963;21:533–551.
200. Checketts MR, Turkyilmaz I, Asar NV. An investigation of the effect of scaling-induced surface roughness on bacterial adhesion in common fixed dental restorative materials. J Prosthet Dent 2014;112:1265–1270.
201. Weishaupt P, Bernimoulin JP, Lange KP, Rothe S, Naumann M, Hägewald S. Clinical and inflammatory effects of galvano-ceramic and metal-ceramic crowns on periodontal tissues. J Oral Rehabil 2007;34:941–947.
202. van Dijken JW, Sjöström S. The effect of glass ionomer cement and composite resin fillings on marginal gingiva. J Clin Periodontol 1991;18:200–203.
203. Konradsson K, Claesson R, van Dijken JW. Dental biofilm, gingivitis and interleukin-1 adjacent to approximal sites of a bonded ceramic. J Clin Periodontol 2007;34:1062–1067.
204. Quirynen M, Marechal M, Busscher HJ, Weerkamp AH, Darius PL, van Steenberghe D. The influence of surface free energy and surface roughness on early plaque formation. An in vivo study in man. J Clin Periodontol 1990;17:138–144.
205. Bollen CM, Lambrechts P, Quirynen M. Comparison of surface roughness of oral hard materials to the threshold surface roughness for bacterial plaque retention: A review of the literature. Dent Mater 1997;13:258–269.

206. Waerhaug J. Histological considerations which govern where the margins of restorations should be located in relation to the gingiva. Dent Clin North Am 1960:161–176.
207. Marcum JS. The effect of crown marginal depth upon gingival tissue. J Prosthet Dent 1967;17:479–487.
208. Sotres LS, Van Huysen G, Gilmore HW. A histologic study of gingival tissue response to amalgam, silicate and resin restorations. J Periodontol 1969;40:543–546.
209. Newcomb GM. The relationship between the location of subgingival crown margins and gingival inflammation. J Periodontol 1974;45:151–154.
210. Waerhaug J. Presence or absence of plaque on subgingival restorations. Scand J Dent Res 1975;83:193–201.
211. Schätzle M, Land NP, Anerud A, Boysen H, Bürgin W, Löe H. The influence of margins of restorations of the periodontal tissues over 26 years. J Clin Periodontol 2001;28:57–64.
212. Wang JC, Lai CH, Listgarten MA. *Porphyromonas gingivalis*, *Prevotella intermedia* and *Bacteroides forsythus* in plaque subjacent to bridge pontics. J Clin Periodontol 1998;25:330–333.
213. Thomas BO. The relationship of operative procedures to the health of the periodontal tissues. J Am Dent Assoc 1949;39:522–532.
214. Ramfjord S. Local factors in periodontal disease. J Am Dent Assoc 1952;44:647–655.
215. Björn AL, Björn H, Grkovic B. Marginal fit of restorations and its relation to peridontal bone level. I. Metal fillings. Odontol Revy 1969;20:311–321.
216. Gilmore N, Sheiham A. Overhanging dental restorations and periodontal disease. J Periodontol 1971;42:8–12.
217. Jeffcoat MK, Howell TH. Alveolar bone destruction due to overhanging amalgam in periodontal disease. J Periodontol 1980;51:599–602.
218. Pack AR, Coxhead LJ, McDonald BW. The prevalence of overhanging margins in posterior amalgam restorations and periodontal consequences. J Clin Periodontol 1990;17:145–152.
219. Jansson L, Ehnevid H, Lindskog S, Blomlöf L. Proximal restorations and periodontal status. J Clin Periodontol 1994;21:577–582.
220. Highfield JE, Powell RN. Effects of removal of posterior overhanging metallic margins of restorations upon the periodontal tissues. J Clin Periodontol 1978;5:169–181.
221. Gorzo I, Newman HN, Strahan JD. Amalgam restorations, plaque removal and periodontal health. J Clin Periodontol 1979;6:98–105.
222. Laurell L, Rylander H, Pettersson B. The effect of different levels of polishing of amalgam restorations on the plaque retention and gingival inflammation. Swed Dent J 1983;7:45–53.
223. Rodriguez-Ferrer HJ, Strahan JD, Newman HN. Effect of gingival health of removing overhanging margins of interproximal subgingival amalgam restorations. J Clin Periodontol 1980;7:457–462.
224. Jernberg GR, Bakdash MB, Keenan KM. Relationship between proximal tooth open contacts and periodontal disease. J Periodontol 1983;54:529–533.
225. O'Leary TJ, Badell MC, Bloomer RS. Interproximal contact and marginal ridge relationships in periodontally healthy young males classified as to orthodontic status. J Periodontol 1975;46:6–9.
226. Geiger AM, Wasserman BH, Turgeon LR. Relationship of occlusion and periodontal disease. 8. Relationship of crowding and spacing to periodontal destruction and gingival inflammation. J Periodontol 1974;45:43–49.
227. Koral SM, Howell TH, Jeffcoat MK. Alveolar bone loss due to open interproximal contacts in periodontal disease. J Periodontol 1981;52:447–450.
228. Larato DC. Relationship of food impaction to interproximal intrabony lesions. J Periodontol 1971;42:237–238.
229. Hancock EB, Mayo CV, Schwab RR, Wirthlin MR. Influence of interdental contacts on periodontal status. J Periodontol 1980;51:445–449.
230. Burch JG. Periodontal considerations in operative dentistry. J Prosthet Dent 1975;34:156–163.
231. Årtun J, Osterberg SK. Periodontal status of teeth facing extraction sites long-term after orthodontic treatment. J Periodontol 1987;58:24–29.
232. Mosteller JH. The etiology of periodontal disease: A review of current literature. J Periodontol 1950;21:168–178.
233. Pihlstrom BL, Anderson KA, Aeppli D, Schaffer EM. Association between signs of trauma from occlusion and periodontitis. J Periodontol 1986;57:1–6.
234. Kepic TJ, O'Leary TJ. Role of marginal ridge relationships as an etiologic factor in periodontal disease. J Periodontol 1978;49:570–575.
235. Alexander AG, Tipnis AK. The effect of irregularity of teeth and the degree of overbite and overjet on the gingival health. A study of 400 subjects. Br Dent J 1970;128:539–544.
236. Hellgren A. The association between crowding of teeth and gingivitis. Trans Eur Orthod Soc, 1956:134–140.
237. Helm S, Petersen PE. Causal relation between malocclusion and periodontal health. Acta Odontol Scand 1989;47:223–228.
238. Wachsman C. Gingivitis in relation to irregularities of the teeth. Paradentologie 1950;4:179–185.
239. Geiger A. Occlusion in periodontal disease. J Periodontol 1965;36:387–393.
240. Geiger AM. Occlusal studies in 188 consecutive cases of periodontal disease. Am J Orthod 1962;48:330–360.
241. Sutcliffe P. Chronic anterior gingivitis. An epidemiological study in school children. Br Dent J 1968;125:47–55.
242. Ainamo J. Relationship between malalignment of the teeth and periodontal disease. Scand J Dent Res 1972;80:104–110.
243. Staufer K, Landmesser H. Effects of crowding in the lower anterior segment: A risk evaluation depending upon the degree of crowding. J Orofac Orthop 2004;65:13–25.
244. Van Kirk LE, Jr. Assessment of malocclusion in population groups. Am J Public Health Nations Health 1959;49:1157–1163.
245. Ingervall B, Jacobsson U, Nyman S. A clinical study of the relationship between crowding of teeth, plaque and gingival condition. J Clin Periodontol 1977;4:214–222.
246. Geiger AM, Wasserman BH, Thompson RH Jr, et al. Relationship of occlusion and periodontal disease. I. A system for evaluating periodontal status. J Periodontol 1971;42:364–370.
247. Wasserman BH, Thompson RH Jr, Geiger AM, et al. Relationship of occlusion and periodontal disease. II. Periodontal status of the study population. J Periodontol 1971;42:371–378.
248. Thompson RH Jr, Geiger AM, Wasserman BH, Turgeon LR. Relationship of occlusion and periodontal disease. 3. Relation of periodontal status to general background characteristics. J Periodontol 1972;43:540–546.
249. Wasserman BH, Geiger AM, Thompson RH Jr, Turgeon LR. Relationship of occlusion and periodontal disease. IV. Relationship of inflammation to general background characteristics and periodontal destruction. J Periodontol 1972;43:547–553.
250. Geiger AM, Wasserman BH, Thompson RH Jr, Turgeon LR. Relationship of occlusion and periodontal disease. V. Relation of classification of occlusion to periodontal status and gingival inflammation. J Periodontol 1972;43:554–560.
251. Geiger AM, Wasserman BH, Turgeon LR. Relationship of occlusion and periodontal disease. VI. Relation of anterior overjet and overbite to periodontal destruction and gingival inflammation. J Periodontol 1973;44:150–157.

252. Wasserman BH, Geiger AM, Turgeon LR. Relationship of occlusion and periodontal disease. VII. Mobility. J Periodontol 1973;44:572–578.
253. Geiger AM, Wasserman BH. Relationship of occlusion and periodontal disease: Part IX—incisor inclination and periodontal status. Angle Orthod 1976;46:99–110.
254. Geiger AM, Wasserman BH. Relationship of occlusion and periodontal disease. Part X. Relation of cross-bite to periodontal status. J Periodontol 1977;48:785–789.
255. Geiger AM, Wasserman BH. Relationship of occlusion and periodontal disease. Part XI. Relation of axial inclination (mesial-distal) and tooth drift to periodontal status. J Periodontol 1980;51:283–290.
256. Poulton DR, Aaronson SA. The relationship between occlusion and periodontal status. Am J Orthod 1961;47:690–699.
257. McCombie F, Stothard D. Relationship between gingivitis and other dental conditions. J Can Dent Assoc 1964;30:506–513.
258. Bilimoria KF. Malocclusion: Its role in the causation of periodontal disease. J All India Dent Assoc 1963;35:293–300.
259. Beagrie GS, James GA. The association of posterior teeth irregularity and periodontal disease. Brit Dent J 1962;113:239.
260. Gould MSE, Picton DCA. The relation between irregularities of the teeth and periodontal disease. Brit Dent J 1966;121:20.
261. Grewe JM, Chadha JM, Hagan D, Zermeno JA. Oral hygiene and occlusal disharmony in Mexican-American children. J Periodontal Res 1969;4:189–192.
262. van Gastel J, Quirynen M, Teughels W, Carels C. The relationships between malocclusion, fixed orthodontic appliances and periodontal disease. A review of the literature. Aust Orthod J 2007;23:121–129.
263. Kugelberg CF. Periodontal healing two and four years after impacted lower third molar surgery. A comparative retrospective study. Int J Oral Maxillofac Surg 1990;19:341–345.
264. Kugelberg CF, Ahlström U, Ericson S, Hugoson A, Kvint S. Periodontal healing after impacted lower third molar surgery in adolescents and adults. A prospective study. Int J Oral Maxillofac Surg 1991;20:18–24.
265. Machtei EE, Zubrey Y, Ben Yehuda A, Soskolne WA. Proximal bone loss adjacent to periodontally "hopeless" teeth with and without extraction. J Periodontol 1989;60:512–515.
266. DeVore CH, Beck FM, Horton JE. Retained "hopeless" teeth. Effects on the proximal periodontium of adjacent teeth. J Periodontol 1988;59:647–651.
267. Wojcik MS, DeVore CH, Beck FM, Horton JE. Retained "hopeless" teeth: Lack of effect periodontally-treated teeth have on the proximal periodontium of adjacent teeth 8-years later. J Periodontol 1992;63:663–666.
268. Machtei EE, Hirsch I. Retention of hopeless teeth: The effect on the adjacent proximal bone following periodontal surgery. J Periodontol 2007;78:2246–2252.

6

OCCLUSAL TRAUMA

Emilio Couso-Queiruga, DDS, MS

Occlusal trauma has been a topic of controversy since 1901 when Karolyi first described an association between traumatic occlusal forces and periodontal disease.[1] Since then, multiple investigations using animal and human models have studied the importance of occlusal therapy and the effects of traumatic forces on the periodontium. However, researchers have shown conflicting evidence with regard to the relationship between traumatic occlusal forces, occlusal therapy, and periodontal breakdown. Therefore, the aim of this chapter is to provide a description of occlusal trauma and its relationship with periodontal diseases, potential contributing factors, diagnostic considerations, and treatment alternatives.

It is important to bear in mind that there is a lack of evidence derived from controlled studies supporting the terms **primary** and **secondary occlusal trauma**. In 1984, a finite element analysis was conducted to calculate the stress exerted upon the periodontal ligament (PDL) following functional occlusal loading in maxillary central incisors. The results suggested that around one-third of the occlusal load associated with primary occlusal trauma is required to generate the stress necessary for the development of secondary occlusal trauma with 60% of bone loss. The magnitude of stress was inversely proportional to bone support, particularly past the 4-mm threshold of supporting bone loss.[6]

Occlusal Trauma and Periodontal Disease

The first association between occlusal forces and periodontal disease was described by Karolyi in 1901 and termed *pyhorrea alveolaris*.[1] Subsequently, different authors suggested an association between traumatic occlusion and failures in periodontal therapy.[4,5,7] Accordingly, Stillman indicated that clinicians must identify and treat occlusal trauma prior to periodontal treatment.[4,5]

Early animal studies supported occlusal trauma as an etiologic factor for periodontal disease.[8,9] On the other hand, investigations from Orban and others pointed to occlusal trauma preceding gingival inflammation or vice versa in the predisposition of periodontal destruction.[10] Macapanpan and

DEFINITIONS AND TERMINOLOGY

Abfraction: The hypothetical process leading to the loss of cervical tooth structure due to a combination of abrasion, erosion, and/or occlusal forces; data supporting this term as a discrete clinical entity are equivocal.

Abrasion: The wearing away of tooth structure or restorative material through an abnormal mechanical process. Examples include gingival and dental abrasions due to incorrect brushing.

Attrition: The physiologic wearing away of a substance or structure, such as the teeth.[2]

Bruxism/tooth grinding: A habit of grinding, clenching, or clamping the teeth. The force so generated may damage both the tooth and the attachment apparatus.[2]

Erosion: An apparent chemical dissolution of enamel and dentin, unrelated to caries, causing a cavity that has a hard, smooth base.[2]

Fremitus: A palpable or visible movement of a tooth when subjected to occlusal forces.[2]

Occlusal adjustment: An intentional mechanical reshaping of occluding tooth surfaces to obtain a more harmonious relationship between teeth, jaws, temporomandibular joint, and muscles of mastication.[2] Also known as *occlusal equilibration* or *selective grinding*.

Occlusal discrepancy: An occlusal scheme that deviates from ideal interactions between occlusal contacts and anatomical components of the craniofacial complex.[2]

Occlusal interference: An undesirable tooth contact that impedes or interferes with harmonious and stable mandibular movements.

Occlusal prematurity: Any contact of opposing teeth that occurs before the desirable intercuspation.

Occlusal trauma: A lesion in the periodontal ligament (PDL), cementum, and adjacent bone caused by traumatic occlusal forces.[3] Formerly known as *trauma from occlusion*.

- **Primary occlusal trauma:** Injury resulting in tissue changes from excessive occlusal forces applied to a tooth or teeth with normal support.[2]
- **Secondary occlusal trauma:** Injury resulting in tissue changes from normal or excessive occlusal forces applied to a tooth or teeth with reduced support.[2]

Splint: Any apparatus, appliance, or device employed to prevent motion or displacement of fractured or movable parts.[2]

Stillman's cleft: A narrow, V-shaped gingival recession on the facial aspect of the tooth.[4,5]

Traumatic occlusal force/excessive occlusal force: Any occlusal force resulting in injury of the teeth and/or the periodontal attachment apparatus.[3]

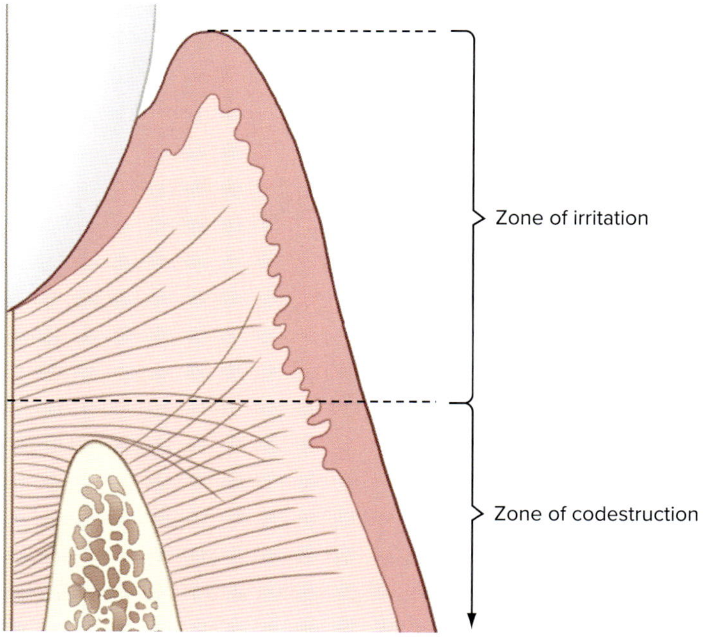

Fig 6-1 Glickman's concept: zone of irritation and zone of codestruction.

Weinmann, also following an animal model, concluded that occlusal trauma will not be the sole cause of periodontal breakdown.[11] Later on, during 1960s and 1970s, two different concepts led by Glickman and Waerhaug emerged concerning the role of occlusal trauma in periodontal disease.

GLICKMAN'S CONCEPT

As part of the theory of codestruction, Glickman suggested the presence of two disease zones,[12] through which he described the effect of **traumatic occlusal forces** on gingival inflammation (Fig 6-1):

- *Zone of irritation:* Comprises the marginal gingival and interdental papillae bounded by the gingival fibers. The presence of gingival inflammation here is the tissue response to local irritants and is unaffected by occlusal forces.
- *Zone of codestruction:* Comprises the PDL, cementum, and alveolar bone, as well as the transseptal interproximal fibers and the alveolar crest fibers. In this area, the presence of inflammation in conjunction with occlusal trauma present a codestructive factor in periodontal disease.

Based on this concept, traumatic occlusal forces do not alter the vascular and cellular features of gingivitis, whereas they do modify *(1)* the environment at the periphery of inflammation, *(2)* the physiologic alignment of the interproximal transseptal fibers, and *(3)* the alveolar crest fibers, gradually resulting in the spread of inflammation directly to the PDL. This alteration results in the development of intrabony pockets and angular osseous defects. However, these lesions are not pathognomonic of occlusal trauma.

When the inflammation remains in the marginal gingiva, within the confines of the gingival and transseptal fibers, it is unaffected by the presence of occlusal trauma. This gingival lesion will initially cause the fragmentation and dissolution of the fibers involving the alveolar bone and gradually arriving at the PDL area, resulting in suprabony pockets and horizontal bone loss.

As a summary of this concept, Glickman stated in 1967 that "trauma from occlusion per se does not cause any type of periodontal pocket. Local irritation is required to initiate the inflammatory changes that lead to periodontal pocket formation."[13]

WAERHAUG'S CONCEPT

Waerhaug conducted an investigation similar to that of Glickman comprising autopsy samples. However, he additionally evaluated the potential association between the depth of migration of the subgingival plaque and the resultant attachment loss through the following measurements[14]:

1. The distance from the plaque to the most apical point of the junctional epithelium.
2. The distance from the plaque to the nearest point of the alveolar crest.

According to these outcome measures, he found no difference between "traumatized" and "nontraumatized" teeth in terms of angular bony defects or intrabony pockets present. However, he described a relationship between the loss of periodontal structure—namely periodontal fiber attachment and alveolar bone—and the downgrowth of the plaque. He argued that an angular defect between two teeth was caused by plaque on one tooth advancing to a more apical level than plaque on the adjacent tooth. This in turn results in deeper attachment loss on one tooth surface than the other. Hence, Waerhaug had concluded that intrabony pockets were invariably associated with this downgrowth of subgingival plaque. Furthermore, no evidence was found to support Glickman's concept.

In the literature, some authors are in agreement with Glickman's concept,[11,15,16] while others support Waerhaug's findings.[14,17,18] What must be acknowledged with regard to these investigations is an inability to draw cause-effect relationships between occlusal trauma and progression of periodontitis, presence of dental plaque, or established periodontal lesions. The inherent limitations of their study designs only allowed the researchers to investigate the presence of an association.

ANIMAL STUDIES

In the 1930s, two animal studies detected an association between occlusal trauma and periodontal disease.[8,9] However, it was not until decades later that the most impactful series of experimental animal investigations were performed. These publications were the results of two distinct research groups publishing out of the Eastman Dental Center (Rochester, NY)[19–26] and the University of Gothenburg (Gothenburg, Sweden).[27–32]

American group

This camp explored the effects of the presence or absence of jiggling-type traumatic forces in healthy and induced periodontitis in a monkey model. In the presence of a traumatic lesion and induced periodontitis, results failed to demonstrate an increase in angular bony defects, additional apical migration of the junctional epithelium, or alveolar bone loss compared with the contralateral side that was not subjected to traumatic injury.[19,20]

Notably, with sustained jiggling forces and zero or minimal clinical signs of inflammation, increased tooth mobility was observed along with widened PDL space, loss in crestal height, and a reduction in the overall alveolar bone. However, no loss of connective tissue attachment was observed, nor its sequelae.[21] When the jiggling forces were interrupted in these teeth with or without minimal signs of inflammation, considerable bone regeneration occurred. Meanwhile, at sites with periodontitis, alveolar bone regeneration and diminished tooth mobility were not observed.[22] On the other hand, after resolution of inflammation in teeth affected with periodontitis and subjected to jiggling forces, decreased tooth mobility and bone repair were observed, even in cases of continued tooth hypermobility without changes in clinical attachment level.[33]

A degree of irreversible crestal alveolar bone loss was also reported due to the interaction between marginal periodontal inflammation and subjacent jiggling trauma, even following elimination of both inflammatory and traumatic factors.[24] This was in addition to the progressively increasing tooth hypermobility in the presence of a healthy but reduced periodontium.[25] The aforementioned findings diminished the emphasis on management of tooth mobility and, in turn, increased the emphasis on resolution of marginal inflammation.[26]

TABLE 6-1 A comparison in experimental design between the American and Scandinavian groups

	American group	Scandinavian group
Supporting concept	Waerhaug's concept[14]	Glickman's concept[12]
Method of occlusal trauma production	Wedge/elevators toward teeth	Cap splint and bar devices
Animal model	Monkey	Dog
Inflammation induction	Cotton floss/silk ligature/toothpick	Cemented band/rubber band/cotton floss ligature with surgically created intrabony defects
Magnitude of force	Light	Heavy
Duration of force	Long	Short
Frequency of force	Low	High
Experimental period	Short	Long

Scandinavian group

This camp evaluated the effects of the presence or absence of continuous traumatic jiggling forces in healthy and experimentally induced periodontitis in beagle dogs. In healthy sites as well as in the presence of gingival inflammation, traumatic occlusal forces produced tooth hypermobility, bone resorption, vascular dilatation, and an increased vascularity. However, no apical migration of the junctional epithelium was observed.[27–29] On the other hand, in the presence of induced periodontitis and traumatic occlusal forces, there was gradually increased horizontal mobility, intrusion of the teeth, angular bone destruction, and apical migration of the junctional epithelium. Nevertheless, comparable horizontal bone loss was observed in the control (without traumatic occlusal forces) and the test group.[28] Other findings included the presence of osteoclastic activity, migration of polymorphonuclear leukocytes, and continued vascular permeability when an established periodontal lesion and jiggling forces were present.[29]

After the jiggling forces were eliminated in the presence of periodontitis, a marked decrease in tooth mobility and diminution in the widened PDL space occurred. However, it is interesting to note that the magnitude of connective tissue attachment loss was similar in the control sites (maintained jiggling forces) and test sites, where jiggling forces were removed. These results suggested that the removal of **occlusal interferences** and reduction in tooth mobility do not have a positive impact in periodontal conditions.[34] Last, in a reduced but healthy periodontium, the presence of tooth hypermobility or jiggling-type forces did not seem to affect the healing following periodontal surgery.[30]

The differences between the two groups are summarized in Table 6-1.[12,14]

As a highlight of the previous animal studies, while bearing in mind the limitations such as the inherent differences between the animal models and the dissimilar types of traumatic occlusal forces, the following conclusions can be drawn:

- Occlusal trauma without the presence of inflammation resulted in increased mobility and loss of bone density, with no clinical attachment loss. When the occlusal forces were removed, the bone volume was recovered.
- Occlusal trauma in the presence of induced periodontitis resulted in increased tooth mobility and greater bone loss. With the American group, clinical attachment loss was found to be similar between groups.[20] With the Scandinavian group, the degree of apical migration of the pocket epithelium was more pronounced in the presence of trauma.[28]

Finally, there is no evidence to support that occlusal trauma initiates gingivitis and/or periodontitis. However, it is evident that it may play a role in accelerating periodontal breakdown in the presence of periodontitis.

CLINICAL STUDIES

An increase in tooth mobility has been described as an important sign of occlusal trauma in a number of studies.[5,7,10,11,14,35] However, this may also be the result of several factors that contribute to a reduction in alveolar bone height.[26,36,37] The role of tooth mobility with regard to the outcomes of periodontal therapy has also been investigated. Rosling et al showed comparable healing following antimicrobial therapy for intrabony pockets located adjacent to both hypermobile and stable teeth.[38] However, other investigations concluded that although mobile teeth can be successfully treated and maintained, the presence of mobility negatively affects the outcomes of periodontal therapy. In this study, nonmobile teeth reported greater attachment gain compared with mobile and extremely mobile teeth, and the latter even demonstrated loss of attachment.[39]

A cross-sectional study evaluated 496 maxillary first molars in 300 individuals in an attempt to identify a potential association between clinical signs of occlusal trauma, disease severity, and radiographic records. From those, only 14 teeth presented with signs of occlusal trauma. In this group, significantly greater probing depths, clinical attachment loss, and less bone support were observed. Hence, the authors demonstrated that teeth with a widened PDL space and mobility had about 10% less osseous support.[40] Similar findings were described in a study by Jin and Cao, reporting a positive correlation between tooth mobility and greater magnitude of periodontal disease.[41] In addition, a study by Wang et al showed that molars that initially exhibited less mobility exhibited greater attachment gain subsequent to periodontal treatment.[42] This was further corroborated in an investigation that associated greater baseline tooth mobility with less clinical attachment gain at 1 year following guided tissue regeneration.[43]

A series of two studies also showed that on a tooth-level basis, occlusal discrepancy acts as an independent risk factor contributing to periodontal disease, demonstrating deeper initial probing depths, worse prognoses, and mobility.[44] As such, teeth with untreated occlusal discrepancies demonstrated deeper probing depths when compared with teeth with initial treatment or teeth without occlusal discrepancies.[45]

Contributing Factors

OCCLUSAL DISCREPANCIES

An **occlusal discrepancy** is defined as an occlusal scheme that deviates from ideal interactions between occlusal contacts and anatomical components of the craniofacial complex.[2]

In 1965, Yuodelis and Mann associated nonworking contacts with periodontal disease and an overall negative impact on the periodontium. Fifty-three percent of the teeth that showed nonworking contacts exhibited greater mobility, bone loss, and increased pocket depths. However, due to the incomplete clinical picture reported in this study, an association between the two entities cannot be drawn.[46] Later, Shefter and McFall reported no influence of occlusal disharmonies on periodontal status.[47] Similarly, Pihlstrom et al observed more clinical attachment loss and increased probing depth in teeth with uneven marginal ridges. However, no differences were found between centric relation, nonworking, working, or protrusive contacts and probing depth, clinical attachment level, or osseous support. Indeed, wear facets were associated with less attachment loss and greater osseous support.[40]

On the other hand, several other studies confirmed the causative impact of occlusal trauma on the periodontal condition over time. Jin and Cao observed deeper probing depths as well as greater clinical attachment and bone loss in teeth with occlusal trauma.[41] Nunn and Harrel, in the first part of a retrospective investigation, observed that teeth with initial occlusal discrepancies showed significantly increased probing depths, increased mobility, and worse long-term prognosis compared to teeth without occlusal discrepancies. As such, the authors considered occlusal discrepancy as an independent risk factor for periodontal disease.[44] In the second part of that study, the results showed that untreated occlusal discrepancies affected the prognosis and accelerated the progression of periodontal disease.[45] In 2009, the same authors described multiple types of occlusal contacts associated with significantly deeper probing depths such as centric relation, posterior protrusive contacts, balancing contacts, combined working and balancing contacts, as well as the length of slide between centric relation and centric occlusion.[48]

BOX 6-1 Clinical and radiographic indicators of occlusal trauma proposed in 2018 by Fan and Caton[55]

- Fremitus
- Tooth mobility
- Occlusal discrepancies
- Wear facets
- Tooth migration
- Fractured tooth
- Thermal sensitivity
- Discomfort/pain on chewing
- Widened PDL space
- Cemental tear
- Root resorption

BRUXISM

In 1980, Budtz-Jørgensen examined **bruxism**-induced periodontal changes. For this investigation, bruxism was experimentally simulated in eight monkeys via occlusal **splint** insertion with simultaneous gingival inflammation.[49] The test side exhibited tight occlusion with the opposing arch, while the control side only exhibited slight occlusal contact. At the end of the study, greater tooth mobility was observed in the test side, although comparable probing depths and alveolar bone loss were seen in all studied teeth. Therefore, the author concluded that there was no association between bruxism and the progression of periodontal disease.[49] In a later publication, the same author reported a potential association between emotional stress and acute occlusal trauma.[50]

In 1981, Ramfjord and Ash pointed out that bruxism may cause primary and secondary occlusal trauma and therefore must be addressed in the prognosis and treatment of periodontitis.[51] Later on, in a human study, it was demonstrated that the occurrence of periodontitis and bruxism within the same individual is an uncommon clinical finding. In this sense, the study group exhibiting bruxism showed a higher frequency of **attrition** while the corresponding periodontitis group showed higher levels of tooth mobility, alveolar bone loss, and overall tooth loss.[52] In 2008, Tokiwa et al concluded that grinding associated with nocturnal bruxism may be a causative factor in the development of dental problems, including tooth mobility, attachment loss, hypersensitivity, and noncarious cervical lesions.[53]

Given the available evidence, occlusal discrepancies and bruxism may both be considered as potential contributors of improper force distribution. However, due to the diverse set of terminology and definitions employed, as well as the differences with regard to study designs, an association cannot be asserted.

Diagnostic Considerations

Occlusal trauma is defined as a histologic lesion; however, some clinical and radiographic indicators have demonstrated diagnostic merit. Clinical signs and symptoms include but are not limited to tooth mobility, **occlusal prematurity**, thermal sensitivity, wear facets, muscle tenderness, fractured teeth, and tooth migration. Additionally, radiographic indicators include thickened lamina dura, widened PDL space, furcation radiolucency, and root resorption.[40,41,51,54] It is important to bear in mind that some of these clinical and radiographic signs and symptoms may be multifactorial and/or indicative of alternative pathologic conditions. Hence, the diagnosis of occlusal trauma should be established based on a comprehensive evaluation of the dentition with clinical and radiographic examinations, rather than based on the mere presence of one of these indicators.

In order to help with the diagnosis of occlusal trauma, two different indices were proposed in 1992 by Jin and Cao: *(1)* the trauma from occlusion index, and *(2)* the adaptability index (ie, a thickened lamina dura and presence of pronounced tooth wear).[41]

SIGNS AND SYMPTOMS OF OCCLUSAL TRAUMA

In 2018, Fan and Caton proposed a series of clinical and radiographic indicators of occlusal trauma to be sought during routine practice (Box 6-1).[55]

Occlusal Trauma and Related Manifestations

OCCLUSAL TRAUMA AND GINGIVAL RECESSION

Stillman was one of the first investigators to suggest the role of traumatic occlusal forces in developing gingival recession. He described a possible association between occlusal trauma and the presence of **Stillman's clefts**, defined as a narrow, V-shaped gingival recession on the facial aspect of the tooth.[4,5] Later, in 1967, Gorman evaluated 4,453 teeth in 164 subjects and investigated the prevalence and incidence of gingival recession, trying to correlate them with various clinical factors. Results demonstrated a causal relationship between malalignment, toothbrush trauma, calculus, and inflammation with gingival recession. However, occlusal trauma was not reported as a significant factor for gingival recession.[56]

In 1977, Bernimoulin and Curilović evaluated the potential relationship between tooth mobility and bone dehiscences in 20 patients with gingival recession. However, the authors failed to identify any relationship between gingival recession or bone dehiscence and tooth mobility.[57] Previous studies are also in concordance with these findings, demonstrating that even in advanced cases of gingival recession, tooth mobility was recorded within normal values.[58,59] In 2004, Harrel and Nunn evaluated the potential role of occlusal discrepancies on changes in the amount of gingiva.[60] Patients were included under the following categories:

- Untreated (n = 30)
- Nonsurgical treatment only (n = 20)
- Both nonsurgical and surgical treatment (n = 41)

The authors failed to identify any significant relationship between initial occlusal discrepancies and initial gingival width, or between occlusal treatment and changes in gingival width.[60] Therefore, there is no solid evidence to support an association between traumatic occlusal forces and gingival recession.

TRAUMATIC OCCLUSAL FORCES AND ABFRACTION

Abfraction is defined as the hypothetical process leading to the loss of cervical tooth structure due to a combination of **abrasion**, **erosion**, and/or occlusal forces.[2]

Some studies in the 1970s demonstrated using finite element analysis that eccentric loads generate stresses that are concentrated in the cervical region.[61–68] Other studies using scanning electron microscopy considered traumatic occlusal forces responsible for angular and deep lesions at the cervical region.[69] Also, noncarious cervical lesions have been associated with bruxism,[70] wear facets,[71–73] occlusion,[74,75] and tensile stress caused by mastication and malocclusion as a primary etiologic factor.[76]

However, given the methodologic inability to detect a causal relationship, cross-sectional studies[77–80] and systematic reviews[81,82] do not provide an elaborate association between bruxism, occlusal factors, and noncarious cervical lesions. In addition, a split-mouth study found that abfraction lesions continued to increase in size regardless of the performance of occlusal adjustment.[83] As such, the association between noncarious cervical lesions and occlusion remains controversial. A plausible explanation for this could be the evident heterogeneity between studies or the differences in the diagnostic criteria for noncarious cervical lesions. On the other hand, a retrospective study found abfraction lesions to be four times more prevalent in patients with bruxism compared to nonbruxers.[84]

Therefore, there is insufficient evidence in support of an association between occlusion and abfraction; however, it can still be speculated to be a theoretic, biomechanically based phenomenon.[3]

Occlusal Trauma and Dental Implants

Some longitudinal studies have attributed the loss of dental implants to repeated episodes of occlusal overloading.[85–88] Similarly, cross-sectional studies associated the presence of wear facets with peri-implantitis,[89] as well as clinical signs of occlusal overload.[90]

Several studies performed in monkeys and employing nonaxial (lateral) traumatic forces supported an association between marginal bone loss and peri-implant disease. Likewise, authors demonstrated that under traumatic occlusal forces, implants could result in eventual loss of osseointegration due to the presence of a surrounding fibrous connective tissue capsule.[91,92] On the other hand, in the presence of peri-implant mucosal health, a dog study by Heitz-Mayfield et al demonstrated no loss of osseointegration or marginal bone loss following 8 months of excessive occlusal load, compared with nonloaded implants.[93] Similar results were reported when early and nonaxial traumatic occlusal forces were applied on implants restored with cantilever-design prostheses.[94] The outcomes were also similar when compared with axial loading.[95,96] However, an adaptive remodeling of the peri-implant bone was observed.[95]

In a series of monkey studies, Miyata et al reported that in healthy peri-implant tissue, no bone resorption was seen following an induced increase in occlusal height by 100 μm. However, when inflammation was present, notable bone resorption was observed around implants.[97] In the second phase of studies, authors explored the same research question with a greater degree of increased occlusal height. Results showed a tendency for bone resorption around implants when the superstructure was more than or equal to 180 μm higher.[98] The final study observed that once a peri-implantitis lesion is established, controlling occlusal and inflammatory factors is not enough to restore peri-implant health.[99]

In a series of dog studies performed by Gotfredsen et al, a lateral static load failed to induce peri-implant bone loss. Interestingly, implants under lateral static forces demonstrated greater bone-to-implant contact than nonloaded implants. This was true even in the presence of peri-implant mucositis or peri-implantitis.[100,101] Kozlovsky et al corroborated these results over a period of 12 weeks. The overload group showed enhanced osseointegration compared with the unloaded group.[102]

In conclusion, there is insufficient evidence to confidently consider occlusal overloading as a risk factor for peri-implantitis in osseointegrated implants[103] or as a precursor of peri-implant soft or hard tissue defects.[104]

Occlusal Treatment

According to the American Academy of Periodontology, the goal of occlusal trauma therapy is to alleviate the etiologic factors, enabling patients to maintain a comfortable and functional dentition. In order to achieve this goal, several therapeutic objectives were suggested[105]:

1. Elimination or reduction of tooth mobility
2. Establishment or maintenance of stable, reproducible intercuspal positions
3. Providing freedom of movement to and from the intercuspal position
4. Providing efficient masticatory function
5. Developing a comfortable occlusion
6. Establishment of an occlusion with acceptable phonation and esthetics
7. Elimination or modification of parafunctional habits

Some treatment modalities in patients with periodontitis and occlusal trauma may include one or more of the following[105]:

1. Occlusal adjustment
2. Management of parafunctional habits
3. Temporary, provisional, or long-term stabilization of mobile teeth with removable or fixed appliances
4. Orthodontic tooth movement
5. Occlusal reconstruction
6. Extraction of select teeth

In the absence of clinical signs or symptoms, occlusal adjustments provide little or no benefit to the patient.[105] As such, occlusal therapy could be beneficial in combination with periodontal treatment as long as clinical indicators of occlusal trauma are present, usually in terms of the patient's comfort and masticatory function.[55] However, there is no strong evidence to support the use of occlusal therapy in routine clinical practice, nor the use of splints in the treatment of occlusal trauma.

OCCLUSAL ADJUSTMENT

Occlusal adjustment is defined as an intentional mechanical reshaping of occluding tooth surfaces to obtain a more harmonious relationship between teeth, jaws, temporomandibular joint, and muscles of mastication.[2]

A randomized controlled trial in 1992 by Burgett et al observed minimal differences in terms of tooth mobility and probing depth between patients with or without occlusal adjustment in combination with periodontal therapy.[106] It is also important to remember that teeth with untreated occlusal discrepancies showed a greater increase in probing depth per year than teeth without initial occlusal discrepancies or teeth with treated occlusal discrepancies.[45] As such, the performance of occlusal adjustment should only be considered in the presence of occlusal discrepancies and/or occlusal trauma.

STABILIZATION OF TEETH

A **splint** is defined as any apparatus, appliance, or device employed to prevent motion or displacement of fractured or movable parts.[2] In the dental field, splinting has been indicated if the mobility disturbs the patient's masticatory function or chewing comfort. Nyman and Lang advocated a fixed splint of cross-arch design as splinting treatment.[107]

Several studies did not find clinical benefits when fixed splinting was used on teeth after initial therapy,[108] surgical periodontal therapy,[109] or before/after nonsurgical periodontal therapy.[110] However, another study reported a decrease in probing depth and clinical attachment gain when teeth were splinted prior to reconstructive surgery.[111] An experimental monkey model showed no force distribution across the splinted teeth when traumatic occlusal forces were applied[112] or an improvement in the mechanical properties of the PDL during healing.[113]

The use of a bite splint or nightguard has been suggested as an adjunctive treatment modality to manage parafunctional habits,[114] as it has been shown to improve the overall prognosis.[115–118] However, it is important to bear in mind that splinting itself does not eliminate the etiology of tooth mobility; once the splints are removed, mobility may resume.

Conclusion

There is strong evidence based on human and animal studies indicating that the presence of traumatic occlusal forces in teeth with a healthy periodontium does not produce periodontal tissue breakdown or loss of connective tissue attachment. However, traumatic occlusal forces could result in permanent or transient increased tooth mobility and alveolar bone loss. On the other hand, traumatic occlusal forces in teeth with periodontitis could increase the rate of the disease progression in some circumstances. Additionally, there is insufficient evidence to prove an association between occlusal trauma and gingival recession or abfraction.

References

1. Karolyi M. Beobachtungen über Pyorrhea Alveolaris. Österr ung Vierteljschrift f Zahnheilk 1901;17:279.
2. American Academy of Periodontology. Glossary of Periodontal Terms. American Academy of Periodontology, 2001.
3. Jepsen S, Caton JG, Albandar JM, et al. Periodontal manifestations of systemic diseases and developmental and acquired conditions: Consensus report of workgroup 3 of the 2017 World Workshop on the Classification of Periodontal and Peri-implant Diseases and Conditions. J Periodontol 2018;89(suppl 1):S237–S248.
4. Stillman PR. The management of pyorrhea. The Dental Cosmos 1917;59:405–414.
5. Stillman PR. Occlusion—The fundamental element in dental science. Int J Orthod Oral Surg Radiogra 1925;11:822–835.
6. Reinhardt RA, Pao YC, Krejci RF. Periodontal ligament stresses in the initiation of occlusal traumatism. J Periodontal Res 1984;19:238–246.
7. McCall JO. Traumatic occlusion. J Am Dent Assoc 1939;26:519–526.
8. Box HK. Experimental traumatogenic occlusion in sheep. Oral Health 1935;25:9–15.
9. Stones HH. An experimental investigation into the association of traumatic occlusion with parodontal disease: (Section of odontology). Proc Roy Soc Med 1938;31:479–495.
10. Orban B. Traumatic occlusion and gum inflammation. J Periodontol 1939;10:39–47.
11. Macapanpan LC, Weinmann JP. The influence of injury to the periodontal membrane on the spread of gingival inflammation. J Dent Res 1954;33:263–272.
12. Glickman I. Inflammation and trauma from occlusion, co-destructive factors in chronic periodontal disease. J Periodontol 1963;34:5–10.
13. Glickman I. Occlusion and the periodontium. J Dent Res 1967;46:53–59.
14. Waerhaug J. The angular bone defect and its relationship to trauma from occlusion and downgrowth of subgingival plaque. J Clin Periodontol 1979;6:61– 82.
15. Glickman I, Smulow JB. Effect of excessive occlusal forces upon the pathway of gingival inflammation in humans. J Periodontol 1965;36:141–147.
16. Posselt U, Emslie RD. Occlusal disharmonies and their effect on periodontal diseases. Int Dent J 1959;9:367–381.
17. Lovdal A, Schei O, Werhaug J, Arno A. Tooth mobility and alveolar bone resorption as a function of occlusal stress and oral hygiene. Acta Odontol Scand 1959;17:61–77.
18. Baer P, Kakehashi S, Littleton NW, White CL, Lieberman JE. Alveolar bone loss and occlusal wear. Periodontics 1963;29:91–98.
19. Polson AM, Kennedy JE, Zander HA. Trauma and progression of marginal periodontitis in squirrel monkeys. I. Co-destructive factors of periodontitis and thermally-produced injury. J Periodontal Res 1974;9:100–107.
20. Polson AM. Trauma and progression of marginal periodontitis in squirrel monkeys. II. Co-destructive factors of periodontitis and mechanically-produced injury. J Periodontal Res 1974;9:108–113.
21. Polson AM, Meitner SW, Zander HA. Trauma and progression of marginal periodontitis in squirrel monkeys. III. Adaption of interproximal alveolar bone to repetitive injury. J Periodontal Res 1976;11:279–289.

22. Polson AM, Meitner SW, Zander HA. Trauma and progression of marginal periodontitis in squirrel monkeys. IV. Reversibility of bone loss due to trauma alone and trauma superimposed upon periodontitis. J Periodontal Res 1976;11:290–298.
23. Polson AM, Zander HA. Effect of periodontal trauma upon intrabony pockets. J Periodontol 1983;54:586–591.
24. Kantor M, Polson AM, Zander HA. Alveolar bone regeneration after removal of inflammatory and traumatic factors. J Periodontol 1976;47:687–695.
25. Perrier M, Polson A. The effect of progressive and increasing tooth hypermobility on reduced but healthy periodontal supporting tissues. J Periodontol 1982;53:152–157.
26. Polson AM. The relative importance of plaque and occlusion in periodontal disease. J Clin Periodontol 1986;13:923–927.
27. Svanberg G, Lindhe J. Experimental tooth hypermobility in the dog. A methodological study. Odontol Revy 1973;24:269–282.
28. Lindhe J, Svanberg G. Influence of trauma from occlusion on progression of experimental periodontitis in the beagle dog. J Clin Periodontol 1974;1:3–14.
29. Svanberg G, Lindhe J. Vascular reactions in the periodontal ligament incident to trauma from occlusion. J Clin Periodontol 1974;1:58–69.
30. Lindhe J, Ericsson I. The influence of trauma from occlusion on reduced but healthy periodontal tissues in dogs. J Clin Periodontol 1976;3:110–122.
31. Ericsson I, Lindhe J. Effect of longstanding jiggling on experimental marginal periodontitis in the beagle dog. J Clin Periodontol 1982;9:497–503.
32. Ericsson I, Lindhe J. Lack of significance of increased tooth mobility in experimental periodontitis. J Periodontol 1984;55:447–452.
33. Polson AM, Adams RA, Zander HA. Osseous repair in the presence of active tooth hypermobility. J Clin Periodontol 1983;10:370–379.
34. Lindhe J, Ericsson I. The effect of elimination of jiggling forces on periodontally exposed teeth in the dog. J Periodontol 1982;53:562–567.
35. Glickman I, Smulow JB. The combined effects of inflammation and trauma from occlusion in periodontitis. Int Dent J 1969;19:393–407.
36. Gher ME. Non-surgical pocket therapy: Dental occlusion. Ann Periodontol 1996;1:567–580.
37. Wentz FM, Jarabak J, Orban B. Experimental occlusal trauma imitating cuspal interferences. J Periodontol 1958;29:117–127.
38. Rosling B, Nyman S, Lindhe J. The effect of systematic plaque control on bone regeneration in infrabony pockets. J Clin Periodontol 1976;3:38–53.
39. Fleszar TJ, Knowles JW, Morrison EC, Burgett FG, Nissle RR, Ramfjord SP. Tooth mobility and periodontal therapy. J Clin Periodontol 1980;7:495–505.
40. Pihlstrom BL, Anderson KA, Aeppli D, Schaffer EM. Association between signs of trauma from occlusion and periodontitis. J Periodontol 1986;57:1–6.
41. Jin LJ, Cao CF. Clinical diagnosis of trauma from occlusion and its relation with severity of periodontitis. J Clin Periodontol 1992;19:92–97.
42. Wang HL, Burgett FG, Shyr Y, Ramfjord S. The influence of molar furcation involvement and mobility on future clinical periodontal attachment loss. J Periodontol 1994;65:25–29.
43. Cortellini P, Tonetti MS, Lang NP, et al. The simplified papilla preservation flap in the regenerative treatment of deep intrabony defects: Clinical outcomes and postoperative morbidity. J Periodontol 2001;72:1702–1712.
44. Nunn ME, Harrel SK. The effect of occlusal discrepancies on periodontitis. I. Relationship of initial occlusal discrepancies to initial clinical parameters. J Periodontol 2001;72:485–494.
45. Harrel SK, Nunn ME. The effect of occlusal discrepancies on periodontitis. II. Relationship of occlusal treatment to the progression of periodontal disease. J Periodontol 2001;72:495–505.
46. Yuodelis RA, Mann WV Jr. The prevalence and possible role of nonworking contacts in periodontal disease. Periodontics 1965;3:219–223.
47. Shefter GJ, McFall WT Jr. Occlusal relations and periodontal status in human adults. J Periodontol 1984;55:368–374.
48. Harrel SK, Nunn ME. The association of occlusal contacts with the presence of increased periodontal probing depth. J Clin Periodontol 2009;36:1035–1042.
49. Budtz-Jørgensen E. Bruxism and trauma from occlusion. An experimental model in Macaca monkeys. J Clin Periodontol 1980;7:149–162.
50. Budtz-Jørgensen E. A 3-month study in monkeys of occlusal dysfunction and stress. Scand J Dent Res 1980;88:171–180.
51. Ramfjord SP, Ash MM Jr. Significance of occlusion in the etiology and treatment of early, moderate, and advanced periodontitis. J Periodontol 1981;52:511–517.
52. Hanamura H, Houston F, Rylander H, Carlsson GE, Haraldson T, Nyman S. Periodontal status and bruxism. A comparative study of patients with periodontal disease and occlusal parafunctions. J Periodontol 1987;58:173–176.
53. Tokiwa O, Park BK, Takezawa Y, Takahashi Y, Sasaguri K, Sato S. Relationship of tooth grinding pattern during sleep bruxism and dental status. Cranio 2008;26:287–293.
54. Hallmon WW. Occlusal trauma: Effect and impact on the periodontium. Ann Periodontol 1999;4:102–108.
55. Fan J, Caton JG. Occlusal trauma and excessive occlusal forces: Narrative review, case definitions, and diagnostic considerations. J Periodontol 2018;89(suppl 1):S214–S222.
56. Gorman WJ. Prevalence and etiology of gingival recession. J Periodontol 1967;38:316–322.
57. Bernimoulin J, Curilović Z. Gingival recession and tooth mobility. J Clin Periodontol 1977;4:107–114.
58. Mühlemann HR. 10 years of tooth-mobility measurements. J Periodontol 1960;31:110–122.
59. Mühlemann HR, Savdir S, Rateitschak KH. Tooth mobility—Its causes and significance. J Periodontol 1965;36:148–153.
60. Harrel SK, Nunn ME. The effect of occlusal discrepancies on gingival width. J Periodontol 2004;75:98–105.
61. Bowen RL, Rodriguez MS. Tensile strength and modulus of elasticity of tooth structure and several restorative materials. J Am Dent Assoc 1962;64:378–387.
62. Goel VK, Khera SC, Ralston JL, Chang KH. Stresses at the dentinoenamel junction of human teeth—A finite element investigation. J Prosthet Dent 1991;66:451–459.
63. McCoy G. On the longevity of teeth. J Oral Implantol 1983;11:248–267.
64. Powers JM, Craig RG, Ludema KC. Frictional behavior and surface failure of human enamel. J Dent Res 1973;52:1327–1331.
65. Rubin C, Krishnamurthy N, Capilouto E, Yi H. Stress analysis of the human tooth using a three-dimensional finite element model. J Dent Res 1983;62:82–86.
66. Selna LG, Shillingburg HT Jr, Kerr PA. Finite element analysis of dental structures—Axisymmetric and plane stress idealizations. J Biomed Mater Res 1975;9:237–252.
67. Thresher RW, Saito GE. The stress analysis of human teeth. J Biomech 1973;6:443–449.

68. Yettram AL, Wright KW, Pickard HM. Finite element stress analysis of the crowns of normal and restored teeth. J Dent Res 1976;55:1004–1011.
69. Brady JM, Woody RD. Scanning microscopy of cervical erosion. J Am Dent Assoc 1977;94:726–729.
70. McCoy G. The etiology of gingival erosion. J Oral Implantol 1982;10:361–362.
71. Kornfeld B. Preliminary report of clinical observations of cervical erosions, a suggested analysis of the cause and the treatment for its relief. Dent Items Interest 1932;54:905–909.
72. Pinto SC, Batitucci RG, Pinheiro MC, Zandim DL, Spin-Neto R, Sampaio JE. Effect of an acid diet allied to sonic toothbrushing on root dentin permeability: An in vitro study. Braz Dent J 2010;21:390–395.
73. Sauro S, Watson TF, Thompson I. Dentine desensitization induced by prophylactic and air-polishing procedures: An in vitro dentine permeability and confocal microscopy study. J Dent 2010;38:411–422.
74. Sawlani K, Lawson NC, Burgess JO, et al. Factors influencing the progression of noncarious cervical lesions: A 5-year prospective clinical evaluation. J Prosthet Dent 2016;115:571–577.
75. Telles D, Pegoraro LF, Pereira JC. Incidence of noncarious cervical lesions and their relation to the presence of wear facets. J Esthet Restor Dent 2006;18:178–183.
76. Lee WC, Eakle WS. Stress-induced cervical lesions: Review of advances in the past 10 years. J Prosthet Dent 1996;75:487–494.
77. Estafan A, Furnari PC, Goldstein G, Hittelman EL. In vivo correlation of noncarious cervical lesions and occlusal wear. J Prosthet Dent 2005;93:221–226.
78. Litonjua LA, Bush PJ, Andreana S, Tobias TS, Cohen RE. Effects of occlusal load on cervical lesions. J Oral Rehabil 2004;31:225–232.
79. Miller N, Penaud J, Ambrosini P, Bisson-Boutelliez C, Briançon S. Analysis of etiologic factors and periodontal conditions involved with 309 abfractions. J Clin Periodontol 2003;30:828–832.
80. Pegoraro LF, Scolaro JM, Conti PC, Telles D, Pegoraro TA. Noncarious cervical lesions in adults: Prevalence and occlusal aspects. J Am Dent Assoc 2005;136:1694–1700.
81. Senna P, Del Bel Cury A, Rösing C. Non-carious cervical lesions and occlusion: A systematic review of clinical studies. J Oral Rehabil 2012;39:450–462.
82. Silva AG, Martins CC, Zina LG, et al. The association between occlusal factors and noncarious cervical lesions: A systematic review. J Dent 2013;41:9–16.
83. Wood ID, Kassir AS, Brunton PA. Effect of lateral excursive movements on the progression of abfraction lesions. Oper Dent 2009;34:273–279.
84. Martinez-Canut P, Llobell A, Romero A. Predictors of long-term outcomes in patients undergoing periodontal maintenance. J Clin Periodontol 2017;44:620–631.
85. Adell R, Lekholm U, Rockler B, Brånemark PI. A 15-year study of osseointegrated implants in the treatment of the edentulous jaw. Int J Oral Surg 1981;10:387–416.
86. Jemt T, Lekholm U, Adell R. Osseointegrated implants in the treatment of partially edentulous patients: A preliminary study on 876 consecutively placed fixtures. Int J Oral Maxillofac Implants 1989;4:211–217.
87. Lindquist LW, Rockler B, Carlsson GE. Bone resorption around fixtures in edentulous patients treated with mandibular fixed tissue-integrated prostheses. J Prosthet Dent 1988;59:59–63.
88. Quirynen M, Naert I, van Steenberghe D. Fixture design and overload influence marginal bone loss and fixture success in the Brånemark system. Clin Oral Implants Res 1992;3:104–111.
89. Dalago HR, Schuldt Filho G, Rodrigues MA, Renvert S, Bianchini MA. Risk indicators for peri-implantitis. A cross-sectional study with 916 implants. Clin Oral Implants Res 2017;28:144–150.
90. Canullo L, Tallarico M, Radovanovic S, Delibasic B, Covani U, Rakic M. Distinguishing predictive profiles for patient-based risk assessment and diagnostics of plaque induced, surgically and prosthetically triggered peri-implantitis. Clin Oral Implants Res 2016;27:1243–1250.
91. Isidor F. Histological evaluation of peri-implant bone at implants subjected to occlusal overload or plaque accumulation. Clin Oral Implants Res 1997;8:1–9.
92. Isidor F. Loss of osseointegration caused by occlusal load of oral implants. A clinical and radiographic study in monkeys. Clin Oral Implants Res 1996;7:143–152.
93. Heitz-Mayfield LJ, Schmid B, Weigel C, et al. Does excessive occlusal load affect osseointegration? An experimental study in the dog. Clin Oral Implants Res 2004;15:259–268.
94. Lima L, Chambrone L, Arajo M, Pannuti CM, Lang NP. Early occlusal overload on SLActive implants restored with cantilever reconstructions. J Dent Res 2010;89:IADR-Abstract 139018.
95. Barbier L, Schepers E. Adaptive bone remodeling around oral implants under axial and nonaxial loading conditions in the dog mandible. Int J Oral Maxillofac Implants 1997;12:215–223.
96. Ogiso M, Tabata T, Kuo PT, Borgese D. A histologic comparison of the functional loading capacity of an occluded dense apatite implant and the natural dentition. J Prosthet Dent 1994;71:581–588.
97. Miyata T, Kobayashi Y, Araki H, Motomura Y, Shin K. The influence of controlled occlusal overload on peri-implant tissue: A histologic study in monkeys. Int J Oral Maxillofac Implants 1998;13:677–683.
98. Miyata T, Kobayashi Y, Araki H, Ohto T, Shin K. The influence of controlled occlusal overload on peri-implant tissue. Part 3: A histologic study in monkeys. Int J Oral Maxillofac Implants 2000;15:425–431.
99. Miyata T, Kobayashi Y, Araki H, Ohto T, Shin K. The influence of controlled occlusal overload on peri-implant tissue. Part 4: A histologic study in monkeys. Int J Oral Maxillofac Implants 2002;17:384–390.
100. Gotfredsen K, Berglundh T, Lindhe J. Bone reactions adjacent to titanium implants with different surface characteristics subjected to static load. A study in the dog (II). Clin Oral Implants Res 2001;12:196–201.
101. Gotfredsen K, Berglundh T, Lindhe J. Bone reactions at implants subjected to experimental peri-implantitis and static load. A study in the dog. J Clin Periodontol 2002;29:144–151.
102. Kozlovsky A, Tal H, Laufer BZ, et al. Impact of implant overloading on the peri-implant bone in inflamed and non-inflamed peri-implant mucosa. Clin Oral Implants Res 2007;18:601–610.
103. Schwarz F, Derks J, Monje A, Wang HL. Peri-implantitis. J Periodontol 2018;89(suppl 1):S267–S290.
104. Hämmerle CHF, Tarnow D. The etiology of hard- and soft-tissue deficiencies at dental implants: A narrative review. J Periodontol 2018;89(suppl 1):S291–S303.
105. Parameter on occlusal traumatism in patients with chronic periodontitis [editorial]. J Periodontol 2000;71(suppl 5S):873–875.
106. Burgett FG, Ramfjord SP, Nissle RR, Morrison EC, Charbeneau TD, Caffesse RG. A randomized trial of occlusal adjustment in the treatment of periodontitis patients. J Clin Periodontol 1992;19:381–387.
107. Nyman SR, Lang NP. Tooth mobility and the biological rationale for splinting teeth. Periodontol 2000 1994;4:15–22.
108. Kegel W, Selipsky H, Phillips C. The effect of splinting on tooth mobility. I. During initial therapy. J Clin Periodontol 1979;6:45–58.

109. Galler C, Selipsky H, Phillips C, Ammons WF Jr. The effect of splinting on tooth mobility. (2) After osseous surgery. J Clin Periodontol 1979;6:317–333.
110. Alkan A, Aykaç Y, Bostanci H. Does temporary splinting before non-surgical therapy eliminate scaling and root planing-induced trauma to the mobile teeth? J Oral Sci 2001;43:249–254.
111. Schulz A, Hilgers RD, Niedermeier W. The effect of splinting of teeth in combination with reconstructive periodontal surgery in humans. Clin Oral Investig 2000;4:98–105.
112. Glickman I, Stein RS, Smulow JB. The effect of increased functional forces upon the periodontium of splinted and non-splinted teeth. J Periodontol 1961;32:290–300.
113. Mandel U, Viidik A. Effect of splinting on the mechanical and histological properties of the healing periodontal ligament in the vervet monkey (*Cercopithecus aethiops*). Arch Oral Biol 1989;34:209–217.
114. Ramfjord SP, Ash MM. Reflections on the Michigan occlusal splint. J Oral Rehabil 1994;21:491–500.
115. Kreiner M, Betancor E, Clark GT. Occlusal stabilization appliances. Evidence of their efficacy. J Am Dent Assoc 2001;132:770–777.
116. McGuire MK, Nunn ME. Prognosis versus actual outcome. III. The effectiveness of clinical parameters in accurately predicting tooth survival. J Periodontol 1996;67:666–674.
117. McGuire MK, Nunn ME. Prognosis versus actual outcome. II. The effectiveness of clinical parameters in developing an accurate prognosis. J Periodontol 1996;67:658–665.
118. Türp JC, Komine F, Hugger A. Efficacy of stabilization splints for the management of patients with masticatory muscle pain: A qualitative systematic review. Clin Oral Investig 2004;8:179–195.

7

PROGNOSIS

Carlos Garaicoa-Pazmiño, DDS, MS

The prediction of disease progression and the anticipation of a specific therapeutic response remain as key elements of every health care profession. In periodontics, **prognosis** plays a key role in the decision-making process for establishing an appropriate treatment plan. This chapter covers different aspects of prognosis in periodontics, including definitions, endpoints, risk/contributing factors, and classification systems.

Endpoints of Prognosis Systems

TOOTH LOSS

Tooth mortality can be predicted based on the presence or absence of several local anatomical and/or contributing factors. Early epidemiologic and retrospective cohort studies evaluated the prevalence of tooth loss and identified risk factors for disease susceptibility (eg, individual teeth, maxilla vs mandible, patient age, and compliance with dental care).[4–7]

Interestingly, the positive correlation between patient age and tooth mortality was remarkably highlighted in two classic studies.[5,7] While Marshall-Day et al reported prevalence of tooth loss in different age groups, Bossert and Marks categorized groups based on the number of teeth affected by periodontal disease and confirmed the risk of age (< 35 years vs ≥ 35 years) with tooth loss (Table 7-1).[4,7,8]

TABLE 7-1 Grouping based on number of lost teeth

Authors	Grouping based on number of lost teeth

Bossert and Marks[7] (1956)	• 1–4 teeth
	• 5–8 teeth
	• 9–32 teeth
	  – 9–16 teeth (≥ one-fourth of dentition)
	  – 17–32 teeth (≥ one-half of dentition)

Hirschfeld and Wasserman[4] (1978), McFall[8] (1982)	• 0–3 teeth (well-maintained) • 4–9 teeth (downhill) • 10–23 teeth (extreme downhill)

DEFINITIONS AND TERMINOLOGY

Prognosis: A prediction as to the progress, course, and outcome of a disease.[1]

- **Diagnostic prognosis:** An evaluation of the course of the disease without treatment.[2]
- **Prosthetic prognosis:** A prediction for the prosthetic restoration after a successful (periodontal) treatment.[2]
- **Therapeutic prognosis:** A prediction of the therapy upon the course of a disease.[2]

Periodontal stability: The prediction of periodontal health after periodontal therapy, measured by a continuous evaluation of signs of inflammation, clinical attachment levels (CALs), and radiographic bone levels.[3]

TABLE 7-2 Tooth loss from two classic longitudinal studies

	Hirschfeld and Wasserman[4] (1978)		McFall[8] (1982)	
Group	Teeth lost	Population	Teeth lost	Population
Well-maintained	2.6%	83.6%	20.5%	77%
Downhill	22.7%	12.6%	35.1%	15%
Extreme downhill	55.4%	4.2%	44.4%	8%

TABLE 7-3 Annual tooth loss based on periodontal therapy rendered

Treatment rendered	Incidence of annual tooth loss (teeth/year)	
	Becker et al[9,12]	Costa et al[11]
Active and supportive periodontal therapy	0.11	0.12
Active periodontal therapy without maintenance	0.22	0.36
No periodontal therapy (active nor supportive)	0.36	NA

NA, not applicable.

A landmark study by Hirschfeld and Wasserman used a similar approach in 600 patients over a period of 22 years and investigated the impact of active and supportive periodontal therapy on tooth loss.[4] The overall rate for teeth lost among the study sample was 7.1%, equivalent to 0.08 teeth per year for each patient. Similarly, McFall repeated Hirschfeld and Wasserman's methodology limited to 100 patients with a follow-up time of 19 years.[8] The distribution of average tooth loss per patient was 0.68, 6.7, and 14.4 for the well-maintained, downhill, and extreme downhill groups, respectively (Table 7-2).[4,8]

Ultimately, a series of studies from Becker et al found a mean incidence for annual tooth loss of 0.11, 0.22, and 0.36 teeth, respectively, for the following groups: treatment and maintenance, treatment without maintenance, and no treatment.[9,10] Conversely, Costa et al reported annual tooth rates of 0.12 and 0.36 per year among regular and irregular compliers, respectively[11] (Table 7-3).[9,11,12]

Patterns of individual tooth loss

The pattern of disease susceptibility for individual teeth was explored among several studies.[4,7,8,13,14] The maxillary dentition is undoubtedly more susceptible to periodontal disease than the mandibular dentition due, at least in part, to the presence of more anatomical factors. A similar pattern was observed comparing posterior and anterior dentition—posterior teeth are more susceptible to disease progression for similar reasons. In this sense, maxillary second molars and mandibular canines are the most and least likely teeth to be lost due to periodontal disease, respectively (Table 7-4).[4]

Prediction of tooth loss vs therapeutic outcomes

Despite these prediction models established to aid clinicians in the decision-making process during treatment planning stages, control of oral hygiene and patient compliance have been proven to be key elements in long-term tooth survival after periodontal therapy. Chace and Low demonstrated that 455 questionable teeth treated with open-flap debridement were able to be retained for an average of 12.4 years (range: 6–40 years) if patient compliance was present and supportive therapy was provided.[15] As such, the anticipation of tooth loss might not be determined solely based on the presence of risk factors, but also taking into consideration the patient and operator's skills to achieve and maintain desirable outcomes after periodontal therapy.

PERIODONTAL STABILITY

Tooth loss–based prognostic systems often provide inconsistent results and showed to be unreliable over time. Therefore, Kwok and Caton denoted the importance of a prognostic system to be based on the intended outcome (periodontal stability), the timing of the projection (short or long term), and the consideration of individual versus

TABLE 7-4 Ranking of individual tooth loss according to Hirschfeld and Wasserman[4] (1978)

Tooth	Well-maintained (n = 292 teeth)	Downhill (n = 366 teeth)	Extreme downhill (n = 309 teeth)
Maxillary second molar	91 (31.1%)	62 (16.9%)	31 (10.0%)
Maxillary first molar	54 (18.4%)	60 (16.4%)	26 (8.4%)
Mandibular second molar	39 (13.3%)	44 (12.0%)	24 (7.8%)
Mandibular first molar	31 (10.6%)	24 (6.6%)	22 (7.1%)
Maxillary second premolar	17 (5.8%)	19 (5.2%)	25 (8.1%)
Mandibular central incisor	12 (4.1%)	31 (8.5%)	30 (9.7%)
Maxillary first premolar	12 (4.1%)	29 (7.9%)	25 (8.1%)
Mandibular second premolar	9 (3.1%)	11 (3.0%)	10 (3.2%)
Maxillary central incisor	8 (2.7%)	22 (6.0%)	30 (9.7%)
Maxillary lateral incisor	7 (2.4%)	24 (6.6%)	30 (9.7%)
Mandibular first premolar	6 (2.1%)	3 (0.8%)	9 (2.9%)
Mandibular lateral incisor	6 (2.1%)	16 (4.4%)	17 (5.5%)
Maxillary canine	0 (0%)	17 (4.6%)	25 (8.1%)
Mandibular canine	0 (0%)	4 (1.1%)	5 (1.6%)

overall prognosis to clarify patient management.[3] **Periodontal stability** can be defined as the prediction of periodontal health after periodontal therapy, measured by a continuous evaluation of signs of inflammation, clinical attachment levels (CALs), and radiographic bone levels.[3]

Determining Factors for Assigning Prognosis

The impact of most of the below-mentioned factors in the pathogenesis of periodontal diseases has been discussed in chapters 3 to 6. Their impact on periodontal disease is supported by different levels of evidence, including but not limited to longitudinal, cross-sectional, and cohort studies. However, the categorization of periodontal prognosis could also be empirical, subject to personal opinion and a clinician's experience. Different prognosis systems have employed very different methods for the creation of the classifications, ranging from opinion-based to different statistical methods after long follow-up periods (Box 7-1).[2,16]

BOX 7-1 Factors for individual vs overall tooth prognosis*

Individual tooth prognosis

- Percentage/distribution of bone loss
- Probing depths
- Presence/depth of furcation involvement
- Mobility
- Crown-to-root ratio
- Root morphology
- Developmental and/or acquired deformities
- Pulpal involvement
- Caries
- Tooth positions and occlusal relationship
- Strategic value
- Provider's knowledge and skills

Overall prognosis

- Age
- Systemic conditions (eg, diabetes)
- Behavioral conditions (eg, smoking)
- Individual tooth prognosis
- Rate of disease progression
- Compliance
- Economic considerations
- Provider's knowledge and skills
- Etiologic factors

*Adapted from Grant et al[2] and McGuire.[16]

Duration of Prognosis (Short- Versus Long-Term)

As reviewed by Kwok and Caton,[3] 5 years was determined arbitrarily by early studies as the threshold to describe short- versus long-term results after periodontal therapy.[4,8,17–19] Furthermore, this cutoff point was justified based on findings from McGuire and Nunn.[20] The 5- to 8-year prediction accuracy of McGuire and Nunn's prognosis system was revealed as 80% overall; however, it decreased to 50% or less when the "good" prognosis category was excluded. It is highly recommended to reassess prognosis at each patient examination during maintenance visits and periodic oral exams.

Classifications

All of the systems listed in Table 7-5 are prognostic classification systems described in the literature to aid clinicians in determining periodontal prognosis.[2–4,8,10,12–15,20–23] Nonetheless, McGuire and Nunn[20] and Kwok and Caton[3] remain as the most widely employed and accepted classifications.

TABLE 7-5 Available classification systems of prognosis

Authors	Categories and case criteria	Endpoint
Hirschfeld and Wasserman,[4] McFall[8]	• Favorable: NA • Questionable: FI, deep PD, extensive BL, Class II mobility or higher	Tooth loss
Becker et al,[12] Becker et al[10]	• Good: NA • Questionable (more than one of the following): – BL close to 50% of root length – 6–8-mm PD – Class II FI with minimal interradicular space or mesial FI of maxillary first premolar – Deep vertical palatal grooves on maxillary incisors – Nonrestorable tooth due to extensive caries • Hopeless (more than one of the following): – BL > 75% of root length – > 8 mm PD – Class III FI – Class III mobility – Poor C:R ratio – Root proximity with minimal interproximal bone – History of repeated periodontal abscess formation	Tooth loss
Grant et al[2]	• Excellent: NA • Very good: NA • Good: NA • Fair: NA • Guarded: NA • Poor: NA • Questionable (doubtful): NA • Hopeless: NA	Tooth loss
Chace and Low[15]	• Questionable: PD > 6 mm, > 0.5 mm of buccolingual mobility, conical root with poor C:R ratio, and Class II or higher FI	Tooth loss (molars only)

NA, not available; BL, bone loss; PD, probing depth; FI, furcation involvement; C:R ratio, crown-to-root ratio; CAL, clinical attachment level; GI, gingival index; PAI, periapical index; TFO, trauma from occlusion; BOP, bleeding on probing; LTO, long-term outcome.

TABLE 7-5 Available classification systems of prognosis *(cont)*

Authors	Categories and case criteria	Endpoint
McGuire and Nunn[20]	• Good (1 or more of the following): – Control of etiologic factors – Adequate periodontal support (clinical and radiographically) to ensure proper maintenance • Fair (1 or more of the following): – < 25% loss of CAL – Class I FI • Poor (1 or more of the following): – < 50% loss of CAL – Class II FI • Questionable (1 or more of the following): – ≥ 50% loss of CAL – Poor C:R ratio – Poor root morphology – Class III FI – Class II FI with difficult access – Class II mobility or greater – Significant root proximity • Hopeless: Inadequate CAL to maintain tooth. Extraction is suggested.	Tooth loss
Checchi et al[13]	• Good: < 50% BL or not fitting in the questionable or hopeless categories • Questionable: 50%–75% BL or presence of bone defect or FI • Hopeless: ≥ 75% BL or with at least two characteristics from the questionable category	Tooth loss
Kwok and Caton[3]	• General variables: Compliance, smoking, diabetes, immunologic dysfunctions, medications known to alter the periodontium, gene polymorphisms, nutrition, hormones, obesity, osteoporosis, alcohol • Local factors: PD, loss of CAL, plaque-retentive factors, TFO, parafunctional habits, mobility – Favorable: Periodontal treatment and maintenance will likely achieve health – Questionable: Periodontal treatment and maintenance may achieve health – Unfavorable: Periodontal treatment and maintenance will unlikely achieve health – Hopeless: Extraction is needed	Periodontal stability
Miller et al[22]	• Age: – < 40 years (score 0) – ≥ 40 years (score 1) • Probing depths: – < 5 mm (score 0) – 5–7 mm (score 1) – 8–10 mm (score 2) – > 10 mm (score 3) • Number of FI (per tooth): – 0 FI (score 0) – 1 FI (score 1) – 2 FI (score 2) – > 3 FI (score 3) – Mandibular through-and-through FI (score 3) • Mobility: – No mobility (score 0) – Class I (score 1) – Class II (score 2) – Class III (score 3) • Molar type: – Mandibular first or second molar (score 0) – Maxillary first molar (score 1) – Maxillary second molar (score 2) • Smoking status: – Nonsmoker (score 0) – Smoker (score 4)	Tooth loss (molars only)

NA, not available; BL, bone loss; PD, probing depth; FI, furcation involvement; C:R ratio, crown-to-root ratio; CAL, clinical attachment level; GI, gingival index; PAI, periapical index; TFO, trauma from occlusion; BOP, bleeding on probing; LTO, long-term outcome. ⟶

TABLE 7-5 Available classification systems of prognosis *(cont)*

Authors	Categories and case criteria	Endpoint
Nibali et al[14]	• Good: < 25% BL • Fair: – < 50% BL – > Class I FI – > Class I mobility – PD > 6 mm • Questionable: – ≥ 50% BL – > Class I FI – > Class I mobility – PD > 6 mm – PAI score 4 • Unfavorable: – ≥ 50% BL – PAI score 4 – Nonrestorable tooth – > Class II FI – > Class II mobility	Tooth loss
McGowan et al[21]	• Variables: – BL/age – PD – FI – Bone defect morphology – Mobility – Anatomical factors – Systemic/behavioral conditions (eg, diabetes, smoking) – BOP • Secure: Stability > 10 years • Doubtful: Stability > 5 years if patient-, tooth- and site-level factors are managed • Poor: Breakdown is expected within 5 years • Irrational to treat: No periodontal support remaining	Periodontal stability
Martinez-Canut and Llobell[23]	• Long-term outcome index • Variables: – Subgingival calculus – GI < 1.7 – Vertical/circumferential bone defects and/or FI – Mean recession > 1.5 mm – Abfractions – Smoking – Bruxism • LTO index 1: One variable • LTO index 2: Two variables • LTO index 3: Three variables • LTO index 4: Four variables • LTO index 5: Five or more variables	Tooth loss

NA, not available; BL, bone loss; PD, probing depth; FI, furcation involvement; C:R ratio, crown-to-root ratio; CAL, clinical attachment level; GI, gingival index; PAI, periapical index; TFO, trauma from occlusion; BOP, bleeding on probing; LTO, long-term outcome.

Miscellaneous

Multivariate analysis and logistic models have been developed to assess a patient's individual prognosis to predict risk for susceptibility or progression of periodontitis.

Lang and Tonetti proposed the periodontal risk assessment, a functional diagram based on percentage of bleeding on probing, prevalence of residual pockets greater than 4 mm, number of teeth lost, loss of periodontal support in relation to patient's age, systemic or genetic conditions, and environmental or behavioral factors (eg, smoking).[24] Each parameter has a scale serving to categorize low-, moderate-, and high-risk profiles. The authors acknowledged that all factors have to be evaluated simultaneously as no single parameter exhibits a predominant role.[24]

Faggion et al developed a multivariate prognostic model to estimate tooth survival after periodontal therapy using systemic conditions (eg, diabetes, coronary heart diseases, infectious diseases, allergies, coagulation disorders), probing depths, tooth mobility, tooth type, plaque index, sulcus bleeding index, alveolar bone level, pulp vitality, and frequency of supportive therapy.[25] It was concluded that this model was able to explain only 14% of variance in tooth loss among treated periodontal patients for 11.8 years but provided survival rate estimates of value during treatment planning.[25]

Lastly, Martinez-Canut et al constructed a multilevel analysis prediction model for tooth loss due to periodontal disease in 500 patients enrolled in 20 years of supportive periodontal therapy.[26] A combination of five patient-related factors (ie, age, severe periodontitis, heavy smoking, bruxism, and number of teeth at baseline) and six tooth-related factors (ie, tooth type, furcation involvement, probing depths, bone loss, mobility, and crown-to-root ratio) were analyzed to determine the usefulness and relevance of the prediction model. High specificity and moderate sensitivity were reported using different intervals of probability, predicting the tooth survival time close to 80% of the cases.[26]

References

1. American Academy of Periodontology. Glossary of Periodontal Terms. American Academy of Periodontology, 2001.
2. Grant DA, Stern IB, Listgarten MA, Orban BJ, Gottlieb B. Periodontics in the Tradition of Gottlieb and Orban, ed 6. St Louis: Mosby, 1988:573–591.
3. Kwok V, Caton JG. Commentary: Prognosis revisited: A system for assigning periodontal prognosis. J Periodontol 2007;78:2063–2071.
4. Hirschfeld L, Wasserman B. A long-term survey of tooth loss in 600 treated periodontal patients. J Periodontol 1978;49:225–237.
5. Marshall-Day CD, Stephens RG, Quigley LF Jr. Periodontal disease: Prevalence and incidence. J Periodontol 1955;26:185–203.
6. Oliver RC. Tooth loss with and without periodontal therapy. Periodontal Abstr 1969;17:8–9.
7. Bossert WA, Marks HH. Prevalence and characteristics of periodontal disease in 12,800 persons under periodic dental observation. J Am Dent Assoc 1956;52:429–442.
8. McFall WT Jr. Tooth loss in 100 treated patients with periodontal disease. A long-term study. J Periodontol 1982;53:539–549.
9. Becker W, Berg L, Becker BE. Untreated periodontal disease: A longitudinal study. J Periodontol 1979;50:234–244.
10. Becker W, Berg L, Becker BE. The long term evaluation of periodontal treatment and maintenance in 95 patients. Int J Periodontics Restorative Dent 1984;4:54–71.
11. Costa FO, Lages EJ, Cota LO, Lorentz TC, Soares RV, Cortelli JR. Tooth loss in individuals under periodontal maintenance therapy: 5-year prospective study. J Periodontal Res 2014;49:121–128.
12. Becker W, Becker BE, Berg LE. Periodontal treatment without maintenance. A retrospective study in 44 patients. J Periodontol 1984;55:505–509.
13. Checchi L, Montevecchi M, Gatto MR, Trombelli L. Retrospective study of tooth loss in 92 treated periodontal patients. J Clin Periodontol 2002;29:651–656.
14. Nibali L, Sun C, Akcalı A, Meng X, Tu YK, Donos N. A retrospective study on periodontal disease progression in private practice. J Clin Periodontol 2017;44:290–297.
15. Chace R Sr, Low SB. Survival characteristics of periodontally-involved teeth: A 40-year study. J Periodontol 1993;64:701–705.
16. McGuire MK. Prognosis versus actual outcome: A long-term survey of 100 treated periodontal patients under maintenance care. J Periodontol 1991;62:51–58.
17. Kaldahl WB, Kalkwarf KL, Patil KD, Molvar MP, Dyer JK. Long-term evaluation of periodontal therapy: I. Response to 4 therapeutic modalities. J Periodontol 1996;67:93–102.
18. Knowles JW, Burgett FG, Nissle RR, Shick RA, Morrison EC, Ramfjord SP. Results of periodontal treatment related to pocket depth and attachment level. Eight years. J Periodontol 1979;50:225–233.
19. Meador HL, Lane JJ, Suddick RP. The long-term effectiveness of periodontal therapy in a clinical practice. J Periodontol 1985;56:253–258.
20. McGuire MK, Nunn ME. Prognosis versus actual outcome. II. The effectiveness of clinical parameters in developing an accurate prognosis. J Periodontol 1996;67:658–665.
21. McGowan T, McGowan K, Ivanovski S. A novel evidence-based periodontal prognosis model. J Evid Based Dent Pract 2017;17:350–360.
22. Miller PD Jr, McEntire ML, Marlow NM, Gellin RG. An evidenced-based scoring index to determine the periodontal prognosis on molars. J Periodontol 2014;85:214–225.
23. Martinez-Canut P, Llobell A. A comprehensive approach to assigning periodontal prognosis. J Clin Periodontol 2018;45:431–439.
24. Lang NP, Tonetti MS. Periodontal risk assessment (PRA) for patients in supportive periodontal therapy (SPT). Oral Health Prev Dent 2003;1:7–16.
25. Faggion CM Jr, Petersilka G, Lange DE, Gerss J, Flemmig TF. Prognostic model for tooth survival in patients treated for periodontitis. J Clin Periodontol 2007;34:226–231.
26. Martinez-Canut P, Alcaraz J, Alcaraz J Jr, et al. Introduction of a prediction model to assigning periodontal prognosis based on survival time. J Clin Periodontol 2018;45:46–55.

8

TREATMENT PLANNING

Carlos Parra Carrasquer, DDS

DEFINITIONS AND TERMINOLOGY

Adjunctive treatment: Supplementary and additional therapeutic procedures. In periodontics, it generally refers to procedures other than scaling and root planing and surgical therapy, such as chemotherapy, occlusal therapy, and restorative care.[1]

Baseline data: 1. Measurements taken at the beginning of treatment with which subsequent measurements are compared. 2. In research, a known quantity or measurement with which subsequent data are compared.[1]

Clinical record: Information comprising a patient's medical and dental history, clinical findings, diagnosis, prognosis, plan of therapy, and progress of treatment.[1]

Treatment plan: The course of therapy and reassessments designed for a patient.[1]

Once an accurate diagnosis, etiology, and prognosis for a patient and/or specific site are established, the next step is to design a tailored treatment plan. Moreover, the ideal **treatment plan** should be comprehensive and consider not only the patient's remaining dental and local factors, but also systemic factors, accounting for environmental and acquired risk factors that the patient may have.

It is also possible that unforeseeable events may occur during treatment that will necessitate improvisation or modification of the initial treatment plan. With the exception of emergency therapy, it is prudent to mitigate all potential events that may arise using adequate consideration and careful planning on a case-by-case basis. Thus, treatment should not start until a carefully constructed treatment plan has been established.

Treatment Goals

The primary goal of periodontal therapy is to treat and correct any pathologic process related to the periodontal tissues. Specifically, the main aims of periodontal therapy are to eliminate gingival inflammation and to correct the conditions derived from it.

Risk factors such as nonmodifiable background factors (eg, age, sex, race/ethnicity, genetics) or environmental, acquired, and behavioral factors (eg, tobacco use, compliance, specific microbiota, diabetes mellitus, HIV, obesity, lifestyle, stress) should also be identified and addressed accordingly.

A comprehensive treatment plan should include short- and long-term goals to create a healthy and functional periodontal environment. The treatment strategy must establish the specific clinical outcome parameters to be reached after therapy:

- Reduction in bleeding on probing (BOP)
  - A full mouth mean BOP < 10%[2]
- Probing depth (PD) < 5 mm[3,4]

- Elimination of degree II and III furcation involvement on multirooted teeth
- Absence of pain

The chief complaint of the patient, esthetics, and long-term maintainability and durability of the treatment should be also considered. Therefore, the ideal treatment plan should establish a blueprint to achieve the best possible biologic, functional, and esthetic outcomes for each individual patient, while maintaining original structural characteristics to the greatest extent possible.

Sequence of Therapeutic Procedures

PRELIMINARY (EMERGENCY) OR SYSTEMIC PHASE

Systemic conditions should be evaluated and corrected as indicated, because they may influence the final outcome of the treatment. This should include tobacco cessation counseling, diet control recommendations, along with other systemic considerations that can be managed. In some circumstances, the presence of certain systemic conditions (eg, tuberculosis) may produce an environment in which dental providers may be exposed to infective agents carried by the patient. In order to alleviate this vulnerability, dental providers may consider referring to the patient's primary care physician or specialists as the need arises. Additionally, it is advisable to refer patients to their physicians in cases of uncontrolled or complex systemic diseases, or if the patient's medications must be updated prior to dental treatment.

The treatment of emergencies (eg, pain, acute infections) that should be performed promptly include but are not limited to dental, periapical, or periodontal pathology. In particular, these include endodontic treatment of infected or abscessed teeth, treatment of periodontal abscesses, treatment of necrotizing periodontal diseases if painful and acute, and extraction of hopeless teeth. In some cases, extraction of hopeless teeth may be postponed to a more convenient time.[5]

INITIAL THERAPY: DISEASE CONTROL (PHASE 1)

The initial phase encompasses the cause-related therapy. The main goal of this phase is to achieve a healthy periodontium by reducing or eliminating inflammation. This will be achieved by eliminating all of the etiologic and contributing or risk factors responsible for inflammation. A tentative treatment plan should be initially established that involves a dynamic series of steps to take place over multiple phases. Moreover, treatment planning should allow for reevaluation and be adjustable to meet the changing preferences, needs, and health conditions of the patient.

The treatment will start by instructing the patient on oral hygiene procedures and providing adequate motivation to perform optimal plaque control. This initial aspect should be reinforced at each subsequent appointment despite the sequence or phase the patient is at.

Furthermore, initial therapy includes removal of plaque and calculus and several other measures such as antimicrobial therapy (local or systemic); correction of defective restorations or carious lesions (provisional or definitive restorative treatment depending on prognosis of tooth and location of caries); and provisionalization if needed. Endodontic therapy, definitive or palliative, may also be completed during this phase, although in some specific cases this can be deferred to later phases of treatment. The chief complaint of the patient, if any, should always be considered and accommodated as soon as possible.

Although the initial phase is nonsurgical, it may necessitate extraction of hopeless, nonrestorable, or nonstrategic teeth, as well as biopsies.

Occlusion and parafunctional habits should be assessed and corrected if necessary by splinting, selective occlusal adjustment, minor orthodontic movement, and/or by use of a mouth guard (either temporary or definitive), depending on the future restorative treatment. It is important to bear in mind that orthodontic treatment is contraindicated until periodontal stability is achieved.

If not performed previously, referral to dental specialists should be completed during this phase. A restorative treatment plan should be formulated, including all interim and/or provisional restorations.

Reevaluation of phase 1 treatment should be carried out 4 to 8 weeks after scaling and root planing.[6] This includes reassessment of the results of initial therapy through a full periodontal examination and periodontal chart, including BOP and plaque scores, assessment of oral hygiene status,

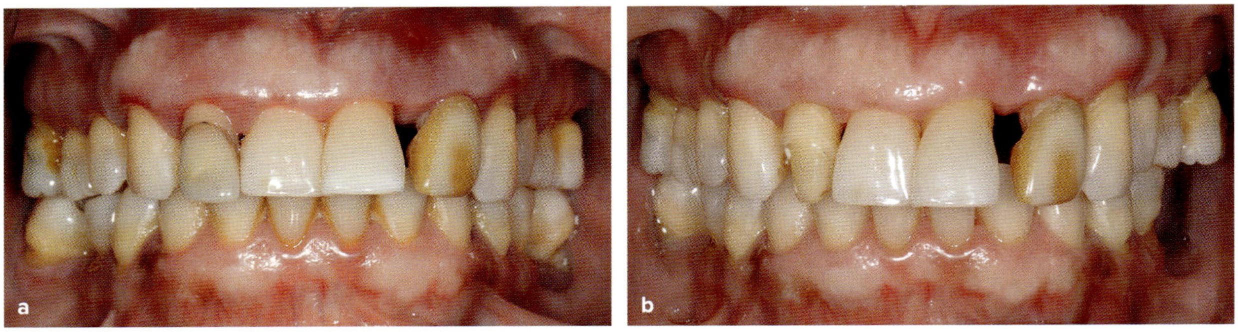

Fig 8-1 Before *(a)* and after *(b)* phase I therapy on a patient with generalized moderate to severe chronic periodontitis.

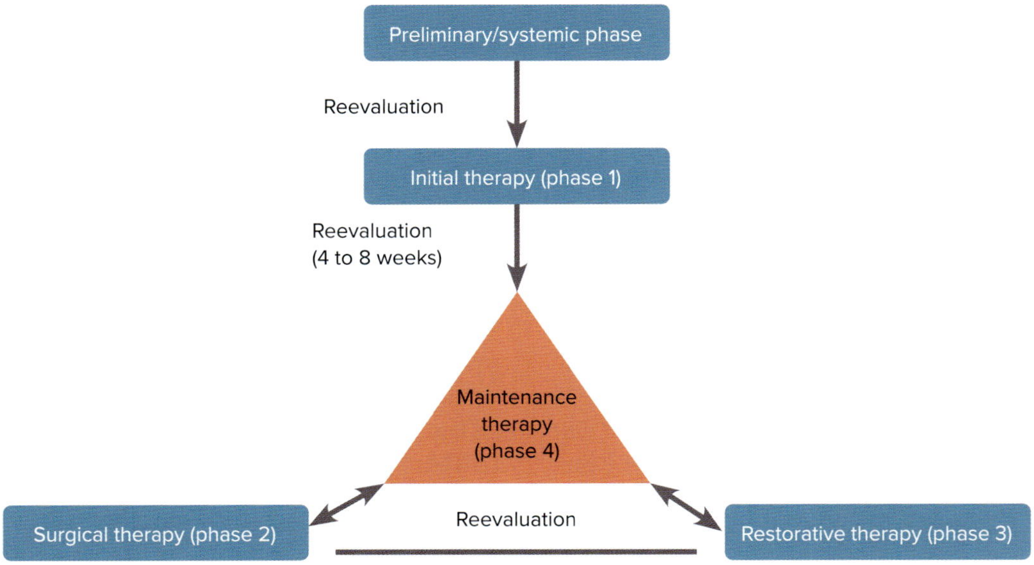

Fig 8-2 Sequence of periodontal phases of treatment.

and reinforcement of oral hygiene instructions and motivation. Additionally, a review of the original diagnosis and prognosis will be performed, as well as modification of the treatment plan if necessary. It is also appropriate at this stage to assess whether further periodontal treatment (either nonsurgical or surgical) is required (Fig 8-1).

At this point in the treatment, the patient should be enrolled in a supportive periodontal therapy (SPT) schedule (phase 4), and all further treatments should be combined with this therapy (Fig 8-2). The patient should not move into surgical therapy until their full-mouth bleeding score (FMBS) is ≤ 20%[7] and full-mouth plaque score (FMPS) is ≤ 20%.[8,9]

SURGICAL THERAPY (PHASE 2)

Periodontal surgery will be performed in this phase to correct or address the sequelae of the disease. This may include, but will not be limited to, the following: resective, regenerative, mucogingival, preprosthetic, preimplant, and/or implant surgeries.

Reevaluation of phase 2 treatment should be carried out at the end of this phase. Different surgical treatments will need different healing times. For example, while a gingivectomy may be reevaluated after 2 months,[10] the reevaluation time frame for a regenerative procedure may be after 6 months or more.[11,12]

RESTORATIVE THERAPY (PHASE 3)

The final restorative plan has to be determined after the evaluation of the cause-related therapy (including both phase 1 and phase 2 of therapy). The patient's ability, motivation, and willingness to collaborate in the whole therapy will determine which type of restorative treatment will be performed. If the patient is not ready for advanced

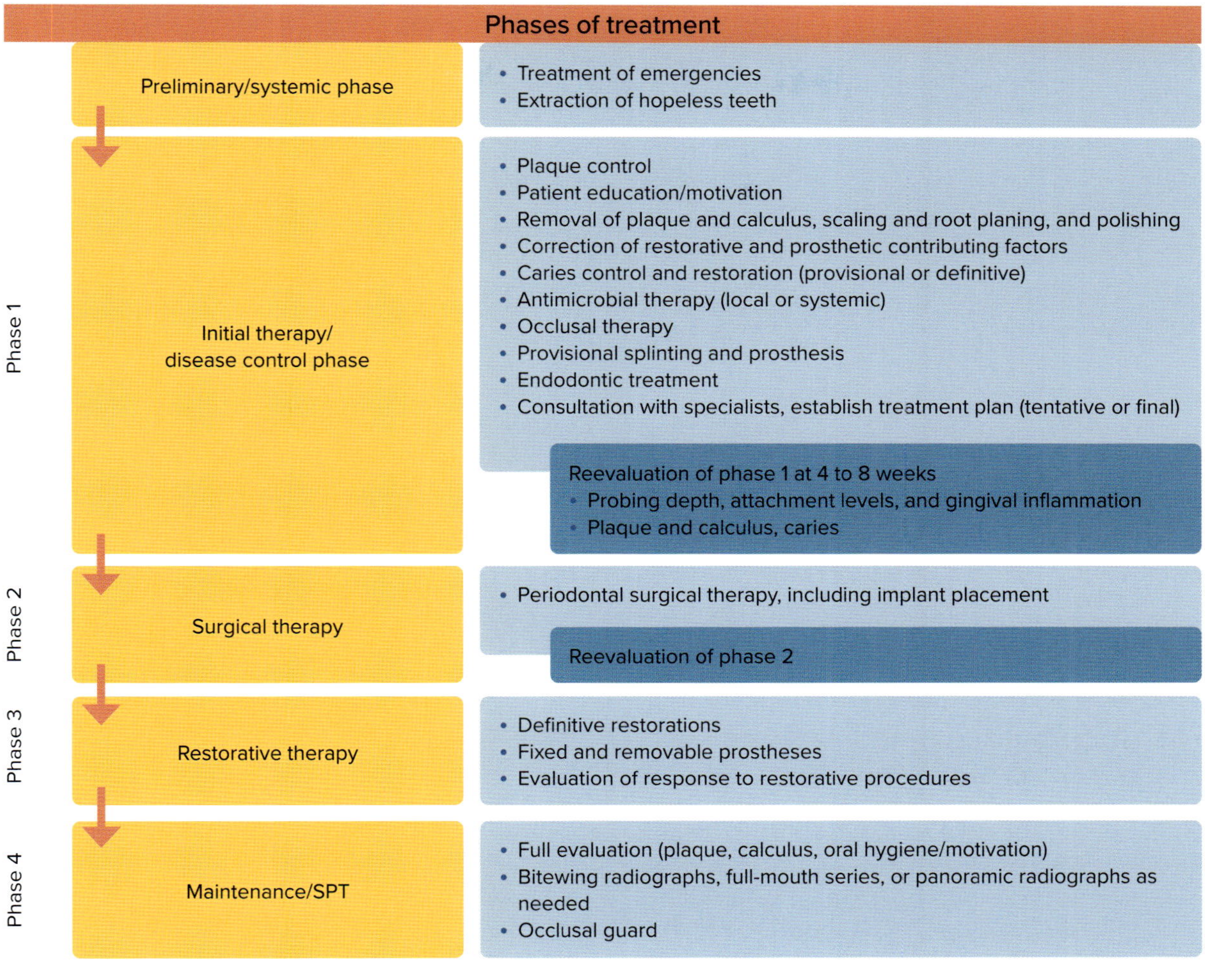

Fig 8-3 Phases of periodontal therapy.

prosthetic treatment because they are not willing to cooperate, they do not comply with maintenance appointments or do not have adequate oral hygiene, among other factors, it may not be advisable to proceed with final and/or complex prosthetic designs that could lead to future complications. This phase will include all fixed or removable prosthodontics and any other types of restorations.

MAINTENANCE PHASE: SPT (PHASE 4)

The main goal of SPT is to preserve the gingival and periodontal health achieved through active therapy, as well as to prevent future reinfection and disease recurrence. The recall interval should be customized for each patient. Each maintenance appointment should include the following steps:

- Create an updated periodontal chart including the periodontal pockets and BOP sites, and perform a cancer screening.
- Emphasize the importance of proper oral hygiene techniques, correcting if necessary, and motivate the patient to perform adequate oral hygiene.
- Debride the dentition and perform instrumentation of deeper sites.
- Polish and apply fluoride.

SPT should also include the evaluation of restorative, orthodontic, and/or endodontic therapies.[13,14] Radiographs may need to be incorporated into the SPT at regular intervals. Figure 8-3 summarizes the different phases of periodontal therapy.

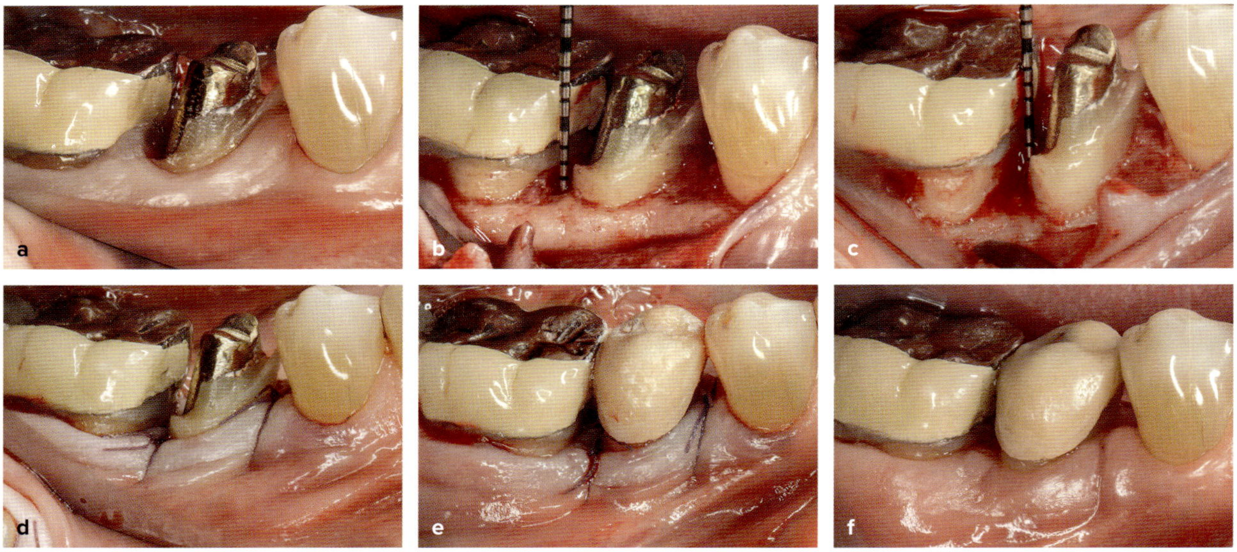

Fig 8-4 Crown-lengthening surgery. *(a)* Violation of supracrestal tissue attachment. *(b)* The osseous crest is 2 mm from the tooth margin. *(c)* Ostectomy and osteoplasty are performed to ensure adequate dimension for supracrestal attached tissue. *(d)* Sutures. *(e)* Provisional restoration. *(f)* Follow-up after 3 weeks.

Periodontal Considerations

RESTORATIVE DENTISTRY

There is a close nexus between periodontal and restorative treatments, and these two should align in harmony to achieve long-term satisfactory outcomes.

The first basic step prior to final restorative work will be achieving clinical health.[15] This will ensure the establishment of stable gingival margins prior to tooth preparation,[16] as well as tooth stabilization[17,18] or spontaneous repositioning of periodontally compromised teeth.[19–21] Preprosthetic periodontal surgery, such as preservation of the morphology of the ridge after extraction/alveolar ridge reconstruction, crown lengthening, and correction of mucogingival deformities, can be performed at this time.

Tooth preparation margins should ideally be placed supragingivally, or in specific cases intracrevicular,[22,23] always considering the supracrestal tissue attachment (formerly referred to as *biologic width*),[24–26] avoiding its violation.[27,28] In case of provisional restorations, it is important to ensure proper surface finish, crown contour, and marginal fit to maintain the health of the periodontal tissues and stability of the gingival margin[29,30] (Fig 8-4).

ENDODONTICS

The dental pulp and the periodontal tissues are in intimate communication. Consequently, severe periodontal disease may initiate or exacerbate inflammatory changes in the pulp. Conversely, persistent infection in the pulp may lead to secondary infection and breakdown of tissues in the periodontium. This mutuality of infection between periodontium and pulp is mediated through physical routes, allowing for communication between the two structures. Rotstein and Simon[31] described the three main avenues of pulp-to-periodontium communication: dentinal tubules, lateral and accessory canals, and apical foramen.

If there is evidence of pulpal pathology and associated periodontal bone loss, the first treatment to be performed should be the endodontic therapy. Next, the tooth should be reevaluated to determine if further periodontal therapy will be needed. Previous root canal treatment does not affect the healing response of deep intrabony defects treated with guided tissue regeneration. Additionally, guided tissue regeneration therapy in deep intrabony defects does not influence tooth vitality.[32] Pulpal infection will need to be addressed early in treatment, during the disease control phase, to avoid any further disease progression or aggravation of the lesion, as long as the tooth is restorable and included in the definitive treatment plan. Pulpectomy can be done in specific cases as a provisional treatment on teeth that will need to be extracted later in the treatment.

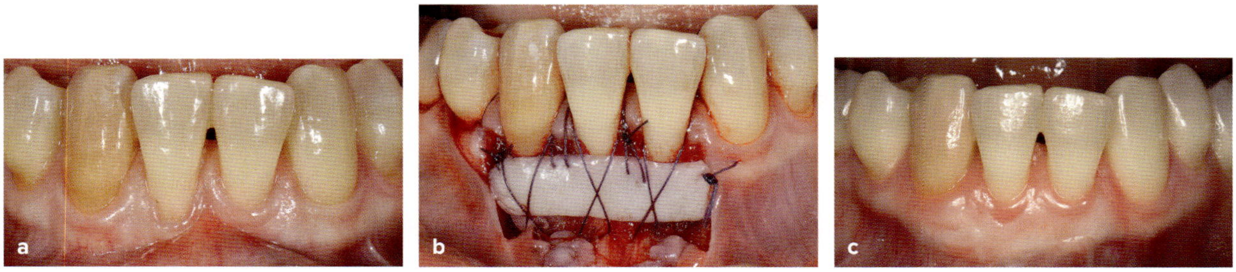

Fig 8-5 *(a)* Baseline situation after orthodontic treatment. There is a 2-mm recession, aberrant frenum, and no attached gingiva. *(b)* A free gingival graft is performed. *(c)* Clinical situation 18 months postoperatively. Note the amount of keratinized tissue and minimal recession.

ORTHODONTICS

Orthodontic treatment may be used in combination with periodontal therapy. It can be performed to correct any sequelae from periodontal disease (eg, tooth drifting, extrusion, black triangles, spacing, preprosthetic/preimplant treatment)[33] or to correct preexisting malocclusion. Orthodontic therapy should only start once adequate plaque control and periodontal stability have been achieved, as orthodontic treatment in periodontally diseased dentitions may contribute to further periodontal destruction.[34] Nevertheless, as long as the dentition is periodontally healthy/stable, teeth with preexisting bone loss may be displaced orthodontically without further attachment loss.[35–38]

Recession of the gingival margin may occur during orthodontic therapy,[39–41] but clinical studies have shown that even a narrow band of gingiva is capable of withstanding the stresses of orthodontic mechanics.[41] Additionally, the direction of the tooth movement is of relevance; while facial movements result in reduced facial gingival dimensions, an increase is seen in lingual tooth movements.[39]

Soft tissue augmentation procedures have been traditionally recommended prophylactically prior to orthodontic therapy in patients with a thin biotype, preexisting recession, minimal bands of keratinized tissue, or facial tooth movements.[42,43] Opposing this concept, some clinicians criticize this approach as an overtreatment and recommend waiting until the potential gingival recession appears. It can then be treated during or after orthodontic treatment (Fig 8-5). In the systematic review by Kloukos et al,[44] the authors concluded that no recommendations could be drawn on the best timing for soft tissue augmentation when a change in the inclination of the incisors is planned during orthodontic movement. Based on current evidence, orthodontic treatment is not contraindicated in patients with a previous history of periodontal tissue destruction. Tooth movement in patients with a reduced but healthy periodontium does not result in significant further loss of attachment.[35,37,45]

DENTAL IMPLANTS

Dental implants are currently the main alternative for partially and completely edentulous patients. If performed appropriately with adequate patient selection, longitudinal studies have shown high long-term survival and success rates.[46,47] Nevertheless, several risk factors/indicators are related to peri-implantitis, such as smoking, previous history of periodontal disease, genetic polymorphism, diabetes mellitus, inadequate oral hygiene, inadequate SPT, specific microbial biofilm composition or iatrogenesis (excessive cement, implant malposition, etc), among others.[48,49] Prior to implant placement, during the initial phases of treatment, those factors have to be adequately identified, communicated to the patient, and addressed as needed.

Implant placement has to be adequately planned early, and it should always be performed in a prosthetically driven approach once periodontal disease and associated inflammation have been treated and controlled. Otherwise, peri-implant bone loss and other biologic complications such as implant loss may occur.[50] A strict SPT is essential to prevent any possible biologic complications[51,52] (see chapter 23 for further considerations).

In conclusion, an adequate treatment plan should be established early, should be dynamic, and should have room for modifications or adjustments. Changes from the original plan are to be expected and should be accommodated as needed. A well-thought-out and well-designed treatment plan will minimize treatment complications or unforeseen events and will ensure durability of the treatment performed.

Case Presentation

Note: The Universal System for tooth numbering is used in the following case.

PATIENT INFORMATION

- Age: 53 years
- Race: Caucasian
- Sex: Female
- Height: 5'1"
- Weight: 123 lbs
- Body mass index: 23.24
- Blood pressure: 129/80 mmHg
- Pulse: 81 bpm
- Chief complaint: "I've been told I have periodontitis, and I want to have it fixed. I also want to have an implant."

MEDICAL HISTORY

- Past medical history
  - Three C-sections
  - Bowel obstruction while pregnant
- Current medical history
  - Osteoarthritis
- Medications
  - No prescription medications
  - Over-the-counter:
    - Fish oil
    - Omega-3 fatty acids
    - Multivitamins
- Allergies
  - No known drug allergies
- Family history
  - Noncontributory
- Social history
  - Former smoker: Quit 15 years ago. Smoked 1 pack/day for approximately 20 years (20 pack-year history)
  - Alcohol: 4 drinks/week (wine)
- Extra oral exam
  - Eyes: WNL
  - Skin: WNL
  - Lips: WNL
  - Temporomandibular joint: Absence of signs and symptoms of disease
  - Lymph nodes: WNL
  - Soft tissue profile: WNL
  - Smile line: High

(WNL, within normal limits.)

DENTAL HISTORY

- Past dental history
  - Last dental visit: 10 years ago
  - Last prophylaxis: 10 years ago
  - Previous periodontal therapy: No
  - Present tooth brushing habits:
    - Electric toothbrush at night and manual in the morning (1-0-1)
    - Floss approximately 4 times/week
    - No mouthwash
    - No interproximal brushes
- Tooth loss history:
  - Extraction of third molars when patient was in her 30s. Mandibular right second premolar was congenitally missing.
- Previous orthodontic therapy: No
- Habits: Not aware of any parafunctional habits. Never used a nightguard.

CLINICAL EXAMINATION

- Dental findings
  - Missing: Teeth 1, 16, 17, 29, 32
  - Decayed: None
  - Defective restorations: None
  - Wear facets: Generalized
  - Open contacts: Teeth 28 to 30
  - Crowding: Moderate in mandibular anterior sextant
  - Fremitus: None
  - Parafunctions habits: Possible bruxism
- Occlusal findings (Fig 8-6)
  - Angle classification: Right and left molar Class II
  - Incisal relationship:
    - Overbite: 3 mm
    - Overjet: 5 mm
  - Protrusion: Anterior guidance. No interferences.
  - Right laterality: Canine guidance. No interferences.
  - Left laterality: Canine guidance + 23. No interferences.
  - Crossbite: None
- Periodontal findings (Fig 8-7)
  - Mobility[53]:
    - Class I: All teeth
  - Plaque control:
    - Plaque score[54]: 75%

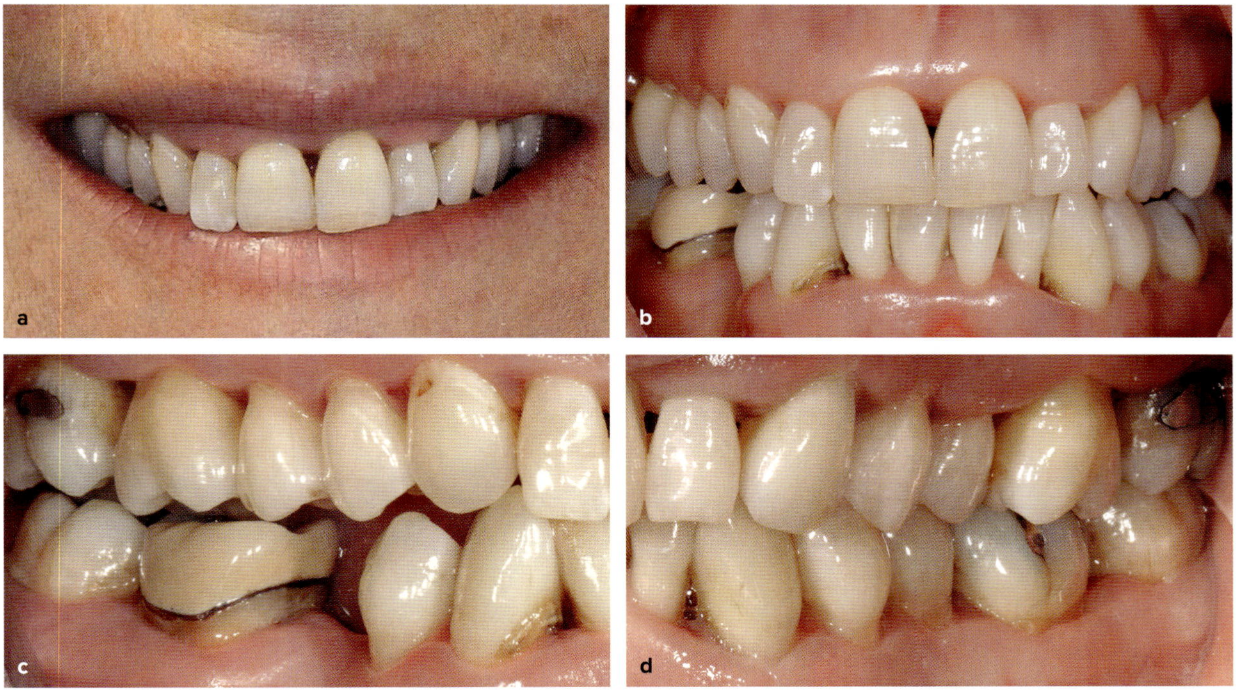

Fig 8-6 *(a)* Smile. *(b)* Frontal view at maximum intercuspation. *(c)* Right side view. *(d)* Left side view.

- Gingival Bleeding Index[55]: 90%
- Biotype: Thick
- Gingival appearance:
  - Color: Pale pink with localized red and dark red–purple areas
  - Size: Normal size with localized enlarged papillae
  - Shape: Edematous gingiva with areas of bulbous and flat papillae
  - Consistency: Firm gingiva with localized soft and edematous areas
  - Surface texture: Smooth shiny gingiva with generalized stippling
  - Gingival margin: Asymmetric gingival margins with generalized recession
- Gingival recession: Generalized
- Lack of keratinized tissue: None
- Probing depths:
  - 4 to 6 mm: Teeth 4, 5, 6, 7, 8, 9, 11, 12, 13, 15, 22, 23, 26, 27, 28
  - 7 to 9 mm: Teeth 2, 3, 10, 14, 19, 20, 21, 30, 31
  - ≥ 10 mm: Tooth 18
- Furcations[56]:
  - Degree I: Teeth 19 and 30
  - Degree II: Teeth 2, 3, 14, 15, 18, 31

- Radiographic findings (Fig 8-8)
  - Bone loss: Presence of generalized horizontal bone loss pattern with generalized absence of crestal lamina dura[3]
  - Furcation: Teeth 2, 3, 14, 15, 18, 19, 30, 31[57,58]
  - Sinus proximity: Maxillary molars in close proximity with maxillary sinuses
  - Calculus: Generalized presence of interproximal calculus
  - Funneling and periodontal ligament widening: Teeth 3, 9, 10, 14, 19, 30

AMERICAN SOCIETY OF ANESTHESIOLOGY (ASA) MEDICAL DIAGNOSIS

- ASA I

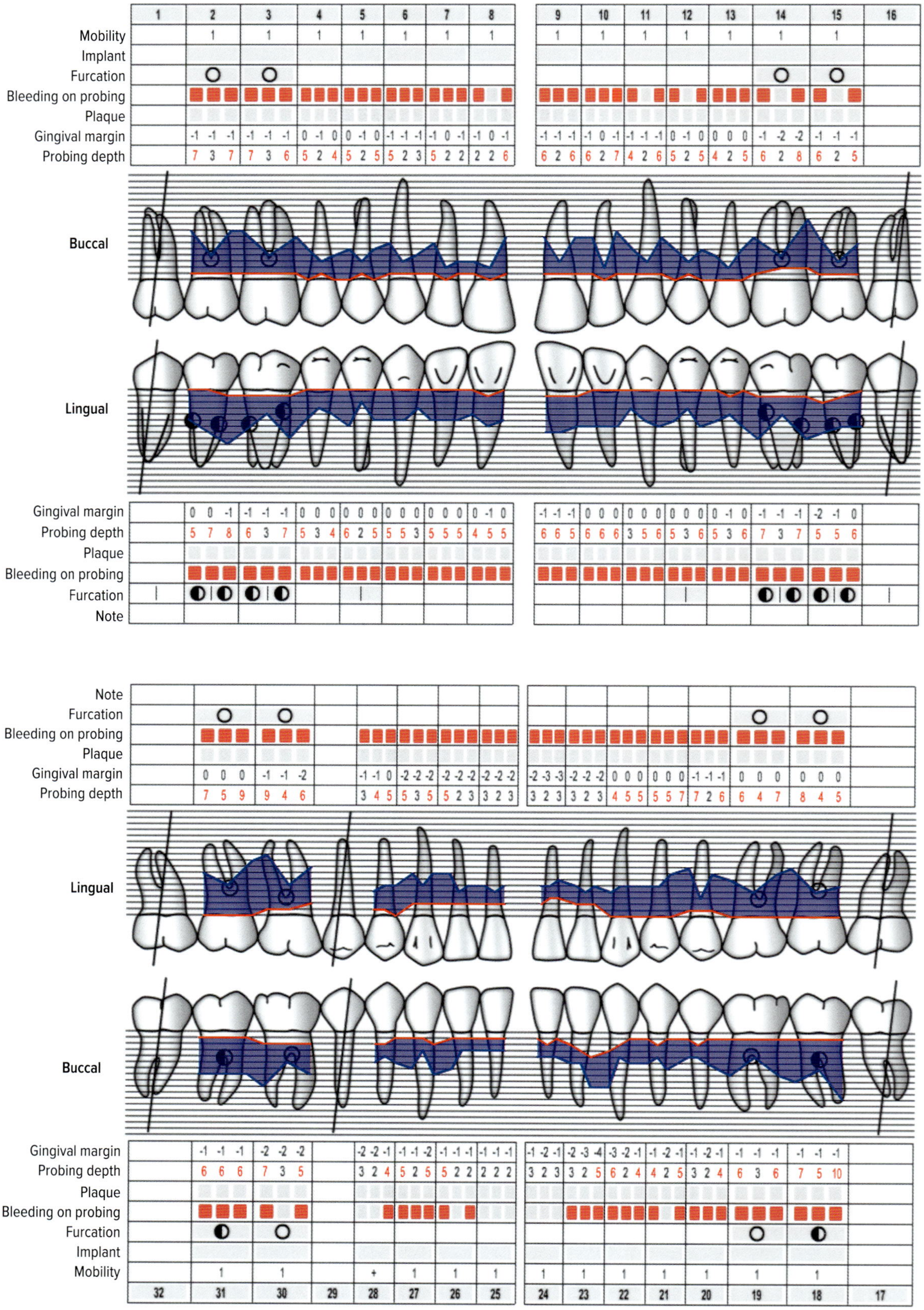

Fig 8-7 Periodontal chart.

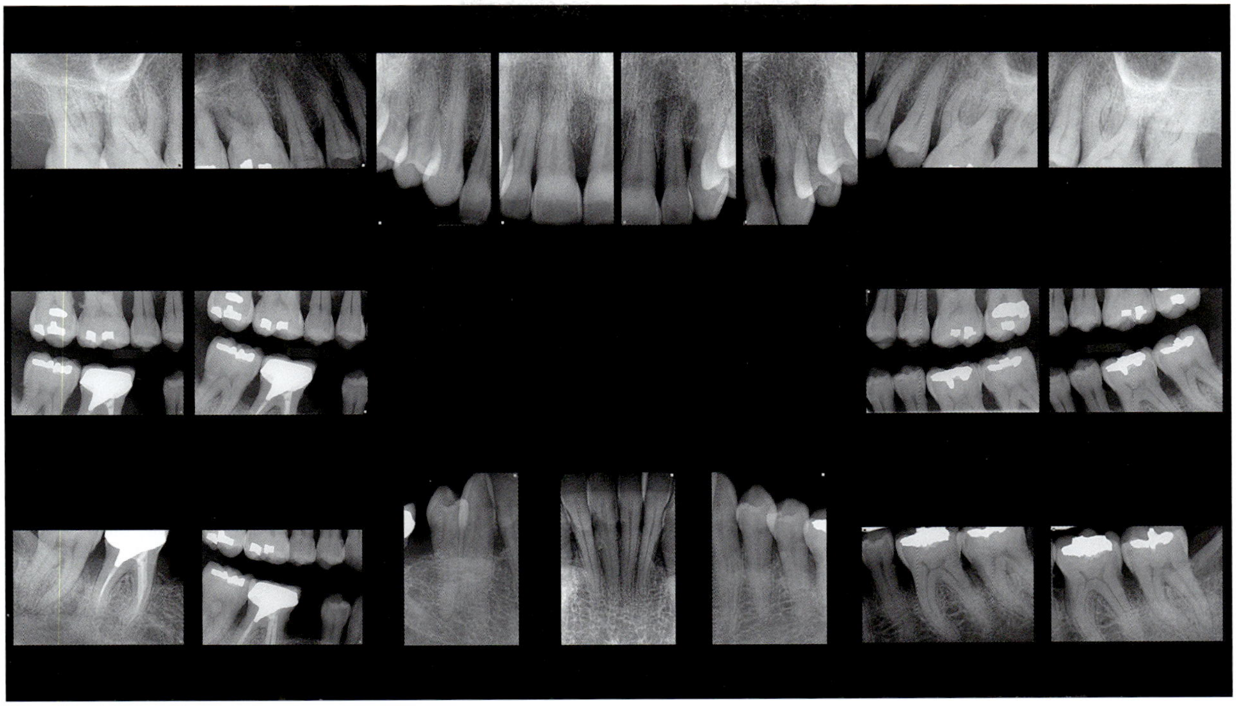

Fig 8-8 Full-mouth radiographic series.

PERIODONTAL DIAGNOSIS

- Based on Armitage[59]
  - Generalized severe chronic periodontitis
  - Developmental or acquired deformities and conditions around teeth
    - Mucogingival deformities and conditions around teeth
      - Soft tissue recession
    - Mucogingival deformities and conditions on edentulous ridges
      - Vertical and horizontal ridge deficiency
    - Occlusal trauma
      - Secondary occlusal trauma
- Based on the 2017 World Workshop on the Classification of Periodontal and Peri-implant Diseases and Conditions[60]
  - Stage III generalized periodontitis with a grade B progression (ie, severe periodontitis with a moderate rate of progression)
  - Mucogingival deformities and conditions around teeth
    - Gingival/soft tissue recession
    - Secondary occlusal trauma
  - Vertical and horizontal hard tissue deficiency
- Etiology
  - Bacterial plaque
- Contributing factors
  - Inadequate oral hygiene
  - Calculus
  - Former smoker
  - Parafunctional habits
  - Traumatic occlusal forces
  - Tooth malposition/malocclusion
  - Loss of attachment
  - Loss of teeth
  - Inflammation

PROGNOSIS

Based on McGuire[61]

- Short term (< 5 years)
  - Good: None
  - Fair: Teeth 4, 5, 6, 8, 9, 10, 11, 12, 13, 20, 21, 22, 24, 25, 26, 27, 28
  - Poor: Teeth 2, 3, 7, 14, 15, 18, 19, 23, 30, 31
  - Questionable: None
  - Hopeless: None
- Long term (> 5 years)
  - Good: None
  - Fair: Teeth 4, 5, 6, 8, 9, 10, 11, 12, 13, 20, 21, 22, 24, 25, 26, 27, 28

- Poor: Teeth 3, 7, 15, 18, 19, 23, 30, 31
- Questionable: Teeth 2 and 14
- Hopeless: None

Based on Kwok and Caton[62]

- Favorable: Teeth 4, 5, 6, 8, 9, 10, 11, 12, 13, 20, 21, 22, 24, 25, 26, 27, 28
- Questionable: Teeth 2, 3, 7, 14, 15, 18, 19, 23, 30, 31
- Unfavorable: None
- Hopeless: None

RECOMMENDED TREATMENT PLAN

- Preliminary/systemic phase
  - None
- Phase 1 therapy (initial)
  - Oral hygiene instructions (OHI)
  - Four quadrants of scaling and root planing and polishing
  - Interdisciplinary consults:
    - Orthodontics consultation to address malocclusion/crowding
    - Implant planning for site 29 (wax-up, radiographic guide, CBCT scan)
  - Occlusal adjustment if/when indicated for selected teeth
  - Reevaluation after 4 to 8 weeks
- Phase 2 therapy (surgical)
  - Four quadrants of periodontal osseous surgery (to be confirmed after reevaluation of phase 1)
  - Surgical placement of implant at site 29
  - Reevaluation of phase 2
- Phase 3 therapy (restorative)
  - Implant-supported crown at 29
- Phase 4 therapy (maintenance):
  - SPT every 3 months
  - Full periodontal evaluation every 12 months
  - New full-mouth radiograph series and panoramic radiograph every 3 to 5 years
  - Nightguard

References

1. American Academy of Periodontology. Glossary of Periodontal Terms. American Academy of Periodontology, 2001.
2. Trombelli L, Farina R, Silva CO, Tatakis DN. Plaque-induced gingivitis: Case definition and diagnostic considerations. J Clin Periodontol 2018;45(suppl 20):S44–S67.
3. Rams TE, Listgarten MA, Slots J. Radiographic alveolar bone morphology and progressive periodontitis. J Periodontol 2018;89:424–430.
4. Claffey N, Egelberg J. Clinical indicators of probing attachment loss following initial periodontal treatment in advanced periodontitis patients. J Clin Periodontol 1995;22:690–696.
5. Azouni KG, Tarakji B. The trimeric model: A new model of periodontal treatment planning. J Clin Diagn Res 2014;8(7):ZE17–ZE20.
6. Segelnick SL, Weinberg MA. Reevaluation of initial therapy: When is the appropriate time? J Periodontol 2006;77:1598–1601.
7. Joss A, Adler R, Lang NP. Bleeding on probing. A parameter for monitoring periodontal conditions in clinical practice. J Clin Periodontol 1994;21:402–408.
8. Cortellini P, Tonetti MS. Focus on intrabony defects: Guided tissue regeneration. Periodontol 2000 2000;22:104–132.
9. Lang NP, Tonetti MS. Periodontal diagnosis in treated periodontitis. Why, when and how to use clinical parameters. J Clin Periodontol 1996;23:240–250.
10. Hatakeyama Y, Uzel MI, Santana RB, Ruben MP. Relationship between position of probe tip and periodontal tissues after periodontal surgery in dogs. Int J Periodontics Restorative Dent 2005;25:247–255.
11. Becker W, Becker BE, Berg L, Prichard J, Caffesse R, Rosenberg E. New attachment after treatment with root isolation procedures: Report for treated Class III and Class II furcations and vertical osseous defects. Int J Periodontics Restorative Dent 1988;8(3):8–23.
12. Hall WB. Decision Making in Periodontology, ed 2. St Louis: Mosby, 1993.
13. Bergenholtz G, Nyman S. Endodontic complications following periodontal and prosthetic treatment of patients with advanced periodontal disease. J Periodontol 1984;55:63–68.
14. Lulic M, Brägger U, Lang NP, Zwahlen M, Salvi GE. Ante's (1926) law revisited: A systematic review on survival rates and complications of fixed dental prostheses (FDPs) on severely reduced periodontal tissue support. Clin Oral Implants Res 2007;18(suppl 3):63–72.
15. Corbet E, Smales R. Oral diagnosis and treatment planning: Part 6. Preventive and treatment planning for periodontal disease. Br Dent J 2012;213:277–284.
16. Lindhe J, Nyman S. Alterations of the position of the marginal soft tissue following periodontal surgery. J Clin Periodontol 1980;7:525–530.
17. Giargia M, Lindhe J. Tooth mobility and periodontal disease. J Clin Periodontol 1997;24:785–795.
18. Kerry GJ, Morrison EC, Ramfjord SP, et al. Effect of periodontal treatment on tooth mobility. J Periodontol 1982;53:635–638.
19. Brunsvold MA. Pathologic tooth migration. J Periodontol 2005;76:859–866.
20. Manor A, Kaffe I, Littner MM. "Spontaneous" repositioning of migrated teeth following periodontal surgery. J Clin Periodontol 1984;11:540–545.
21. Sato S, Ujiie H, Ito K. Spontaneous correction of pathologic tooth migration and reduced infrabony pockets following nonsurgical periodontal therapy: A case report. Int J Periodontics Restorative Dent 2004;24:456–461.
22. Kois JC. The restorative-periodontal interface: Biological parameters. Periodontol 2000 1996;11:29–38.
23. Nevins M, Skurow HM. The intracrevicular restorative margin, the biologic width, and the maintenance of the gingival margin. Int J Periodontics Restorative Dent 1984;4(3):30–49.

24. Jepsen S, Caton JG, Albandar JM, et al. Periodontal manifestations of systemic diseases and developmental and acquired conditions: Consensus report of workgroup 3 of the 2017 World Workshop on the Classification of Periodontal and Peri-implant Diseases and Conditions. J Periodontol 2018;89(suppl 1):S237–S248.
25. Gargiulo AW, Wentz FM, Orban B. Mitotic activity of human oral epithelium exposed to 30 per cent hydrogen peroxide. Oral Surg Oral Med Oral Pathol 1961;14:474–492.
26. Vacek JS, Gher ME, Assad DA, Richardson AC, Giambarresi LI. The dimensions of the human dentogingival junction. Int J Periodontics Restorative Dent 1994;14:154–165.
27. Ingber JS, Rose LF, Coslet JG. The "biologic width"—A concept in periodontics and restorative dentistry. Alpha Omegan 1977;70:62–65.
28. Maynard JG Jr, Wilson RD. Physiologic dimensions of the periodontium significant to the restorative dentist. J Periodontol 1979;50:170–174.
29. Amsterdam M, Fox L. Provisional splinting: Principles and techniques. Dent Clin North Am 1959;4:73–99.
30. Yuodelis RA, Faucher R. Provisional restorations: An integrated approach to periodontics and restorative dentistry. Dent Clin North Am 1980;24:285–303.
31. Rotstein I, Simon JH. Diagnosis, prognosis and decision-making in the treatment of combined periodontal-endodontic lesions. Periodontol 2000 2004;34:165–203.
32. Cortellini P, Tonetti MS. Evaluation of the effect of tooth vitality on regenerative outcomes in infrabony defects. J Clin Periodontol 2001;28:672–679.
33. Kokich VG. Esthetics: The orthodontic-periodontic restorative connection. Semin Orthod 1996;2:21–30.
34. Ericsson I, Thilander B, Lindhe J, Okamoto H. The effect of orthodontic tilting movements on the periodontal tissues of infected and non-infected dentitions in dogs. J Clin Periodontol 1977;4:278–293.
35. Boyd RL, Leggott PJ, Quinn RS, Eakle WS, Chambers D. Periodontal implications of orthodontic treatment in adults with reduced or normal periodontal tissues versus those of adolescents. Am J Orthod Dentofacial Orthop 1989;96:191–198.
36. Nelson PA, Artun J. Alveolar bone loss of maxillary anterior teeth in adult orthodontic patients. Am J Orthod Dentofacial Orthop 1997;111:328–334.
37. Polson AM, Reed BE. Long-term effect of orthodontic treatment on crestal alveolar bone levels. J Periodontol 1984;55:28–34.
38. Re S, Corrente G, Abundo R, Cardaropoli D. Orthodontic treatment in periodontally compromised patients: 12-year report. Int J Periodontics Restorative Dent 2000;20:31–39.
39. Andlin-Sobocki A, Bodin L. Dimensional alterations of the gingiva related to changes of facial/lingual tooth position in permanent anterior teeth of children. A 2-year longitudinal study. J Clin Periodontol 1993;20:219–224.
40. Joss-Vassalli I, Grebenstein C, Topouzelis N, Sculean A, Katsaros C. Orthodontic therapy and gingival recession: A systematic review. Orthod Craniofac Res 2010;13:127–141.
41. Maynard JG Jr, Ochsenbein C. Mucogingival problems, prevalence and therapy in children. J Periodontol 1975;46:543–552.
42. Coatoam GW, Behrents RG, Bissada NF. The width of keratinized gingiva during orthodontic treatment: Its significance and impact on periodontal status. J Periodontol 1981;52:307–313.
43. Maynard JG. The rationale for mucogingival therapy in the child and adolescent. Int J Periodontics Restorative Dent 1987;7:36–51.
44. Kloukos D, Eliades T, Sculean A, Katsaros C. Indication and timing of soft tissue augmentation at maxillary and mandibular incisors in orthodontic patients. A systematic review. Eur J Orthod 2014;36:442–449.
45. Polson A, Caton J, Polson AP, Nyman S, Novak J, Reed B. Periodontal response after tooth movement into intrabony defects. J Periodontol 1984;55:197–202.
46. Adell R, Eriksson B, Lekholm U, Brånemark PI, Jemt T. Long-term follow-up study of osseointegrated implants in the treatment of totally edentulous jaws. Int J Oral Maxillofac Implants 1990;5:347–359.
47. Simonis P, Dufour T, Tenenbaum H. Long-term implant survival and success: A 10–16-year follow-up of non-submerged dental implants. Clin Oral Implants Res 2010;21:772–777.
48. Renvert S, Quirynen M. Risk indicators for peri-implantitis. A narrative review. Clin Oral Implants Res 2015;26(suppl 11):15–44.
49. Stacchi C, Berton F, Perinetti G, et al. Risk factors for peri-implantitis: Effect of history of periodontal disease and smoking habits. A systematic review and meta-analysis. J Oral Maxillofac Res 2016;7(3):e3.
50. Roccuzzo M, De Angelis N, Bonino L, Aglietta M. Ten-year results of a three-arm prospective cohort study on implants in periodontally compromised patients. Part 1: Implant loss and radiographic bone loss. Clin Oral Implants Res 2010;21:490–496.
51. Roccuzzo M, Bonino F, Aglietta M, Dalmasso P. Ten-year results of a three arms prospective cohort study on implants in periodontally compromised patients. Part 2: Clinical results. Clin Oral Implants Res 2012;23:389–395.
52. Roccuzzo M, Bonino L, Dalmasso P, Aglietta M. Long-term results of a three arms prospective cohort study on implants in periodontally compromised patients: 10-year data around sandblasted and acid-etched (SLA) surface. Clin Oral Implants Res 2014;25:1105–1112.
53. Miller SC. Textbook of Periodontia, ed 3. Philadelphia: Blakiston, 1950.
54. O'Leary TJ, Drake RB, Naylor JE. The plaque control record. J Periodontol 1972;43:38.
55. Ainamo J, Bay I. Periodontal indexes for and in practice [in Danish]. Tandlaegebladet 1976;80:149–152.
56. Hamp SE, Nyman S, Lindhe J. Periodontal treatment of multirooted teeth. Results after 5 years. J Clin Periodontol 1975;2:126–135.
57. Hardekopf JD, Dunlap RM, Ahl DR, Pelleu GB Jr. The "furcation arrow." A reliable radiographic image? J Periodontol 1987;58:258–261.
58. Deas DE, Moritz AJ, Mealey BL, McDonnell HT, Powell CA. Clinical reliability of the "furcation arrow" as a diagnostic marker. J Periodontol 2006;77:1436–1441.
59. Armitage GC. Development of a classification system for periodontal diseases and conditions. Ann Periodontol 1999;4:1–6.
60. Caton JG, Armitage G, Berglundh T, et al. A new classification scheme for periodontal and peri-implant diseases and conditions—Introduction and key changes from the 1999 classification. J Periodontol 2018;89(suppl 1):S1–S8.
61. McGuire MK. Prognosis versus actual outcome: A long-term survey of 100 treated periodontal patients under maintenance care. J Periodontol 1991;62:51–58.
62. Kwok V, Caton JG. Commentary: Prognosis revisited: A system for assigning periodontal prognosis. J Periodontol 2007;78:2063–2071.

9

NONSURGICAL THERAPY

Federico Ausenda, DDS, MS

DEFINITIONS AND TERMINOLOGY

Laser: Acronym for "light amplification by stimulated emission of radiation." A device that transforms light of various set frequencies into an extremely intense, small, and nearly nondivergent beam of monochromatic radiation in the visible region with all the waves in-phase. Capable of mobilizing immense heat and power when focused at close range, it is used as a tool in surgical procedures, diagnosis, and physiologic studies.[2]

Root planing: A treatment procedure designed to remove cementum or surface dentin that is rough, impregnated with calculus, or contaminated with toxins or microorganisms.[3]

Scaler: An instrument for removing calculus or other deposits from the surfaces of teeth.[2]

Scaling: Instrumentation of the crown and root of the teeth to remove plaque, calculus, and stains from these surfaces.[3]

It is estimated that 46% of U.S. adults, representing 64.7 million people, have periodontitis.[1] Nonsurgical therapy is the first step of periodontal treatment and therefore is one of the most commonly performed procedures. Aims of nonsurgical periodontal therapy include eliminating or reducing inflammation of the gingival tissues through the removal of calculus, biofilm, and endotoxins that are present on the crown and root surfaces.[2] It consists of oral hygiene instructions (OHI), supra- and subgingival **scaling** and **root planing** (SRP), use of chemicals and antibiotics, extraction of hopeless teeth, correction of defective restorations, and occlusal adjustment.

Oral Hygiene Instructions and Devices

In the prevention and treatment of periodontitis, professional instrumentation is of little value if performed without proper OHI.[4] There is no clear evidence to identify which brushing technique is the most effective; however, the Bass[5] method seems to be the most appropriate in the prevention of gingival inflammation because positioning the brush at a 45-degree angle allows the bristle tips to penetrate subgingivally.

The use of an electric toothbrush provides a significant benefit compared to a manual toothbrush according to a meta-analysis by Yaacob et al.[6] This study found a plaque reduction according to the Quigley Hein Index (Turesky) of 11% in the short term and 21% in the long term. This pattern is also consistent with a reduction in gingivitis for the Löe and Silness Index of 6% in the short term and 11% in the long term.

The use of interproximal devices as an adjunct to tooth brushing has also been investigated. A review by Sälzer et al[7] found moderate evidence that interproximal devices in combination with tooth brushing reduce plaque and gingivitis, but found low evidence of the effectiveness of floss in plaque removal. A network meta-analysis by Kotsakis et al[8] evaluated different interproximal devices and found interdental brushes and water jets to be the most effective devices for reducing gingival bleeding, while toothpicks and floss were the least effective methods.

TABLE 9-1 Characteristics of different mechanical instruments

	Sonic	Ultrasonic	
		Magnetostrictive	Piezoelectric
Power	Compressed air	Electricity	Electricity
Vibration frequency	2–8 KHz	20–50 KHz	20–50 KHz
Stroke pattern	Elliptic/circular	Elliptic/circular	Linear
Working surfaces	4	4	2

Instruments

MANUAL, SONIC, AND ULTRASONIC

Nonsurgical therapy is performed with both manual (eg, Gracey curettes, chisels, hoe **scalers**, sickle scalers, Hirschfeld file scalers, and mini curettes) and mechanical instruments. There is not clear evidence to claim one instrument over another as superior in terms of treatment outcomes.[4,9,10] Similarly, manual and ultrasonic instruments are equally efficient in the removal of biofilm, calculus, and endotoxins,[11,12] so they are often used together in clinical practice. The different types of mechanical instruments are summarized in Table 9-1.

Both curettes and ultrasonic instruments have improved in recent decades. Classic investigations by Kerry[13] and Nishmine and O'Leary[14] were in favor of manual instrumentation, finding that root surfaces were smoother after hand instrumentation than instrumentation with ultrasonic devices. Also, hand instruments were able to remove eight times more endotoxins than ultrasonic instruments. On the other hand, Gellin et al[15] compared sonic scalers with curettes and found them equally effective when used alone; however, the combination of hand and mechanical instruments was the most effective modality for calculus removal. In the instrumentation of furcations, ultrasonic tips have been considered more effective than manual curettes.[16]

A systematic review by the Hallmon and Rees[17] in 2003 reported the findings of 9 studies with a total of 129 subjects. This investigation concluded that manual and mechanical instrumentation are comparable in affecting clinical parameters. Also, instrumentation time was comparable, and the adjunct use of subgingival irrigants resulted in similar outcomes.

Removal of Contaminated Cementum

It was initially thought[18] that removal of contaminated cementum was necessary in order to achieve satisfactory outcomes after performing SRP. However, in a clinical trial comparing roots that were aggressively planed and others that received only calculus debridement, Mombelli et al[19] showed that 1 year after therapy, the improvements observed for both test and control groups were similar. It was also demonstrated that the reduction of select gram-negative microorganisms was more important than the removal of contaminated cementum. Similarly, in 1988, Nyman et al[20] demonstrated that the intentional excessive removal of cementum is unnecessary to achieve health.

Adjunctive Therapy

IRRIGATION

A position paper by the American Academy of Periodontology[21] found that there is insufficient evidence to support the use of subgingival irrigation as monotherapy. There may be a benefit if used over multiple appointments; however, substantivity remains as the major challenge. The use of subgingival irrigation as an adjunct to SRP is also controversial; there is insufficient evidence to support its use even with some studies showing a synergistic effect with minimal improvements.

ANTIBIOTICS

Systemic antimicrobials against the subgingival biofilm should not be delivered as monotherapy. They should be used as an adjunct to mechanical debridement, and administration should start the day of debridement completion.[22]

Haffaje et al[23] in a systematic review found that adjunctive use of systemic antibiotics leads to greater clinical attachment gain. The greatest improvements were seen when treating aggressive periodontitis; however, no specific antibiotic was clearly shown as superior. The selection of the type of antibiotic must be performed on a case-by-case basis.

With regard to locally delivered antibiotics, similar conclusions were found in another systematic review by Hanes and Purvis.[24] This study showed greater clinical attachment gain and reduction in probing depths (PDs) with minocycline gel, chlorhexidine chips, and doxycycline gel in conjunction with SRP compared to SRP alone.

LASERS

The use of different types of **lasers** (eg, argon, carbon dioxide, diode, Nd:YAG, Er:YAG) in nonsurgical therapy has also been investigated, although the clinical benefits remain controversial. A statement by the American Academy of Periodontology[25] indicates that there is minimal evidence to support the use of a laser for the purpose of subgingival debridement, either as a monotherapy or adjunctive to SRP. There is also conflicting evidence to support that lasers as a group can reduce subgingival microbial loads beyond what can be achieved by SRP alone. Slot et al[26] examined the evidence on the effect of diode lasers in nonsurgical therapy and found that there was a significant difference in gingival index and bleeding score when the diode laser was used as an adjunct to SRP. However, the adjunctive use of the diode laser with SRP had an effect comparable with that of SRP alone. Zhao et al[27] in a systematic review and meta-analysis on the use of the Er:YAG laser as an alternative or in conjunction with SRP found that the Er:YAG laser led to a significantly greater short-term reduction in PD compared with SRP alone. However, the clinical efficacy of Er:YAG was similar to that of SRP alone after 3 months.

PHOTODYNAMIC THERAPY

Photodynamic therapy (PDT) consists of the use of low-power lasers at adequate wavelengths that use a dye to generate free radicals that can eliminate bacteria. Bassir et al[28] conducted a clinical trial investigating the effects of PDT at different wavelengths in 16 patients with moderate to severe chronic periodontitis. Results demonstrated an improvement for all clinical parameters at 1 and 3 months. However, there was no additional benefit in clinical parameters for sites treated with PDT compared with those that received only SRP. Similarly, in a randomized controlled trial (RCT) comparing 20 healthy control patients and 40 periodontitis patients treated with SRP or with SRP + PDT, Segarra-Vidal et al[29] found that in patients with moderate to severe chronic periodontitis, the additional use of PDT leads only to a significantly greater reduction of *Aggregatibacter actinomycetemcomitans* and no other additional improvement compared with SRP alone.

POWDERS

Several air polishing devices have been employed in the attempt to remove biofilm from the root surfaces. The mechanism of action is based on the ability of the jet of air, water, and powder, made of microscopic solid particles of different diameters (sodium bicarbonate, glycine powder, erythritol), to hit the root, causing biofilm removal and leaving a smoother surface.[30]

Wennström et al[31] conducted a split-mouth study on 20 patients with PDs of 5 to 8 mm. Two quadrants were treated with SRP alone and two with SRP and air polishing with glycine powder. Both treatments resulted in improvements in bleeding on probing (BOP), PD, and clinical attachment level (CAL), but there were no additional benefits from air polishing at 2 months. Flemming et al[32] also investigated the efficacy and safety of glycine powder air polishing in moderate to deep pockets in 30 patients. It was found that the subgingival adjunctive use of glycine powder air polish led to significantly lower total bacterial counts at 10 days and lower total *Porphyromonas gingivalis* count at 90 days compared with SRP alone.

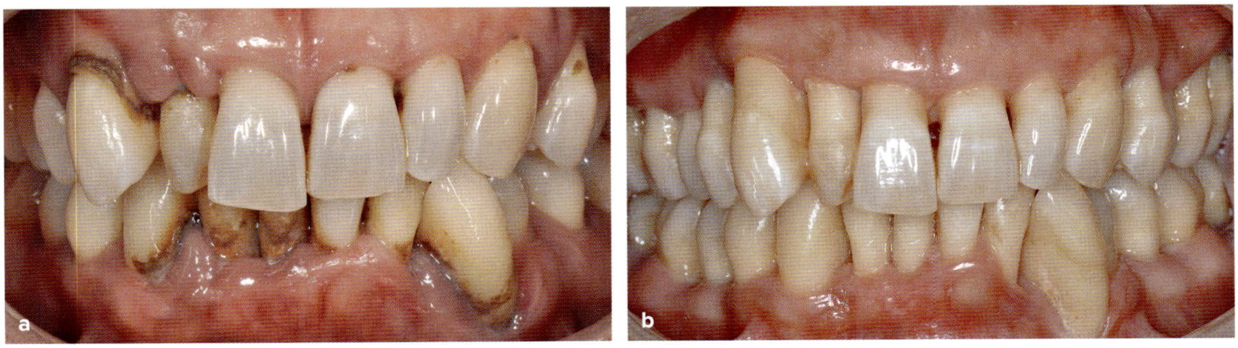

Fig 9-1 *(a)* Baseline: supra- and subgingival calculus and inflamed periodontal tissues. *(b)* Reevaluation: Calculus has been removed and inflammation is significantly reduced.

BOX 9-1 Comparison of different approaches for nonsurgical therapy

SRP by quadrant
- SRP performed quadrant by quadrant in four sessions (one per week)
- Oral hygiene instructions

FMD*
- SRP of the entire dentition within 24 h
- One or two sessions in 24 h
  - Brushing the tongue for 1 minute with chlorhexidine gel 1%
  - Mouthrinse twice for 1 minute with chlorhexidine 0.2% and gargling the last 10 seconds to reach the tonsils
  - Subgingival irrigation with chlorhexidine gel 1% in all pockets
- Oral hygiene instructions
  - At-home rinses with 2% chlorhexidine mouthwash twice a day for 2 weeks

*According to Quirynen et al.[37]

Operative Considerations

THERAPEUTIC OBJECTIVES

The expected endpoints of nonsurgical therapy are the following[33–36] (Fig 9-1):

- Reduction in BOP
- Reduction in PD
- Gain in CAL

TECHNIQUE SELECTION

Nonsurgical therapy can be carried out by the following different modalities (Box 9-1)[37]:

- SRP by quadrant: Usually consists of weekly sessions in which OHI is given and instrumentation is performed with manual and ultrasonic instruments one or two quadrants at a time.
- Full-mouth SRP (FMSRP): Consists of SRP that is performed for the entire dentition in one session.
- Full-mouth disinfection (FMD): One or two sessions in a period of time shorter than 24 hours in which OHI is given and calculus and biofilm are removed from the oral cavity along with local application of antiseptics and the utilization of chlorhexidine mouthrinse for 2 weeks.[37–43]

Several authors have investigated the differences between a full-mouth approach and quadrant by quadrant. According to Koshy et al,[42] the benefits of a single-stage full-mouth approach include a reduction in the risk of contamination between treated and untreated sites, the concomitant use of chlorhexidine, and the enhanced effect of systemic antibiotics when needed. However, some

TABLE 9-2 Studies comparing different modalities of nonsurgical therapy

Study	Groups	Methods	Results
Quirynen et al[37] (1995)	10 patients, 2 groups	Quad SRP vs FMD	1 month: FMD showed greater PD reduction compared with quad SRP 2 months: FMD showed greater reduction in spirochetes and motile rods compared with quad SRP
Quirynen et al[40] (2000)	36 patients, 3 groups	Quad SRP vs FMSRP vs FMD	FMSRP and FMD groups had greater PD reduction and lower spirochetes and motile rods compared with SRP by quad
Apatzidou et al[47] (2004)	44 patients, 2 groups	Quad SRP vs FMSRP	Improvements with both treatments, equal clinical and microbiologic efficacy
Swierkot et al[51] (2009)	28 patients, 3 groups	Quad SRP vs FMSRP vs FMD	No differences in clinical and microbiologic parameters at 8 months
Santuchi et al[45] (2016)	90 patients, 2 groups	Quad SRP vs FMD	No significant differences between groups

Quad, quadrant.

authors[43–45] have demonstrated that there is no clear superiority at a clinical level between the classic approach and the single-stage full-mouth approach. Nevertheless, there is evidence[46–48] showing that when systemic antibiotics are needed, FMD may be the treatment modality of choice. Also, a single-stage approach may be recommended when the patient has time limitations.[49,50]

QUADRANT SRP VERSUS FMD

Table 9-2[37,40,45,47,51] summarizes several investigations comparing the different modalities for nonsurgical therapy.

To date, the clinical superiority of any of these approaches remains controversial. Eberhard et al[49] in a Cochrane review evaluated seven RCTs and found that there are slightly better outcomes for PD reduction and gain in attachment with FMD compared with control groups. However, these were modest additional improvements, and there was a very limited number of studies for comparison. This was later confirmed in a commentary by Greenstein[50] reporting that FMD saves time and has no adverse effects; however, there is a need for more RCTs to test if relevant advantages exist. Lang et al[43] also conducted a systematic review studying the effects of FMSRP, FMD, and quadrant SRP. Results indicated that although PD reduction was significantly greater with FMSRP and FMD than with quadrant SRP (0.2 mm), full-mouth approaches do not provide advantages that are clinically relevant. Hence, all three modalities can be used as initial treatment for patients with periodontitis.

Limitations of Nonsurgical Therapy

The percentage of remaining plaque and calculus on the root surfaces after nonsurgical therapy is greater in deeper pockets and teeth with furcation involvement (Table 9-3).[52–55]

In a classic study, Waerhaug[52] instrumented and extracted 84 teeth with at least one surface with more than 3 mm PD. Overall, 212 supra- and subgingival tooth surfaces were analyzed. Of these, only 44% were free of plaque. Removal of all subgingival plaque was achieved in 83% of the surfaces when PD was less than 3 mm. When PDs were between 3 and 5 mm, there was a good chance of leaving calculus after instrumentation. Lastly, when PD was greater than 5 mm, there was a high chance of leaving calculus; in fact, only 11% of these surfaces were found to be plaque free after instrumentation.

In a study by Stambaugh et al,[53] the presence of residual plaque and calculus was evaluated on extracted teeth after performing SRP for periodontal pockets ranging from 1 to 10 mm (mean: 7.69 mm). As a result, the authors demonstrated that curette efficiency (ie, depth of pocket where

TABLE 9-3 Studies comparing different modalities and outcomes of nonsurgical therapy.

Author	Groups	Methods	Results
Brayer et al[55] (1989)	114 single-rooted teeth	Open vs closed SRP with different levels of operator experience	• Moderate to deep pockets are better reached with open approach • More experienced operators produced a significantly greater number of calculus-free root surfaces than less experienced ones
Waerhaug[52] (1978)	84 extracted teeth	SRP + immediate extraction; SRP + flap; multiple SRP	90% chance of leaving calculus on root after SRP in pockets greater than 5 mm
Stambaugh et al[53] (1981)	7 extracted teeth	SRP	• 3.73 mm = curette efficacy • 6.21 mm = curette limit
Rabbani et al[54] (1981)	199 extracted teeth	62 scaled teeth and 57 controls	• PD < 3 mm easiest for SRP • PD 3–5 mm more difficult for SRP • PD > 5 mm most difficult for SRP

the tooth was instrumented to a plaque- and calculus-free surface) was 3.73 mm on average. On the other hand, the instrument limit (maximum PD with evidence of instrumentation on the root surface) was 5.52 mm on average, with a maximum of 6.21 mm.

In addition, Rabbani et al[54] studied the effectiveness of SRP on 199 teeth that were later extracted. Results demonstrated a significant correlation between the PD and the amount of residual calculus. In concordance with previous studies, this investigation also showed that the deeper the pocket, the more difficult to scale, and residual calculus is more likely to be found in deeper pockets, with no significant differences between anterior and posterior teeth.

Later, Badersten et al[56] in a split-mouth prospective study showed that repeated sessions of SRP every 3 months did not lead to any clinical improvements after the first three cycles. On the other hand, König et al[57] showed that a second round of nonsurgical therapy 5 months later leads to even more CAL gain and reduces the need for surgical intervention.

NONSURGICAL VERSUS SURGICAL

There are no significant differences between surgical and nonsurgical therapy in the treatment of pockets with PDs up to 4 mm.[36,58–65] On the other hand, a clinical trial by Brayer et al[55] involving 114 single-rooted teeth showed that in medium (4 to 6 mm PD) to deep (> 6 mm PD) pockets when performing SRP, a higher percentage of calculus-free root surfaces is achieved with an open approach independently of operator experience. In a longitudinal study comparing SRP, osseous surgery, and modified Widman flap (MWF), Becker et al[61] found after 5 years that all methods led to significant decreases in PD and gingival and plaque scores, and no method showed a significant difference. A meta-analysis by Heitz-Mayfield et al[66] showed that when PDs are between 4 and 6 mm, nonsurgical therapy leads to less PD reduction and more CAL gain than surgical therapy. For PDs 6 mm or greater, surgical therapy leads to higher PD reduction and CAL gain than nonsurgical therapy. Lastly, in a clinical study with 21 patients, Caffesse et al[67] investigated the effectiveness of SRP alone versus SRP with a flap. Results showed that the roots had greater calculus and plaque when SRP was performed alone and also if there were grooves, fossae, or furcations (Table 9-4).

TABLE 9-4 Percentage of calculus-free surfaces with scaling alone vs scaling and flap*

Approach	PD = 1 to 3 mm	PD = 4 to 6 mm	PD = > 6 mm
No flap	86%	43%	32%
Flap	86%	76%	50%

*Data from Caffesse et al.[67]

CRITICAL PROBING DEPTH

In a split-mouth study on 15 patients comparing SRP alone and SRP with MWF, Lindhe et al[68] found that for PDs less than 2.9 mm, SRP will likely lead to CAL loss. Also, for PDs less than 4.2 mm, SRP in conjunction with MWF will likely lead to CAL loss.

When further analyzing the data from both SRP and MWF groups, it was later noted that another critical probing depth value could be identified.[69] In fact, for PDs 5.4 mm or greater, MWF leads to more pronounced CAL gain than SRP alone. This study concluded that for PDs between 2.9 mm and 5.4 mm, nonsurgical therapy is preferred, while for PDs 5.4 mm or greater, surgical therapy is preferred.

MULTIROOTED TEETH

Given the presence of a variety of local anatomical and contributing factors, multirooted teeth present with more challenges for nonsurgical therapy than do single-rooted teeth. As such, many authors have studied the performance of manual and ultrasonic instruments in furcation areas. Parashis et al[16] found that a flap approach with the use of rotary burs was effective for calculus removal in furcation areas. Loos et al[70] found that 2 years after full-mouth SRP, more loss of attachment was observed in molar furcation sites (25%) than molar flat sites (10%) and nonmolar sites (7%). Fleischer et al[71] in a clinical study on 50 teeth treated by experienced and inexperienced operators with SRP or with SRP + flap found that the experience level was significantly correlated with a higher percentage of calculus removal. Also, results indicated that adding a flap increased the performance of both experienced and unexperienced operators. However, in furcations, even experienced operators had a calculus-free surface only 68% of the time.

THE POSTPROPHYLAXIS ABSCESS

Even after meticulous nonsurgical therapy, there is a risk of leaving undetected subgingival deposits that could progressively lead to recurrence of inflammation.[72] If adequate instrumentation of the coronal part of a deep pocket is performed, healing and reattachment can occur around this coronal aspect even when biofilm is still present in the deeper portion. When this occurs, the biofilm can cause inflammation and exudate that may cause a periodontal abscess if unable to drain though the pocket.[73] Although this phenomenon rarely occurs, the treatment often requires flap elevation to drain the abscess and obtain proper access for root surface instrumentation.

Reevaluation

The reevaluation of the nonsurgical phase is a critical step in periodontal therapy. It allows the clinician to assess the improvements after initial therapy, evaluate the patient's compliance and motivation, evaluate the tissue conditions, and identify if additional treatment is necessary. The correct timing for the reevaluation appointment is paramount: Reevaluating too soon could result in overtreatment, and waiting too long may lead to disease progression and return to pathogenic flora. In a prospective clinical trial involving 10 patients, Caton et al[74] evaluated 128 pockets after a single episode of root planing at 1, 2, 4, 8, and 16 weeks and found significant reduction in plaque, BOP, and PD and increase in CAL up to 4 weeks. The favorable changes could be maintained until the 16-week time interval. Segelnick and Weinberg[75] concluded that reevaluation at 2 weeks is too early because the reestablishment of the junctional epithelium is still occurring, and the repair of the connective tissue continues for 4 to 8 weeks. Pocket repopulation occurs around 2 months after instrumentation, and a longer waiting period may cause repopulation by periodontal pathogenic bacteria. For these reasons, a reevaluation after at least 8 weeks is recommended.

References

1. Eke PI, Dye BA, Wei L, et al. Update on prevalence of periodontitis in adults in the United States: NHANES 2009 to 2012. J Periodontol 2015;85:611–622.
2. American Academy of Periodontology. Glossary of Periodontal Terms. American Academy of Periodontology, 2001.
3. Van der Weijden GA, Timmerman MF. A systematic review on the clinical efficacy of subgingival debridement in the treatment of chronic periodontitis. J Clin Periodontol 2002;29(suppl 3):55–71.
4. Needleman I, Nibali L, Di Iorio A. Professional mechanical plaque removal for prevention of periodontal diseases in adults—Systematic review update. J Clin Periodontol 2015;42(suppl 16):S12–S35.
5. Bass CC. The necessary personal oral hygiene for prevention of caries and periodontoclasia. New Orleans Med Surg J 1948;101:52–70.
6. Yaacob M, Worthington HV, Deacon SA, et al. Powered versus manual toothbrushing for oral health. Cochrane Database Syst Rev 2014;(6):CD002281.
7. Sälzer S, Slot DE, Van der Weijden FA, Dörfer CE. Efficacy of interdental mechanical plaque control in managing gingivitis—A meta-review. J Clin Periodontol 2015;42(suppl 16):S92–S105.
8. Kotsakis GA, Lian Q, Ioannou AL, Michalowicz BS, John MT, Chu H. A network meta-analysis of interproximal oral hygiene methods in the reduction of clinical indices of inflammation. J Periodontol 2018;89:558–570.
9. Tunkel J, Heinecke A, Flemmig TF. A systematic review of efficacy of machine-driven and manual subgingival debridement in the treatment of chronic periodontitis. J Clin Periodontol 2002;29(suppl 3):72–81.
10. Walmsley AD, Lea SC, Landini G, Moses AJ. Advances in power driven pocket/root instrumentation. J Clin Periodontol 2008;35(8 suppl):22–28.
11. Drisko CL, Cochran DL, Blieden T, et al. Position paper: Sonic and ultrasonic scalers in periodontics. Research, Science and Therapy Committee of the American Academy of Periodontology. J Periodontol 2000;71:1792–1801.
12. Dahiya P, Kamal R, Gupta R, Pandit N. Comparative evaluation of hand and power-driven instruments on root surface characteristics: A scanning electron microscopy study. Contemp Clin Dent 2011;2:79–83.
13. Kerry GJ. Roughness of root surfaces after use of ultrasonic instruments and hand curettes. J Periodontol 1967;38:340–346.
14. Nishimine D, O'Leary TJ. Hand instrumentation versus ultrasonics in the removal of endotoxins from root surfaces. J Periodontol 1979;50:345–349.
15. Gellin RG, Miller MC, Javed T, Engler WO, Mishkin DJ. The effectiveness of the Titan-S sonic scaler versus curettes in the removal of subgingival calculus. A human surgical evaluation. J Periodontol 1986;57:672–680.
16. Parashis AO, Anagnou-Vareltzides A, Demetriou N. Calculus removal from multirooted teeth with and without surgical access. II. Comparison between external and furcation surfaces and effect of furcation entrance width. J Clin Periodontol 1993;20:294–298.
17. Hallmon WW, Rees TD. Local anti-infective therapy: Mechanical and physical approaches. A systematic review. Ann Periodontol 2003;8:99–114.
18. Daly CG, Kieser JB, Corbet EF, Seymourt GJ. Cementum involved in periodontal disease: A review of its features and clinical management. J Dent 1979;7:185–193.
19. Mombelli A, Nyman S, Brägger U, Wennström J, Lang NP. Clinical and microbiological changes associated with an altered subgingival environment induced by periodontal pocket reduction. J Clin Periodontol 1995;22:780–787.
20. Nyman S, Westfelt E, Sarhed G, Karring T. Role of "diseased" root cementum in healing following treatment of periodontal disease. A clinical study. J Clin Periodontol 1988;15:464–468.
21. Greenstein G; Research, Science and Therapy Committee of the American Academy of Periodontology. Position Paper: The role of supra- and subgingival irrigation in the treatment of periodontal diseases. J Periodontol 2005;76:2015–2027.
22. Herrera D, Alonso B, León R, Roldán S, Sanz M. Antimicrobiol therapy in periodontitis: The use of systemic antimicrobials against the subgingival biofilm. J Clin Periodontol 2008;35(8 suppl):45–66.
23. Haffajee AD, Socransky SS, Gunsolley JC. Systemic anti-infective periodontal therapy. A systematic review. Ann Periodontol 2003;8:115–181.
24. Hanes PJ, Purvis JP. Local anti-infective therapy: Pharmacological agents. A systematic review. Ann Periodontol 2003;8:79–98.
25. American Academy of Periodontology. American Academy of Periodontology statement on the efficacy of lasers in the non-surgical treatment of inflammatory periodontal disease. J Periodontol 2011;82:513–514.
26. Slot DE, Jorritsma KH, Cobb CM, Van der Weijden FA. The effect of the thermal diode laser (wavelength 808–980 nm) in non-surgical periodontal therapy: A systematic review and meta-analysis. J Clin Periodontol 2014;41:681–692.
27. Zhao Y, Yin Y, Tao L, Nie P, Tang Y, Zhu M. Er:YAG laser versus scaling and root planing as alternative or adjuvant for chronic periodontitis treatment: A systematic review. J Clin Periodontol 2014;41:1069–1079.
28. Bassir SH, Moslemi N, Jamali R, et al. Photoactivated disinfection using light-emitting diode as an adjunct in the management of chronic periodontitis: A pilot double-blind split-mouth randomized clinical trial. J Clin Periodontol 2013;40:65–72.
29. Segarra-Vidal M, Guerra-Ojeda S, Vallés LS, et al. Effects of photodynamic therapy in periodontal treatment: A randomized, controlled clinical trial. J Clin Periodontol 2017;44:915–925.
30. Petersilka GJ. Subgingival air-polishing in the treatment of periodontal biofilm infections. Periodontol 2000 2011;55:124–142.
31. Wennström JL, Dahlén G, Ramberg P. Subgingival debridement of periodontal pockets by air polishing in comparison with ultrasonic instrumentation during maintenance therapy. J Clin Periodontol 2011;38:820–827.
32. Flemmig TF, Arushanov D, Daubert D, Rothen M, Mueller G, Leroux BG. Randomized controlled trial assessing efficacy and safety of glycine powder air polishing in moderate-to-deep periodontal pockets. J Periodontol 2012;83:444–452.
33. Badersten A, Nilveus R, Egelberg J. Effect of nonsurgical periodontal therapy. II. Severely advanced periodontitis. J Clin Periodontol 1984;11:63–76.
34. Kaldahl WB, Kalkwarf KL, Patil KD, Dyer JK, Bates RE Jr. Evaluation of four modalities of periodontal therapy. Mean probing depth, probing attachment level and recession changes. J Periodontol 1988;59:783–793.
35. Lindhe J, Westfelt E, Nyman S, Socransky SS, Heijl L, Bratthall G. Healing following surgical/non-surgical treatment of periodontal disease. A clinical study. J Clin Periodontol 1982;9:115–128.
36. Suvan JE. Effectiveness of mechanical nonsurgical pocket therapy. Periodontol 2000 2005;37:48–71.

37. Quirynen M, Bollen CM, Vandekerckhove BN, Dekeyser C, Papaioannou W, Eyssen H. Full- vs partial-mouth disinfection in the treatment of periodontal infections: Short-term clinical and microbiological observations. J Dent Res 1995;74:1459–1467.
38. Quirynen M, Teughels W, van Steenberghe D. Impact of antiseptics on one-stage, full-mouth disinfection. J Clin Periodontol 2006;33:49–52.
39. Quirynen M, Zhao H, Soers C, et al. The impact of periodontal therapy and the adjunctive effect of antiseptics on breath odor-related outcome variables: A double-blind randomized study. J Periodontol 2005;76:705–712.
40. Quirynen M, Mongardini C, De Soete M, et al. The role of chlorhexidine in the one-stage full-mouth disinfection treatment of patients with advanced adult periodontitis. Long-term clinical and microbiological observations. J Clin Periodontol 2000;27:578–589.
41. Quirynen M, De Soete M, Boschmans G, et al. Benefit of "one-stage full-mouth disinfection" is explained by disinfection and root planing within 24 hours: A randomized controlled trial. J Clin Periodontol 2006;33:639–647.
42. Koshy G, Corbet EF, Ishikawa I. A full-mouth disinfection approach to nonsurgical periodontal therapy—Prevention of reinfection from bacterial reservoirs. Periodontol 2000 2004;36:166–178.
43. Lang NP, Tan WC, Krähenmann MA, Zwahlen M. A systematic review of the effects of full-mouth debridement with and without antiseptics in patients with chronic periodontitis. J Clin Periodontol 2008;35(8 suppl):8–21.
44. Sanz M, Teughels W; Group A of European Workshop on Periodontology. Innovations in non-surgical periodontal therapy: Consensus report of the sixth European Workshop on Periodontology. J Clin Periodontol 2008;35(8 suppl):3–7.
45. Santuchi CC, Cortelli JR, Cortelli SC, et al. Scaling and root planing per quadrant versus one-stage full-mouth disinfection: Assessment of the impact of chronic periodontitis treatment on quality of life—A clinical randomized, controlled trial. J Periodontol 2016;87:114–123.
46. Gomi K, Yashima A, Nagano T, Kanazashi M, Maeda N, Arai T. Effects of full-mouth scaling and root planing in conjunction with systemically administered azithromycin. J Periodontol 2007;78:422–429.
47. Apatzidou DA, Riggio MP, Kinane DF. Quadrant root planing versus same-day full-mouth root planing. II. Microbiological findings. J Clin Periodontol 2004;31:141–148.
48. Jervøe-Storm PM, AlAhdab H, Semaan E, Fimmers R, Jepsen S. Microbiolgical outcomes of quadrant versus full-mouth root planing as monitored by real-time PCR. J Clin Periodontol 2007;34:156–163.
49. Eberhard J, Jepsen S, Jervøe-Storm PM, Needleman I, Worthington HV. Full-mouth disinfection for the treatment of adult chronic periodontitis. Cochrane Database Syst Rev 2008;(1):CD004622.
50. Greenstein G. Full-mouth therapy versus individual quadrant root planing: A critical commentary. J Periodontol 2002;73:797–812.
51. Swierkot K, Nonnenmacher CI, Mutters R, Flores-de-Jacoby L, Mengel R. One-stage full-mouth disinfection versus quadrant and full-mouth root planing. J Clin Periodontol 2009;36:240–249.
52. Waerhaug J. Healing of the dento-epithelial junction following subgingival plaque control. II: As observed on extracted teeth. J Periodontol 1978;49:119–134.
53. Stambaugh RV, Dragoo M, Smith DM, Carasali L. The limits of subgingival scaling. Int J Periodontics Restorative Dent 1981;1:30–41.
54. Rabbani GM, Ash MM Jr, Caffesse RG. The effectiveness of subgingival scaling and root planing in calculus removal. J Periodontol 1981;52:119–23.
55. Brayer WK, Mellonig JT, Dunlap RM, Marinak KW, Carson RE. Scaling and root planing effectiveness: The effect of root surface access and operator experience. J Periodontol 1989;60:67–72.
56. Badersten A, Nilveus R, Egelberg J. Effect of nonsurgical periodontal therapy. III. Single versus repeated instrumentation. J Clin Periodontol 1984;11:114–124.
57. König J, Schwahn C, Fanghänel J, Plötz J, Hoffmann T, Kocher T. Repeated scaling versus surgery in young adults with generalized advanced periodontitis. J Periodontol 2008;79:1006–1013.
58. Isidor F, Karring T. Long-term effect of surgical and non-surgical periodontal treatment. A 5-year clinical study. J Periodontal Res 1986;21:462–472.
59. Isidor F, Karring T, Attström R. The effect of root planing as compared to that of surgical treatment. J Clin Periodontol 1984;11:669–681.
60. Becker W, Becker BE, Ochsenbein C, et al. A longitudinal study comparing scaling, osseous surgery, and modified Widman procedures. Results after one year. J Periodontol 1988;59:351–365.
61. Becker W, Becker BE, Caffesse R, et al. A longitudinal study comparing scaling, osseous surgery, and modified Widman procedures: Results after 5 years. J Periodontol 2001;72:1675–1684.
62. Ramfjord SP, Nissle RR, Shick RA, Cooper H Jr. Subgingival curettage versus surgical elimination of periodontal pockets. J Periodontol 1968;39:167–175.
63. Ramfjord SP, Knowles JW, Nissle RR, Burgett FG, Shick RA. Results following three modalities of periodontal therapy. J Periodontol 1975;46:522–526.
64. Ramfjord SP, Caffesse RG, Morrison EC, et al. 4 modalities of periodontal treatment compared over 5 years. J Clin Periodontol 1987;14:445–452.
65. Lindhe J, Westfelt E, Nyman S, Socransky SS, Haffajee AD. Long-term effect of surgical/non-surgical treatment of periodontal disease. J Clin Periodontol 1984;11:448–458.
66. Heitz-Mayfield LJ, Trombelli L, Heitz F, Needleman I, Moles D. A systematic review of the effect of surgical debridement vs non-surgical debridement for the treatment of chronic periodontitis. J Clin Periodontol 2002;29(suppl 3):92–102.
67. Caffesse RG, Sweeney PL, Smith BA. Scaling and root planing with and without periodontal flap surgery. J Clin Periodontol 1986;13:205–210.
68. Lindhe J, Socransky SS, Nyman S, Haffajee A, Westfeld E. "Critical probing depths" in periodontal therapy. J Clin Periodontol 1982;9:323–336.
69. Heitz-Mayfield LJ, Lang NP. Surgical and nonsurgical periodontal therapy. Learned and unlearned concepts. Periodontol 2000 2013;62:218–231.
70. Loos B, Nylund K, Claffey N, Egelberg J. Clinical effects of root debridement in molar and non-molar teeth. A 2-year follow-up. J Clin Periodontol 1989;16:498–504.
71. Fleischer HC, Mellonig JT, Brayer WK, Gray JL, Barnett JD. Scaling and root planing efficacy in multirooted teeth. J Periodontol 1989;60:402–409.
72. Waerhaug J. Healing of the dento-epithelial junction following subgingival plaque control. I. As observed in human biopsy material. J Periodontol 1978;49:1–8.
73. Dello Russo NM. The post-prophylaxis periodontal abscess: Etiology and treatment. Int J Periodontics Restorative Dent 1985;5:28–37.
74. Caton J, Proye M, Polson A. Maintenance of healed periodontal pockets after a single episode of root planing. J Periodontol 1982;53:420–424.
75. Segelnick SL, Weinberg MA. Reevaluation of initial therapy: When is the appropriate time? J Periodontol 2006;77:1598–1601.

10

SURGICAL NONREGENERATIVE THERAPY

Anusha Reddy Etikala, BDS, MS

The field of periodontics encompasses a great variety of surgical approaches with a long and well-investigated body of evidence. In particular, surgical nonregenerative therapies have been extensively studied by leading academic groups around the world in a prospective longitudinal model. Long-term follow-ups from these randomized controlled clinical studies comparing various nonsurgical and surgical nonregenerative therapies played a pivotal role in the evolution of the periodontal field. These groups along with the most relevant studies are reviewed in this chapter (Table 10-1).[1–5]

DEFINITIONS AND TERMINOLOGY

Curettage: open curettage: A surgical procedure involving the debridement of tooth roots and removal of infected sulcular epithelium (granulation tissue) after flap reflection. Usually accomplished using sharp instruments, such as curettes or surgical debridement burs.[6]

Ostectomy: The excision or removal of alveolar bone proper (tooth-supporting bone) in osseous resective and/or crown lengthening surgery. Often performed in order to establish positive bony architecture.[6]

TABLE 10-1 Historic perspective of different flap designs and surgical techniques

Flap operation	Publication	Goal	Incisions		Remarks
			Horizontal	Releasing	
Original Widman flap	Widman[1] (1918)	Pocket elimination	1-mm scalloped	Extending beyond MGJ	APF with interproximal bone left denuded
Neumann flap	Neumann[2] (1912)	Pocket elimination	Intrasulcular	Sectional	APF with closed interproximal sites by flap adaptation
Kirkland flap	Kirkland[3] (1931)	Pocket reduction	Intrasulcular	Only for flap retraction	Original flap position
Friedman flap	Friedman[4] (1962)	Pocket elimination	Scalloped as indicated	Extending to MGJ	APF without bone denudation
Frisch flap	Frisch et al[5] (1967)	Pocket reduction	Lingual scalloped, buccal double interproximal	NA	Total retention of labial gingiva

MGJ, mucogingival junction; APF, apically positioned flap; NA, not applicable.

TABLE 10-2 Summary of clinical findings from longitudinal studies on ENAP

Publication	Months from baseline	Mean PD reduction (mm)	Recession (mm)	New attachment (mm)
Yukna et al[11] (1976)	12	2.7	0.6	2.1
Yukna[12] (1978)	36	2.3	0.6	1.85
Yukna and Williams[13] (1980)	60	1.8	0.3	1.5

Techniques

MODIFIED WIDMAN FLAP

The modified Widman flap (MWF) technique was published in 1974 by Ramfjord and Nissle. The main goal of this procedure is to access the root surface for instrumentation purposes and decrease pocket depths.[7] Only minimal bone recontouring and soft tissue removal is indicated for proper postoperative flap adaptation.

OSSEOUS SURGERY

In 1949, Schluger conceived and described the principles of osseous resection.[8] Next, in 1958, Goldman and Cohen proposed the intrabony pocket classification and treatment recommendations according to the location and number of osseous walls.[9] Later, in 1964, Ochsenbein and Bohannan classified interdental craters and suggested osseous surgical treatment approaches with the primary objective of removing the minimal amount of bone necessary that will meet the needs of an adequate architectural form.[10]

EXCISIONAL NEW ATTACHMENT PROCEDURE

The excisional new attachment procedure (ENAP) is a definitive subgingival **curettage** performed with a surgical knife. The main goal is elimination of the pocket lining with secondary goals including soft tissue preparation, gaining better access, and new attachment to the root surface. Yukna et al longitudinally evaluated the healing following ENAP in 9 human subjects, and their results are summarized in Table 10-2.[11–13]

LASER-ASSISTED NEW ATTACHMENT PROCEDURE

The laser-assisted new attachment procedure (LANAP) is a patented protocol using a PerioLase MVP-7 Nd:YAG laser (Millennium Dental Technologies).[14] This is an FDA-cleared laser treatment[15] indicated (according to the manufacturer) in patients with moderate to deep probing depths (PDs) with visible bony defects and infection in the gingival tissue and when there are esthetic considerations. The inflamed sulcular and pocket epithelium is excised without substantial removal of connective tissue.

With regard to the use of lasers as an adjunct to periodontal therapy, a recent meta-analysis including nine studies of surgical periodontal therapy with and without the use of lasers showed no statistically significant difference between the experimental groups.[16] The authors concluded that there is insufficient evidence to support the effectiveness of dental lasers as an adjunct to resective or regenerative surgical periodontal therapy.[16] In addition, an American Academy of Periodontology 2018 best evidence review reported that in patients with moderate to severe periodontitis, nonsurgical treatment by scaling and root planing (SRP) and infrared diode laser, and the surgical treatment by Er:YAG laser alone, may promote relatively small (< 1 mm) but significant improvements in PD and clinical attachment level (CAL).[17]

Longitudinal Studies

MICHIGAN STUDIES

The earliest of the longitudinal studies was developed at the University of Michigan by Ramfjord et al.[18] The study principles and methodology were first described in 1968. Both single- and multirooted teeth were studied. PD measurements were performed at four sites per

TABLE 10-3 Summary of Michigan studies

Publication	Number of participants	Follow-up (y)	Treatment modalities	Main outcomes
Ramfjord et al[18] (1968)	32	2	CR	Significant CAL gain in deep pockets
			PE	Slight loss of attachment
Ramfjord et al[19] (1975)	79	5	CR	Greatest CAL gain during first 3 years, least PD reduction
			PE	Initial PD reduction but overall CAL loss
			MWF	Slight CAL gain during first year, but CAL loss thereafter
Knowles et al[22] (1979)	43	8	CR	Long-term significant PD reduction in 4–6-mm pockets, less PD reduction in ≥ 7-mm pockets
			PE	Greater PD reduction in 4–6-mm pockets
			MWF	Greatest PD reduction in ≥ 7-mm pockets
Hill et al[20] (1981)	90	2	CR, PE, MWF, SRP	1–3-mm PD: Overall minimal PD reduction and CAL loss. 4–6-mm PD: Greater PD reduction after PE, MWF. CAL gain after SRP; CAL lost for PE, MWF and CR. ≥ 7-mm PD: Greater PD reduction after PE, similar CAL loss in all groups.
Ramfjord et al[21] (1987)	90	5	CR, PE, MWF, SRP	1–3-mm PD: No change in PDs but similar loss of CAL across all groups. 4–6-mm PD: Similar PD reduction in all groups, CAL loss from greatest to least was PE > MWF > SRP > CR. ≥ 7-mm PD: Both PD reduction and CAL loss in order of greatest to least was PE > MWF > SRP > CR.

CR, curettage; PE, surgical pocket elimination; SC, subgingival curettage.

tooth at the line angles. Initial therapy consisted of oral hygiene instructions (OHI) and SRP. Occlusal adjustment was also performed as indicated. Following active periodontal therapy, patients were enrolled in recall appointments at 3-month intervals. In the first study, patients received either curettage or surgical pocket elimination, consisting of gingivectomy/flap surgery and osseous recontouring.[18] A split-mouth design was later incorporated into the study design where curettage was compared with MWF and pocket elimination in 82 patients.[19] In the subsequent longitudinal studies, four different treatment modalities were assigned randomly to each quadrant in a split-mouth design.[20,21] In these investigations, pockets of 1 to 3 mm were considered *shallow*, pockets of 4 to 6 mm were *moderate*, and pockets ≥ 7 mm were *deep*. Results from the Michigan studies are summarized in Table 10-3.[18–22]

Maintenance care

The role of personal plaque control and periodontal maintenance care was evaluated in the 1982 publication by Ramfjord et al.[23] There were 78 patients who were enrolled in 3-month-interval maintenance recalls for over 8 years following surgery. Also, the 25% of the sample with the lowest plaque scores was compared against the 25% of individuals with the highest plaque scores. Results from this investigation concluded that although proper personal oral hygiene is key for successful long-term outcomes, the role of personal home care was not critical for the maintenance of posttreatment PD and CALs as long as patients had professional maintenance appointments every 3 months.[23] Subsequent clinical observations also highlighted the importance of maintenance care every 3 to 4 months in the long-term prognosis of treated periodontitis patients.[24]

TABLE 10-4 Summary of Minnesota studies

Publication	Number of participants	Follow-up (y)	Treatment modalities	Main outcomes
Pihlstrom et al[26] (1981)	17	4	SRP, SRP + MWF	1–3-mm PD: Slight loss of attachment with both therapies. 4–6-mm PD: PD reduction along with sustained CAL gain with both therapies. ≥ 7-mm PD: Greatest PD reduction and CAL gain with both therapies, but with a difference in PD reduction of 0.9 mm in favor of SRP + MWF.
Pihlstrom et al[27] (1983)	17	6.5	SRP, SRP + MWF	1–3-mm PD: Not reported. 4–6-mm PD: Equally effective sustained PD reduction with both treatments. ≥ 7-mm PD: Initially more PD reduction with MWF, but no difference in CAL between the two treatments.

Tooth mobility

The data from the 8-year longitudinal studies demonstrated that there is a significant relationship between initial tooth mobility and change in levels of attachment following treatment. As such, pockets associated with teeth with grade 2 or 3 mobility did not respond as favorably to periodontal treatment as those with minimal to no mobility.[25]

Conclusions from Michigan longitudinal studies

- Final PD reduction was proportional to initial PD.
- Greater PD reduction and CAL gain were observed in interproximal sites.
- Thorough debridement of root surfaces with proper access is more important than specific treatment modalities.

MINNESOTA STUDIES

Pihlstrom et al conducted a series of studies to compare long-term effectiveness of SRP alone and SRP followed by surgical therapy.[26] Both molars and nonmolars were included. Following initial SRP and OHI, MWF was randomly performed for only one-half of the dentition. Maintenance was performed three to four times per year. The main drawback of these studies is the small sample size as well as the high dropout rate over the years. Results from Minnesota studies are summarized in Table 10-4.[26,27]

Molar and nonmolar comparison

A further comparison with respect to tooth type—molars versus nonmolars—revealed that for PDs of 4 to 6 mm, there was greater PD reduction and CAL loss on molars than nonmolars treated by either method of therapy. For PDs 7 mm or more, a greater effect of PD reduction on nonmolars with MWF procedure was observed. However, there was no difference between tooth types for CAL with either treatment method for PDs 7 mm or greater.[28]

Conclusions from Minnesota longitudinal studies

- SRP alone and in combination with MWF are effective in treating periodontitis.
- MWF resulted in greater PD reduction for deeper PDs.

NEBRASKA STUDIES

In these investigations, Kaldahl et al compared the effects of nonsurgical and surgical therapy in a series of longitudinal studies.[29–32] Following initial therapy, a split-mouth design was applied where each quadrant randomly received either coronal scaling (CS), root planing, MWF, or osseous surgery with an apically positioned flap. During initial therapy, teeth that were designated to receive CS were scaled with no subgingival instrumentation. Periodontal maintenance was performed every 3 months.

Results of the long-term evaluation of these four therapies were published in 1996. Incidence of sites breaking

TABLE 10-5 Summary of Nebraska studies

Publication	Number of participants	Follow-up (y)	Treatment modalities	Main outcomes
Kaldahl et al[30] (1988)	82	2	CS, RP, MWF, FO	1–4-mm PD: FO resulted in loss of attachment. 5–6-mm PD: RP and MWF resulted in greatest CAL gain. PD reduction in order of greatest to least was FO > MWF > RP > CS. ≥ 7-mm PD: RP, MWF, and FO produced similar gains. PD reduction in order of greatest to least was FO > MWF > RP > CS.
Kaldahl et al[31] (1996)	82	7	CS, RP, MWF, FO	1–4-mm PD: No differences between the therapies at the end of year 2. 5–6-mm PD: No differences in PD reduction between RP and MWF at the end of year 3. ≥ 7-mm PD: No differences in PD reduction between RP and MWF at the end of year 5. Similar CAL gain by RP, MWF, and FO. Recession noted in order of greatest to least was FO > MWF > RP > CS.

RP, root planing; FO, apically positioned flap with osseous surgery.

down (≥ 3 mm from baseline) was analyzed, and it was reported that CS resulted in higher incidence of breakdown compared with other therapies during the first year after treatment. Breakdown incidences were also greater with increasing PD severities. There was no further loss of CAL 1 year after retreatment in 88% of sites.[29] Results from the Nebraska studies are summarized in Table 10-5.[30,31]

Effects of smoking

The Nebraska studies classified the subjects into heavy smokers (≥ 20 cigarettes/day), light smokers (< 20 cigarettes/day), past smokers, and nonsmokers. Analysis of these results showed that heavy and light smokers had less PD reduction and less CAL gain than past smokers and nonsmokers. However, there were no differences in BOP among the four groups. It was also concluded that heavy and light smokers responded less favorably to therapy than past smokers and nonsmokers, and past history of smoking was not deleterious to the response to therapy.[32] Subjects with higher breakdown incidences also tended to be smokers at the initial exam.[29]

Conclusions from Nebraska longitudinal studies

- The deeper the initial PD, the greater the postoperative reduction.
- The deeper the PD, the more likely to have disease recurrence.
- Smokers have a higher incidence of breakdown.

LOMA LINDA–LUND STUDIES

A series of longitudinal studies were conducted in collaboration between Lund University in Sweden and Loma Linda University in California. These studies mainly evaluated the response of single-rooted teeth to nonsurgical therapy. Repeated instrumentation was considered at 2 and 6 months following initial therapy.[33] Results from the Loma Linda–Lund studies are summarized in Table 10-6.[33–41]

Oral hygiene

Cercek et al[42] evaluated the effects of plaque control and instrumentation over a 2-year period in seven patients with chronic periodontitis. Supragingival plaque control was compared with subgingival plaque control and SRP, separately. Results demonstrated that a minimal effect on pocket reduction was derived from the patient's self-performed plaque control, and most of the effect was derived from professional SRP.[42]

The reproducibility of probing attachment level measurements was also evaluated in nonmolars. The results showed that approximately 90% of the recordings could be reproduced within ± 1.0-mm difference.[43]

TABLE 10-6 Summary of Loma Linda–Lund studies

Publication	Number of participants	Teeth	PD range (mm)	Follow-up	Treatment modalities and study objectives	Main outcomes
Badersten et al[33] (1981)	15	Nonmolars	4–7	13 m	Hand vs ultrasonic instrumentation	Similar improvements in plaque scores, BOP, PD reduction, and CAL changes for both treatments.
Badersten et al[34] (1984)	16	Nonmolars	Up to 12	2 y	Hand vs ultrasonic instrumentation	Nonsurgical therapy showed improvement for all initial PD values. No difference in results between the two treatments. Deep residual PD sites are more likely to bleed on probing.
Badersten et al[35] (1984)	13	Nonmolars	Up to 11	2 y	Single vs repeated instrumentation	Gradual and marked improvement during the first 9 months, no further changes in PD and CAL after. No differences between single and repeated SRP.
Badersten et al[36] (1985)	20	Nonmolars	Up to 11	2 y	Operator variability	Negligible variability between sites treated by six different operators (1 periodontist and 5 hygienists).
Badersten et al[37] (1985)	33	Nonmolars	Up to 12	2 y	Nonresponding sites	Linear and gradual pattern of CAL loss seen in 73% of nonresponding sites over 24 months. Shallower sites showed early loss followed by stabilization; deeper pockets showed gradual loss.
Badersten et al[38] (1985)	49	Nonmolars	Up to 12	2 y	Localization of sites with CAL loss	CAL loss was most frequent for < 7-mm PD sites than ≥ 7-mm PD sites. Buccal surfaces showed higher CAL loss than proximal or lingual surfaces.
Badersten et al[39] (1987)	49	Nonmolars	Up to 12 (only proximal surfaces)	2 y	Probing attachment changes	Subjects with higher proportion of sites with CAL gain had lower proportion of sites with CAL loss. Sites with deep initial PDs showed high incidence of CAL gain.
Badersten et al[40] (1987)	46	Nonmolars	Up to 12	4 y	Long-term effects of nonsurgical therapy	Minimal changes in BOP, PD, and CAL levels between 24 to 48 months. Both deep and shallow PDs can be maintained over 4 years.
Nordland et al[41] (1987)	19	Nonmolars and molars	NR	2 y	Effects of plaque control and SRP	≥ 4-mm PD: Molar furcations responded less favorably than other sites. ≥ 7-mm PD: 21% of molar furcations, 7% of flat molar surfaces, and 11% of nonmolar sites showed CAL loss.

NR, not reported.

TABLE 10-7 Summary of Arizona studies

Publication	Number of participants	Follow-up	Treatment modalities	Main outcomes
Becker et al[44] (1988)	16	12 m	SRP, MWF, OS	1–3-mm PD: MWF and OS resulted in greater CAL loss. 4–6-mm PD: MWF and OS resulted in greater PD reduction than SRP. ≥ 7-mm PD: MWF and OS resulted in greater PD reduction than SRP.
Becker et al[45] (2001)	16	5 y	SRP, MWF, OS	1–3-mm PD: All therapies produced significant CAL loss. 4–6-mm PD: All therapies produced significant PD reduction, no significant differences between methods. ≥ 7-mm PD: All therapies produced significant PD reduction, no significant differences between methods.

OS, osseous surgery with apically positioned flap.

Conclusions from Loma Linda–Lund longitudinal studies

- Shallow pockets resulted in slight loss of CAL, while deeper pockets showed high incidence of CAL gain.
- Attachment loss was due to trauma associated with SRP rather than loss as a result of continuing inflammatory disease process.
- There is no certain value of initial PD where nonsurgical periodontal therapy is no longer effective.
- BOP, PD, and CAL have low diagnostic sensitivity and predictability.

ARIZONA STUDIES

Becker et al conducted longitudinal studies in a private practice setting in Tucson, Arizona. These investigations were performed in cooperation with the University of Michigan.[44,45] Following oral hygiene instructions and initial SRP, a split-mouth design was applied to compare SRP, MWF, and apically positioned flap (APF) with osseous surgery in posterior teeth. Anterior teeth were excluded from the study. Patients were enrolled in a 3-month maintenance program. Results from the Arizona studies are summarized in Table 10-7.[44,45]

Mean annual tooth loss rate in periodontitis patients

Prior to the longitudinal studies, Becker et al reported the mean annual adjusted tooth loss rate from their retrospective studies (Table 10-8).[46–48]

Conclusions from Arizona longitudinal studies

- SRP was effective at maintaining CALs but not in reducing PD.
- At 5 years, APF with osseous surgery had the greatest number of sites losing > 2 mm CAL compared with SRP and MWF.
- All procedures produced gingival recession. However, more recession occurred on sites treated with APF with osseous surgery.

WASHINGTON STUDIES

Smith et al conducted a split-mouth study evaluating the posterior teeth of patients with bilaterally similar periodontitis.[49] Nonsurgical therapy was followed by randomly assigned osseous recontouring or flap curettage treatments in a cross-arch fashion. Patients were enrolled in a 6-month recall for the first 2 years, followed by a recall program every 3 months.[49] Results from the Washington studies are summarized in Table 10-9.[49,50]

Conclusions from Washington longitudinal studies

- Osseous recontouring resulted in a net loss of attachment, whereas flap curettage produced a net gain, especially in deeper pockets.
- Deeper pockets had greater PD reduction, more so with osseous recontouring.

TABLE 10-8 Tooth loss rate

Publication	Participant population (periodontitis patients)	Mean annual adjusted tooth loss rate	Number of participants	Average follow-up (y)
Becker et al[46] (1984)	Treatment: Yes Maintenance: Yes	0.11	44	5.25
Becker et al[47] (1984)	Treatment: Yes Maintenance: No	0.22	16	6.58
Becker et al[48] (1979)	Treatment: No Maintenance: No	0.36	100	3.7

TABLE 10-9 Summary of Washington studies

Publication	Number of participants	Follow-up	Treatment modalities	Main outcomes
Smith et al[49] (1980)	12	6 m	FC, OS	Both techniques showed similar PD reduction in deeper pockets with intrabony defects. PD reduction from OS maintained over 6 months. Pockets recurred after FC. OS resulted in a net CAL loss; FC produced net CAL gain in deeper pockets.
Olsen et al[50] (1985)	12	5 y	FC, OS	PDs in FC sites returned to preoperative values, PDs with OS remained reduced at 5 years specially in interproximal areas.

FC, open-flap curettage; OS, osseous recontouring surgery.

SWEDISH STUDIES

Rosling et al compared the effectiveness of different surgical approaches. After therapy, all subjects received OHI and professional cleanings every 2 weeks for 2 years.[51] Later, Lindhe's group started a series of studies comparing long-term effectiveness of surgical and nonsurgical procedures. Patients received SRP alone or in combination with MWF in a split-mouth study followed by maintenance every 2 weeks for the first 6 months and then 3-month recalls for up to 24 months.[52] Results from the Swedish studies are summarized in Table 10-10.[51–54]

Lang et al published a 50-year follow up study in 2009 demonstrating that gingival inflammation is a risk factor for tooth loss.[55] As such, sites with consistent bleeding (gingival index [GI] = 2) had 70% more attachment loss than sites that were consistently noninflamed (GI = 0). Also, teeth with sites that were consistently noninflamed had a 50-year survival rate of 99.5%, while teeth with consistently inflamed gingiva had a 50-year survival rate of 63.4%.[51]

Critical probing depth

Using regression analysis from data from their previous studies, Lindhe et al determined the so-called critical probing depth (CPD) for SRP and MWF.[56] PDs shallower than CPD tend to lose attachment after the procedure. On the other hand, PDs above the CPD wouldn't cause further damage, and it favors CAL gain. The results showed that this value for the SRP group was 2.9 mm ± 0.4 and for the MWF group was 4.2 mm ± 0.2.[56] Later, Heitz-Mayfield and Lang further analyzed the data from SRP and access flap surgery and proposed another CPD of 5.4 mm, indicating that flap surgery is recommended mainly when PD is ≥ 5.4 mm, while SRP is preferred between 2.9 mm and 5.4 mm.[57]

Conclusions from Swedish longitudinal studies

- Adequate levels of oral hygiene maintained by the patients are more critical than the mode of therapy used.
- An equal response can be achieved for sites with initial PD > 3 mm with both surgical and nonsurgical therapy.

TABLE 10-10 Summary of Swedish studies

Publication	Number of participants	Follow-up (y)	Treatment modalities	Main outcomes
Rosling et al[51] (1976)	50	2	APF/WF with or without OS, GV	Most favorable healing in sites without bone resection and when there was complete bone coverage. Better OH resulted in more CAL gain.
Rosling[53] (1983)	50	4	APF/WF with or without OS, GV	Periodontal status could be maintained over time regardless of initial surgical approach if vigorous plaque control was maintained.
Lindhe et al[52] (1982)	15	2	SRP, SRP + MWF	CAL improved after SRP at 6 and 12 months but returned to baseline at 24 months. Single-rooted teeth had better results than multirooted teeth. Greater CAL gain in deeper pockets with MWF.
Lindhe et al[54] (1984)	15	5	SRP, SRP + MWF	No differences in PD reduction or CAL gain between the two groups. Patients with good OH had more reduction in PD and greater CAL gain.

WF, Widman flap; OS, ostectomy; GV, gingivectomy; OH, oral hygiene.

TABLE 10-11 Summary of Denmark studies

Publication	Number of participants	Follow-up	Treatment modalities	Main outcomes
Isidor et al[58] (1984)	17	6 m	SRP, MWF, APF	SRP showed some PD reduction, surgery resulted in more PD reduction. Slightly more CAL gain with SRP than with surgical treatment.
Isidor and Karring[59] (1986)	16	5 y	SRP, MWF, APF	PD reduction maintained with all treatments. Slight CAL loss (0–0.2 mm) seen in surgically treated sites, slight CAL gain (0.3 mm) in SRP sites over 5 years.

DENMARK STUDIES

Isidor et al studied the effects of SRP, MWF, and APF in single-rooted teeth with a split-mouth design and followed the patients for 5 years. During the first 6 months, patients were recalled every 2 weeks after surgery. At 6 months, SRP resulted in considerable reduction in PD, but surgical treatments resulted in more shallow pockets.[58] Results from the Denmark studies are summarized in Table 10-11.[58,59]

Conclusions from Denmark longitudinal studies

- At 1-year follow-up, only MWF resulted in coronal regrowth of bone in angular bony defects (0.5 mm).
- Scaling at frequent recalls is an important factor in arresting the progression of the disease. No correlation was found between oral hygiene and recurrence of periodontitis.

Conclusions

Most longitudinal studies discussed in this chapter support and validate that excellent clinical results can be achieved with SRP and many modalities of surgical treatment. Also, these results can be maintained in the long term with regular maintenance recalls. As highlighted in the Swedish studies, the patient's oral hygiene and plaque control play a major role in maintaining periodontal stability. It is important to mention that although these studies presented with several limitations, the bulk of evidence collected during the conduction of these investigations significantly influenced and defined the progression of the field of periodontology. To date, these investigations continue serving as a guide for treatment planning and proper selection of therapeutic approach.

References

1. Widman L. The operative treatment of pyorrhea alveolaris: A new surgical method. Sven. Tandlakar Tidske Suppl 1918;338:853–860.
2. Neumann R. Die Alveolar-Pyorrhoe und ihre Behandlung: Erfahrungen und therapeutische. Winke aus der Praxis. Berlin: Meusser, 1912.
3. Kirkland O. The suppurative periodontal pus pocket; its treatment by the modified flap operation. J Am Dent Assoc 1931;18:1462–1470.
4. Friedman N. Mucogingival Surgery: The apically repositioned flap. J Periodontol 1962;33:328–340.
5. Frisch J, Jones RA, Bhaskar SN. Conservation of maxillary anterior esthetics: A modified surgical approach. J Periodontol 1967;38:11–17.
6. American Academy of Periodontology. Glossary of Periodontal Terms. American Academy of Periodontology, 2001.
7. Ramfjord SP, Nissle RR. The modified Widman flap. J Periodontol 1974;45:601–607.
8. Schluger S. Osseous resection; a basic principle in periodontal surgery. Oral Surg Oral Med Oral Pathol 1949;2:316–325.
9. Goldman H, Cohen DW. The infrabony pocket: Classification and treatment. J Periodontol 1958;29:272–291.
10. Ochsenbein C, Bohannan HM. The palatal approach to osseous surgery II. Clinical application. J Periodontol 1964;35:54–68.
11. Yukna RA, Bowers GM, Lawrence JJ, Fedi PF Jr. A clinical study of healing in humans following the excisional new attachment procedure. J Periodontol 1976;47:696–700.
12. Yukna RA. Longitudinal evaluation of the excisional new attachment procedure in humans. J Periodontol 1978;49:142–144.
13. Yukna RA, Williams JE Jr. Five year evaluation of the excisional new attachment procedure. J Periodontol 1980;51:382–385.
14. Gregg RH II, McCarthy DK [inventors]. Millennium Dental Technologies, assignee. Laser excisional new attachment procedure. US patent 5,642,997. 1 July 1997.
15. Gregg RH, McCarthy DK. Laser ENAP for periodontal bone regeneration. Dent Today 1998;17:88–91.
16. Behdin S, Monje A, Lin GH, Edwards B, Othman A, Wang HL. Effectiveness of laser application for periodontal surgical therapy: Systematic review and meta-analysis. J Periodontol 2015;86:1352–1363.
17. Chambrone L, Ramos UD, Reynolds MA. Infrared lasers for the treatment of moderate to severe periodontitis: An American Academy of Periodontology best evidence review. J Periodontol 2018;89:743–765.
18. Ramfjord SP, Nissle RR, Shick RA, Cooper H Jr. Subgingival curettage versus surgical elimination of periodontal pockets. J Periodontol 1968;39:167–175.
19. Ramfjord SP, Knowles JW, Nissle RR, Burgett FG, Shick RA. Results following three modalities of periodontal therapy. J Periodontol 1975;46:522–526.
20. Hill RW, Ramfjord SP, Morrison EC, et al. Four types of periodontal treatment compared over two years. J Periodontol 1981;52:655–662.
21. Ramfjord SP, Caffesse RG, Morrison EC, et al. 4 modalities of periodontal treatment compared over 5 years. J Clin Periodontol 1987;14:445–452.
22. Knowles JW, Burgett FG, Nissle RR, Shick RA, Morrison EC, Ramfjord SP. Results of periodontal treatment related to pocket depth and attachment level. Eight years. J Periodontol 1979;50:225–233.
23. Ramfjord SP, Morrison EC, Burgett FG, et al. Oral hygiene and maintenance of periodontal support. J Periodontol 1982;53:26–30.
24. Ramfjord SP. Maintenance care for treated periodontitis patients. J Clin Periodontol 1987;14:433–437.
25. Fleszar TJ, Knowles JW, Morrison EC, Burgett FG, Nissle RR, Ramfjord SP. Tooth mobility and periodontal therapy. J Clin Periodontol 1980;7:495–505.
26. Pihlstrom BL, Ortiz-Campos C, McHugh RB. A randomized four-years study of periodontal therapy. J Periodontol 1981;52:227–242.
27. Pihlstrom BL, McHugh RB, Oliphant TH, Ortiz-Campos C. Comparison of surgical and nonsurgical treatment of periodontal disease. A review of current studies and additional results after 6½ years. J Clin Periodontol 1983;10:524–541.
28. Pihlstrom BL, Oliphant TH, McHugh RB. Molar and nonmolar teeth compared over 6½ years following two methods of periodontal therapy. J Periodontol 1984;55:499–504.
29. Kaldahl WB, Kalkwarf KL, Patil KD, Molvar MP, Dyer JK. Long-term evaluation of periodontal therapy: II. Incidence of sites breaking down. J Periodontol 1996;67:103–108.
30. Kaldahl WB, Kalkwarf KL, Patil KD, Dyer JK, Bates RE Jr. Evaluation of four modalities of periodontal therapy. Mean probing depth, probing attachment level and recession changes. J Periodontol 1988;59:783–793.
31. Kaldahl WB, Kalkwarf KL, Patil KD, Molvar MP, Dyer JK. Long-term evaluation of periodontal therapy: I. Response to 4 therapeutic modalities. J Periodontol 1996;67:93–102.
32. Kaldahl WB, Johnson GK, Patil KD, Kalkwarf KL. Levels of cigarette consumption and response to periodontal therapy. J Periodontol 1996;67:675–681.
33. Badersten A, Nilvéus R, Egelberg J. Effect of nonsurgical periodontal therapy. I. Moderately advanced periodontitis. J Clin Periodontol 1981;8:57–72.
34. Badersten A, Nilvéus R, Egelberg J. Effect of nonsurgical periodontal therapy. II. Severely advanced periodontitis. J Clin Periodontol 1984;11:63–76.
35. Badersten A, Nilvéus R, Egelberg J. Effect of nonsurgical periodontal therapy. III. Single versus repeated instrumentation. J Clin Periodontol 1984;11:114–124.
36. Badersten A, Nilvéus R, Egelberg J. Effect of non-surgical periodontal therapy (IV). Operator variability. J Clin Periodontol 1985;12:190–200.
37. Badersten A, Nilvéus R, Egelberg J. Effect of nonsurgical periodontal therapy. V. Patterns of probing attachment loss in nonresponding sites. J Clin Periodontol 1985;12:270–282.
38. Badersten A, Nilvéus R, Egelberg J. Effect of non-surgical periodontal therapy. VI. Localization of sites with probing attachment loss. J Clin Periodontol 1985;12:351–359.
39. Badersten A, Nilvéus R, Egelberg J. Effect of nonsurgical periodontal therapy (VIII). Probing attachment changes related to clinical charactersitcs. J Clin Periodontol 1987;14:425–432.
40. Badersten A, Nivéus R, Egelberg J. 4-year observations of basic periodontal therapy. J Clin Periodontol 1987;14:438–444.
41. Nordland P, Garrett S, Kiger R, Vanooteghem R, Hutchens LH, Egelberg J. The effect of plaque control and root debridement in molar teeth. J Clin Periodontol 1987;14:231–236.
42. Cercek JF, Kiger RD, Garrett S, Egelberg J. Relative effects of plaque control and instrumentation on the clinical parameters of human periodontal disease. J Clin Periodontol 1983;10:46–56.
43. Badersten A, Nilvéus R, Egelberg J. Reproducibility of probing attachment level measurements. J Clin Periodontol 1984;11:475–485.

44. Becker W, Becker BE, Ochsenbein C, et al. A longitudinal study comparing scaling, osseous surgery and modified Widman procedures. Results after one year. J Periodontol 1988;59:351–365.
45. Becker W, Becker BE, Caffesse R, et al. A longitudinal study comparing scaling, osseous surgery, and modified Widman procedures: Results after 5 years. J Periodontol 2001;72:1675–1684.
46. Becker W, Berg L, Becker BE. The long term evaluation of periodontal treatment and maintenance in 95 patients. Int J Periodontics Restorative Dent 1984;4:54–71.
47. Becker W, Becker BE, Berg LE. Periodontal treatment without maintenance. A retrospective study in 44 patients. J Periodontol 1984;55:505–509.
48. Becker W, Berg L, Becker BE. Untreated periodontal disease: A longitudinal study. J Periodontol 1979;50:234–244.
49. Smith DH, Ammons WF Jr, Van Belle G. A longitudinal study of periodontal status comparing osseous recontouring with flap curettage. I. Results after 6 months. J Periodontol 1980;51:367–375.
50. Olsen CT, Ammons WF, van Belle G. A longitudinal study comparing apically repositioned flaps, with and without osseous surgery. Int J Periodontics Restorative Dent 1985;5:10–33.
51. Rosling B, Nyman S, Lindhe J, Jern B. The healing potential of the periodontal tissues following different techniques of periodontal surgery in plaque-free dentitions. A 2-year clinical study. J Clin Periodontol 1976;3:233–250.
52. Lindhe J, Westfelt E, Nyman S, Socransky SS, Heijl L, Bratthall G. Healing following surgical/non-surgical treatment of periodontal disease. A clinical study. J Clin Periodontol 1982;9:115–128.
53. Rosling B. Periodontally treated dentitions: Their maintenance and prognosis. Int Dent J 1983;33:147–151.
54. Lindhe J, Westfelt E, Nyman S, Socransky SS, Haffajee AD. Long-term effect of surgical/non-surgical treatment of periodontal disease. J Clin Periodontol 1984;11:448–458.
55. Lang NP, Schätzle MA, Löe H. Gingivitis as a risk factor in periodontal disease. J Clin Periodontol 2009;36(suppl 10):3–8.
56. Lindhe J, Socransky SS, Nyman S, Haffajee A, Westfelt E. "Critical probing depths" in periodontal therapy. J Clin Periodontol 1982;9:323–336.
57. Heitz-Mayfield LJA, Lang NP. Surgical and nonsurgical periodontal therapy. Learned and unlearned concepts. Periodontol 2000 2013;62:218–231.
58. Isidor F, Karring T, Attström R. The effect of root planing as compared to that of surgical treatment. J Clin Periodontol 1984;11:669–681.
59. Isidor F, Karring T. Long-term effect of surgical and non-surgical periodontal treatment. A 5-year clinical study. J Periodontal Res 1986;21:462–472.

11

SURGICAL REGENERATIVE THERAPY

Mustafa Tattan, BDS

DEFINITIONS AND TERMINOLOGY

Bone fill: The restoration of bone tissue in a treated periodontal alveolar bone defect. Bone fill may be indirectly assessed clinically by increased resistance to probing and radiodensity as compared with pretreatment measurements. Bone fill does not address the presence or absence of new cementum, periodontal ligament, or alveolar bone, histologically.[14]

Graft: Any allograft, alloplast, autograft, or xenograft material placed with the intention of repair, augmentation, or regeneration of a defect or deficiency.[14]

Guided tissue regeneration: A surgical procedure with the goal of achieving new bone, cementum, and periodontal ligament (PDL) attachment to a periodontally diseased tooth, using barrier devices or membranes to provide space maintenance, epithelial exclusion, and wound stabilization.[14]

Osseous defect: A reduction or deficiency of the bony architecture around teeth and implants caused by disease or trauma; can be intrabony or interradicular in nature.[14]

When periodontal tissues are lost to destructive disease processes, a compound of structures and cellular entities are involved. These correspond to the complex connective tissue structure of the periodontium, comprised of the gingival lamina propria, periodontal ligament (PDL), cementum, and alveolar bone. As such, it is imperative for the clinician to have a comprehensive understanding of the individual cellular players prior to contemplating a regenerative strategy. This will allow the clinician to best manipulate the behavioral properties of each component for the purpose of periodontal regeneration.

Decades ago, it was discovered that compartmentalizing the various cell sources within the periodontium during regenerative procedures would best serve the wound healing process, resulting in a resemblance as close as possible to the natural periodontal architecture. Based on this, in 1976, Melcher reported on the varying migratory profiles of the gingival, osteogenic, and PDL cells and proposed that, given the gingival cells' capacity to beat the osteogenic cells restricting the process of bone formation, regeneration of all periodontal components by wound compartmentalization would not be overoptimistic.[1] Later on, in the 1980s, a number of studies pioneered the exploration of this phenomenon, often referred to as *controlled repopulation*. With the use of animal models and a handful of case reports, these investigations frequently observed a considerable amount of new attachment.[2–13] It was through identifying differences in cellular characteristics, and the pivotal role that they play in ensuring attachment apparatus regeneration, that the surgical technique known as **guided tissue regeneration** (GTR) was born (Fig 11-1).

Criteria and Rationale for GTR

The basic concept behind GTR is enabling the regeneration of the desired tissues accompanied by simultaneous prevention of unwanted cellular infiltration. When an exposed root surface is repopulated with cells, those of epithelial origin result in the formation of a long junctional epithelium,

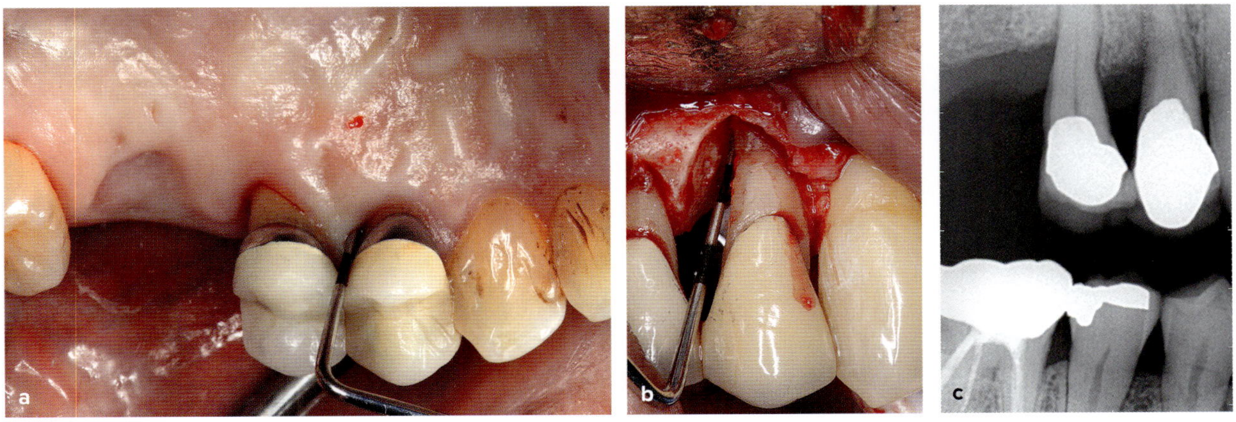

Fig 11-1 Guided tissue regeneration. *(a)* Preoperative probing depth. *(b)* Intraoperative photograph illustrating the depth of the defect. *(c)* Radiographic evaluation at 6-month follow-up. (Courtesy of Dr Vahid Khoshkam.)

those of gingival connective tissue origin result in root resorption, those of osseous origin result in ankylosis, and those of PDL origin result in regenerated attachment.[15]

In periodontics, the knowledge acquired about cellular behavior in this capacity is the result of research experimenting with a great number of diverse biologic environments (Table 11-1).[2,5,6,8,9] Nyman et al introduced the use of a barrier membrane for periodontal regeneration (known as the *Millipore filter* at the time).[6,8] In these investigations, as well as others that followed,[2,9,11,13] new connective tissue attachment—often associated with cementum deposition and fiber insertion—was regenerated with the use of a barrier membrane.

One of the questions addressed by these early studies had been whether or not new connective tissue attachment could be regenerated on surfaces that previously harbored plaque. In 1984, Gottlow et al designed an experimental animal model whereby alveolar bone buccal to the roots was removed to a level that constituted 50% to 75% of their total length.[2] Later, the overlying soft tissue flap was repositioned in a manner that would permit exposure of the roots to plaque accumulation for the following 6 months. When the plaque-accumulation phase was completed, the roots were thoroughly scaled and cleared of the cemental layer, their corresponding crowns resected, and their canals filled. Prior to submerging all the roots below the extended buccal soft tissue flap, a barrier membrane was used to blanket the experimental group while the control group was left in direct contact with the inner surface of the flap. The findings revealed that regenerating new attachment can surely be achieved on former plaque-harboring surfaces, and more so with the use of a barrier membrane (0.9 to 6.8 mm) than without it (0.0 to 2.5 mm). Notably, the authors reported a higher frequency and magnitude of root resorption associated with the control group, emphasized by the presence of multinucleated cells and resorption cavities under microscopic magnification.[2]

It was not long after initiating this series of investigations that the same research group tested the promising findings of animal models on a clinical root surface inflicted with periodontitis.[9] The selected case was a mandibular incisor with a deep angular defect. Following adequate instrumentation of the root surface, a Millipore filter was coronally stabilized to the facial enamel with resin and positioned between the exposed root surface and the flap. The authors observed substantial amounts of bone within the angular defect site as well as a layer of newly formed cementum—with inserting collagen fibers—well beyond the most apical boundary of prior instrumentation.

These early discoveries had illuminated the path toward the clinical applicability of GTR, setting the foundation for subsequent research that would broaden the understanding of periodontal regeneration and improve technique efficacy over the next decades. Research today has expanded the previously limited window to periodontal regeneration by characterizing clinical indications, such as intrabony[16] and furcation[17] defects, as well as technique diversification with the use of peptides/proteins, scaffold systems, lasers, stem cells, and gene therapy.[18] The most fundamental component of GTR is the barrier membrane (Fig 11-2), while other constituents (eg, bone **grafts** and biologics) have been added with technique development.

TABLE 11-1 Landmark investigations that provided early insight into GTR at previously diseased and nondiseased root surfaces

Year	Authors	Sample	Barrier type	Main findings
1980	Nyman et al[6]	1 dog + 2 monkeys	NA (root embedded within bone and CT)	No new fibrous attachment on previously exposed root surface in contact with CT. Fibrous reattachment on previously exposed root surface with preserved PDL tissue.
1980	Karring et al[5]	3 dogs	NA (root embedded within bone and CT)	No new CT attachment on previously exposed root surface. Instead, healing occurred via root resorption and ankylosis. Functional attachment apparatus reformed on previously exposed root surface with preserved PDL tissue.
1982	Nyman et al[8]	3 monkeys	Millipore filter	New cementum with inserted collagen fibers at the middle and apical regions of curetted surfaces. CT adhesion with no new cementum at the coronal region of the surfaces.
1982	Nyman et al[9]	1 human	Millipore filter	New cementum with inserted collagen fibers on previously periodontally diseased root surface.
1984	Gottlow et al[2]	3 monkeys	Millipore filter	New cementum with inserted collagen fibers on previously exposed root surface. Considerably greater attachment occurred below a Millipore filter compared with a flap alone.

CT, connective tissue; NA, not applicable.

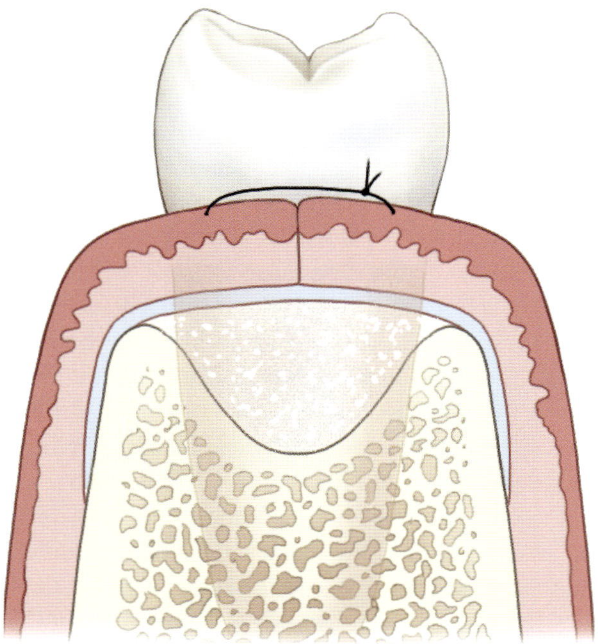

Fig 11-2 Illustration of GTR and the pivotal role of the barrier membrane.

Barrier Membranes

Barrier membranes in GTR have progressively evolved since the utilization of cellulose ester Millipore filters. While the primary role of a membrane—maximizing the natural potential for regeneration by preventing unwanted cellular infiltration—is often served by all the different types available, some secondary, scenario-specific roles remain contingent on the material composition or construct of the membrane.

Broadly speaking, the barrier membrane composition can be classified into synthetic or nonsynthetic and absorbable or nonabsorbable. These categorizing terms refer to material source for synthetic/nonsynthetic and degradational interaction within bodily tissues for absorbable/nonabsorbable. Based on these general characteristics, the membrane of choice pertaining to varying clinical scenarios will be at the operator's discretion based on benefits and limitations associated with each type of membrane. The different aspects to be considered are enumerated in Table 11-2. Generally, in an extensive number of clinical investigations, membrane usage has demonstrated considerable clinical advantages in the treatment of furcation and intrabony defects.[16,17]

TABLE 11-2 Key characteristics of absorbable and nonabsorbable membranes used for GTR

	Nonabsorbable	Absorbable
Examples	• Millipore filter • PTFE • ePTFE • Titanium mesh	• Collagen membrane • PLA/PGA • Acellular dermal matrix • Allografts
Space-making capability	Greater	Poor
Bacterial resistance	Greater	Lesser
Cell attachment and proliferation	Lesser	Greater
Biologic properties	Biocompatible	Biocompatible
	Biologically inert	Biologically interactive
	Requires second surgery for membrane retrieval	Enables biodegradability
Incidence of postoperative exposure	Greater	Lesser
Sources	Synthetic and nonsynthetic	
Other	NA	Modifiable properties through additional chemical treatment

PTFE, polytetrafluoroethylene; ePTFE, expanded polytetrafluoroethylene; PLA, polylactic acid; PGA; polyglycolic acid; NA, not applicable. *Green*, advantages; *Red*, disadvantages.

Despite inherent differences due to the source and degradation properties, a set of requisite characteristics correspond to any membrane that is to be considered clinically viable. Briefly, these include biocompatibility[19]; maintenance of vascularity[20,21]; cell occlusiveness at the membrane superstratum[21]; cell migration, attachment, proliferation, and differentiation at the membrane substratum[20]; bacterial resistance[22]; and space-making capability.[23] Apart from these main membrane properties that apply to absorbable and nonabsorbable membranes alike, a more discrete set of traits entails each class.

NONABSORBABLE MEMBRANES

Although the Millipore filter was the first employed membrane and was able to support bone and cementum with inserting collagen fibers in the unprecedented phase of GTR research,[9] it has not remained as the most commonly used nonabsorbable membrane. First introduced in 1985 as a plausible alternative to Millipore filters, expanded polytetrafluoroethylene (ePTFE) has since become the most well-documented nonabsorbable membrane. As such, when research showed that the permucosally placed filters were readily contaminated and did not present the correct porosity to allow for epithelial ingrowth and wound stability, ePTFE rose to the occasion.[23]

These ePTFE membranes were used in an early case series and were reportedly associated with mean bone and attachment gain of 5.1 and 5.6 mm, respectively.[12] Though limited to a sample size of only 12 patients, Gottlow et al demonstrated proof-of-principle findings in two distinct clinical scenarios: angular and furcation defects.[12] Similar outcomes were substantiated by robust clinical research, indicating 4 to more than 6 mm of attachment gain and significant **bone fill** in the treatment of intrabony defects.[24,25] With regard to furcation defects, Kinaia et al[26] reported in a 2011 meta-analysis that the use of nonabsorbable membranes in GTR at Class II furcation defects was superior to open flap debridement (OFD). The authors reported differences of 1.41 ± 0.46 mm, 1.16 ± 0.29 mm, and 0.58 ± 0.11 mm in vertical clinical attachment gain, horizontal bone fill, and vertical bone fill, respectively.[26]

The ePTFE membrane also presents with a modified form known as the *titanium-reinforced ePTFE*, wherein a pliable titanium framework is embedded within the ePTFE material. The malleability of the titanium allows for greater adaptation of the membrane to certain defects. Although these are not as common, they can be used in cases of wide and/or nonsupportive defects to provide better space-maintaining capabilities.[27]

Given the limitations that present with the use of nonabsorbable membranes—namely the need for a second surgical procedure and greater incidence of postoperative complications—absorbable membranes have become the more popular option for GTR today.

ABSORBABLE MEMBRANES

Membranes characterized by their interactive, degradational nature within biologic environments, also known as *absorbable membranes*, were developed when certain limitations of nonabsorbable membranes were encountered.[27,28] The primary drawback of nonabsorbable membranes is the need for a second surgery, which may potentially jeopardize newly formed tissues.[29,30]

Absorbable membranes were initially classified into *collagen-based* and *polymer-based* membranes. Collagen membranes are commonly derived from bovine or porcine origin, while polymers are chemically synthesized aliphatic polyesters.[19] With collagen, the degradation process is the result of host collagenase activity elicited subsequent to membrane implantation. Experimental advancements have allowed for the treatment of these biomaterials in order to diminish antigenicity and reduce collagenase activity (thereby modifying degradation kinetics).[19,31]

Conversely, polymer-based membranes are absorbed into bodily tissues as a result of hydrolytic activity.[19] Polymers used to make absorbable membranes include polyglycolic acid (PGA) and polylactic acid (PLA).[32,33] A PGA-PLA copolymer, commonly referred to as *polyglactin 910* due to the 9:1 PGA:PLA ratio, was also later developed.[34–36] Advantages of polymer-based membranes over collagen membranes include a wider range of potentially manufacturable properties, reproducibility due to finely controlled conditions, and relatively undemanding large-scale production.

Some of the more recently presented absorbable materials for GTR include allografts, such as an acellular dermal matrix (ADM)[37] and amniotic membrane,[38,39] as well as xenogeneic pericardium.[40,41] Apart from being easily manipulated and adapted to periodontal defects, absorbable membranes have demonstrated regenerative applicability; both collagen[3,42–45] and polymer-based membranes[46–51] alike. A substantial amount of clinical attachment level (CAL) gain at intrabony defects has been reported to reach up to 3.6 ± 1.5 mm when absorbable membranes are used.[27] It is noteworthy to mention that, in this report, polymers had achieved superior outcomes compared to collagen membranes (CAL gain of 4.1 ± 1.6 mm vs 3.0 ± 1.7).[27] As for furcation—and specifically the predictable Class II—defects, although the adaptability of absorbable membranes may pose some difficulty depending on the defect morphology,[17] systematic reviews have confirmed considerable attachment gain associated with their use.[26,52] A CAL gain of 1.39 mm, horizontal bone fill of 1.85 mm, and vertical bone fill of 1.49 mm was reported when absorbable membranes were used for Class II furcation defects.[26]

Bone Grafting Materials

In addition to barrier membranes, the use of biomaterials, including bone grafts, has been integrated into GTR since the conception of the technique. A diverse set of bone grafts has been employed with varying degrees of clinical outcomes.[17,53] The biologic rationale behind using bone grafts with GTR is to maximize the regenerative potential via osteoinduction and/or osteoconduction and blood clot stabilization.[30] The most commonly used and well-documented grafting materials are discussed in the following sections and summarized in Table 11-3.[54–73] (See also the "Grafting Alternatives" section in chapter 20.)

AUTOGRAFTS

An osseous *autograft*, or autogenous bone, refers to bone that is transferred from one site to another within the same individual for the purpose of grafting. Though autogenous bone bears several limitations, it is considered the gold standard because it is osteogenic, osteoinductive, and osteoconductive.

Early on, autogenous bone that was used for periodontal defect regeneration was harvested from extraoral sites, such as the tibia, iliac crest, rib, and calvarium.[74–77] Despite having demonstrated some clinical success,[78] these sources have become obsolete due to impracticality and cost as well as the more reasonable alternative that had emerged: intraoral sites.

Bone has been harvested from several intraoral sites, including maxillary tuberosities, the mandibular ramus and symphysis, exostoses, postextraction sites, and edentulous ridges.[55,79–81] Varying methods[82] through which these grafts were procured and prepared have been reported, namely as cortical bone chips via osteoplasty or ostectomy,[54] osseous coagulum (cortical bone chips mixed in the patient's blood),[81] a mix of harvested cortical and cancellous bone,[83] and via bone swaging.[84] Several studies have demonstrated successful use of

TABLE 11-3 Bone grafting materials used in combination with GTR procedures

Type	Sources/subtypes	Brand name (manufacturer)	Evidence
Autograft	• Tibia • Iliac crest • Rib • Calvarium • Maxillary tuberosity • Mandibular ramus • Exostoses • Alveolar ridge • Mental symphysis	NA	• Nabers and O'Leary[54] (1965) • Hiatt and Schallhorn[55] (1973) • Rosenberg[56] (1971)
Allograft	• Freeze-dried bone allograft • Demineralized freeze-dried bone allograft	• Puros (Zimmer Biomet) • MinerOss (Biohorizons) • Creos allo.gain (Nobel Biocare) • AlloOss (ACE Surgical Supply)	• Dragoo and Kaldahl[57] (1983) • Sanders et al[58] (1983) • Mellonig[59] (1991) • Bowers et al[60–62] (1989) • Rummelhart et al[63] (1989)
Xenograft	• Bovine • Porcine • Equine	• Bio-Oss (Geistlich) • Creos xenogain (Nobel Biocare) • NuOss (ACE Surgical Supply)	• Skoglund et al[64] (1997) • Richardson et al[65] (1999)
Alloplast	• Hydroxyapatite • β-tricalcium phosphate • Calcium sulfate • Bioactive glass • Polymers	• Pro Osteon (Zimmer Biomet) • PerioGlas (NovaBone) • Biogran (Zimmer Biomet) • SynthoGraft (Bicon) • IngeniOs (Zimmer Biomet) • GraftSet (Salvin) • CalMatrix (Lifecore Biomedical) • Symbios OsteoGraf (Dentsply Sirona) • Biocoral (Biocoral)	• AlGhamdi et al[66] (2010) • Meffert et al[67] (1985) • Bowen et al[68] (1989) • Stahl and Froum[69] (1987) • Stahl and Froum[70] (1986) • Nery and Lynch[71] (1978) • Ong et al[72] (1998) • Nevins et al[73] (2000)

NA, not applicable.

autogenous bone for periodontal regeneration, reporting notable bone fill,[55,56] and its use remains in practice today, often combined with allogeneic and xenogeneic grafts.

ALLOGRAFTS

An osseous *allograft* refers to bone that is transferred from one individual to another within the same species for the purpose of grafting. All types of allografts are osteoconductive, while only a distinct class—demineralized freeze-dried bone allografts (DFDBA)—may potentially possess osteoinductive properties as well.[85,86] Grafts that are harvested from other individuals are treated and preserved in a manner that nearly eliminates all potential for disease transfer.[87–90] The two primary classes of allografts are the following[85]:

- *Freeze-dried bone allografts (FDBA):* This class of allografts loses cell viability during preparation and hence only acts as a scaffold for cellular infiltration that is later replaced by new bone. Due to its mineral content, it appears radiopaque in radiographic assessments.[85] Early reports have suggested that the use of FDBA results in formation of long junctional epithelium as opposed to true periodontal regeneration.[57] Despite this, studies have repeatedly demonstrated defect fill using this allograft, obtaining even better outcomes when used in combination with autogenous bone.[58,59]
- *Demineralized freeze-dried bone allografts (DFDBA):* This class of allografts also lacks cell viability; however, in the demineralization process, it releases a growth factor known as *bone morphogenetic protein (BMP)*, among others.[91,92] First discovered in 1965, and further

researched in 1971, BMPs actively recruit pluripotent cells and stimulate their differentiation into bone-forming cellular profiles.[93–95] Whether or not DFDBA can predictably induce bone formation has been questioned because of several factors: *(1)* the influence of age on its function,[96] *(2)* an insufficient amount of BMP release in light of the clinical demand, and *(3)* varying degrees of bone formation between different commercially available DFDBAs.[97–99] A series of investigations by Bowers et al histologically verified true periodontal regeneration at intrabony defects using DFDBA,[60–62] rendering their use in surgical regenerative therapy viable.

The clinical performance of FDBA and DFDBA have been directly compared with each other, yielding similar outcomes.[63] The mean **osseous defect** repair observed between the two materials was 1.7 mm for DFDBA and 2.4 for FDBA. Similarly, mean CAL gain attributed to DFDBA was 1.7 mm, compared to 2.0 mm ascribed to FDBA.[63]

XENOGRAFTS

An osseous *xenograft* refers to bone that is transferred from an individual of a different species for the purpose of grafting. Xenografts are merely osteoconductive, serving as scaffolds that allow for bone formation in their vicinity but not to be replaced by newly formed bone.[64] These are of bovine or porcine origin and undergo treatment in order to eliminate disease transmission and graft rejection. Although xenografts have previously obtained pocket reduction, attachment gain, and bone fill comparable with that achieved by DFDBA when treating intrabony defects,[65] there is a lack of evidence that true periodontal regeneration is exhibited.

ALLOPLASTS

An osseous *alloplast* refers to a synthetic material that is employed as a space filler within an osseous defect for the purpose of defect repair. It is generally evidenced that alloplasts do not possess any innate regenerative capacity; they only act as a readily available biologic filler that promotes repair as opposed to regeneration.[66,100] Common examples of such agents include hydroxyapatite (HA) products,[67–69,101] β-tricalcium phosphate (β-TCP),[70,71,102] bioactive glass,[72,73] and certain polymers. These materials are not typically used in routine practice, and evidence concerning their clinical performance remains limited.

Biologics

The most recent additions to GTR are biologics. In essence, these materials are reservoirs of human cytokines, growth factors, and/or other protein products that are expected to improve early wound healing and overall tissue regeneration. These occur as a result of a given agent facilitating different cellular processes—mainly differentiation, proliferation, and migration. While many biologics with this claim have surfaced across the market today, among the most commonly used and researched are platelet-rich plasma (PRP), recombinant human platelet-derived growth factor (rhPDGF), synthetic peptide binding protein P-15, and enamel matrix derivative (EMD). Overall, these biologics are extensively used in GTR today.

In terms of rhPDGF, although initial evidence presented promising potential,[103,104] a reliable quantity of data supporting superior clinical outcomes remains scarce. One multicenter randomized controlled trial showed better clinical outcomes with rhPDGF, yielding up to 4.3 mm of CAL gain.[105] EMD has also demonstrated significantly superior CAL gain when compared to OFD; however, the beneficial impact was diminished when compared to EMD with grafting material and/or a barrier membrane.[18]

Clinical Considerations and Outcomes

With GTR being applied to multiple clinical scenarios and coupled with various materials, technique applicability and outcome predictability come with a multitude of clinical considerations. For both intrabony and furcation defects, alternative techniques to GTR as well as varying GTR approaches have been compared and investigated in the literature. In 2011, Bashutski et al published a decision tree that aids with intrabony defect treatment planning based on defect angle, depth, and number of remaining walls. Additionally, the authors recommended treatment of Class II furcation defects based on interproximal bone, vertical and horizontal defect depth, and interradicular separation.[106] A more recent decision tree for the assessment of intrabony defects was published by Kao et al, following the 2015 American Academy of Periodontology Regeneration Workshop. This decision tree, however, mainly focused on arriving at treatment selection between a regenerative approach instead of nonsurgical management, osseous surgery with resection, or tooth replacement.[16]

Concerning intrabony defects treated with GTR, the collection of all clinical evidence until 1997, summarized in a systematic review,[27] demonstrated attachment gain of 3.86 ± 1.69 mm. The conclusions of those investigations indicated that deeper defects benefited most from GTR procedures, with defects deeper than 3 mm consistently culminating in superior clinical gains than their shallower counterparts.[27] Additionally, defect dimensions of 25 degrees or smaller were deemed most plausible in achieving positive outcomes following regenerative therapy.[16]

In contrast with intrabony defects, little evidence is available advocating clinical and/or histologic success as periodontal destruction progresses past a Class II furcation. However, sufficient evidence is available from histologic and clinical investigations regarding the success of regenerative procedures in the treatment of maxillary (facial or interproximal) and mandibular (facial or lingual) Class II furcation defects.[17]

GTR VERSUS OFD

Intrabony defects

A 2003 systematic review reported significantly superior clinical outcomes pertaining to GTR over OFD. The primary outcomes reported were CAL gain, probing depth (PD) reduction, and gingival recession (REC) reduction.[52] These superior outcomes of GTR compared to OFD were later validated in a 2006 Cochrane systematic review and meta-analysis reporting a CAL gain difference of 1.22 mm, PD reduction difference of 1.21 mm, and postoperative REC difference of 0.26 mm favoring GTR over OFD.[107] Both these reviews are in concordance with the findings of Cortellini and Tonetti, who reported CAL gains of 3.4 ± 1.8 mm and 1.8 ± 1.4 mm for GTR and OFD, respectively.[27] These conclusions were also corroborated by the 2015 systematic review following the American Academy of Periodontology Regeneration Workshop, deeming GTR superior to OFD with regard to PD reduction, CAL gain, and REC reduction.[16] Moreover, GTR was also presented as a viable option in the treatment of defects that are noncontained or possess an unfavorable architecture.[108] When compared with OFD, the usage of GTR in noncontained defects resulted in significantly better outcomes, bearing a mean 2.89 mm of CAL gain.

Furcation defects

In 2015, Avila-Ortiz et al[17] evaluated the outcomes of previous systematic reviews, all showing results in favor of GTR over OFD in the treatment of maxillary and mandibular Class II furcation defects,[26,52,100,109–111] with limited evidence deeming regenerative therapy in Class III furcation defects a viable therapeutic approach. The difference in outcome measures between GTR and OFD were estimated to be 0.73 ± 0.92 mm in vertical PD reduction, 0.62 ± 1.53 mm in vertical probing attachment level gain, 0.72 ± 1.55 mm in horizontal bone fill, and 0.58 ± 1.46 mm in vertical bone fill.[26,52,109,111] This American Academy of Periodontology Regeneration Workshop systematic review substantiated the conclusion of GTR being superior to OFD, also highlighting that therapeutic success can be achieved in cases of Class I furcation defects via nonregenerative approaches.[17]

GTR WITH ABSORBABLE VERSUS NONABSORBABLE MEMBRANES

Intrabony defects

In the year 2000, a review reported weighted means of CAL gain equivalent to 3.7 ± 1.8 mm and 3.6 ± 1.5 mm attributed to GTR with nonabsorbable and absorbable membranes, respectively. This report, the result of 592 intrabony defects pooled from 17 studies, had highlighted comparable predictability between the use of either membrane type.[27] A long-term clinical investigation and two reviews also reported comparable outcomes for *(1)* PLA and polyglactin 910 versus ePTFE,[52] *(2)* polylactic-polyglycolic acid (PLG/PLA) and collagen versus ePTFE,[112] *(3)* and PLG/PLA versus collagen versus ePTFE[113] membranes. These outcomes were based on CAL gain,[52,112,113] PD reduction, and resultant REC.[52,113]

Furcation defects

This comparison was closely evaluated by two meta-analyses.[26,52] In the earlier of the two studies by Murphy and Gunsolley, absorbable membranes demonstrated significantly better outcomes in vertical probing attachment level for the treatment of Class II furcation defects but comparable outcomes in terms of vertical PD. The authors reported these aforementioned findings with no overall difference between the barrier types.[52] Similarly, in the treatment of Class II furcation defects, Kinaia et al[26] reported "modest" superiority for absorbable over nonabsorbable membranes: 0.25 mm vertical PD reduction, 0.39 mm CAL gain, 0.29 mm horizontal bone fill, and 0.77 mm vertical bone fill. The expected clinical outcomes according to this meta-analysis are 2.07 mm vertical PD reduction, 1.39 mm CAL gain, 1.85 mm horizontal bone fill, and 1.49 mm vertical bone fill via absorbable membranes. And, correspondingly, 1.77 mm vertical PD reduction, 1.35 mm CAL gain, 1.54 mm horizontal bone fill, and 0.75 mm vertical bone fill are expected via nonabsorbable membranes.[26] These findings once again support that the use of both types of membranes in the regeneration of Class II furcation defects report comparable results with regard to clinical outcomes.

GTR WITH OR WITHOUT GRAFTING MATERIAL

Intrabony defects

Following the conduction of two systematic reviews[100,114] based on the limited available evidence, the use of bone grafts with barrier membranes for GTR seemed to not provide any additional benefit over barrier membranes alone in deep defects. However, the addition of bone grafting can be useful to create a scaffold and maintain space.[30] These outcomes have also been reported by a previous meta-analysis on the topic, reporting no further enhancements in intrabony defect outcomes.[52] On the other hand, despite these general findings, the nature of the defect (contained versus noncontained) may significantly influence the potential benefit of adding bone grafting materials to the intrabony defect. For example, it may be especially useful for noncontained defects or when several walls are missing. Most studies regarding the use of bone grafts in combination with GTR have compared this approach to OFD, wherein the clinical outcomes are largely in favor of GTR with bone grafts.

Furcation defects

Most research investigating GTR with grafting materials compared to OFD for furcation defects reported superiority for the former over the latter.[17] In terms of GTR with or without grafting, Chen et al found that there is evident overall advantage attributed to GTR with grafting over GTR alone and/or OFD in the treatment of maxillary and mandibular Class II furcation defects.[111] Similar superior outcomes when using grafting materials were reported in two previous meta-analyses, deeming their use beneficial in GTR of Class II furcations.[26,52]

Determining Factors

Despite the reported predictability of periodontal regenerative procedures, it remains absolutely essential to practice proper case selection. Clinical success, although predictably achievable, is delicately contingent on many patient-related, defect-related, and technique-related factors. A plethora of evidence supports the impact of such factors on distinct elements of the overall clinical outcome. The most evidenced and clinically relevant of these factors, as well as the ramifications they bear, are discussed in the following sections.

PATIENT-RELATED FACTORS

Patients exhibit a combination of physiologic, environmental, behavioral, and genetic components, all of which accompany some liability for GTR outcomes.[27]

Oral hygiene

One of the prime factors influencing the outcomes of GTR is compliance with adequate oral hygiene.[16,30] Many investigations have highlighted the direct impact that the perpetual presence of plaque, bleeding on probing, and a pathogenic microbial challenge (ie, the presence of pathogenic bacteria might hinder ideal healing) have on poor clinical outcomes.[115,116] A study designed to evaluate the influence of oral hygiene in this regard[117] reported that patients who had 3-month maintenance visits exhibited stable attachment levels at 4 years. Meanwhile, the corresponding group of patients who had sporadic care lost approximately 2.8 mm of the attachment level gained across the same observational period, demonstrating a 50-fold increased risk of attachment loss compared with the former study group. More specifically with furcation defects, there is a general indication for the regenerative and nonregenerative correction of these defects when cleansability is unachievable.[110] Hence, this will also entail the necessity for adequate postsurgical oral hygiene to avoid impaired wound healing and poor long-term prognosis.[100]

Smoking

Throughout the literature on intrabony and furcation defects, cigarette smoking is highlighted as a modifiable factor that is associated with compromised clinical outcomes of regenerative procedures.[16,17] One study reported a significant difference in attachment level gained across a 1-year observational period between nonsmokers

(5.2 ± 1.9 mm) and smokers (2.1 ± 1.2 mm).[116] While there is sufficient data indicating smoking as a negative influencer of regeneration, some authors have suggested that, with appropriate postsurgical anti-infective therapy, the anticipated poor clinical outcomes can be compensated. This anti-infective therapy protocol constitutes applying 25% metronidazole gel on the outer surface of the membrane, chlorhexidine use as long as the membrane is in place, antibiotic consumption 6 to 8 weeks postoperatively, and more frequent prophylactic visits.[118]

Miscellaneous

Other factors that may negatively influence the regenerative capacity include uncontrolled diseases, such as diabetes mellitus, immunodeficiencies, and stress. However, evidence is not concrete for all such factors.[16,17,30] An additional, mildly evidenced factor is interleukin-1 gene polymorphism, reported to be uninfluencing at 1 year but greatly impacting long-term outcomes.[119]

DEFECT-RELATED FACTORS

Prior to examining defect morphology, the anatomical characteristics surrounding the defect should be carefully evaluated because these may play a role in periodontal regeneration. The amount of keratinized gingiva, as well as the gingival thickness corresponding to the region of interest, have been documented as important factors to be considered. Gingival thickness of more than 1 mm is regarded as the minimal necessary limit to achieve consistent clinical outcomes in terms of minimal resultant recession, CAL gain, and bone fill.[27,120] Similarly, baseline tooth mobility—particularly of grade III—is deleterious to periodontal regeneration and has been associated with reduced expected CAL gain.[30,121]

Intrabony defects

The baseline morphology of the defect plays a pivotal role in the final outcome of the regenerative procedure. This factor includes the depth of the defect, where a greater magnitude of improvement is expected in deeper defects. Despite superior attachment gain being anticipated in deeper defects, both shallow and deep defects possess the potential of regeneration to a level that corrects the intrabony portion.[30] An equally important morphologic feature of a defect is the width. A reported defect angle of 25 degrees or smaller was considered most plausible for predictable attachment gain than those of greater than 37 degrees.[16,30] Finally, the remaining bony walls—and more accurately the containment—is associated with greater predictability, particularly for gel formulations of biologics that would require certain containment to remain at the site of anticipated regeneration.[30]

Furcation defects

The primary factor associated with furcation defects is the extent of the furcation involvement. Additional morphologic characteristics include the root trunk length (longer trunks exhibit slightly more furcation closure), the root divergence (limiting or enabling access to the defect), as well as the vertical and horizontal dimensions of the furcation entrance in terms of remaining adjacent bone levels.[17,122]

TECHNIQUE-RELATED FACTORS

Some aspects of the operator's technique have also demonstrated a significant impact on the outcomes of regenerative procedures. Broadly, these include nonsterile technique, inadequate surgical technique, and membrane instability, among others.[123] With regard to surgical technique, Tonetti et al[116] have demonstrated that flap design can greatly influence the regenerative outcomes by showing that a modified papilla preservation[124] technique resulted in significantly greater attachment gain than a simply supracrestally positioned membrane and modified Widman flap. This flap design contributes to minimal trauma and greater wound stability. Also, maintaining a submerged membrane during the wound healing phase is crucial to maximize the regenerative capacity and avoid bacterial contamination and infection.

Postoperative Considerations

Postoperative complications are not uncommon with GTR procedures, and they include infection, pain, swelling, and suppuration.[27] However, the most frequent of all complications is certainly membrane exposure,[30] reported to occur after almost 50% of regenerative procedures in one study.[125] Several other investigations have reported the prevalence of membrane exposure and associated infection ranging between 20% to 87%.[126–130] Membrane exposure may also be a significant factor for the resultant CAL gain, where a mean difference of 0.47 mm was reported by a meta-analysis.[125] Another investigation reported no CAL gain and substantially more gingival recession associated with 26% of cases with membrane exposures within a total of 30 treated intrabony defects.[131] These effects have been attributed to bacterial colonization following exposure to the oral cavity.[115,132–136]

Another factor that has classically been associated with preventing membrane exposure is the surrounding connective tissue that fills into and anchors the external surface of the membrane.[134] This is commonly considered a result of tension-free flap adaptation and wound stability during the early phases of healing. As such, it has been suggested that flap design, and specifically the papilla preservation technique, amply reduces the incidence of membrane exposure.[126,137]

Management of membrane exposures primarily comprises adopting an anti-infective regimen. This may include antibiotic administration, antibacterial mouthrinses, and adequate infection control practice.[138] Additionally, it is recommended to retrieve a nonabsorbable membrane after exposure as a preventive measure to avoid further bacterial colonization.[106]

Conclusion

While GTR is a powerful therapeutic approach, it is nonetheless a complex process that depends on a variety of local and systemic factors. After adequate case selection based on patient and defect characteristics, favorable clinical outcomes are to be expected. Subsequently, technique selection becomes secondarily essential. Many variations of GTR, utilizing different grafting materials, biologics, and flap designs, have become popular and demonstrated clinical benefit. However, despite the employment of adequate materials and techniques, it remains crucial to respect the biologic limits of regeneration.

References

1. Melcher AH. On the repair potential of periodontal tissues. J Periodontol 1976;47:256–260.
2. Gottlow J, Nyman S, Karring T, Lindhe J. New attachment formation as the result of controlled tissue regeneration. J Clin Periodontol 1984;11:494–503.
3. Blumenthal NM. The use of collagen membranes to guide regeneration of new connective tissue attachment in dogs. J Periodontol 1988;59:830–836.
4. Caton J, Nyman S, Zander H. Histometric evaluation of periodontal surgery. II. Connective tissue attachment levels after four regenerative procedures. J Clin Periodontol 1980;7:224–231.
5. Karring T, Nyman S, Lindhe J. Healing following implantation of periodontitis affected roots into bone tissue. J Clin Periodontol 1980;7:96–105.
6. Nyman S, Karring T, Lindhe J, Plantén S. Healing following implantation of periodontitis-affected roots into gingival connective tissue. J Clin Periodontol 1980;7:394–401.
7. Boyko GA, Melcher AH, Brunette DM. Formation of new periodontal ligament by periodontal ligament cells implanted in vivo after culture in vitro. A preliminary study of transplanted roots in the dog. J Periodontal Res 1981;16:73–88.
8. Nyman S, Gottlow J, Karring T, Lindhe J. The regenerative potential of the periodontal ligament. An experimental study in the monkey. J Clin Periodontol 1982;9:257–265.
9. Nyman S, Lindhe J, Karring T, Rylander H. New attachment following surgical treatment of human periodontal disease. J Clin Periodontol 1982;9:290–296.
10. Polson AM, Caton J. Factors influencing periodontal repair and regeneration. J Periodontol 1982;53:617–625.
11. Aukhil I, Simpson DM, Schaberg TV. An experimental study of new attachment procedure in beagle dogs. J Periodontal Res 1983;18:643–654.
12. Gottlow J, Nyman S, Lindhe J, Karring T, Wennström J. New attachment formation in the human periodontium by guided tissue regeneration. Case reports. J Clin Periodontol 1986;13:604–616.
13. Caffesse RG, Smith BA, Castelli WA, Nasjleti CE. New attachment achieved by guided tissue regeneration in beagle dogs. J Periodontol 1988;59:589–594.
14. American Academy of Periodontology. Glossary of Periodontal Terms. American Academy of Periodontology, 2001.
15. Caffesse RG, Becker W. Principles and techniques of guided tissue regeneration. Dent Clin North Am 1991;35:479–494.
16. Kao RT, Nares S, Reynolds MA. Periodontal regeneration—Intrabony defects: A systematic review from the AAP Regeneration Workshop. J Periodontol 2015;86(2 suppl):S77–S104.
17. Avila-Ortiz G, De Buitrago JG, Reddy MS. Periodontal regeneration—Furcation defects: A systematic review from the AAP Regeneration Workshop. J Periodontol 2015;86(2 suppl):S108–S130.
18. Lin Z, Rios HF, Cochran DL. Emerging regenerative approaches for periodontal reconstruction: A systematic review from the AAP Regeneration Workshop. J Periodontol 2015;86(2 suppl):S134–S152.
19. Hutmacher D, Hürzeler MB, Schliephake H. A review of material properties of biodegradable and bioresorbable polymers and devices for GTR and GBR applications. Int J Oral Maxillofac Implants 1996;11:667–678.
20. Takata T, Wang HL, Miyauchi M. Attachment, proliferation and differentiation of periodontal ligament cells on various guided tissue regeneration membranes. J Periodontal Res 2001;36:322–327.
21. Hutmacher DW, Kirsch A, Ackermann KL, Hürzeler MB. A tissue engineered cell-occlusive device for hard tissue regeneration—A preliminary report. Int J Periodontics Restorative Dent 2001;21:49–59.
22. Hung SL, Lin YW, Wang YH, Chen YT, Su CY, Ling LJ. Permeability of *Streptococcus mutans* and *Actinobacillus actinomycetemcomitans* through guided tissue regeneration membranes and their effects on attachment of periodontal ligament cells. J Periodontol 2002;73:843–851.
23. Scantlebury TV. 1982–1992: A decade of technology development for guided tissue regeneration. J Periodontol 1993;64(11 suppl):1129–1137.
24. Döri F, Huszár T, Nikolidakis D, Arweiler NB, Gera I, Sculean A. Effect of platelet-rich plasma on the healing of intrabony defects treated with an anorganic bovine bone mineral and expanded polytetrafluoroethylene membranes. J Periodontol 2007;78:983–990.

25. Cortellini P, Carnevale G, Sanz M, Tonetti MS. Treatment of deep and shallow intrabony defects. A multicenter randomized controlled clinical trial. J Clin Periodontol 1998;25:981–987.
26. Kinaia BM, Steiger J, Neely AL, Shah M, Bhola M. Treatment of Class II molar furcation involvement: Meta-analyses of reentry results. J Periodontol 2011;82:413–428.
27. Cortellini P, Tonetti MS. Focus on intrabony defects: Guided tissue regeneration. Periodontol 2000 2000;22:104–132.
28. Hardwick R, Hayes BK, Flynn C. Devices for dentoalveolar regeneration: An up-to-date literature review. J Periodontol 1995;66:495–505.
29. Stoecklin-Wasmer C, Rutjes AWS, da Costa BR, Salvi GE, Jüni P, Sculean A. Absorbable collagen membranes for periodontal regeneration: A systematic review. J Dent Res 2013;92:773–781.
30. Cortellini P, Tonetti MS. Clinical concepts for regenerative therapy in intrabony defects. Periodontol 2000 2015;68:282–307.
31. Brunel G, Piantoni P, Elharar F, Benqué E, Marin P, Zahedi S. Regeneration of rat calvarial defects using a bioabsorbable membrane technique: Influence of collagen cross-linking. J Periodontol 1996;67:1342–1348.
32. Frazza EJ, Schmitt EE. A new absorbable suture. J Biomed Mater Res 1971;5:43–58.
33. Kulkarni RK, Pani KC, Neuman C, Leonard F. Polylactic acid for surgical implants. Arch Surg 1966;93:839–843.
34. Reed AM, Gilding DK. Biodegradable polymers for use in surgery—Poly(glycolic)/poly(lactic acid) homo and copolymers: 2. In vitro degradation. Polymer 1981;22:494–498.
35. Gilding DK, Reed AM. Biodegradable polymers for use in surgery—Polyglycolic/poly(actic acid) homo- and copolymers: 1. Polymer 1979;20:1459–1464.
36. Craig PH, Williams JA, Davis KW, et al. A biologic comparison of polyglactin 910 and polyglycolic acid synthetic absorbable sutures. Surg Gynecol Obstet 1975;141:1–10.
37. De Andrade PF, de Souza SLS, de Oliveira Macedo G, et al. Acellular dermal matrix as a membrane for guided tissue regeneration in the treatment of Class II furcation lesions: A histometric and clinical study in dogs. J Periodontol 2007;78:1288–1299.
38. Kiany F, Moloudi F. Amnion membrane as a novel barrier in the treatment of intrabony defects: A controlled clinical trial. Int J Oral Maxillofac Implants 2015;30:639–647.
39. Kothiwale SV, Anuroopa P, Gajiwala AL. A clinical and radiological evaluation of DFDBA with amniotic membrane versus bovine derived xenograft with amniotic membrane in human periodontal Grade II furcation defects. Cell Tissue Bank 2009;10:317–326.
40. Rothamel D, Schwarz F, Fienitz T, et al. Biocompatibility and biodegradation of a native porcine pericardium membrane: Results of in vitro and in vivo examinations. Int J Oral Maxillofac Implants 2012;27:146–154.
41. Stavropoulos A, Chiantella G, Costa D, Steigmann M, Windisch P, Sculean A. Clinical and histologic evaluation of a granular bovine bone biomaterial used as an adjunct to GTR with a bioresorbable bovine pericardium collagen membrane in the treatment of intrabony defects. J Periodontol 2011;82:462–470.
42. Camelo M, Nevins ML, Schenk RK, et al. Clinical, radiographic, and histologic evaluation of human periodontal defects treated with Bio-Oss and Bio-Gide. Int J Periodontics Restorative Dent 1998;18:321–331.
43. Paul BF, Mellonig JT, Towle HJ 3rd, Gray JL. Use of a collagen barrier to enhance healing in human periodontal furcation defects. Int J Periodontics Restorative Dent 1992;12:123–131.
44. Tanner MG, Solt CW, Vuddhakanok S. An evaluation of new attachment formation using a microfibrillar collagen barrier. J Periodontol 1988;59:524–530.
45. Wang HL, O'Neal RB, Thomas CL, Shyr Y, MacNeil RL. Evaluation of an absorbable collagen membrane in treating Class II furcation defects. J Periodontol 1994;65:1029–1036.
46. Caffesse RG, Nasjleti CE, Morrison EC, Sanchez R. Guided tissue regeneration: Comparison of bioabsorbable and non-bioabsorbable membranes. Histologic and histometric study in dogs. J Periodontol 1994;65:583–591.
47. Caton J, Greenstein G, Zappa U. Synthetic bioabsorbable barrier for regeneration in human periodontal defects. J Periodontol 1994;65:1037–1045.
48. Cortellini P, Pini Prato G, Tonetti MS. Periodontal regeneration of human intrabony defects with bioresorbable membranes. A controlled clinical trial. J Periodontol 1996;67:217–223.
49. Laurell L, Falk H, Fornell J, Johard G, Gottlow J. Clinical use of a bioresorbable matrix barrier in guided tissue regeneration therapy. Case series. J Periodontol 1994;65:967–975.
50. Gottlow J, Laurell L, Lundgren D, et al. Periodontal tissue response to a new bioresorbable guided tissue regeneration device: A longitudinal study in monkeys. Int J Periodontics Restorative Dent 1994;14:436–449.
51. Tonetti MS, Cortellini P, Suvan JE, et al. Generalizability of the added benefits of guided tissue regeneration in the treatment of deep intrabony defects. Evaluation in a multi-center randomized controlled clinical trial. J Periodontol 1998;69:1183–1192.
52. Murphy KG, Gunsolley JC. Guided tissue regeneration for the treatment of periodontal intrabony and furcation defects. A systematic review. Ann Periodontol 2003;8:266–302.
53. Sculean A, Nikolidakis D, Nikou G, Ivanovic A, Chapple ILC, Stavropoulos A. Biomaterials for promoting periodontal regeneration in human intrabony defects: A systematic review. Periodontol 2000 2015;68:182–216.
54. Nabers CL, O'Leary TJ. Autogenous bone transplants in the treatment of osseous defects. J Periodontol 1965;36:5–14.
55. Hiatt WH, Schallhorn RG. Intraoral transplants of cancellous bone and marrow in periodontal lesions. J Periodontol 1973;44:194–208.
56. Rosenberg MM. Free osseous tissue autografts as a predictable procedure. J Periodontol 1971;42:195–209.
57. Dragoo MR, Kaldahl WB. Clinical and histological evaluation of alloplasts and allografts in regenerative periodontal surgery in humans. Int J Periodontics Restorative Dent 1983;3(2):8–29.
58. Sanders JJ, Sepe WW, Bowers GM, et al. Clinical evaluation of freeze-dried bone allografts in periodontal osseous defects. Part III. Composite freeze-dried bone allografts with and without autogenous bone grafts. J Periodontol 1983;54:1–8.
59. Mellonig JT. Freeze-dried bone allografts in periodontal reconstructive surgery. Dent Clin North Am 1991;35:505–520.
60. Bowers GM, Chadroff B, Carnevale R, et al. Histologic evaluation of new attachment apparatus formation in humans. Part III. J Periodontol 1989;60:683–693.
61. Bowers GM, Chadroff B, Carnevale R, et al. Histologic evaluation of new attachment apparatus formation in humans. Part II. J Periodontol 1989;60:675–682.
62. Bowers GM, Chadroff B, Carnevale R, et al. Histologic evaluation of new attachment apparatus formation in humans. Part I. J Periodontol 1989;60:664–674.
63. Rummelhart JM, Mellonig JT, Gray JL, Towle HJ. A comparison of freeze-dried bone allograft and demineralized freeze-dried bone allograft in human periodontal osseous defects. J Periodontol 1989;60:655–663.
64. Skoglund A, Hising P, Young C. A clinical and histologic examination in humans of the osseous response to implanted natural bone mineral. Int J Oral Maxillofac Implants 1997;12:194–199.

65. Richardson CR, Mellonig JT, Brunsvold MA, McDonnell HT, Cochran DL. Clinical evaluation of Bio-Oss: A bovine-derived xenograft for the treatment of periodontal osseous defects in humans. J Clin Periodontol 1999;26:421–428.
66. AlGhamdi AS, Shibly O, Ciancio SG. Osseous grafting part II: Xenografts and alloplasts for periodontal regeneration—A literature review. J Int Acad Periodontol 2010;12:39–44.
67. Meffert RM, Thomas JR, Hamilton KM, Brownstein CN. Hydroxylapatite as an alloplastic graft in the treatment of human periodontal osseous defects. J Periodontol 1985;56:63–73.
68. Bowen JA, Mellonig JT, Gray JL, Towle HT. Comparison of decalcified freeze-dried bone allograft and porous particulate hydroxyapatite in human periodontal osseous defects. J Periodontol 1989;60:647–654.
69. Stahl SS, Froum SJ. Histologic and clinical responses to porous hydroxylapatite implants in human periodontal defects. Three to twelve months postimplantation. J Periodontol 1987;58:689–695.
70. Stahl SS, Froum S. Histological evaluation of human intraosseous healing responses to the placement of tricalcium phosphate ceramic implants. I. Three to eight months. J Periodontol 1986;57:211–217.
71. Nery EB, Lynch KL. Preliminary clinical studies of bioceramic in periodontal osseous defects. J Periodontol 1978;49:523–527.
72. Ong MM, Eber RM, Korsnes MI, et al. Evaluation of a bioactive glass alloplast in treating periodontal intrabony defects. J Periodontol 1998;69:1346–1354.
73. Nevins ML, Camelo M, Nevins M, et al. Human histologic evaluation of bioactive ceramic in the treatment of periodontal osseous defects. Int J Periodontics Restorative Dent 2000;20:458–467.
74. AlGhamdi AS, Shibly O, Ciancio SG. Osseous grafting part I: Autografts and allografts for periodontal regeneration—A literature review. J Int Acad Periodontol 2010;12(2):34–38.
75. Schallhorn RG. The use of autogenous hip marrow biopsy implants for bony crater defects. J Periodontol 1968;39:145–147.
76. Schallhorn RG. Eradication of bifurcation defects utilizing frozen autogenous hip marrow implants. J Ont Dent Assoc 1968;45:18–22.
77. Schallhorn RG, Hiatt WH, Boyce W. Iliac transplants in periodontal therapy. J Periodontol 1970;41:566–580.
78. Schallhorn RG, Hiatt WH. Human allografts of iliac cancellous bone and marrow in periodontal osseous defects. II. Clinical observations. J Periodontol 1972;43:67–81.
79. Misch CM. Comparison of intraoral donor sites for onlay grafting prior to implant placement. Int J Oral Maxillofac Implants 1997;12:767–776.
80. Halliday DG. The grafting of newly formed autogenous bone in the treatment of osseous defects. J Periodontol 1969;40:511–514.
81. Robinson E. Osseous coagulum for bone induction. J Periodontol 1969;40:503–510.
82. Schallhorn RG. Present status of osseous grafting procedures. J Periodontol 1977;48:570–576.
83. Diem CR, Bowers GM, Moffitt WC. Bone blending: A technique for osseous implants. J Periodontol 1972;43:295–297.
84. Ewen SJ. Bone swaging. J Periodontol 1965;36:57–63.
85. Wang HL, Cooke J. Periodontal regeneration techniques for treatment of periodontal diseases. Dent Clin North Am 2005;49:637–659.
86. Miron RJ, Sculean A, Shuang Y, et al. Osteoinductive potential of a novel biphasic calcium phosphate bone graft in comparison with autographs, xenografts, and DFDBA. Clin Oral Implants Res 2016;27:668–675.
87. Buck BE, Malinin TI, Brown MD. Bone transplantation and human immunodeficiency virus. An estimate of risk of acquired immunodeficiency syndrome (AIDS). Clin Orthop Relat Res 1989;240:129–136.
88. Buck BE, Resnick L, Shah SM, Malinin TI. Human immunodeficiency virus cultured from bone. Implications for transplantation. Clin Orthop Relat Res 1990;251:249–253.
89. Mellonig JT. Autogenous and allogeneic bone grafts in periodontal therapy. Crit Rev Oral Biol Med 1992;3:333–352.
90. Scarborough NL, White EM, Hughes JV, Manrique AJ, Poser JW. Allograft safety: Viral inactivation with bone demineralization. Contemp Orthop 1995;31:257–261.
91. Urist MR. Surface-decalcified allogeneic bone (SDAB) implants. A preliminary report of 10 cases and 25 comparable operations with undecalcified lyophilized bone implants. Clin Orthop Relat Res 1968;56:37–50.
92. Urist MR, Strates BS. Bone formation in implants of partially and wholly demineralized bone matrix. Including observations on acetone-fixed intra and extracellular proteins. Clin Orthop Relat Res 1970;71:271–278.
93. Urist MR. Bone: Formation by autoinduction. Science 1965;150:893–899.
94. Urist MR, Strates BS. Bone morphogenetic protein. J Dent Res 1971;50:1392–1406.
95. Urist MR, Jurist JM Jr, Dubuc FL, Strates BS. Quantitation of new bone formation in intramuscular implants of bone matrix in rabbits. Clin Orthop Relat Res 1970;68:279–293.
96. Zhang M, Powers RM Jr, Wolfinbarger L Jr. Effect(s) of the demineralization process on the osteoinductivity of demineralized bone matrix. J Periodontol 1997;68:1085–1092.
97. Becker W, Becker BE, Caffesse R. A comparison of demineralized freeze-dried bone and autologous bone to induce bone formation in human extraction sockets. J Periodontol 1994;65:1128–1133.
98. Becker W, Urist MR, Tucker LM, Becker BE, Ochsenbein C. Human demineralized freeze-dried bone: Inadequate induced bone formation in athymic mice. A preliminary report. J Periodontol 1995;66:822–828.
99. Schwartz Z, Mellonig JT, Carnes DL Jr, et al. Ability of commercial demineralized freeze-dried bone allograft to induce new bone formation. J Periodontol 1996;67:918–926.
100. Reynolds MA, Aichelmann-Reidy ME, Branch-Mays GL, Gunsolley JC. The efficacy of bone replacement grafts in the treatment of periodontal osseous defects. A systematic review. Ann Periodontol 2003;8:227–265.
101. Sapkos SW. The use of Periograf in periodontal defects. Histologic findings. J Periodontol 1986;57:7–13.
102. Strub JR, Gaberthüel TW, Firestone AR. Comparison of tricalcium phosphate and frozen allogenic bone implants in man. J Periodontol 1979;50:624–629.
103. McGuire MK, Kao RT, Nevins M, Lynch SE. rhPDGF-BB promotes healing of periodontal defects: 24-month clinical and radiographic observations. Int J Periodontics Restorative Dent 2006;26:223–231.
104. Nevins M, Giannobile WV, McGuire MK, et al. Platelet-derived growth factor stimulates bone fill and rate of attachment level gain: Results of a large multicenter randomized controlled trial. J Periodontol 2005;76:2205–2215.
105. Jayakumar A, Rajababu P, Rohini S, et al. Multi-centre, randomized clinical trial on the efficacy and safety of recombinant human platelet-derived growth factor with β-tricalcium phosphate in human intra-osseous periodontal defects. J Clin Periodontol 2011;38:163–172.

106. Bashutski J, Oh TJ, Chan HL, Wang HL. Guided tissue regeneration: A decision-making model. J Int Acad Periodontol 2011;13:48–57.
107. Needleman IG, Worthington HV, Giedrys-Leeper E, Tucker RJ. Guided tissue regeneration for periodontal infra-bony defects. Cochrane Database Syst Rev 2006;(2):CD001724.
108. Aimetti M, Romano F, Pigella E, Pranzini F, Debernardi C. Treatment of wide, shallow, and predominantly 1-wall intrabony defects with a bioabsorbable membrane: A randomized controlled clinical trial. J Periodontol 2005;76:1354–1361.
109. Jepsen S, Eberhard J, Herrera D, Needleman I. A systematic review of guided tissue regeneration for periodontal furcation defects. What is the effect of guided tissue regeneration compared with surgical debridement in the treatment of furcation defects? J Clin Periodontol 2002;29(suppl 3):103–116.
110. Huynh-Ba G, Kuonen P, Hofer D, Schmid J, Lang NP, Salvi GE. The effect of periodontal therapy on the survival rate and incidence of complications of multirooted teeth with furcation involvement after an observation period of at least 5 years: A systematic review. J Clin Periodontol 2009;36:164–176.
111. Chen TH, Tu YK, Yen CC, Lu HK. A systematic review and meta-analysis of guided tissue regeneration/osseous grafting for the treatment of Class II furcation defects. J Dent Sci 2013;8:209–224.
112. Parrish LC, Miyamoto T, Fong N, Mattson JS, Cerutis DR. Non-bioabsorbable vs bioabsorbable membrane: Assessment of their clinical efficacy in guided tissue regeneration technique. A systematic review. J Oral Sci 2009;51:383–400.
113. Silvestri M, Rasperini G, Milani S. 120 infrabony defects treated with regenerative therapy: Long-term results. J Periodontol 2011;82:668–675.
114. Trombelli L, Heitz-Mayfield LJA, Needleman I, Moles D, Scabbia A. A systematic review of graft materials and biological agents for periodontal intraosseous defects. J Clin Periodontol 2002;29(suppl 3):117–135.
115. Machtei EE, Cho MI, Dunford R, Norderyd J, Zambon JJ, Genco RJ. Clinical, microbiological, and histological factors which influence the success of regenerative periodontal therapy. J Periodontol 1994;65:154–161.
116. Tonetti MS, Prato GP, Cortellini P. Factors affecting the healing response of intrabony defects following guided tissue regeneration and access flap surgery. J Clin Periodontol 1996;23:548–556.
117. Cortellini P, Pini-Prato G, Tonetti M. Periodontal regeneration of human infrabony defects (V). Effect of oral hygiene on long-term stability. J Clin Periodontol 1994;21:606–610.
118. Machtei EE, Oettinger-Barak O, Peled M. Guided tissue regeneration in smokers: Effect of aggressive anti-infective therapy in Class II furcation defects. J Periodontol 2003;74:579–584.
119. De Sanctis M, Zucchelli G. Interleukin-1 gene polymorphisms and long-term stability following guided tissue regeneration therapy. J Periodontol 2000;71:606–613.
120. Anderegg CR, Martin SJ, Gray JL, Mellonig JT, Gher ME. Clinical evaluation of the use of decalcified freeze-dried bone allograft with guided tissue regeneration in the treatment of molar furcation invasions. J Periodontol 1991;62:264–268.
121. Cortellini P, Tonetti MS, Lang NP, et al. The simplified papilla preservation flap in the regenerative treatment of deep intrabony defects: Clinical outcomes and postoperative morbidity. J Periodontol 2001;72:1702–1712.
122. Bowers GM, Schallhorn RG, McClain PK, Morrison GM, Morgan R, Reynolds MA. Factors influencing the outcome of regenerative therapy in mandibular Class II furcations: Part I. J Periodontol 2003;74:1255–1268.
123. Wang HL, MacNeil RL. Guided tissue regeneration. Absorbable barriers. Dent Clin North Am 1998;42:505–522.
124. Cortellini P, Pini Prato G, Tonetti MS. The modified papilla preservation technique with bioresorbable barrier membranes in the treatment of intrabony defects. Case reports. Int J Periodontics Restorative Dent 1996;16:546–559.
125. Machtei EE. The effect of membrane exposure on the outcome of regenerative procedures in humans: A meta-analysis. J Periodontol 2001;72:512–516.
126. Cortellini P, Prato GP, Tonetti MS. The modified papilla preservation technique. A new surgical approach for interproximal regenerative procedures. J Periodontol 1995;66:261–266.
127. Mayfield L, Söderholm G, Hallström H, et al. Guided tissue regeneration for the treatment of intraosseous defects using a biabsorbable membrane. A controlled clinical study. J Clin Periodontol 1998;25:585–595.
128. Mora F, Etienne D, Ouhayoun JP. Treatment of interproximal angular defects by guided tissue regeneration: 1 year follow-up. J Oral Rehabil 1996;23:599–606.
129. Murphy KG. Postoperative healing complications associated with Gore-Tex periodontal material. Part I. Incidence and characterization. Int J Periodontics Restorative Dent 1995;15:363–375.
130. Zucchelli G, Bernardi F, Montebugnoli L, De Sanctis M. Enamel matrix proteins and guided tissue regeneration with titanium-reinforced expanded polytetrafluoroethylene membranes in the treatment of infrabony defects: A comparative controlled clinical trial. J Periodontol 2002;73:3–12.
131. Ling LJ, Hung SL, Lee CF, Chen YT, Wu KM. The influence of membrane exposure on the outcomes of guided tissue regeneration: Clinical and microbiological aspects. J Periodontal Res 2003;38:57–63.
132. De Sanctis M, Zucchelli G, Clauser C. Bacterial colonization of bioabsorbable barrier material and periodontal regeneration. J Periodontol 1996;67:1193–1200.
133. De Sanctis M, Zucchelli G, Clauser C. Bacterial colonization of barrier material and periodontal regeneration. J Clin Periodontol 1996;23:1039–1046.
134. Zucchelli G, De Sanctis M, Clauser C. Integrated connective tissue in bioabsorbable barrier material and periodontal regeneration. J Periodontol 1997;68:996–1004.
135. Nowzari H, Slots J. Microorganisms in polytetrafluoroethylene barrier membranes for guided tissue regeneration. J Clin Periodontol 1994;21:203–210.
136. Nowzari H, Matian F, Slots J. Periodontal pathogens on polytetrafluoroethylene membrane for guided tissue regeneration inhibit healing. J Clin Periodontol 1995;22:469–474.
137. Cortellini P, Pini Prato G, Tonetti MS. Periodontal regeneration of human intrabony defects with titanium reinforced membranes. A controlled clinical trial. J Periodontol 1995;66:797–803.
138. Christgau M, Schmalz G, Wenzel A, Hiller KA. Periodontal regeneration of intrabony defects with resorbable and non-resorbable membranes: 30-month results. J Clin Periodontol 1997;24:17–27.

12

TISSUE ENGINEERING

Juan C. Rodríguez, DDS, MS
Miguel Romero Bustillos, DDS, PhD

DEFINITIONS AND TERMINOLOGY

Chemotaxis: The migration of cells along a concentration gradient of an attractant.[2]

Fibroblast growth factor: A family of growth factors with mitogenic properties for fibroblasts and mesoderm-derived cell types.[2]

Growth factors: A diverse group of polypeptides that have important roles in regulation of growth and development of a variety of organs.[2]

Progenitor cell: An undifferentiated cell that gives rise to one or more types of more specialized cells.[2]

Tissue engineering: A technique to utilize a combination of cells, signaling molecules and scaffolds in an effort to regenerate tissues, thereby restoring biological function and structures.[2]

The main focus of most periodontal therapies is to cease the destruction of the periodontium (ie, gingiva, bone, cementum, and periodontal ligament [PDL]) and to regenerate or repair the damaged or lost structures. In periodontics, **tissue engineering** aims at mimicking the preexistent micro and macro structures in hopes of guiding tissue formation in a synchronized manner in order to achieve regeneration. However, given that *regeneration* is a histologic term, the success is typically measured by radiographic and functional parameters (ie, reduction in mobility or attachment gain) that can be quantified clinically.

Tissue engineering is a multidisciplinary field that involves the application of the principles and methods of engineering and life sciences to help in the development of biologic substitutes to restore, maintain, or improve the function of damaged tissues and organs.[1] Tissue engineering in periodontology applies the principles of engineering and life sciences toward the development of biologic techniques that can restore lost alveolar bone, PDL, and root cementum.[1]

Biomimetic implantable materials such as bone grafts, membranes, protein derivatives, and protein super concentrates, and their application into periodontal wounds, are the main characters in the ever-progressing field of periodontal tissue engineering. This chapter describes the role of different biomaterials and tissue engineering techniques as well as new advances in applied clinical sciences.

Periodontal Tissue Engineering

The main goal of tissue engineering is to harness the body's own capacity to regenerate functionally active periodontal tissues that physiologically respond to metabolic cues and stimuli. The following factors must be considered in order to achieve this goal (Fig 12-1)[3]:

- *Cells:* The presence of appropriate numbers of responsive **progenitor cells** that will create the new hybrid periodontal tissues.

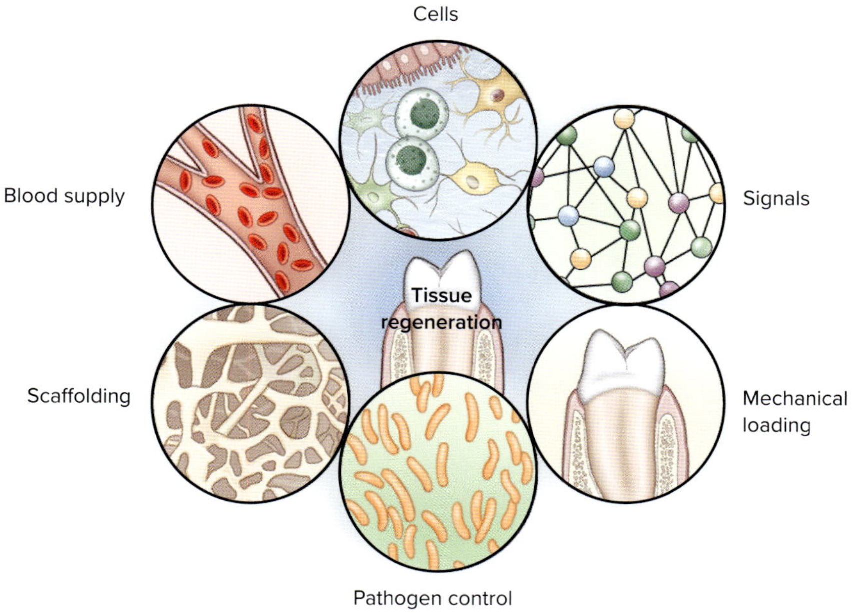

Fig 12-1 Critical components of periodontal tissue engineering.

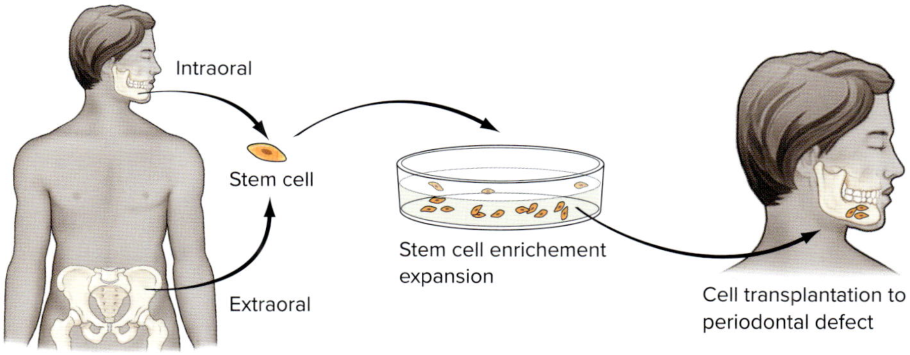

Fig 12-2 Example of cell-based therapy.

- *Signals:* Appropriate levels and sequencing of regulatory signals (signaling molecules) that instruct the cells to form the multiple tissue types in the periodontium.
- *Scaffolds:* An appropriate extracellular matrix or carrier construct to act as a scaffold to hold the cells.
- *Blood supply:* New vascular networks promoted by angiogenic signals provide the nutritional base for tissue growth and homeostasis.
- *Mechanical loading:* Appropriate mechanical loading is essential for the development of highly organized, functional PDL fibers.
- *Pathogen control:* Due to the microbial load at the periodontal lesion, strategies to control infection and host response are required to optimize periodontal regeneration.

When all of these factors are present simultaneously in periodontal therapy, the possibility of achieving successful regeneration of the lost or injured tissues increases. The principle of delivering specific cells to periodontal defects to reconstruct target sites is known as *cell-based tissue engineering*. Once cells are in their target area, they will aid in regeneration, acting as carriers to deliver growth signals or differentiate to multiple cell types promoting regeneration.[4,5] The cell types used in periodontal tissue engineering can be further divided into autogenous (same individual), allogeneic (different individual from the same species), and xenogeneic (different species)[6] (Fig 12-2).

TABLE 12-1 Preclinical applications of cell therapies for periodontal tissue engineering, divided by cell type, source, and pertinence[3,9]

Cell type	Graft type	Defect type
Bone marrow stromal cells	Autograft	Class III furcation involvement Periodontal fenestration Osteotomy
Adipose stromal cells	Autograft	Periodontal palatal defects
PDL cells	Autograft Allograft Xenograft	Class II furcation involvement Periodontal fenestration
PDL stem cells	Autograft Allograft	Ectopic Periodontal defect Periodontal fenestration
Cementoblasts	Allograft	Ectopic Periodontal fenestration
Dental follicle cells	Allograft	Ectopic Periodontal fenestration

Cell-Based Therapy

In periodontics, autogenous cells are often preferred over allogeneic and xenogeneic sources. Stem cells can be classified depending on the potency for differentiation. *Totipotent* means that the cell has the ability to differentiate to all cell types, such as in a zygote. Other stem cell types include *pluripotent* stem cells, which can differentiate into almost all cell types; *multipotent* cells, which can differentiate into cells of the same family; *oligopotent* cells such as those that differentiate into few related cells; and *unipotent*, which are the cells that can generate cells of the same type. Based on the source, the stem cells can also be classified as *embryonic stem cells*, *adult stem cells*, or *induced pluripotent stem cells*.[4,7]

Cell-based therapy involves transferring new cells into tissues affected by a disease or disorder—in this case, periodontitis and peri-implantitis.[6] These cells are used to enhance periodontal regeneration by delivering molecular signals and differentiating into multiple cell types. *Mesenchymal stem cells (MSCs)* are self-renewable cells that are capable of differentiating into cells which comprise a specific tissue or organ.[4,8,9] In addition, cell-based therapy can be divided based on the source, as extraoral and intraoral (Table 12-1).[3,9]

EXTRAORAL MSCs

Several authors have described the use of extraoral tissue-derived MSCs in periodontal tissue engineering, reporting different degrees of success.[10–12] In particular, *bone marrow MSCs (BMSCs)*, which are the cells isolated from bone marrow and with the capacity to differentiate to produce bone, cartilage, and adipose tissue, have been widely described and used in animal and human clinical models with promising results. In 2004, Kawaguchi et al[12] showed that autotransplantation with BMSCs promoted periodontal regeneration in experimentally induced Class III furcation defects in dogs. In addition, BMSCs have been shown to differentiate into key cells to obtain periodontal regeneration, such as cementoblasts, PDL cells, fibroblasts, and osteoblasts.[12,13] The application of BMSCs in preprosthetic reconstructions of alveolar sockets and sinus floor augmentation procedures have also shown increased bone formation and accelerated healing.[14–16] Researchers have used BMSCs and platelet-rich plasma (PRP) in intrabony defects and showed probing depth (PD) reduction and resolution of bleeding on probing (BOP) and mobility. Its use has also been explored as autogenous scaffolds with expanded BMSCs in implant therapy with the goal of enhancing osteogenesis.[11,17–19]

TABLE 12-2 Gene delivery with viral and nonviral vectors[9]

Vector	Advantages	Type
Adenovirus	• High transduction rate • Transfection of wide range of cell types	Viral
Lentivirus	• Nonimmunogenic • Sustained gene expression	Viral
Adeno-associated virus	• Transduction in both dividing and nondividing cells • Sustained gene expression	Viral
Plasmid	• Nonimmunogenic • Transfection • Localized gene expression	Nonviral
Nucleic acid/polymer complexes	• Targeted downregulation of gene expression	Nonviral

INTRAORAL MSCs

Limiting surgical exposure to the oral cavity has several advantages over extraoral harvesting, due in part to a reduced morbidity and ease of access. In this sense, animal studies have shown the potential of using PDL fibroblasts for periodontal regeneration.[20,21] PDL stem cells have been shown to promote true periodontal regeneration with formation of new cementum, alveolar bone, and a functionally oriented ligament space.[21,22] When evaluating the feasibility of utilizing alveolar bone MSCs from marrow aspirates and bone core samples of edentulous sites, Mason et al found that alveolar bone MSCs exhibited multipotency, genetic stability over time, and the ability to form de novo bone when implanted subcutaneously.[23]

Gene-Delivery Therapy

Gene-delivery therapy aims to transfer genetic information to manipulate, induce, or suppress specific genes that are used for therapeutic goals.[24] Gene delivery uses a variety of viral (eg, retroviruses, adenoviruses, lentiviruses, adeno-associated viruses) and nonviral vectors to modulate host response, in both defense and repair or regeneration (Table 12-2).[3,9] Gene expression following a viral transfection is generally efficacious and sustainable.[25,26] As such, in contrast to recombinant proteins used in tissue regeneration, the effects of which usually range from several hours to days, viral vector genes can be expressed in vivo from weeks to years, depending on the type of viral vector transfection and the targeted tissue.[9]

Early research in the field of gene delivery for periodontal tissue regeneration showed that the application of growth factors[27,28] or cytokine receptors by gene transfer provides a greater sustainability than single protein application. Thus, gene therapy may achieve greater bioavailability of growth factors within periodontal wounds and provide a greater regenerative potential.[29]

Nonviral gene therapy relies on the combination of nucleic acids with synthetic or natural vectors, as well as physical forces to deliver genetic information to a target cell population.[9,30] One of the major advantages of nonviral gene therapy includes the delivery of significantly larger fragments of genetic information and lack of risk for immunogenicity and infection. Some of the most notable advantages of gene therapy over other tissue engineering modalities include the following[3,9]:

- Greater sustainability than the application of a single protein or compound.
- Reduction of technical challenges related to ex vivo protein expression and purifications.
- Transient and controlled delivery of genetic sequences encoding regenerative factors.
- When combined with other tissue engineering strategies, it offers a strong potential for regeneration in a 3D aspect at the tooth-ligament-bone interface.

TABLE 12-3 Growth factors in periodontal tissue engineering[9,32–34]

Growth factor	Effect
Platelet-derived growth factor (PDGF)	Migration, proliferation, and noncollagenous matrix synthesis of MSCs
Bone morphogenetic protein (BMP)	Proliferation, differentiation of osteoblasts, and differentiation of PDL cells into osteoblasts
Enamel matrix derivative (EMD)	Proliferation, protein synthesis, and mineral nodule formation in PDL cells, osteoblasts, and cementoblasts
Teriparatide	Acts on preosteoblasts to increase proliferation and on osteoblasts to decrease apoptosis
Growth and differentiation factor 5 (GDF-5)	MSC differentiation and stimulation of human PDL cell proliferation
Fibroblast growth factor 2 (FGF-2)	Proliferation and attachment of endothelial and PDL cells
Platelet-rich concentrates	Enhancement of wound healing as well as cell adhesion, proliferation, and migration

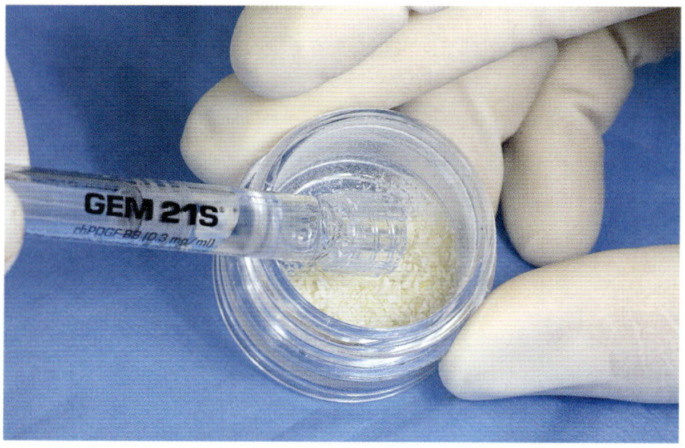

Fig 12-3 Application of recombinant human PDGF-BB over allogeneic bone graft. (Courtesy of Dr Gonzalo Blasi.)

Signaling Molecules

Growth factors are a diverse group of polypeptides that represent a class of biologic mediators of critical cellular activities, including migration, proliferation, differentiation, and matrix synthesis.[31] The periodontal literature has investigated a multitude of players in the field of signaling molecules and biologic agents, some of which are used in clinical practice and others that are showing promising findings (Table 12-3).[9,32–34]

PLATELET-DERIVED GROWTH FACTORS

Platelet-derived growth factors (PDGFs) play an essential role in periodontal tissue repair by promoting PDL, fibroblast, and cementum proliferation and have been extensively used in vitro and in vivo.[35] In large animal models, the application of PDGF is often combined with insulinlike growth factor (IGF). In periodontal regeneration models, the utilization of PDGF often resulted in increased bone, cementum, and PDL formation.[36–38] Similarly, in complex regeneration scenarios such as Class III furcation defects, guided tissue regeneration (GTR) with PDGF-BB and expanded polytetrafluoroethylene (ePTFE) membranes stimulated PDL formation in early stages followed by total periodontal regeneration.[39] The utilization of PDGF/IGF-1 for guided bone regeneration (GBR) at implants placed into extraction sockets also showed increased early (3-week) histologic and clinical bone formation.[40,41]

PDGF-BB is approved by the U.S. Food and Drug Administration (FDA) for periodontal regeneration (eg, intrabony defects, furcation lesions, and gingival recessions), and it is commercially available in the United States (Fig 12-3). Long-term evaluations have shown promising results and improved treatment outcomes in periodontal regeneration.[35,42] Also, long-term stable clinical and radiographic improvement of localized periodontal defects was shown in a randomized controlled clinical trial (RCT) using recombinant human PDGF-BB protein in combination with β-tricalcium phosphate (β-TCP).[43] In this clinical study, results showed that with use of PDGF-BB at a concentration of 0.3 mg/mL, intrabony defects improved in terms of clinical attachment gain (≥ 2.7 mm) and linear bone gain (≥ 1.1 mm) in 87% of the cases at 36 months compared to 53.8% for the group treated with β-TCP alone.

For the treatment of mucogingival recessions, a split-mouth RCT evaluated the outcomes of Miller Class II gingival recessions treated by either 0.3 mg/mL recombinant human PDGF-BB + β-TCP + bioabsorbable collagen wound-healing dressing or connective tissue graft (CTG), both groups in combination with a coronally advanced flap (CAF). At the end of the investigation (6 months postsurgery), both groups demonstrated significant improvements; however, the CTG group showed statistically significant superior outcomes for recession depth and width reduction, as well as root coverage. On the other hand, the PDGF group demonstrated statistically significant superior outcomes for PD reduction. In addition, this study evaluated the outcomes of the same treatment modalities by means of histologic and microcomputer tomography in six teeth planned for extraction. Interestingly, the sites treated with CTG didn't show evidence of periodontal regeneration, whereas all teeth treated with PDGF + β-TCP demonstrated new cementum, PDL, and alveolar bone.[44]

BONE MORPHOGENETIC PROTEINS

Bone morphogenetic proteins (BMPs) are a group of proteins that belong to the transforming growth factor family and are capable of inducing cartilage, bone, and marrow formation.[45] Preclinical and clinical studies have shown that BMPs possess the ability to promote formation of normal physiologic bone, assuming the morphology of the surrounding osseous structures.[46,47] Multiple BMPs have been evaluated for clinical use, including BMP-2 (osteoinductive), BMP-5 (chondrogenic), and BMP-7 (osteoinductive). All these have been used alone or in combination with other signaling molecules to increase bone production and hopefully periodontal regeneration. When BMP-2 is grafted with autogenous bone, it seems to increase cell activity, osteoid lines, and vascular supply.[48] Contrasting these findings, Kao et al showed that when BMP-2 was blended with bovine-derived xenograft, less bone formation was obtained.[49]

Currently, the use of BMP-2 (commercially available as Infuse Bone Graft, Medtronic) is approved by the FDA as an alternative to autogenous bone grafting for sinus augmentation and ridge preservation procedures owing to its osteoinductive potential.[46,48,50]

Negative aspects of BMPs described in the literature are mainly cost, increased risk of ankylosis when used next to natural dentition, osteoclast-mediated bone resorption, and increased postoperative inflammation.[51]

FIBROBLAST GROWTH FACTOR 2

Fibroblast growth factor 2 (FGF-2) is an important element in wound-healing and angiogenic processes. FGF-2 inhibits osteogenic differentiation of PDL cells, maintaining their differentiation potential and increasing cellular proliferation.[9] As shown in a recent systematic review, this factor has the potential to improve bone fill in periodontal regeneration.[42] In a clinical trial evaluating the treatment of intrabony defects, periodontal regeneration and bone fill were significantly improved with FGF-2 when compared to flap debridement and enamel matrix derivatives (EMD).[52] The results from this investigation showed more favorable outcomes for the FGF-2 group with regard to radiographic bone fill as well as clinical attachment gains (1.7 mm in the flap debridement group, 2.3 mm in the EMD group, and 2.7 mm in the FGF-2 group). As of 2020, it has not been cleared by the FDA for use in the United States or Canada.

GROWTH AND DIFFERENTIATION FACTOR 5

Growth and differentiation factor 5 (GDF-5) has been used for periodontal regeneration as well as alveolar bone and sinus augmentation procedures. GDF-5 is a member of the transforming growth factor β (TGF-β) superfamily. With regard to its use in periodontal regeneration, both in vitro and in vivo studies have demonstrated its ability to stimulate PDL cell proliferation, osteoblast differentiation, and extracellular matrix synthesis. A randomized clinical pilot study was conducted to study the effect of GDF-5 embedded in β-TCP for intrabony defects in chronic periodontitis patients. Six months after therapy, the clinical attachment gain for the test group was almost double the level gained in the control group (3.2 mm vs 1.7 mm), although this was not statistically significant.[53,54] Similar to other growth factors, a higher degree of bone augmentation was observed when GDF-5 was combined with β-TCP.[55]

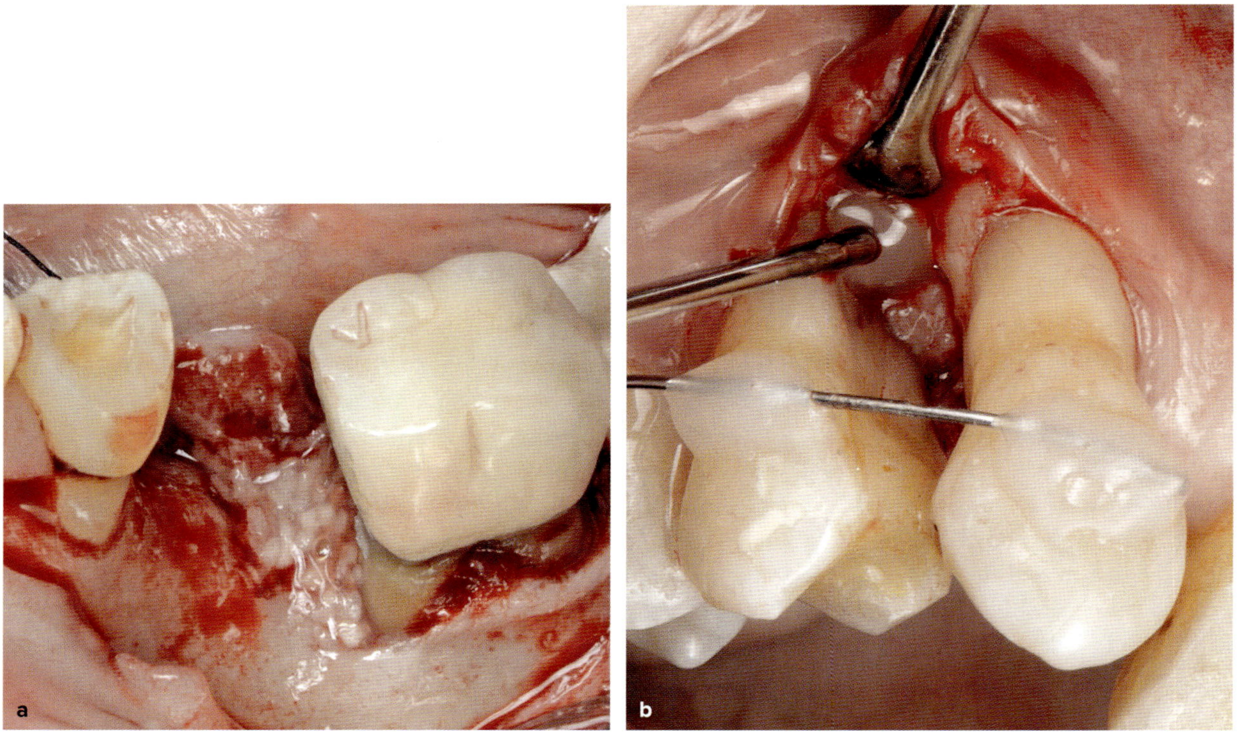

Fig 12-4 *(a)* EMD in combination with allogeneic bone graft for the treatment of an intrabony defect. *(b)* EMD application on an intrabony defect. (Courtesy of Dr Gonzalo Blasi.)

ENAMEL MATRIX DERIVATIVES

EMD primarily consists of amelogenins obtained from porcine tooth buds[56–58] and also contains proteins such as enamelin, tuftelin, and ameloblastin, among others. EMD is commercialized under the name Emdogain (Straumann), and it is FDA approved as an adjunct to bone grafting, for periodontal regeneration, and for the treatment of mucogingival recessions (Fig 12-4a). Like other signaling molecules, EMD has the potential to promote formation of new cementum, PDL, and alveolar bone.[59,60] EMD has been studied in different fields of periodontology, but it is mainly applied for intrabony and furcation defects as well as gingival recession coverage (Fig 12-4b). Histologic and clinical studies treating intrabony defects have shown regeneration of the periodontal tissues with the use of EMD.[60] Tonetti et al[61] performed a multicenter RCT to compare the performance of a minimally invasive papilla preservation flap with or without the adjunctive use of EMD. Results from this investigation reported that EMD-treated defects gained 3.1 ± 1.5 mm of clinical attachment level, while control defects yielded a clinical attachment level gain of 2.5 ± 1.5 mm.[61]

More recently, its use has been evaluated in patients with compromised healing potential such as smokers and diabetic patients.[62,63] In 2006, Castellanos et al[64] conducted a prospective RCT comparing CAF for the treatment of gingival recessions with or without EMD. Results after 1 year showed that the EMD group obtained a mean defect reduction of 2.32 ± 1.03 mm versus 1.41 ± 0.57 mm on control sites. Also, keratinized tissue gain favored the sites treated with EMD (0.82 ± 0.2 mm vs 0.04 ± 0.01 mm).[64]

PLATELET-RICH CONCENTRATES

In the early 1990s, a novel platelet gel was formulated and utilized in surgery as an autologous, blood-derived product to seal wounds and stimulate healing.[65,66] This gel was named PRP. PRP, as the name implies, is mainly composed of platelets, which actively secrete growth factors for initiating wound healing and enhancing cell adhesion, proliferation, and migration of various cell types.[67,68] In order to achieve the desired end product, the PRP process required the addition of bovine thrombin and calcium chloride to the blood.[65] This cell product was later modified and renamed platelet rich in growth factors

(PRGF) by Eduardo Anitua.[69] These two platelet-rich products, PRP and PRGF, are considered first-generation concentrates, and they were not utilized as mainstream clinical adjuvants mainly because they were time consuming, they required multiple steps and a higher cost, and they relied on extrinsic anticoagulants.

Platelet-rich fibrin (PRF) was considered an evolution from PRP because it no longer required external additives and remained 100% autologous; it is considered a second-generation platelet concentrate[70] (Fig 12-5). A stable fibrin matrix in PRF allows the blood concentrate to create a 3D structure that holds a number of growth factors and cytokines, including PDGF, TGF-β1, IGF, and vascular endothelial growth factor.[70] When growth factor release rates were compared in an in vitro study by Kobayashi et al, PRP showed a release of significantly higher proteins at earlier time points, whereas PRF displayed a continual and steady release of growth factors over a 10-day period.[71]

One of the main considerations when analyzing and interpreting data in the literature from platelet-rich concentrates or PRF is the wide variability in protocols and hardware (centrifuges, spinning rates and times, as well as collection tubes) used to obtain these products. These variabilities could be responsible for some of the heterogeneity observed in the study outcomes. Collectively though, the use of PRF and its variants have demonstrated their effectiveness for enhancing bone and soft tissue healing,[72–74] especially when applied for socket grafting, recession coverage, GTR, and sinus augmentation procedures. Some of the most robust evidence for the application of PRF substrates is in regard to intrabony and furcation treatment. A recent systematic review reported that there is a notable benefit when adding PRF to conventional open flap debridement.[73] Another potential application for PRF is the treatment of the donor site after CTG harvesting is performed. Studies have shown decreased postoperative pain and enhanced wound healing[75,76] (Fig 12-6).

TERIPARATIDE

Teriparatide consists of the first 34 amino acids of the parathyroid hormone. It has been shown to influence survival of PDL cells and to cause osteoblast-like behavior with increased osteoprotegerin expression.[77] As such, the FDA approved teriparatide for the treatment of osteoporosis, and it is commercially available as Forteo (Lilly) and dosed as a daily parenteral injection.

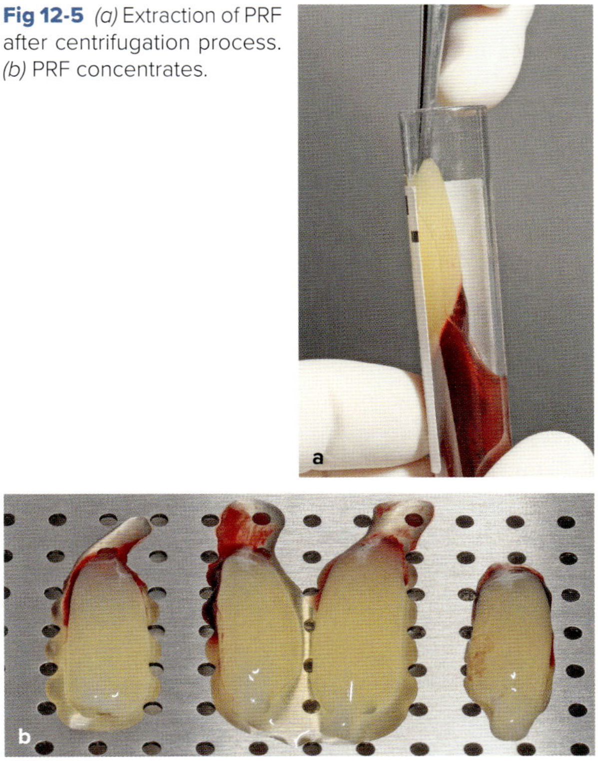

Fig 12-5 *(a)* Extraction of PRF after centrifugation process. *(b)* PRF concentrates.

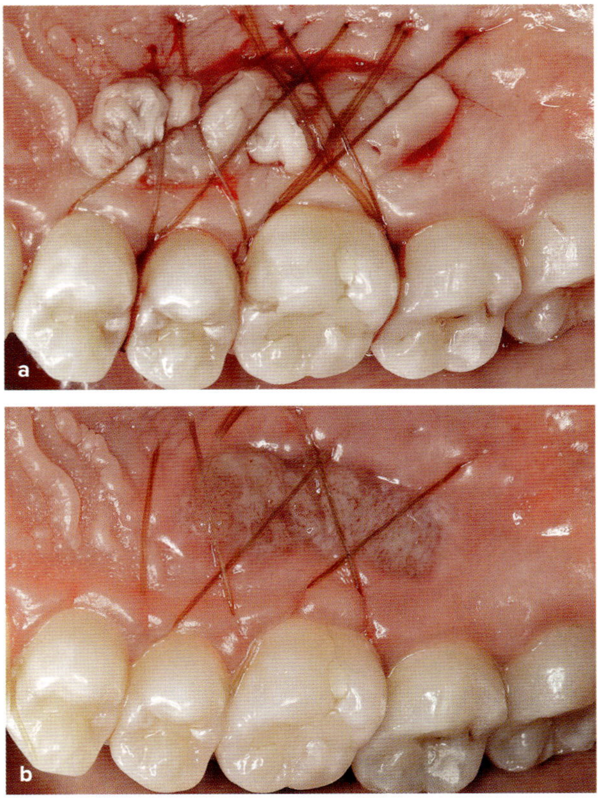

Fig 12-6 Application of L-PRF on palatal donor site after free gingival graft harvesting. *(a)* Postoperative view. *(b)* Follow-up at 1 week. (Courtesy of Dr Vahid Khoshkam.)

Clinical evaluations have found substantial evidence of increasing bone formation in extraction sockets and around dental implants.[78] It is suggested that patients with metabolic bone diseases would benefit the most from a teriparatide-based treatment,[34] given its ability to reduce osteoblast apoptosis while increasing preosteoblast proliferation. A clinical trial evaluating the effect of teriparatide on patients following periodontal surgery found improved clinical outcomes compared with placebo.[79] Clinical outcomes measured included PD reduction at 12 months (2.42 mm in the test group vs 1.32 mm in the control group), clinical attachment level gain at 12 months (1.58 mm in the test group vs 0.42 mm in the control group), and BOP reduction (28% in the test group vs 39% in the control group).[79]

Scaffolding Matrices

As previously mentioned, one of the most important components of tissue engineering is a 3D template provided by scaffolds. These frameworks act as a defined supporting structure that allows the settlement and guidance of cells and proteins for tissue growth in the target area. As such, this concept has been used in GTR for decades. Generally, all scaffolds share a variety of common characteristics,[3] such as the following:

- Providing a 3D architecture that supports a desired volume, shape, and mechanical strength
- Consisting of a high porosity and surface-to-volume ratio with a well-interconnected open pore structure
- Biocompatibility
- Degrading at a controlled pattern, which allows adequate support until tissue defects are fully regrown

PREFABRICATED SCAFFOLDS

The use of naturally derived and synthetic polymeric prefabricated scaffolds in periodontal regeneration has undergone significant evolution throughout the years.[6]

Autografts, allografts, xenografts, and hydroxyapatite particles represent naturally derived scaffolds, whereas alloplasts and polymers like poly(lactide-co-glycolide) are synthetic scaffolds.[80]

Autogenous bone grafts are considered the gold standard for periodontal regeneration because they possess several key characteristics. Most importantly, bone transplanted from the same patient is native to its host environment and provides a preestablished population of viable cells and growth factors necessary for osteogenesis.[9] However, due to increased morbidity and clinical outcomes comparable with alternative grafting substitutes, the use of allografts and xenografts has become more common in daily practice.

Different materials used as a scaffold have different physical properties and rates of degradation based on their origin and/or processing. By taking into consideration the fact that scaffolds stimulate cell behavior, the rate of material degradation plays a fundamental role on the initiation of regenerative procedures.[80] A scaffold can provide a suitable environment for targeted cells and controls the dynamic release of entrapped biologics. β-TCP is an example that has been used in periodontal regeneration as a delivery system with growth factors like PDGF-BB and GDF-5.[3,9]

INJECTABLE SCAFFOLDS

Biocompatible and biodegradable polyhydroxy esters, such as polyglycolide, polylactide, and their copolymers, have been extensively investigated. However, similar to conventional bone grafting, a surgical intervention is needed for the implantation of a preshaped device. Therefore, an injectable hydrogel could represent an alternative approach to encapsulate cells with minimal invasiveness.[81] In this sense, a wide range of the hydrogels have been developed for specific applications (eg, water-soluble chitosan derivatives, chitosan-graft-glycolic acid, and phloretic acid) showing high potential as an injectable biomaterial for cartilage tissue engineering. Nevertheless, the use of injectable scaffolds remains very limited in the periodontal field.[6]

COMPUTER-BASED DESIGNED AND FABRICATED SCAFFOLDS

Computer-based applications in tissue engineering represent some of the most recent developments in scaffold design and fabrication. This type of technology has been used in recent years to define virtual 3D models for surgical planning by using data from several imaging sources. Specifically, computed tomography (CT) or magnetic resonance imaging (MRI) data are used to create the 3D anatomical geometry of a defect that can later be used as a scaffold. One major advantage of this 3D-printed scaffold is that because it is produced from the 3D model, it should fill the defect space precisely.[3] A recent single case report by Rasperini et al[82] used CBCT to design a customized polycaprolactone scaffold fabricated via selective laser sintering for the treatment of a periodontal defect. The scaffold consisted of *(1)* an internal region with pegs to support PDL regeneration and the delivery of recombinant human PDGF-BB and *(2)* a layered external region that would resorb over time with subsequent replacement by alveolar bone.[82] This careful structural arrangement aimed to create different areas or zones tailored to promote specific tissue formation in an organized pattern that would mimic the host's natural tissues. Even though this case showed great potential for future applications, more research is needed to further develop this particular approach.

Conclusions

Arguably the most challenging aspect of tissue engineering is achieving regeneration by restoring all periodontal components to the same structure and function. Complete 3D reconstruction of the lost periodontal structures is still unpredictable, and this field remains highly productive in terms of materials science, engineering, and cell biology. Tissue engineering has made promising advances in the last decades, and it seems to go hand in hand with advances in technology and biologic understandings. Future challenges include the fabrication of personalized scaffolds that adapt and evolve within the targeted sites, providing structural support, and gene or protein guidance to growth factors to repair and replace lost or damaged tissues.

References

1. Dabra S, Chhina K, Soni N, Bhatnagar R. Tissue engineering in periodontal regeneration: A brief review. Dent Res J (Isfahan) 2012;9:671–680.
2. American Academy of Periodontology. Glossary of Periodontal Terms. American Academy of Periodontology, 2001.
3. Rios HF, Lin Z, Oh B, Park CH, Giannobile WV. Cell- and gene-based therapeutic strategies for periodontal regenerative medicine. J Periodontol 2011;82:1223–1237.
4. Mao JJ, Giannobile WV, Helms JA, et al. Craniofacial tissue engineering by stem cells. J Dent Res 2006;85:966–979.
5. Discher DE, Mooney DJ, Zandstra PW. Growth factors, matrices, and forces combine and control stem cells. Science 2009;324:1673–1677.
6. Chen FM, Liu X. Advancing biomaterials of human origin for tissue engineering. Prog Polym Sci 2016;53:86–168.
7. Kolios G, Moodley Y. Introduction to stem cells and regenerative medicine. Respiration 2013;85:3–10.
8. Ullah I, Subbarao RB, Rho GJ. Human mesenchymal stem cells: Current trends and future prospective. Biosci Rep 2015;35:e00191.
9. Pilipchuk SP, Plonka AB, Monje A, et al. Tissue engineering for bone regeneration and osseointegration in the oral cavity. Dent Mater 2015;31:317–338.
10. Kaigler D, Pagni G, Park CH, et al. Stem cell therapy for craniofacial bone regeneration: A randomized, controlled feasibility trial. Cell Transplant 2013;22:767–777.
11. Yamada Y, Ueda M, Hibi H, Nagasaka T. Translational research for injectable tissue-engineered bone regeneration using mesenchymal stem cells and platelet-rich plasma: From basic research to clinical case study. Cell Transplant 2004;13:343–355.
12. Kawaguchi H, Hirachi A, Hasegawa N, et al. Enhancement of periodontal tissue regeneration by transplantation of bone marrow mesenchymal stem cells. J Periodontol 2004;75:1281–1287.
13. Hasegawa N, Kawaguchi H, Hirachi A, et al. Behavior of transplanted bone marrow-derived mesenchymal stem cells in periodontal defects. J Periodontol 2006;77:1003–1007.
14. Kaigler D, Pagni G, Park CH, Tarle SA, Bartel RL, Giannobile WV. Angiogenic and osteogenic potential of bone repair cells for craniofacial regeneration. Tissue Eng Part A 2010;16:2809–2820.
15. Kaigler D, Silva EA, Mooney DJ. Guided bone regeneration using injectable vascular endothelial growth factor delivery gel. J Periodontol 2013;84:230–238.
16. Pagni G, Kaigler D, Rasperini G, Avila-Ortiz G, Bartel R, Giannobile WV. Bone repair cells for craniofacial regeneration. Adv Drug Deliv Rev 2012;64:1310–1319.
17. Ito K, Yamada Y, Naiki T, Ueda M. Simultaneous implant placement and bone regeneration around dental implants using tissue-engineered bone with fibrin glue, mesenchymal stem cells and platelet-rich plasma. Clin Oral Implants Res 2006;17:579–586.
18. Yamada Y, Ueda M, Naiki T, Takahashi M, Hata K, Nagasaka T. Autogenous injectable bone for regeneration with mesenchymal stem cells and platelet-rich plasma: Tissue-engineered bone regeneration. Tissue Eng 2004;10:955–964.
19. Yamada Y, Ueda M, Hibi H, Baba S. A novel approach to periodontal tissue regeneration with mesenchymal stem cells and platelet-rich plasma using tissue engineering technology: A clinical case report. Int J Periodontics Restorative Dent 2006;26:363–369.
20. Shimono M, Ishikawa T, Ishikawa H, et al. Regulatory mechanisms of periodontal regeneration. Microsc Res Tech 2003;60:491–502.
21. Akizuki T, Oda S, Komaki M, et al. Application of periodontal ligament cell sheet for periodontal regeneration: A pilot study in beagle dogs. J Periodontal Res 2005;40:245–251.
22. Lekic PC, Rajshankar D, Chen H, Tenenbaum H, McCulloch CA. Transplantation of labeled periodontal ligament cells promotes regeneration of alveolar bone. Anat Rec 2001;262:193–202.
23. Mason S, Tarle SA, Osibin W, Kinfu Y, Kaigler D. Standardization and safety of alveolar bone-derived stem cell isolation. J Dent Res 2014;93:55–61.
24. Ditto AJ, Shah PN, Yun YH. Non-viral gene delivery using nanoparticles. Expert Opin Drug Deliv 2009;6:1149–1160.
25. Walther P, Wang L, Liessem S, Frascaroli G. Viral infection of cells in culture: Approaches for electron microscopy. Methods Cell Biol 2010;96:603–618.
26. Kim TK, Eberwine JH. Mammalian cell transfection: The present and the future. Anal Bioanal Chem 2010;397:3173–3178.
27. Jin Q, Anusaksathien O, Webb SA, Printz MA, Giannobile WV. Engineering of tooth-supporting structures by delivery of PDGF gene therapy vectors. Mol Ther 2004;9:519–526.

28. Franceschi RT, Wang D, Krebsbach PH, Rutherford RB. Gene therapy for bone formation: In vitro and in vivo osteogenic activity of an adenovirus expressing BMP7. J Cell Biochem 2000;78:476–486.
29. Ramseier CA, Rasperini G, Batia S, Giannobile WV. Advanced reconstructive technologies for periodontal tissue repair. Periodontol 2000 2012;59:185–202.
30. Al-Dosari MS, Gao X. Nonviral gene delivery: Principle, limitations, and recent progress. AAPS J 2009;11:671–681.
31. Huang Z, Ryu W, Ren P, Fasching R, Goodman SB. Controlled release of growth factors on allograft bone in vitro. Clin Orthop Relat Res 2008;466:1905–1911.
32. Ramseier CA, Abramson ZR, Jin Q, Giannobile WV. Gene therapeutics for periodontal regenerative medicine. Dent Clin North Am 2006;50:245–263.
33. Lee J, Wikesjö UM. Growth/differentiation factor-5: Pre-clinical and clinical evaluations of periodontal regeneration and alveolar augmentation—Review. J Clin Periodontol 2014;41:797–805.
34. Rios HF, Bashutski JD, McAllister BS, et al. Emerging regenerative approaches for periodontal reconstruction: Practical applications from the AAP Regeneration Workshop. Clin Adv Periodontics 2015;5:40–46.
35. Khoshkam V, Chan HL, Lin GH, et al. Outcomes of regenerative treatment with rhPDGF-BB and rhFGF-2 for periodontal intrabony defects: A systematic review and meta-analysis. J Clin Periodontol 2015;42:272–280.
36. Lynch SE, Williams RC, Polson AM, et al. A combination of platelet-derived and insulin-like growth factors enhances periodontal regeneration. J Clin Periodontol 1989;16:545–548.
37. Park JB, Matsuura M, Han KY, et al. Periodontal regeneration in Class III furcation defects of beagle dogs using guided tissue regenerative therapy with platelet-derived growth factor. J Periodontol 1995;66:462–477.
38. Giannobile WV, Hernandez RA, Finkelman RD, et al. Comparative effects of platelet-derived growth factor-BB and insulin-like growth factor-I, individually and in combination, on periodontal regeneration in *Macaca fascicularis*. J Periodontal Res 1996;31:301–312.
39. Cho MI, Lin WL, Genco RJ. Platelet-derived growth factor-modulated guided tissue regenerative therapy. J Periodontol 1995;66:522–530.
40. Becker W, Lynch SE, Lekholm U, et al. A comparison of ePTFE membranes alone or in combination with platelet-derived growth factors and insulin-like growth factor-I or demineralized freeze-dried bone in promoting bone formation around immediate extraction socket implants. J Periodontol 1992;63:929–940.
41. Stefani CM, Machado MA, Sallum EA, Sallum AW, Toledo S, Nociti H Jr. Platelet-derived growth factor/insulin-like growth factor-1 combination and bone regeneration around implants placed into extraction sockets: A histometric study in dogs. Implant Dent 2000;9:126–131.
42. Lin Z, Rios HF, Cochran DL. Emerging regenerative approaches for periodontal reconstruction: A systematic review from the AAP Regeneration Workshop. J Periodontol 2015;86(2 suppl):134S–152S.
43. Nevins M, Kao RT, McGuire MK, et al. Platelet-derived growth factor promotes periodontal regeneration in localized osseous defects: 36-month extension results from a randomized, controlled, double-masked clinical trial. J Periodontol 2013;84:456–464.
44. McGuire MK, Scheyer ET, Schupbach P. Growth factor-mediated treatment of recession defects: A randomized controlled trial and histologic and microcomputed tomography examination. J Periodontol 2009;80:550–564.
45. Urist MR, Strates BS. Bone morphogenetic protein. J Dent Res 1971;50:1392–1406.
46. Fiorellini JP, Howell TH, Cochran D, et al. Randomized study evaluating recombinant human bone morphogenetic protein-2 for extraction socket augmentation. J Periodontol 2005;76:605–613.
47. Ripamonti U, Crooks J, Petit JC, Rueger DC. Periodontal tissue regeneration by combined applications of recombinant human osteogenic protein-1 and bone morphogenetic protein-2. A pilot study in Chacma baboons (*Papio ursinus*). Eur J Oral Sci 2001;109:241–248.
48. Triplett RG, Nevins M, Marx RE, et al. Pivotal, randomized, parallel evaluation of recombinant human bone morphogenetic protein-2/absorbable collagen sponge and autogenous bone graft for maxillary sinus floor augmentation. J Oral Maxillofac Surg 2009;67:1947–1960.
49. Kao DW, Kubota A, Nevins M, Fiorellini JP. The negative effect of combining rhBMP-2 and Bio-Oss on bone formation for maxillary sinus augmentation. Int J Periodontics Restorative Dent 2012;32:61–67.
50. Boyne PJ, Marx RE, Nevins M, et al. A feasibility study evaluating rhBMP-2/absorbable collagen sponge for maxillary sinus floor augmentation. Int J Periodontics Restorative Dent 1997;17:11–25.
51. James AW, LaChaud G, Shen J, et al. A review of the clinical side effects of bone morphogenetic protein-2. Tissue Eng Part B Rev 2016;22:284–297.
52. Kitamura M, Akamatsu M, Kawanami M, et al. Randomized placebo-controlled and controlled non-inferiority phase III trials comparing trafermin, a recombinant human fibroblast growth factor 2, and enamel matrix derivative in periodontal regeneration in intrabony defects. J Bone Miner Res 2016;31:806–814.
53. Stavropoulos A, Windisch P, Gera I, Capsius B, Sculean A, Wikesjö UM. A phase IIa randomized controlled clinical and histological pilot study evaluating rhGDF-5/beta-TCP for periodontal regeneration. J Clin Periodontol 2011;38:1044–1054.
54. Windisch P, Stavropoulos A, Molnar B, et al. A phase IIa randomized controlled pilot study evaluating the safety and clinical outcomes following the use of rhGDF-5/beta-TCP in regenerative periodontal therapy. Clin Oral Investig 2012;16:1181–1189.
55. Koch FP, Becker J, Terheyden H, Capsius B, Wagner W. A prospective, randomized pilot study on the safety and efficacy of recombinant human growth and differentiation factor-5 coated onto beta-tricalcium phosphate for sinus lift augmentation. Clin Oral Implants Res 2010;21:1301–1308.
56. Zetterström O, Andersson C, Eriksson L, et al. Clinical safety of enamel matrix derivative (Emdogain) in the treatment of periodontal defects. J Clin Periodontol 1997;24:697–704.
57. Gestrelius S, Andersson C, Johansson AC, et al. Formulation of enamel matrix derivative for surface coating. Kinetics and cell colonization. J Clin Periodontol 1997;24(9 Pt 2):678–684.
58. Gestrelius S, Andersson C, Lidström D, Hammarström L, Somerman M. In vitro studies on periodontal ligament cells and enamel matrix derivative. J Clin Periodontol 1997;24(9 Pt 2):685–692.
59. Shin SH, Cueva MA, Kerns DG, Hallmon WW, Rivera-Hidalgo F, Nunn ME. A comparative study of root coverage using acellular dermal matrix with and without enamel matrix derivative. J Periodontol 2007;78:411–421.

60. Sculean A, Chiantella GC, Windisch P, Donos N. Clinical and histologic evaluation of human intrabony defects treated with an enamel matrix protein derivative (Emdogain). Int J Periodontics Restorative Dent 2000;20:374–381.
61. Tonetti MS, Lang NP, Cortellini P, et al. Enamel matrix proteins in the regenerative therapy of deep intrabony defects. J Clin Periodontol 2002;29:317–325.
62. Takeda K, Mizutani K, Matsuura T, et al. Periodontal regenerative effect of enamel matrix derivative in diabetes. PLoS One 2018;13:e0207201.
63. Trombelli L, Farina R, Minenna L, Toselli L, Simonelli A. Regenerative periodontal treatment with the single flap approach in smokers and nonsmokers. Int J Periodontics Restorative Dent 2018;38:e59–e67.
64. Castellanos A, de la Rosa M, de la Garza M, Caffesse RG. Enamel matrix derivative and coronal flaps to cover marginal tissue recessions. J Periodontol 2006;77:7–14.
65. Whitman DH, Berry RL, Green DM. Platelet gel: An autologous alternative to fibrin glue with applications in oral and maxillofacial surgery. J Oral Maxillofac Surg 1997;55:1294–1299.
66. Jameson C. Autologous platelet concentrate for the production of platelet gel. Lab Med 2007;38:39–42.
67. Marx RE. Platelet-rich plasma: Evidence to support its use. J Oral Maxillofac Surg 2004;62:489–496.
68. Cromack DT, Porras-Reyes B, Mustoe TA. Current concepts in wound healing: Growth factor and macrophage interaction. J Trauma 1990;30(12 suppl):S129–S133.
69. Anitua E. Plasma rich in growth factors: Preliminary results of use in the preparation of future sites for implants. Int J Oral Maxillofac Implants 1999;14:529–535.
70. Dohan Ehrenfest DM, Del Corso M, Diss A, Mouhyi J, Charrier JB. Three-dimensional architecture and cell composition of a Choukroun's platelet-rich fibrin clot and membrane. J Periodontol 2010;81:546–555.
71. Kobayashi E, Flückiger L, Fujioka-Kobayashi M, et al. Comparative release of growth factors from PRP, PRF, and advanced-PRF. Clin Oral Investig 2016;20:2353–2360.
72. Marx RE, Carlson ER, Eichstaedt RM, Schimmele SR, Strauss JE, Georgeff KR. Platelet-rich plasma: Growth factor enhancement for bone grafts. Oral Surg Oral Med Oral Pathol Oral Radiol Endod 1998;85:638–646.
73. Miron RJ, Zucchelli G, Pikos MA, et al. Use of platelet-rich fibrin in regenerative dentistry: A systematic review. Clin Oral Investig 2017;21:1913–1927.
74. Miron RJ, Fujioka-Kobayashi M, Bishara M, Zhang Y, Hernandez M, Choukroun J. Platelet-rich fibrin and soft tissue wound healing: A systematic review. Tissue Eng Part B Rev 2017;23:83–99.
75. Jankovic S, Aleksic Z, Klokkevold P, et al. Use of platelet-rich fibrin membrane following treatment of gingival recession: A randomized clinical trial. Int J Periodontics Restorative Dent 2012;32:e41–e50.
76. Sousa F, Machado V, Botelho J, Proença L, Mendes JJ, Alves R. Effect of A-PRF application on palatal wound healing after free gingival graft harvesting: A prospective randomized study. Eur J Dent 2020;14:63–69.
77. Lossdörfer S, Götz W, Jäger A. PTH(1-34) affects osteoprotegerin production in human PDL cells in vitro. J Dent Res 2005;84:634–638.
78. Kuchler U, Luvizuto ER, Tangl S, Watzek G, Gruber R. Short-term teriparatide delivery and osseointegration: A clinical feasibility study. J Dent Res 2011;90:1001–1006.
79. Bashutski JD, Eber RM, Kinney JS, et al. Teriparatide and osseous regeneration in the oral cavity. N Engl J Med 2010;363:2396–2405.
80. Taba M Jr, Jin Q, Sugai JV, Giannobile WV. Current concepts in periodontal bioengineering. Orthod Craniofac Res 2005;8:292–302.
81. Yu L, Ding J. Injectable hydrogels as unique biomedical materials. Chem Soc Rev 2008;37:1473–1481.
82. Rasperini G, Pilipchuk SP, Flanagan CL, et al. 3D-printed bioresorbable scaffold for periodontal repair. J Dent Res 2015;94(9 suppl):153S–157S.

13

PERIODONTAL CHEMOTHERAPEUTICS

Andrea Ravidà, DDS, MS
Lorenzo Tavelli, DDS, MS

DEFINITIONS AND TERMINOLOGY

Adjunctive treatment: Supplementary and additional therapeutic procedures. In periodontics, it generally refers to procedures other than scaling and root planing and surgical therapy, such as chemotherapy and occlusal therapy.[5]

Antimicrobial therapy: The use of specific agents for the control or destruction of microorganisms, either systemically or at specific sites.[5]

Antiseptic: An agent that inhibits the growth and development of microorganisms.[5]

Chemotherapy: The treatment or control of a disease by chemical agents.[5]

Periodontal disease is caused by bacterial plaque and its by-products in a susceptible host. Thus, both the development and progression of this inflammatory condition are strongly associated with bacterial pathogens and the host immune response.

Soon after the removal of plaque and calculus from the dental surfaces, bacteria again initiate the formation of a biofilm that gradually becomes more complex. This biofilm will continuously increase in size, becoming more pathogenic, motile, and mainly composed of gram-negative anaerobic bacteria. In 1998, Socransky et al classified the microbial species involved in subgingival plaque into complexes, grouping together the species most associated with periodontal breakdown in the *red complex*. The red complex bacterial species—*Porphyromonas gingivalis*, *Treponema denticola*, and *Tannerella forsythia*—are now the most widely studied pathogens associated with periodontitis.[1] The presence of these species has been associated with an increased risk for periodontal breakdown, while their elimination results in improved clinical outcomes.[2] As such, when treating the different forms of periodontal disease, several **adjunctive treatments** (eg, antibiotics) can be applied. However, the mechanical removal of the etiologic and contributing factors is always required. Indeed, Haffajee et al, in a systematic review and the following consensus report, concluded that there was no evidence to support the use of systemic antibiotics as monotherapy without manual instrumentation of the root surfaces.[3] These results were corroborated a year later in an American Academy of Periodontology position paper.[4]

The adjunctive effect of periodontal chemotherapeutics (Fig 13-1) has been used to limit the bacterial growth, target putative pathogens, and modulate the host response to prevent tissue destruction and bone loss associated with periodontitis.

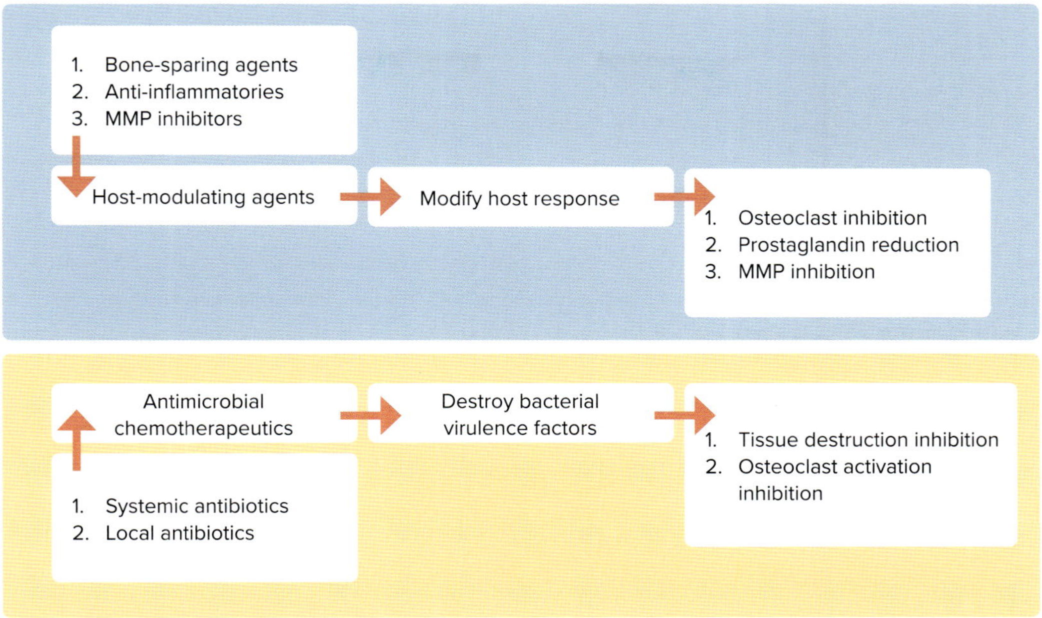

Fig 13-1 Periodontal chemotherapeutics. MMP, matrix metalloproteinase.

Systemic Antibiotics

INDICATIONS

Not all periodontal patients are good candidates to receive systemic antibiotics. Indeed, the effectiveness of the systemic administration of antibiotics may depend on the periodontal status (eg, pocket depths, degree of inflammation) and the presence or absence of etiologic/contributory factors. Moreover, before administering adjunctive periodontal therapy, several factors such as a patient's age, allergies, or other medical conditions must be taken into consideration. The risks and benefits of administering antibiotics should always be weighed for each particular individual before initiating therapy.

It has been reported that the following patients are good candidates to receive systemic antibiotics:

1. Patients who exhibit continuing breakdown of periodontal attachment despite conventional mechanical therapy.[6]
2. Patients with acute or severe periodontal infection (eg, acute necrotizing periodontal diseases, periodontal abscess).[7]
3. Patients with recurrent or refractory periodontitis related to persistent subgingival pathogens and possible impaired host resistance.
4. Patients with aggressive types of periodontitis.[8]
5. Patients with compromised medical conditions or poor host defense mechanisms.[9]
6. Patients with severe chronic periodontitis.[10,11]
7. Patients with diabetes mellitus[12] and smokers.[13]
8. Medically compromised patients as prophylaxis.
9. Patients receiving surgical or nonsurgical therapy, as an adjunct.

Moreover, in specific clinical scenarios, such as patients with progressive or active disease and deep pockets, the **antimicrobial therapy** in addition to scaling and root planing (SRP) could provide the patient with greater benefits and clinically relevant improvements.[14]

TIMING OF ANTIBIOTIC ADMINISTRATION

It has been reported that antibiotic administration after SRP could reduce the number of patients who undergo periodontal surgery, decreasing the need for further procedures.[15] To define guidelines and select the most appropriate timing for antibiotic administration, a careful evaluation of the scientific literature is paramount. So far, only a limited number of studies have investigated the most appropriate timing for systemic antibiotic administration.

The first question to be asked is: "Should we prescribe antibiotics following the first or last session of SRP?" A lack of high-quality evidence does not allow for strong conclusions to answer this question. In 1994, Loesche and Giordano[16] reanalyzed data from two previous clinical studies, one administering antibiotics after the first session of SRP[17] and the other study after the last session.[18] The final clinical outcomes reported better results in favor of the latter, suggesting that the use of antimicrobials is more effective when the majority of the biofilm has been disaggregated.

The second question is: "Should systemic antibiotics be prescribed following the last session of SRP or only at reevaluation after further reinstrumentation?" In a retrospective study, Kaner et al[19] compared two groups of patients with generalized aggressive periodontitis who were previously treated in two different studies by two different investigators.[20,21] The test group received systemic amoxicillin (AMX) and metronidazole (MTZ) immediately after SRP, while the control group received the same regimen 3 months after SRP (and following subgingival reinstrumentation). After 6 months of follow-up, in initially deep sites (probing depth > 6 mm at baseline), probing depth (PD) reduction and clinical attachment level (CAL) gain were significantly higher when the antibiotic was prescribed immediately after the last session of SRP. Furthermore, Guerrero et al performed a 6-month randomized clinical trial (RCT) in patients with generalized aggressive periodontitis comparing SRP with placebo versus SRP plus 500 mg AMX/500 mg MTZ.[22] At the end of this study, the authors continued investigating the same cohort of patients. This time, both groups underwent further instrumentation, taking as an adjunct the opposite medication as previously received (ie, patients who initially received placebo were given antibiotics while patients who initially received antibiotics were given placebo). This study design allowed the investigators to assess not only the clinical value of the antibiotic administration, but also the best timing for administration.[23] As a result, patients who received antibiotics at the initial therapy had a significant improvement in clinical parameters such as PD reduction and percentage of sites improving above clinically relevant thresholds, compared with patients who received antibiotics at retreatment. In summary, data from the available literature suggest that the best timing for the use of antimicrobials is immediately after the last session of SRP.

AZITHROMYCIN

Azithromycin (AZM) is a macrolide that binds to the 50S subunit of bacterial ribosome inhibiting protein synthesis. It is generally bacteriostatic but can be bactericidal in high concentrations. The higher resistance to the gastric acid is the main advantage of AZM because it increases its oral absorption to higher than other antibiotics in the azalides group. Furthermore, AZM has the potential of reaching very high concentrations in the tissue (100 times higher than serum AZM concentration). This includes infected tissue where it is preferentially carried on by phagocytes.[24] It is effective against a wide variety of oral bacteria,[25,26] particularly benzoyl-DL-arginine-naphthylamide (BANA) positive, red-complex species.[27] Another potential advantage is the higher patient compliance due to its short regimen.

The impact of adjunctive systemic AZM administration used together with periodontal therapy has yielded mixed results. Mascarenhas et al reported that the utilization of AZM in combination with SRP improves the efficacy of nonsurgical periodontal therapy in reducing PD and improving CAL in smokers.[27] Similar results were reported by Haffajee et al.[28] However, Sampaio et al found no adjunctive benefit of AZM in the treatment of generalized chronic periodontitis.[29] The adjunctive effects of systemic AZM in combination with periodontal pocket reduction surgery was also explored in the treatment of chronic periodontitis in smokers. The results showed that it did not significantly enhance PD reduction or CAL gain.[30] Overall, there is enough evidence to conclude that the systemic employment of AZM increases the therapeutic efficacy of SRP in patients with either chronic or aggressive periodontitis.[31,32] In particular, certain groups of patients (diabetic patients and smokers) seem to benefit the most from the administration of AZM. However, further studies are needed to present more solid evidence. Table 13-1 outlines all the RCTs comparing SRP + AZM versus SRP with or without placebo.[10,27,28,33–43]

METRONIDAZOLE

MTZ is a narrow-spectrum bactericidal antibiotic specific for anaerobes[44] that acts by disrupting bacterial DNA synthesis. This antibiotic has a half-life of 6 to 14 hours and is cleared by the liver. Adverse events are rare, but attention must be paid to the drug interaction between MTZ and warfarin or alcohol. The first study in periodontology using systemically administered MTZ was carried out in animals (mongrel dogs) to study the effect of this antibacterial substance on the quantity and quality of the dental plaque when signs of gingivitis were present. In this 1979 study, Listgarten et al reported that MTZ administration

TABLE 13-1 Randomized clinical trials comparing SRP + AZM versus SRP with or without placebo

Study	Disease	Posology	n test/n control	Intervention	Follow-up (m)	Main findings
Smith et al[33] (2002)	ChP (smokers and nonsmokers)	500 mg/3 days	23/21	Test: SRP + AZM Control: SRP + placebo	6	SRP + AZM useful in deep PD
Mascarenhas et al[27] (2005)	ChP (smokers)	500 mg/1 day 250 mg/4 days	15/15	Test: SRP + AZM Control: SRP alone	6	SRP + AZM reduced PD, increased CAL gain
Gomi et al[34] (2007)	ChP (nonsmokers)	500 mg/3 days	17/17	Test: SRP + AZM Control: SRP alone	6	SRP + AZM reduced PD, increased CAL gain
Haffajee et al[28] (2007)	ChP (smokers and nonsmokers)	500 mg/3 days	25/23	Test: SRP + AZM Control: SRP alone	12	SRP + AZM useful in deep PD
Haas et al[35] (2008)	AP (smokers and nonsmokers)	500 mg/3 days	12/12	Test: SRP + AZM Control: SRP + placebo	1	SRP + AZM reduced PD, increased CAL gain
Oteo et al[36] (2010)	ChP (smokers and nonsmokers)	500 mg/3 days	15/13	Test: SRP + AZM Control: SRP + placebo	6	SRP + AZM reduced PD, increased CAL gain
Han et al[10] (2012)	ChP (smokers and nonsmokers)	500 mg/3 days	14/14	Test: SRP + AZM Control: SRP + placebo	6	NSSD
Emingil et al[37] (2012)	AP (smokers and nonsmokers)	500 mg/3 days	16/16	Test: SRP + AZM Control: SRP + placebo	6	SRP + AZM reduced PD
Botero et al[38] (2013)	Diabetic patients with ChP (smokers and nonsmokers)	500 mg/3 days	31/28	Test: SRP + AZM Control: SRP + placebo	9	SRP + AZM reduced PD, increased CAL gain
Hincapié et al[39] (2014)	ChP (diabetic)	500 mg/3 days	33/37/35	Test: SRP + AZM Control 1: SRP + placebo Control 2: Supragingival prophylaxis with AZM	9	AZM no effect in frequency of detection of red complex bacteria
Fonseca et al[40] (2015)	ChP (smokers and nonsmokers)	500 mg/3 days	15/15	Test: SRP + AZM Control: SRP alone	6	NSSD
Martande et al[41] (2016)	ChP (nonsmokers)	500 mg/3 days	35/35	Test: SRP + AZM Control: SRP + placebo	12	SRP + AZM reduced PD, increased CAL gain
Saleh et al[42] (2016)	ChP (nonsmokers)	500 mg/3 days	11/10	Test: SRP + AZM Control: SRP alone	3	SRP + AZM reduced PD
Morales et al[43] (2018)	ChP (smokers and nonsmokers)	500 mg/3 days	16/15	Test: SRP + AZM Control: SRP + placebo	9	NSSD

ChP, chronic periodontitis; AP, aggressive periodontitis; NSSD, no statistically significant difference.

throughout a period of 4 weeks radically changed the composition of the microbial flora, reducing both plaque and gingival index scores, but did not eliminate gingivitis.[45] These results were later confirmed by Heijl and Lindhe in a similarly designed study during a period of 28 days.[46] Later on, due to the promising results in animal models, clinical trials were conducted in humans.

Loesche was the first investigator who suggested the use of MTZ for the treatment of chronic periodontal disease. Five patients with periodontitis were treated with 250 mg of MTZ for 1 week, and two of them received additional SRP. After the treatment, the percentage of spirochetes present in the periodontal pockets decreased for up to 6 months and an improvement in the clinical parameters was observed, especially in those sites having deep pockets or attachment loss ≥ 5 mm. A few years later, the same research group performed an RCT focused on whether or not MTZ could reduce the necessity of surgery after SRP. In this RCT, patients with BANA-positive results in ≥ 2 pockets or patients with elevated proportions of spirochetes were randomly assigned to MTZ (250 mg 3 times per day for 1 week, n = 15) or placebo (n = 18) after nonsurgical therapy. At the end of the study, the test group showed a statistically significant reduction in probing depth and attachment gain in moderate to deep pockets. In addition, the number of teeth in need of surgery reduced dramatically in the test group (from 14.9 to 6.0), while the control group only exhibited a modest reduction (from 14.3 to 11.0).[18] Although it is possible to find studies comparing SRP alone versus SRP + MTZ[13,28,47–52] this antibiotic is more often used in combination with AMX due to its poor efficacy against *Aggregatibacter actinomycetemcomitans*. For patients allergic to AMX, it could be combined with cefuroxime axetil or ciprofloxacin.[53]

COMBINATION THERAPY: METRONIDAZOLE AND AMOXICILLIN

Combination therapy refers to the simultaneous use of antibiotics from different drug classes to target a wide range of bacterial species. In periodontics, the most commonly employed antibiotic combination therapy is MTZ and AMX. Both drugs are bactericidal and provide a synergistic increase in activity.[54] It has been demonstrated that this combination therapy is effective against *A actinomycetemcomitans* in patients with various forms of periodontal disease by eliminating this bacterial strain in 114 out of 118 (96.6%) patients who had microbial tests positive for *A actinomycetemcomitans*.[55] In addition, its effectiveness has been confirmed clinically in systematic reviews and meta-analyses. In 2012, Sgolastra et al demonstrated that in patients with chronic periodontitis, MTZ and AMX increased CAL and decreased PD when compared with SRP alone. However, benefits were not significantly different between SRP and SRP with combination therapy for bleeding on probing (BOP), suppuration, or the reduction of microbial pathogens.[56] The same authors performed a similar meta-analysis in patients with aggressive periodontitis, reporting statistically significant PD reduction and CAL gain in the combination therapy group.[56]

Despite the vast number of articles reporting the clinical benefit of the adjunctive use of AMX + MTZ for the treatment of periodontal disease (Table 13-2),[14,56–58] only recently has the optimal dose and duration been addressed. McGowan et al performed a meta-analysis including 18 randomized placebo-controlled trials and concluded that after 3 months, there was no clinical difference between different doses or duration of the antibiotics. Hence, without clear superiority of one regimen, they recommended the use of the highest dose (500/500 mg or 500/400 mg) three times daily for the shortest duration of time (7 days) to reduce the risk of antibiotic resistance.[58] Finally, direct clinical comparison of MTZ + AMX versus MTZ alone has been conducted in a series of studies that have reported a tendency toward overall greater benefits for the MTZ + AMX regimen[13,50,59] with no statistically significant differences between groups.

TETRACYCLINE

Tetracyclines are a group of bacteriostatic antibiotics that act by binding to the 30S ribosomal subunit, which in turn prevents the binding of the tRNA and mRNA ribosomal complex. In addition, it has been demonstrated that they are able to inhibit collagenase activity due to the inhibition of matrix metalloproteinase (MMP) activity.[60,61] Tetracyclines are effective against many anaerobic bacteria and more efficient against gram-positive than gram-negative bacteria. The drug class includes tetracycline as well as the semi-synthetics minocycline and doxycycline. Doxycycline (50- or 100-mg capsule) has the longest half-life and the highest protein binding capacity,[4] while minocycline has the best tissue penetration (absorption). The effectiveness of the tetracyclines in the treatment of periodontal disease was initially attributed to its concentration in the crevicular fluid being two to four times higher than in the blood.[62] However, in contrast to the earliest findings,

TABLE 13-2 Systematic reviews evaluating MTZ and AMX

Study	Type of periodontitis	Main conclusion
Herrera et al[14] (2002)	Chronic and aggressive	SRP + Atb: greater CAL and PD change than SRP alone and reduced risk of additional CAL loss; AMX + MTZ greatest CAL change in deep pockets
Sgolastra et al[57] (2012)	Chronic	AMX + MTZ + SRP more effective than SRP alone in chronic periodontitis (CAL gain and PD reduction); no differences in BOP reduction or suppuration
Sgolastra et al[56] (2012)	Aggressive	AMX + MTZ + SRP more effective than SRP alone in aggressive periodontitis (CAL gain and PD reduction); no significant adverse event
McGowan et al[58] (2018)	Chronic and aggressive	No difference between different doses or duration of AMX + MTZ at 3 months; 7-day regimen of 500/500 mg or 500/400 mg three times daily of AMX + MTZ was recommended

Atb, antibiotics.

Sakellari et al reported that tetracycline concentration in the gingival crevicular fluid seems to be less than in the plasma with variability among different individuals.[63] A variety of side effects have been associated with this antibiotic, including dizziness, headache, increased blood urea nitrogen, gastrointestinal disorders, and tooth discoloration in children, as well as increased bacterial resistance of up to 77% of the cultivable subgingival microflora.[64] Hence, while systemic tetracycline therapy was formerly very common, the use of MTZ and AMX is now preferred to avoid such complications and side effects.

Local Antimicrobials

Antimicrobials can be delivered locally through several vehicles, including chips, trays, polymers, and fibers. Although it is possible to find classic studies performing full-mouth treatment,[65,66] the employment of local antimicrobials is currently restricted to patients with localized periodontal lesions and patients with refractory periodontitis undergoing maintenance therapy. The advantages of the local over the systemic administration are the reduced side effects, bacterial resistance, and development of superinfections. Furthermore, local antimicrobials demonstrated higher local availability and low plasma levels,[67] as well as controlled release for several days. However, the available evidence has shown very controversial results, raising several questions on their usage. The drugs investigated for local application include minocycline, azithromycin, doxycycline, tetracycline, and MTZ (Table 13-3). Today, the use of locally delivered antibiotics is gaining popularity for the treatment of implant diseases.

MINOCYCLINE MICROSPHERES AND OINTMENT

Two different forms of subgingivally administrating minocycline have been reported in the literature. The first one as a 2% ointment (Dentomycin, Cyanamid) and the second as microspheres in a dry powder with a bioabsorbable polymer in a 1:3 ratio (1 mg microsphere + 3 mg polymer = 4 mg total), via a syringe, under the trade name Arestin (Bausch Health). When the microspheres and the polymer contact moisture inside the pocket, the antibiotic is released. It has been shown that gradual release allowed for the presence of minocycline in the gingival crevicular fluid with a concentration up to 34 mg/mL for up to 14 days.[68] In 2001, Williams et al conducted a multicenter RCT to study the efficacy and safety of minocycline microspheres when administered as an adjunct to nonsurgical therapy in patients with moderate or advanced periodontitis. PD reductions after 9 months were significantly higher for the combined therapy group, showing a 22% greater therapeutic effect when compared with SRP alone.[68] Furthermore, when the same comparison was performed in smokers, minocycline microspheres demonstrated a 32% greater PD reduction than SRP alone at 9 months.[69] Higher PD reduction in favor of SRP with minocycline has been consistently reported in several clinical trials.[70–74] However, this pattern was not always valid for BOP and CAL.

TABLE 13-3 Examples of locally delivered antibiotics

Brand name (manufacturer)	Antibiotic	Carrier	Dosage or concentration	Characteristic	Administration
Arestin (Bausch Health)	Minocycline hydrochloride	Microspheres	1 mg	Bactericidal, absorbable	1 application
Atridox (DenMat)	Doxycycline hyclate	Flowable polymer	10%	Bactericidal, absorbable	1 application
Actisite (Alza)*	Tetracycline	Nonabsorbable fibers	12.7 mg	Bactericidal, nonabsorbable	1 application (remove after 10 days)

*No longer available in the United States.

AZITHROMYCIN GEL

Locally delivered 0.5% azithromycin (indigenously prepared bioabsorbable controlled-release gel) as an adjunct to nonsurgical treatment has been studied in multiple clinical trials and demonstrated to be effective in the treatment of chronic periodontitis. A recent meta-analysis evaluating the effect of locally delivered azithromycin plus SRP compared with SRP alone reported statistically significant reduction in PD by 0.99 mm (95% confidence interval 0.42–1.57) and increased attachment level by 1.12 mm (95% confidence interval 0.31–1.92) in favor of the combined therapy.[31] Another study[75] was performed in patients with chronic periodontitis and type 2 diabetes. The results were in line with that of the meta-analysis showing enhanced reductions in PD and gain in CAL over 9 months for the group where the antibiotic was applied.[75]

DOXYCYCLINE

Doxycycline hyclate, with the trade name Atridox (DenMat), is a gel administered via syringe, mixing two components: *(1)* the active 10% doxycycline gel and *(2)* the delivery vehicle, a flowable bioabsorbable carrier. This controlled-release drug in the gingival fluid reaches concentrations that range from over 1,900 mg/mL during the first day of administration to about 300 mg/mL after 1 week.[76] The efficacy of this drug delivery system was first evaluated as a monotherapy in two classic articles.[77,78] In the first article, it showed superior results when compared with placebo and oral hygiene, and equal results when compared with SRP. In the second study, similar results were found when comparing Atridox alone and SRP alone. The same group reported that in patients with chronic periodontitis in the posterior dentition, Atridox administered with 45 minutes of debridement showed better results than 4 hours of SRP alone at the 3-month follow-up. However, at the 6-month examination, no statistically significant differences in PD or CAL were found between the two treatment groups.[79] Furthermore, Walker et al[80,81] showed that a treatment with doxycycline reduced the anaerobic population/red-complex bacteria and did not lead to antibiotic resistance. At least six other articles have studied doxycycline hyclate in addition to SRP,[82–87] reporting better short-term PD and CAL reduction than with SRP alone. However, this trend was not found for BOP and plaque levels. It must be remembered that the use of doxycycline or any other locally delivered antibiotic is only recommended as an adjunctive therapy to SRP and/or maintenance in isolated sites.

TETRACYCLINE FIBER

Nonabsorbable tetracycline HCl (12.7 mg) in a 23-mm length and 0.5-mm diameter fiber (trade name: Actisite, Alza) was the first locally delivered antibiotic with FDA approval. However, this product is no longer available in the United States. When positioned in the pocket, the fibers are retained for 10 days (not absorbable) and usually wrapped with cyanoacrylate to maintain them into the pocket.

Several researchers have studied Actisite as adjunctive therapy for SRP. A two-part study by Goodson et al reported that tetracycline fibers used after SRP decreased PD and increased CAL compared to SRP alone in patients with chronic periodontitis.[88,89] However, Drisko et al reported no difference between test and control groups after 12 months.[90] Newman et al performed the same comparison in periodontal maintenance patients with localized areas of recurrent periodontitis. The results showed better CAL gain (1.81 mm vs 1.08 mm) and PD reduction (1.56 mm vs 1.08 mm) in patients with SRP combined with Actisite adjunctive therapy after 6 months.[91] Furthermore, Actisite showed a reduction in PD, especially in deep pockets (reduction of 3.2 mm in sites with PD of ≥ 7 mm) after 6 months in patients with refractory periodontitis.[92] Finally, rinsing with 0.12% chlorhexidine after tetracycline fiber placement could have a synergistic effect, decreasing the number of bacterial pathogens.[93] Multiple other investigations studied the efficacy of tetracycline in this vehicle,[94–99] reporting similar findings in favor of tetracycline fiber administration in addition to SRP compared with SRP alone in terms of PD, CAL, and BOP.

METRONIDAZOLE GEL

For the local delivery of MTZ, it was developed as a gel formed of 40% MTZ benzoate corresponding to 25% MTZ in a mixture of glycerol mono-oleate and sesame oil. A gradual release of the antibiotic takes place from the gel matrix and after 1 day exceeds the minimum inhibitory concentration in half of the patients.[100] Lie et al compared the effect of SRP and MTZ gel versus SRP alone versus SRP plus topical tetracycline in 18 patients with chronic periodontitis. All of the treatment groups showed a significant change from baseline after 3 and 6 months ($P < .01$). However, no differences for PD and relative attachment level between the treatment groups were reported.[101] In a similar study, Kinane and Radvar compared SRP alone (20 patients) versus three different combination treatments: SRP in conjunction with *(1)* 25% tetracycline fibers (19 patients); *(2)* 2% minocycline gel (21 patients); and *(3)* 25% MTZ gel (19 patients). All treatment groups presented better clinical parameters than the control group (SRP alone). In addition, tetracycline fiber applications showed significant improvement in PD over SRP and MTZ at 3 months (1.5 mm vs 0.9 mm), but not at 6 months (1.38 mm vs 0.93 mm).[97] Finally, results from other investigations studying the performance of this gel consistently favored SRP with MTZ over SRP alone.[23,102–104]

Host-Modulating Agents

Host modulation was first introduced to dentistry in 1990.[105] The main goal of this approach is to modify the host response by downregulating damaging factors and events and regulating regenerative or defensive responses. Today, there are multiple human and animal studies evaluating the pharmacologic agents modulating the host response and their effectiveness to reduce the consequences of periodontal disease.

MATRIX METALLOPROTEINASE INHIBITORS

MMPs are endopeptidases responsible for the degradation of collagen and other proteins in the extracellular matrix. In numerous pathologic conditions such as periodontitis, MMPs are the important mediators associated with tissue destruction and progression of the disease. Depending on their location of production, MMPs can be divided into bacteria-derived and host-derived. In the first group, MMPs are produced by periodontal pathogens,[106] while in the second, by host cells (eg, macrophages and neutrophils). The main goal of host modulation therapy is to increase MMP inhibitors and therefore decrease extracellular collagen destruction. In 1984, Golub et al showed that tetracycline antibiotics possess the ability to inhibit collagenase activity.[107] Subantimicrobial doses (eg, 20 mg) of doxycycline, for example, showed an improved periodontal condition when administered over a 9-month period. Caton et al compared the effects in chronic periodontitis patients who received SRP alone and patients who received SRP in conjunction with 20 mg of doxycycline. Statistically significant CAL gain and PD reduction were reported in the group receiving doxycycline compared with the control group after 3 months of treatment. Furthermore, additional improvements were seen at 6 and 9 months. This study showed the following about long-term subantimicrobial doses of doxycycline[108]:

- Do not lead to antibiotic resistance
- Decrease the number of spirochetes without altering the number of other cellular morphotypes
- Are more effective in more compromised sites

Out of the initial 181 patients, 146 were included in the follow-up study, which included an additional 3-month recall. This study revealed that although PDs remained significantly reduced, the CALs were no longer significantly improved.[109] More recently, Tüter et al reported greater improvement for PD, gingival index, and gingival crevicular fluid levels of MMP-8 when using SRP plus a subantimicrobial dose of doxycycline compared with SRP plus placebo.[110] Furthermore, Preshaw et al studied its usage in a population of patients who smoked, reporting 21% greater CAL gain and 26% greater reduction of PD in smokers who received a subantimicrobial dose of doxycycline than those who received a placebo.[111] Nowadays, the commercially available form of subantimicrobial doses of doxycycline is called Periostat (Pharmaceutical Manufacturing Research Services) and is the only available agent approved by the FDA to use as a host modulation agent.

ANTI-INFLAMMATORY THERAPIES

Nonsteroidal anti-inflammatory drugs (NSAIDs) are commonly used to decrease pain and reduce chronic or acute inflammation. The capacity of NSAIDs to decrease the amount of bone loss in patients with periodontal disease has also been studied. This is accomplished through the inhibition of the enzymes cyclooxygenase 1 (COX-1) and COX-2 (enzymes involved in the inflammatory process) that synthetize arachidonic acid metabolites. One particular metabolite, prostaglandin E2 (PGE2), has been found in the gingival crevicular fluid and has been associated with periodontal destruction.[112] NSAIDs have the capacity to inhibit the lipoxygenase and COX enzymes, thereby suppressing the production of leukotrienes, thromboxane, prostaglandins, and prostacyclin. However, their administration during periodontal treatment is not suggested due to the adverse effects of the nonselective inhibition of COX-1 and COX-2[113] such as hemorrhage, renal and hepatic impairment, as well as damage to the mucosa of the gastrointestinal tract. For this reason, NSAIDs have not be approved by the FDA for the treatment of periodontitis.

BONE-SPARING AGENTS

Bisphosphonates are chemically stable analogs of pyrophosphates.[114] They can control mineralization and bone resorption in vivo and calcium phosphate formation and dissolution in vitro.[115] They are frequently used as a treatment of bone diseases such as osteoporosis, Paget disease of bone, bone metastasis, and multiple myeloma. In periodontics, the published studies have reported promising results by modifying the host response and reducing bone loss in patients taking bisphosphonates when compared with control subjects. Rocha et al performed an RCT to study the effect of alendronate on periodontal bone loss in patients with type 2 diabetes mellitus. The results showed that the additional use of alendronate resulted in significantly more improvement in alveolar bone crest height than placebo therapy after 6 months of treatment.[116] Bashutski et al reported that the employment of teriparatide was associated with a greater resolution of alveolar bone defects than placebo in humans and may offer therapeutic potential for localized bone defects.[117] Furthermore, other articles reported a decrease in PD and tooth mobility in patients taking bisphosphonates (etidronate) after SRP.[118,119] On the other hand, some trials failed to show a significant improvement in humans,[120] while others even reported greater periodontal destruction in the group receiving bisphosphonates.[121] Today, bisphosphonates are not routinely used in the treatment of periodontitis, and no bisphosphonate-related medication is approved by the FDA for treatment of periodontal diseases. In addition, the use of bisphosphonates could lead to undesired side effects and complications.[122]

Conclusions

It has been demonstrated that, generally speaking, the administration of systemically or locally delivered antibiotics can improve the outcomes of nonsurgical therapy. Nevertheless, case selection and weighing the potential risks and benefits must always be considered. Similarly, depending on the local and systemic conditions of the patient, antibiotics may be more or less effective. For example, patients with deep pockets, smokers, or cases of aggressive disease may benefit the most from this adjunctive therapy. However, to limit their overuse, potentially leading to the development of bacterial resistance, routine prescription for all patients is not recommended. At the moment, the highest dose (500/500 mg or 500/400 mg) of systemic combination therapy (AMX and MTZ) for the shortest duration (7-day regimen) as an adjunct to SRP is the most documented form of administered antibiotics in periodontal therapy.

References

1. Socransky SS, Haffajee AD, Cugini MA, Smith C, Kent RL Jr. Microbial complexes in subgingival plaque. J Clin Periodontol 1998;25:134–144.
2. Haffajee AD, Socransky SS, Patel MR, Song X. Microbial complexes in supragingival plaque. Oral Microbiol Immunol 2008;23:196–205.
3. Haffajee AD, Socransky SS, Gunsolley JC. Systemic anti-infective periodontal therapy. A systematic review. Ann Periodontol 2003;8:115–181.
4. Slots J, Greenwell H, Fiorellini J, Giannobile W, Offenbacher S, Salkin L. Systemic antibiotics in periodontics. J Periodontol 2004;75:1553–1565.
5. American Academy of Periodontology. Glossary of Periodontal Terms. American Academy of Periodontology, 2001.
6. Slots J, Rams TE. New views on periodontal microbiota in special patient categories. J Clin Periodontol 1991;18:411–420.
7. Johnson BD, Engel D. Acute necrotizing ulcerative gingivitis. A review of diagnosis, etiology and treatment. J Periodontol 1986;57:141–150.
8. Schenkein HA, Van Dyke TE. Early-onset periodontitis: Systemic aspects of etiology and pathogenesis. Periodontol 2000 1994;6:7–25.
9. Special patient categories. Periodontol 2000 1994;6:1–124.
10. Han B, Emingil G, Özdemir G, et al. Azithromycin as an adjunctive treatment of generalized severe chronic periodontitis: Clinical, microbiologic, and biochemical parameters. J Periodontol 2012;83:1480–1491.
11. Borges I, Faveri M, Figueiredo LC, et al. Different antibiotic protocols in the treatment of severe chronic periodontitis: A 1-year randomized trial. J Clin Periodontol 2017;44:822–832.
12. Tamashiro NS, Duarte PM, Miranda TS, et al. Amoxicillin plus metronidazole therapy for patients with periodontitis and type 2 diabetes: A 2-year randomized controlled trial. J Dent Res 2016;95:829–836.
13. Matarazzo F, Figueiredo LC, Cruz SE, Faveri M, Feres M. Clinical and microbiological benefits of systemic metronidazole and amoxicillin in the treatment of smokers with chronic periodontitis: A randomized placebo-controlled study. J Clin Periodontol 2008;35:885–896.
14. Herrera D, Sanz M, Jepsen S, Needleman I, Roldán S. A systematic review on the effect of systemic antimicrobials as an adjunct to scaling and root planing in periodontitis patients. J Clin Periodontol 2002;29(3 suppl):136–159.
15. Walters J, Lai PC. Should antibiotics be prescribed to treat chronic periodontitis? Dent Clin North Am 2015;59:919–933.
16. Loesche WJ, Giordano JR. Metronidazole in periodontitis V: Debridement should precede medication. Compendium 1994;15:1198–1203.
17. Loesche WJ, Schmidt E, Smith BA, Morrison EC, Caffesse R, Hujoel PP. Effects of metronidazole on periodontal treatment needs. J Periodontol 1991;62:247–257.
18. Loesche WJ, Giordano JR, Hujoel P, Schwarcz J, Smith BA. Metronidazole in periodontitis: Reduced need for surgery. J Clin Periodontol 1992;19:103–112.
19. Kaner D, Christan C, Dietrich T, Bernimoulin JP, Kleber BM, Friedmann A. Timing affects the clinical outcome of adjunctive systemic antibiotic therapy for generalized aggressive periodontitis. J Periodontol 2007;78:1201–1208.
20. Christan C, Dietrich T, Hägewald S, Kage A, Bernimoulin JP. White blood cell count in generalized aggressive periodontitis after non-surgical therapy. J Clin Periodontol 2002;29:201–206.
21. Kaner D, Bernimoulin JP, Kleber BM, Heizmann WR, Friedmann A. Gingival crevicular fluid levels of calprotectin and myeloperoxidase during therapy for generalized aggressive periodontitis. J Periodontal Res 2006;41:132–139.
22. Guerrero A, Griffiths GS, Nibali L, et al. Adjunctive benefits of systemic amoxicillin and metronidazole in non-surgical treatment of generalized aggressive periodontitis: A randomized placebo-controlled clinical trial. J Clin Periodontol 2005;32:1096–1107.
23. Griffiths GS, Ayob R, Guerrero A, et al. Amoxicillin and metronidazole as an adjunctive treatment in generalized aggressive periodontitis at initial therapy or re-treatment: A randomized controlled clinical trial. J Clin Periodontol 2011;38:43–49.
24. Gladue RP, Bright GM, Isaacson RE, Newborg MF. In vitro and in vivo uptake of azithromycin (CP-62,993) by phagocytic cells: Possible mechanism of delivery and release at sites of infection. Antimicrob Agents Chemother 1989;33:277–282.
25. Position Paper: Systemic antibiotics in periodontics. J Periodontol 2004;75:1553–1565.
26. Blandizzi C, Malizia T, Lupetti A, et al. Periodontal tissue disposition of azithromycin in patients affected by chronic inflammatory periodontal diseases. J Periodontol 1999;70:960–966.
27. Mascarenhas P, Gapski R, Al-Shammari K, et al. Clinical response of azithromycin as an adjunct to non-surgical periodontal therapy in smokers. J Periodontol 2005;76:426–436.
28. Haffajee AD, Torresyap G, Socransky SS. Clinical changes following four different periodontal therapies for the treatment of chronic periodontitis: 1-year results. J Clin Periodontol 2007;34:243–253.
29. Sampaio E, Rocha M, Figueiredo LC, et al. Clinical and microbiological effects of azithromycin in the treatment of generalized chronic periodontitis: A randomized placebo-controlled clinical trial. J Clin Periodontol 2011;38:838–846.
30. Dastoor SF, Travan S, Neiva RF, Rayburn LA, Giannobile WV, Wang HL. Effect of adjunctive systemic azithromycin with periodontal surgery in the treatment of chronic periodontitis in smokers: A pilot study. J Periodontol 2007;78:1887–1896.
31. Zhang Z, Zheng Y, Bian X. Clinical effect of azithromycin as an adjunct to non-surgical treatment of chronic periodontitis: A meta-analysis of randomized controlled clinical trials. J Periodontal Res 2016;51:275–283.
32. Buset SL, Zitzmann NU, Weiger R, Walter C. Non-surgical periodontal therapy supplemented with systemically administered azithromycin: A systematic review of RCTs. Clin Oral Investig 2015;19:1763–1775.
33. Smith SR, Foyle DM, Daniels J, et al. A double-blind placebo-controlled trial of azithromycin as an adjunct to non-surgical treatment of periodontitis in adults: Clinical results. J Clin Periodontol 2002;29:54–61.
34. Gomi K, Yashima A, Nagano T, Kanazashi M, Maeda N, Arai T. Effects of full-mouth scaling and root planing in conjunction with systemically administered azithromycin. J Periodontol 2007;78:422–429.
35. Haas AN, de Castro GD, Moreno T, et al. Azithromycin as an adjunctive treatment of aggressive periodontitis: 12-months randomized clinical trial. J Clin Periodontol 2008;35:696–704.
36. Oteo A, Herrera D, Figuero E, O'Connor A, Gonzalez I, Sanz M. Azithromycin as an adjunct to scaling and root planing in the treatment of *Porphyromonas gingivalis*-associated periodontitis: A pilot study. J Clin Periodontol 2010;37:1005–1015.
37. Emingil G, Han B, Ozdemir G, et al. Effect of azithromycin, as an adjunct to nonsurgical periodontal treatment, on microbiological parameters and gingival crevicular fluid biomarkers in generalized aggressive periodontitis. J Periodontal Res 2012;47:729–739.

38. Botero JE, Yepes FL, Ochoa SP, et al. Effects of periodontal non-surgical therapy plus azithromycin on glycemic control in patients with diabetes: A randomized clinical trial. J Periodontal Res 2013;48:706–712.
39. Hincapié JP, Castrillón CA, Yepes FL, et al. Microbiological effects of periodontal therapy plus azithromycin in patients with diabetes: Results from a randomized clinical trial. Acta Odontol Latinoam 2014;27:89–95.
40. Fonseca DC, Cortelli JR, Cortelli SC, et al. Clinical and microbiologic evaluation of scaling and root planing per quadrant and one-stage full-mouth disinfection associated with azithromycin or chlorhexidine: A clinical randomized controlled trial. J Periodontol 2015;86:1340–1351.
41. Martande SS, Pradeep AR, Singh SP, et al. Clinical and microbiological effects of systemic azithromycin in adjunct to nonsurgical periodontal therapy in treatment of *Aggregatibacter actinomycetemcomitans* associated periodontitis: A randomized placebo-controlled clinical trial. J Investig Clin Dent 2016;7:72–80.
42. Saleh A, Rincon J, Tan A, Firth M. Comparison of adjunctive azithromycin and amoxicillin/metronidazole for patients with chronic periodontitis: Preliminary randomized control trial. Aust Dent J 2016;61:469–481.
43. Morales A, Gandolfo A, Bravo J, et al. Microbiological and clinical effects of probiotics and antibiotics on nonsurgical treatment of chronic periodontitis: A randomized placebo-controlled trial with 9-month follow-up. J Appl Oral Sci 2018;26:e20170075.
44. Tally FP, Sutter VL, Finegold SM. Treatment of anaerobic infections with metronidazole. Antimicrob Agents Chemother 1975;7:672–675.
45. Listgarten MA, Lindhe J, Parodi R. The effect of systemic antimicrobial therapy on plaque and gingivitis in dogs. J Periodontal Res 1979;14:65–75.
46. Heijl L, Lindhe J. The effect of metronidazole on the development of plaque and gingivitis in the beagle dog. J Clin Periodontol 1979;6:197–209.
47. Carvalho LH, D'Avila GB, Leão A, Haffajee AD, Socransky SS, Feres M. Scaling and root planing, systemic metronidazole and professional plaque removal in the treatment of chronic periodontitis in a Brazilian population. I. Clinical results. J Clin Periodontol 2004;31:1070–1076.
48. Rooney J, Wade WG, Sprague SV, Newcombe RG, Addy M. Adjunctive effects to non-surgical periodontal therapy of systemic metronidazole and amoxycillin alone and combined. A placebo controlled study. J Clin Periodontol 2002;29:342–350.
49. Palmer RM, Matthews JP, Wilson RF. Non-surgical periodontal treatment with and without adjunctive metronidazole in smokers and non-smokers. J Clin Periodontol 1999;26:158–163.
50. Feres M, Soares GM, Mendes JA, et al. Metronidazole alone or with amoxicillin as adjuncts to non-surgical treatment of chronic periodontitis: A 1-year double-blinded, placebo-controlled, randomized clinical trial. J Clin Periodontol 2012;39:1149–1158.
51. Preus HR, Gunleiksrud TM, Sandvik L, Gjermo P, Baelum V. A randomized, double-masked clinical trial comparing four periodontitis treatment strategies: 1-year clinical results. J Periodontol 2013;84:1075–1086.
52. Sigusch B, Beier M, Klinger G, Pfister W, Glockmann E. A 2-step non-surgical procedure and systemic antibiotics in the treatment of rapidly progressive periodontitis. J Periodontol 2001;72:275–283.
53. van Winkelhoff AJ, Winkel EG. Microbiological diagnostics in periodontics: Biological significance and clinical validity. Periodontol 2000 2005;39:40–52.
54. Pavicić MJ, van Winkelhoff AJ, de Graaff J. Synergistic effects between amoxicillin, metronidazole, and the hydroxymetabolite of metronidazole against *Actinobacillus actinomycetemcomitans*. Antimicrob Agents Chemother 1991;35:961–966.
55. van Winkelhoff AJ, Tijhof CJ, de Graaff J. Microbiological and clinical results of metronidazole plus amoxicillin therapy in *Actinobacillus actinomycetemcomitans*-associated periodontitis. J Periodontol 1992;63:52–57.
56. Sgolastra F, Petrucci A, Gatto R, Monaco A. Effectiveness of systemic amoxicillin/metronidazole as an adjunctive therapy to full-mouth scaling and root planing in the treatment of aggressive periodontitis: A systematic review and meta-analysis. J Periodontol 2012;83:731–743.
57. Sgolastra F, Gatto R, Petrucci A, Monaco A. Effectiveness of systemic amoxicillin/metronidazole as adjunctive therapy to scaling and root planing in the treatment of chronic periodontitis: A systematic review and meta-analysis. J Periodontol 2012;83:1257–1269.
58. McGowan K, McGowan T, Ivanovski S. Optimal dose and duration of amoxicillin-plus-metronidazole as an adjunct to non-surgical periodontal therapy: A systematic review and meta-analysis of randomized, placebo-controlled trials. J Clin Periodontol 2018;45:56–67.
59. Silva MP, Feres M, Sirotto TA, et al. Clinical and microbiological benefits of metronidazole alone or with amoxicillin as adjuncts in the treatment of chronic periodontitis: A randomized placebo-controlled clinical trial. J Clin Periodontol 2011;38:828–837.
60. Golub LM, Wolff M, Lee HM, et al. Further evidence that tetracyclines inhibit collagenase activity in human crevicular fluid and from other mammalian sources. J Periodontal Res 1985;20:12–23.
61. Burns FR, Stack MS, Gray RD, Paterson CA. Inhibition of purified collagenase from alkali-burned rabbit corneas. Invest Ophthalmol Vis Sci 1989;30:1569–1575.
62. Gordon JM, Walker CB, Murphy JC, Goodson JM, Socransky SS. Tetracycline: Levels achievable in gingival crevice fluid and in vitro effect on subgingival organisms. Part I. Concentrations in crevicular fluid after repeated doses. J Periodontol 1981;52:609–612.
63. Sakellari D, Goodson JM, Kolokotronis A, Konstantinidis A. Concentration of 3 tetracyclines in plasma, gingival crevice fluid and saliva. J Clin Periodontol 2000;27:53–60.
64. Kornman KS, Karl EH. The effect of long-term low-dose tetracycline therapy on the subgingival microflora in refractory adult periodontitis. J Periodontol 1982;53:604–610.
65. Fourmousis I, Tonetti MS, Mombelli A, Lehmann B, Lang NP, Brägger U. Evaluation of tetracycline fiber therapy with digital image analysis. J Clin Periodontol 1998;25:737–745.
66. Mombelli A, Lehmann B, Tonetti M, Lang NP. Clinical response to local delivery of tetracycline in relation to overall and local periodontal conditions. J Clin Periodontol 1997;24:470–477.
67. Southard GL, Dunn RL, Garrett S. The drug delivery and biomaterial attributes of the Atrigel technology in the treatment of periodontal disease. Expert Opin Investig Drugs 1998;7:1483–1491.
68. Williams RC, Paquette DW, Offenbacher S, et al. Treatment of periodontitis by local administration of minocycline microspheres: A controlled trial. J Periodontol 2001;72:1535–1544.
69. Paquette D, Oringer R, Lessem J, et al. Locally delivered minocycline microspheres for the treatment of periodontitis in smokers. J Clin Periodontol 2003;30:787–794.
70. Nakagawa T, Yamada S, Oosuka Y, et al. Clinical and microbiological study of local minocycline delivery (Periocline) following scaling and root planing in recurrent periodontal pockets. Bull Tokyo Dent Coll 1991;32:63–70.

71. Henderson RJ, Boyens JV, Holborow DW, Pack AR. Scaling and root-planing treatment with adjunctive subgingival minocycline. A clinical pilot study over six months, of sites adjacent to and remote from the antibiotic application. J Int Acad Periodontol 2002;4:77–87.
72. Graça MA, Watts TL, Wilson RF, Palmer RM. A randomized controlled trial of a 2% minocycline gel as an adjunct to non-surgical periodontal treatment, using a design with multiple matching criteria. J Clin Periodontol 1997;24:249–253.
73. Bland PS, Goodson JM, Gunsolley JC, et al. Association of antimicrobial and clinical efficacy: Periodontitis therapy with minocycline microspheres. J Int Acad Periodontol 2010;12:11–19.
74. Goodson JM, Gunsolley JC, Grossi SG, et al. Minocycline HCl microspheres reduce red-complex bacteria in periodontal disease therapy. J Periodontol 2007;78:1568–1579.
75. Agarwal E, Bajaj P, Naik SB, Pradeep AR. Locally delivered 0.5% azithromycin as an adjunct to non-surgical treatment in patients with chronic periodontitis with type 2 diabetes: A randomized controlled clinical trial. J Periodontol 2017;88:1281–1287.
76. Stoller NH, Johnson LR, Trapnell S, Harrold CQ, Garrett S. The pharmacokinetic profile of a biodegradable controlled-release delivery system containing doxycycline compared to systemically delivered doxycycline in gingival crevicular fluid, saliva, and serum. J Periodontol 1998;69:1085–1091.
77. Garrett S, Johnson L, Drisko CH, et al. Two multi-center studies evaluating locally delivered doxycycline hyclate, placebo control, oral hygiene, and scaling and root planing in the treatment of periodontitis. J Periodontol 1999;70:490–503.
78. Garrett S, Adams DF, Bogle G, et al. The effect of locally delivered controlled-release doxycycline or scaling and root planing on periodontal maintenance patients over 9 months. J Periodontol 2000;71:22–30.
79. Wennström JL, Newman HN, MacNeill SR, et al. Utilisation of locally delivered doxycycline in non-surgical treatment of chronic periodontitis. A comparative multi-centre trial of 2 treatment approaches. J Clin Periodontol 2001;28:753–761.
80. Walker CB, Godowski KC, Garrett S, Wesselman C. Reduction of two red complex bacteria by sustained-release doxycycline and correlation to improvement in mean pocket depth. Compend Contin Educ Dent 2011;32:e32–e37.
81. Walker CB, Godowski KC, Borden L, et al. The effects of sustained release doxycycline on the anaerobic flora and antibiotic-resistant patterns in subgingival plaque and saliva. J Periodontol 2000;71:768–774.
82. Eickholz P, Kim TS, Bürklin T, et al. Non-surgical periodontal therapy with adjunctive topical doxycycline: A double-blind randomized controlled multicenter study. J Clin Periodontol 2002;29:108–117.
83. Akalin FA, Baltacioğlu E, Sengün D, et al. A comparative evaluation of the clinical effects of systemic and local doxycycline in the treatment of chronic periodontitis. J Oral Sci 2004;46:25–35.
84. Machion L, Andia DC, Lecio G, et al. Locally delivered doxycycline as an adjunctive therapy to scaling and root planing in the treatment of smokers: A 2-year follow-up. J Periodontol 2006;77:606–613.
85. Ağan S, Sönmez S, Serdar M. The effect of topical doxycycline usage on gingival crevicular fluid MMP-8 levels of chronic and aggressive periodontitis patients: A pilot study. Int J Dent Hyg 2006;4:114–121.
86. Bogren A, Teles RP, Torresyap G, Haffajee AD, Socransky SS, Wennström JL. Locally delivered doxycycline during supportive periodontal therapy: A 3-year study. J Periodontol 2008;79:827–835.
87. Gupta R, Pandit N, Aggarwal S, Verma A. Comparative evaluation of subgingivally delivered 10% doxycycline hyclate and xanthan-based chlorhexidine gels in the treatment of chronic periodontitis. J Contemp Dent Pract 2008;9:25–32.
88. Goodson JM, Cugini MA, Kent RL, et al. Multicenter evaluation of tetracycline fiber therapy: II. Clinical response. J Periodontal Res 1991;26:371–379.
89. Goodson JM, Cugini MA, Kent RL, et al. Multicenter evaluation of tetracycline fiber therapy: I. Experimental design, methods, and baseline data. J Periodontal Res 1991;26:361–370.
90. Drisko CL, Cobb CM, Killoy WJ, et al. Evaluation of periodontal treatments using controlled-release tetracycline fibers: Clinical response. J Periodontol 1995;66:692–699.
91. Newman MG, Kornman KS, Doherty FM. A 6-month multi-center evaluation of adjunctive tetracycline fiber therapy used in conjunction with scaling and root planing in maintenance patients: Clinical results. J Periodontol 1994;65:685–691.
92. Vandekerckhove BN, Quirynen M, van Steenberghe D. The use of tetracycline-containing controlled-release fibers in the treatment of refractory periodontitis. J Periodontol 1997;68:353–361.
93. Morrison SL, Cobb CM, Kazakos GM, Killoy WJ. Root surface characteristics associated with subgingival placement of monolithic tetracycline-impregnated fibers. J Periodontol 1992;63:137–143.
94. Minabe M, Takeuchi K, Nishimura T, Hori T, Umemoto T. Therapeutic effects of combined treatment using tetracycline-immobilized collagen film and root planing in periodontal furcation pockets. J Clin Periodontol 1991;18:287–290.
95. Tonetti M, Cugini MA, Goodson JM. Zero-order delivery with periodontal placement of tetracycline-loaded ethylene vinyl acetate fibers. J Periodontal Res 1990;25:243–249.
96. Wong MY, Lu CL, Liu CM, Hou LT, Chang WK. Clinical response of localized recurrent periodontitis treated with scaling, root planing, and tetracycline fiber. J Formos Med Assoc 1998;97:490–497.
97. Kinane DF, Radvar M. A six-month comparison of three periodontal local antimicrobial therapies in persistent periodontal pockets. J Periodontol 1999;70:1–7.
98. Yalcin F, Demirel K, Onan U. Evaluation of adjunctive tetracycline fiber therapy with scaling and root planing: Short-term clinical results. Periodontal Clin Investig 1999;21:23–27.
99. Aimetti M, Romano F, Torta I, Cirillo D, Caposio P, Romagnoli R. Debridement and local application of tetracycline-loaded fibres in the management of persistent periodontitis: Results after 12 months. J Clin Periodontol 2004;31:166–172.
100. Stoltze K. Concentration of metronidazole in periodontal pockets after application of a metronidazole 25% dental gel. J Clin Periodontol 1992;19(9 Pt 2):698–701.
101. Lie T, Bruun G, Böe OE. Effects of topical metronidazole and tetracycline in treatment of adult periodontitis. J Periodontol 1998;69:819–827.
102. Palmer RM, Matthews JP, Wilson RF. Adjunctive systemic and locally delivered metronidazole in the treatment of periodontitis: A controlled clinical study. Br Dent J 1998;184:548–552.
103. Stelzel M, Florès-de-Jacoby L. Topical metronidazole application as an adjunct to scaling and root planing. J Clin Periodontol 2000;27:447–452.
104. Riep B, Purucker P, Bernimoulin JP. Repeated local metronidazole-therapy as adjunct to scaling and root planing in maintenance patients. J Clin Periodontol 1999;26:710–715.
105. Williams RC. Periodontal disease. N Engl J Med 1990;322:373–382.
106. Grenier D, Roy E, Mayrand D. Modulation of *Porphyromonas gingivalis* proteinase activity by suboptimal doses of antimicrobial agents. J Periodontol 2003;74:1316–1319.

107. Golub LM, Ramamurthy N, McNamara TF, et al. Tetracyclines inhibit tissue collagenase activity. A new mechanism in the treatment of periodontal disease. J Periodontal Res 1984;19:651–655.
108. Caton JG, Ciancio SG, Blieden TM, et al. Treatment with subantimicrobial dose doxycycline improves the efficacy of scaling and root planing in patients with adult periodontitis. J Periodontol 2000;71:521–532.
109. Caton JG, Ciancio SG, Blieden TM, et al. Subantimicrobial dose doxycycline as an adjunct to scaling and root planing: Post-treatment effects. J Clin Periodontol 2001;28:782–789.
110. Tüter G, Serdar M, Kurtiş B, et al. Effects of scaling and root planing and subantimicrobial dose doxycycline on gingival crevicular fluid levels of matrix metalloproteinase-8, -13 and serum levels of hsCRP in patients with chronic periodontitis. J Periodontol 2010;81:1132–1139.
111. Preshaw PM, Hefti AF, Bradshaw MH. Adjunctive subantimicrobial dose doxycycline in smokers and non-smokers with chronic periodontitis. J Clin Periodontol 2005;32:610–616.
112. Noguchi K, Ishikawa I. The roles of cyclooxygenase-2 and prostaglandin E2 in periodontal disease. Periodontol 2000 2007;43:85–101.
113. Greenwell H, Bissada NF. Emerging concepts in periodontal therapy. Drugs 2002;62:2581–2587.
114. Rogers MJ, Gordon S, Benford HL, et al. Cellular and molecular mechanisms of action of bisphosphonates. Cancer 2000;88(suppl 12):2961–2978.
115. Fleisch H, Russell RG, Francis MD. Diphosphonates inhibit hydroxyapatite dissolution in vitro and bone resorption in tissue culture and in vivo. Science 1969;165:1262–1264.
116. Rocha M, Nava LE, Vázquez de la Torre C, Sánchez-Márin F, Garay-Sevilla ME, Malacara JM. Clinical and radiological improvement of periodontal disease in patients with type 2 diabetes mellitus treated with alendronate: A randomized, placebo-controlled trial. J Periodontol 2001;72:204–209.
117. Bashutski JD, Eber RM, Kinney JS, et al. Teriparatide and osseous regeneration in the oral cavity. N Engl J Med 2010;363:2396–2405.
118. Takaishi Y, Ikeo T, Miki T, Nishizawa Y, Morii H. Suppression of alveolar bone resorption by etidronate treatment for periodontal disease: 4- to 5-year follow-up of four patients. J Int Med Res 2003;31:575–584.
119. Takaishi Y, Miki T, Nishizawa Y, Morii H. Clinical effect of etidronate on alveolar pyorrhoea associated with chronic marginal periodontitis: Report of four cases. J Int Med Res 2001;29:355–365.
120. El-Shinnawi UM, El-Tantawy SI. The effect of alendronate sodium on alveolar bone loss in periodontitis (clinical trial). J Int Acad Periodontol 2003;5:5–10.
121. Weinreb M, Quartuccio H, Seedor JG, et al. Histomorphometrical analysis of the effects of the bisphosphonate alendronate on bone loss caused by experimental periodontitis in monkeys. J Periodontal Res 1994;29:35–40.
122. Farrugia MC, Summerlin DJ, Krowiak E, et al. Osteonecrosis of the mandible or maxilla associated with the use of new generation bisphosphonates. Laryngoscope 2006;116:115–120.

14

PERIODONTAL WOUND HEALING

Lorenzo Tavelli, DDS, MS
Andrea Ravidà, DDS, MS

Principles of Wound Healing

The response of the body to a pathologic and/or traumatic event is defined as **wound healing**. In periodontology, this process can result in different **healing** patterns: **repair**, **new attachment**, or **regeneration**.[1] While periodontal *repair* can frequently be achieved, periodontal *regeneration* remains a challenge.[2]

Periodontal **wound** healing shares principles with healing in nonoral sites, with the first event represented by the hemorrhage of the capillaries and the formation of a blood clot. On the other hand, one unique feature of periodontal wound healing is that mucoperiosteal flaps are often repositioned over a root surface deprived of its original attachment, and therefore, healing occurs between a vascularized surface (ie, flap) and a mineralized nonvascular area.[3]

While wound healing involves several phases (ie, hemostasis, inflammatory, proliferative, and maturation phase) regardless of the type of surgery performed (Table 14-1), this chapter focuses on wound-healing events following the main periodontal procedures. Indeed, the healing mechanism and the surgical outcomes are mainly dictated by the soft and hard tissues that were exposed to the injury (gingiva, alveolar bone, cementum, and/or periodontal ligament [PDL]).

Factors Affecting Wound Healing

Multiple factors play key roles in the wound-healing process. Among these, infection control is considered one of the most important because it allows the transition from the inflammatory to the proliferative phase.[4] Guo and DiPietro outlined the most significant factors related to cutaneous wound healing[5] (Box 14-1), which seem to follow a similar pattern to oral mucosal healing.[4,6]

In particular, periodontal wound healing seems to benefit from dietary supplements, such as B vitamins, vitamin D, and calcium.[7–9] Furthermore, the patient's psychosocial factors, such as anxiety, depression, and stress, can affect the postoperative pain, the analgesic use, and the overall healing process

DEFINITIONS AND TERMINOLOGY

Healing: The process of repair or regeneration of injured, lost, or surgically treated tissue.[1]

- **Healing by first intention:** Primary union of a wound in which the incised tissue edges are held in close approximation until union occurs.[1] Also referred to as *healing by primary intention*.
- **Healing by second intention:** Wound closure wherein the edges remain separated and the wound heals from the base and sides via the formation of granulation tissue.[1]
- **Healing by third intention:** Also known as *delayed primary closure* or *tertiary wound healing*. A method to manage heavily infected or contaminated wounds in which the wound is left open several days following tissue injury. Primary closure is not achieved until the reduction of inflammation and bacterial count is observed.[1]

New attachment: The union of connective tissue or epithelium with a root surface that has been deprived of its original attachment apparatus. This new attachment may be epithelial adhesion and/or connective adaptation or attachment. May also include new cementum.[1]

TABLE 14-1 Wound-healing phases

Phase	Timing	Events
Hemostasis	1 day	• Platelet plug formation • Stable fibrin clot
Inflammatory	2–4 days	• Neutrophil migration • Phagocytosis • Release of inflammatory cytokines • Removal of bacteria and cellular debris
Proliferative	4–21 days	• Growth factor release by macrophages • Fibroblast proliferation • Reepithelialization • Angiogenesis by endothelial cells • Neovascularization • Granulation tissue formation
Maturation/ remodeling	21 days to months	• Collagen fiber maturation • Collagen type I replaces collagen type III

Reattachment: To attach again. The reunion of epithelial and connective tissue with a root surface following separation by incision or physical injury (not by disease). Not to be confused with *new attachment*.[1]

Regeneration: Reproduction or reconstitution of a lost or injured part in a manner similar or identical to its original form. In periodontics, refers to the formation of new bone, cementum, and a functionally oriented periodontal ligament at a site deprived of its original attachment apparatus. In edentulous spaces, refers to the surgical augmentation of a resorbed ridge.[1]

Repair: Healing of a wound by tissue that does not fully restore the architecture or the function of the part.[1]

Wound: An injury to living tissue; a forcible interruption of the continuity of any tissue.[1]

Wound healing: A process involving a cascade of cellular and molecular changes occurred after tissue injury, resulting in either tissue repair or tissue regeneration. The types of wound healing include healing by primary, secondary, and third intention.[1]

BOX 14-1 Local and systemic factors affecting wound-healing events

Local factors
- Oxygenation
- Infection
- Foreign body
- Venous sufficiency

Systemic factors
- Age
- Sex
- Sex hormones
- Stress
- Ischemia
- Disease (eg, diabetes, hereditary healing disorders)
- Obesity
- Medications (eg, glucocorticoid steroids, chemotherapy)
- Alcoholism
- Smoking
- Immunocompromised conditions
- Nutrition

following periodontal surgery.[10] Lastly, the detrimental effect of smoking on periodontal wound healing has been widely investigated, reporting a variety of detrimental effects in procedures including but not limited to guided tissue regeneration[11] (GTR) and periodontal plastic surgery[12,13] (Fig 14-1).

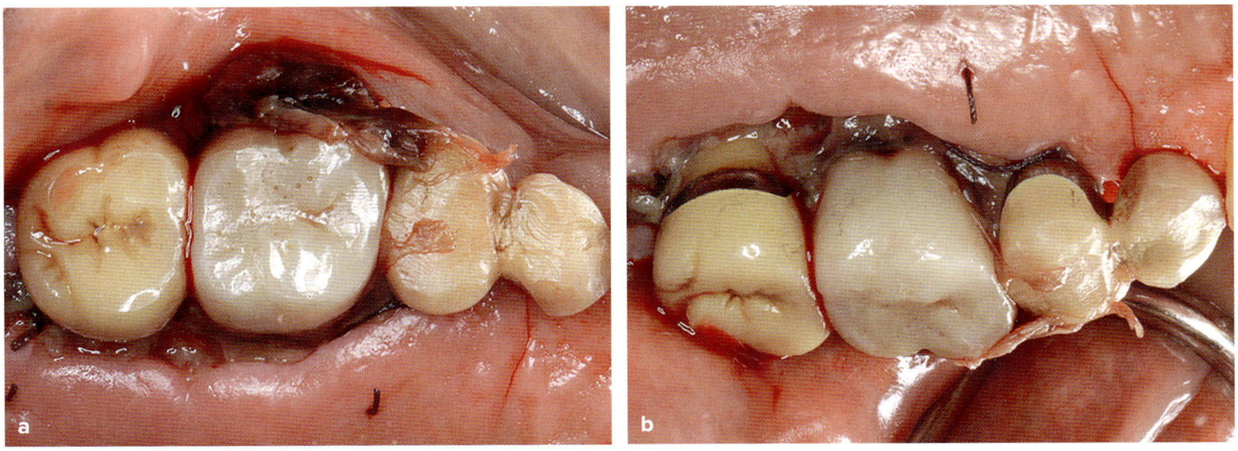

Fig 14-1 Complication following GTR procedure at 2 weeks follow-up in smoker. *(a)* Occlusal view. *(b)* Palatal view.

Healing Following Periodontal Procedures

NONSURGICAL THERAPY

The healing following scaling and root planing (SRP) has been extensively studied, both in animal and human models.[14–16] In a human study, Stahl et al showed that the epithelialization of the pocket following subgingival curettage and root planing is complete within 1 week and that the inflammatory infiltrate is similar to the control sites after 8 weeks.[14] It has been suggested that the bleeding washes out most of the remaining bacteria, plaque, and calculus following the subgingival scaling,[17] while some of the remaining pocket epithelium will give rise to the reformation of the junctional epithelium.[15] According to Waerhaug, this process is completed within 2 weeks.[15] The initial pocket depth reduction following SRP (about 1 week) is related to increased gingival recession, while the secondary pocket reduction (after 3 weeks) is due to clinical attachment gain.[18]

In an animal study, Caton and Zander showed that the healing following periodic root planing, subgingival curettage, and plaque control was accomplished by the formation of a long junctional epithelium (LJE) rather than new connective tissue (CT) attachment.[16] However, this LJE was demonstrated to be no different in resistance to plaque or disease progression.[19,20]

GINGIVECTOMY

Orban was the first to discuss the principles and the healing events occurring after gingivectomy.[21] Later on, animal studies were conducted to further investigate wound healing following this procedure. In particular, by using a combined radioautographic and histologic method, Engler et al and Ramfjord et al evaluated the dynamics of epithelial and CT healing after gingivectomy (Table 14-2).[22,23] It was observed that the migratory velocity of epithelial cells was approximately 0.5 mm/day and that the complete healing of the outer surface occurred after 2 weeks (Fig 14-2). However, the healing of the new gingival sulcus required 4 to 5 weeks.

Further studies confirmed that complete epithelialization following gingivectomy occurred in 7 to 14 days[24] and that after 12 days, new epithelial attachment is regenerated against the enamel and root cementum.[25] On the other hand, it has been shown that the regeneration of the free gingiva takes 3 to 9 days, while the maturation and functional orientation of the CT needs more than 5 weeks.[26]

FLAPS

The healing following different types of periodontal flaps has been studied in terms of type of attachment,[27,28] revascularization,[29] and strength needed to separate the flap from the tooth surface,[30] among others aspects. In addition, the influence of incision design[31] and the

TABLE 14-2 Healing phases following gingivectomy as described by Engler et al[22] and Ramfjord et al[23]

Healing time	Events
2 hours	• Wound covered by blood clot • Acute inflammation and dilated vessels • PMN infiltration • Thin layer (0.2 mm) of CT beneath the incision • Thin layer of degenerating cells adjacent to the incision
5–9 hours	• Well-defined clot • Thin layer of degenerating cells become filled with PMNs
9 hours	• Band of basophilic cells
13 hours	• Migration of basophilic cells • Band of PMNs covering the wound • Minor signs of inflammation • Loss of the continuity of osteoblasts on outer surface of alveolar crest
24 hours	• Increased DNA synthesis in the epithelium at the wound margin • Increase in number of labeled CT cells • Most CT cells located 0.3–0.5 mm below the PMN band covering the wound
36 hours	• Decreased synthesis of DNA
48 hours	• Most synthesis of DNA occurring at the epithelial cells of the wound edge • Increased number of labeled endothelial and perivascular cells 0.3–0.5 mm below PMN band • Inflammatory cells • Few cementoblasts
2–5 days	• Epithelium migrating slowly toward the tooth surface • Presence of rete pegs • Labeled endothelial cells and fibroblasts 0.3–0.5 mm below PMN band
5–7 days	• Epithelium migrating apically to form the sulcus • Wound partially covered with a thin layer of epithelium that separates the layer of PMNs and debris from the underlying CT • Labeled CT cells immediately under the newly formed epithelial layer covering the wound
7–14 days	• Newly formed marginal gingiva • New free gingiva formed as a result of CT proliferation • Outer gingiva completely epithelialized, beginning of the epithelialization of the sulcus • Several osteoblasts on the alveolar crest surface • Inflammation from the new gingival sulcus to the alveolar crest • Sulcus lined with epithelium • Increase of collagen bundles in the free gingiva • 9 days: Intense osteoclastic activity • 14 days: No more osteoclasts at the alveolar crest, osteoblastic layer well defined
21 days	• Outer surface of the marginal gingiva with normal appearance • Diffuse inflammation in the newly epithelialized sulcus • CT well organized in distinct collagen bundles
35 days	• Well-organized epithelium in the gingival sulcus • Complete epithelialization of the marginal gingiva and sulcus • CT indistinguishable from the control

PMN, polymorphonuclear leukocyte.

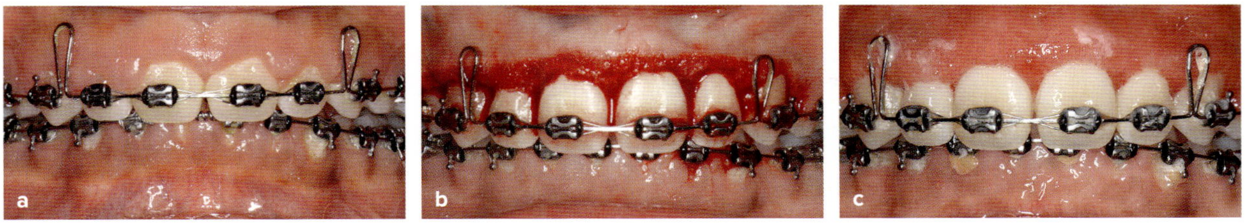

Fig 14-2 Gingivectomy. *(a)* Preoperative view of the maxillary anterior sextant. *(b)* Immediate postoperative view. *(c)* Healing after 2 weeks. (Courtesy of Dr Carlos Garaicoa Pazmiño.)

TABLE 14-3 Outcomes following partial- or full-thickness flap elevation

Study	Design	Sample size	Partial-thickness flap	Full-thickness flap
Donnenfeld et al[43] (1964)	Human	13 patients	NA	BL: 0.63 mm
Pfeifer[40] (1965)	Human	1 patient	Very minor osteoclastic activity	Osteoclastic activity
Pfeifer and Heller[42] (1971)	Human	2 patients	Healing by LJE	Healing by LJE in the coronal half and CT in the apical half
Wood et al[41] (1972)	Human	7 patients	BL: 0.98 mm	BL: 0.62 mm
Fickl et al[44] (2011)	Animal (dog)	5 dogs	BL: 0.12 ± 0.38 mm	BL: 0.64 ± 0.14 mm

NA, not applicable; BL, bone loss.

removal or preservation of pocket epithelium has been also investigated.[32]

At wound closure, the space between the root surface and the mucoperiosteal flap will immediately fill with blood. Then, plasma proteins will precipitate onto the wound surfaces within seconds and provide an initial basis for adherence of the blood clot.[33] However, the initial adhesion of the flap to the root surface mediated by the blood clot does not seem to be able to maintain them together.[30,34] Hiatt et al showed that the tensile strength of the tooth–soft tissue interface was still vulnerable to mechanical trauma at 7 days postsurgery, while functional stability between the denuded root and soft tissue is achieved after approximately 14 days.[30]

It has also been reported that the healing following open flap debridement, lateral positioned flap, and coronally advanced flap results in new attachment with formation of LJE (increased by approximately 20%) and CT with fibers parallel to the root surface.[27,28,35,36]

According to Wilderman and Wentz, the following healing phases can be identified when a pedicle flap is performed: *(1)* adaptation (within 4 days), *(2)* proliferation (4–21 days), *(3)* attachment (21–28 days), and *(4)* maturation (28 days–6 months).[28]

During the early wound healing, wound stability plays a key role on the final outcomes, and excessive tensile forces can violate the integrity of the blood clot that adheres to the root surface, resulting in wound rupture between the root surface and the mucoperiosteal flap.[37]

SPLIT- VERSUS FULL-THICKNESS FLAP

Wilderman et al demonstrated that loss of alveolar support occurs following flap surgeries.[38] This observation was further corroborated by other studies showing that flap elevation, whether partial- or split-thickness (leaving the periosteum over the bone) or full-thickness (periosteum with the flap), induces bone resorption[39] (Table 14-3).[40–44]

In a pilot study involving two patients, Pfeifer and Heller evaluated the influence of split- or full-thickness lateral sliding flap on bone loss.[42] After 8 months, the histologic analysis showed LJE and CT attachment in the sites that received a full-thickness flap, while in sites treated with a split-thickness flap, only LJE attachment was observed. It was suggested that the osteogenic potential of the periosteum may have played a role in inducing the CT attachment in the full-thickness flap, while dissecting vessels and thus reducing the blood supply may represent a disadvantage of the partial-thickness flap.[42]

According to Wood et al, the key factor in determining bone loss following flap reflection is the thickness of supporting tissues (bone and gingival CT).[41] Therefore, they suggested performing a full-thickness flap when gingival tissue is thin to minimize crestal bone loss.[41]

On the other hand, an animal investigation by Fickl et al challenged this conclusion, showing that a partial-thickness flap was related to less vertical bone loss and osteoclastic activity than a full-thickness flap. However, these results should be evaluated with caution because they are based on the exclusion of an outlier, in which split-thickness flap elevation induced more bone loss and osteoclastic activity than the full-thickness flap.[44]

A possible explanation of the controversial results provided in the literature regarding the association between partial- or full-thickness flaps and bone loss may be the different split-thickness flap preparation among clinicians. When no CT (or a minimal thickness) is left on the periosteum, the protection of the underlying bone may not be adequate. Indeed, the remaining portion of the CT on the bone can prevent the necrosis of the periosteum.[44]

In conclusion, there is not enough evidence to support one approach as superior. Nevertheless, it is well established that elevating a flap causes osteoclastic activity and bone resorption, which are probably related to several factors, such as individual characteristics as well as bone and soft tissue thicknesses.

APICALLY POSITIONED FLAP

Pfeifer investigated the healing following an apically repositioned flap leaving 2 to 3 mm of denuded bone. He described an initial healing phase (from 2 to 10 postoperative days) with the formation of a "young proliferative tissue," primarily from the mesenchymal cells of the PDL, and a second stage ("phase of function") that results in the formation of attached gingiva. Osteoclastic activity was observed from the 4th to the 10th day and resulted in minimal bone loss.[45] However, in a similar investigation, Costich and Ramfjord reported a more severe and prolonged reaction that included bone loss and cemental resorption in a few cases, leading the authors to suggest avoiding bone denudation as much as possible. In this study, bone resorption was still occurring 6 weeks after the surgery.[46]

Donnenfeld et al assessed the clinical results following an apically positioned flap, showing its effectiveness in eliminating periodontal pockets and increasing the width of the attached gingiva. However, bone loss and gingival recession are the main drawbacks of this procedure. In particular, the mean bone loss was found to be 0.63 mm, while the mean apical migration from the CEJ of the epithelial attachment was 0.69 mm during the 12 weeks of follow-up.[43]

OSSEOUS SURGERY

Wilderman et al described the healing events following osseous surgery in humans.[47] In the early phases of healing, a fibrin clot was established between the flap and the underlaying structures (bone and tooth). Then, the formation of young CT, collagen, and collagen fiber was observed. The complete maturation of new collagen fibers required 6 months. Interestingly, more bone loss and less bone repair were found in thin alveolar bone compared with thick alveolar bone. The peak of bone repair was seen at 3 to 4 weeks, especially in thin bone. Immature bone was replaced by intermediate bone at 6 months and then mature bone at 18 months. The authors reported an initial crestal bone loss of 1.2 mm followed by 0.4 mm of new bone apposition, resulting in an average crestal bone height reduction of 0.8 mm. In addition, they observed that osteoblastic activity was still present 1 year after the osseous surgery.[47]

Moghaddas and Stahl observed an average resorption in the alveolar crestal height at 6 months of 0.23 mm, 0.55 mm, and 0.8 mm at the interradicular, radicular, and furcation sites, respectively.[48] According to Selipsky, removal of buccal or lingual bone has a smaller impact on tooth support than removal of interproximal bone, which may be responsible for the increased mobility observed following osseous surgery that returned to the presurgical status within 1 year.[49]

In an animal study, Caton and Nyman investigated the effect of osseous surgery in eliminating angular bony defects. They found that resection of the osseous walls of angular bony defects not only led to alveolar bone height reduction but also to CT attachment loss. In addition, elimination of the angular bony defects as well

TABLE 14-4 Wound-healing phases following FGG according to Oliver et al[56]

Phase	Connective tissue	Epithelium
Initial (0–3 days)	• Thin layer of fibrin separating periosteum and graft. • No evidence of blood vessels from the bed to the graft. • "Plasmatic" circulation: Nutrition is provided only by the exudate spreading through the graft from the periosteum.	• Degeneration • Desquamation of the outer layers • Leukocytes
Revascularization (4–11 days)	• Minimal alveolar crest resorption, periosteum intact with no resorption. • 4th day: Fibroblasts in the area between the graft and the periosteum. Vessels appeared in the graft. • 7th day: Dense network of capillary budding throughout the graft. Epithelialized marginal gingiva. • 11th day: Fibrous union between graft and periosteum. Free gingiva observed. New marginal gingiva formed from granulation tissue from PDL.	• 5th day: Epithelium degenerated and desquamated. • Deepest portion of epithelial ridges contributed to reepithelialization of the graft. • Thin layer of epithelium from adjacent tissues proliferated over the graft. • 11th day: Complete epithelialization.
Maturation (11–42 days)	14th day: Increased density and further orientation of the connective tissue fibers at the periosteum–graft interface.	• Increased thickness. • 14th day: Epithelial ridges fully developed. • 28th day: Keratinization starts.

as reduction in the height of the interdental soft tissue were observed.[50]

SOFT TISSUE GRAFTING

Free gingival graft

The free gingival graft (FGG) harvesting technique was first introduced by Björn for replacing alveolar mucosa.[51] Later on, this procedure was also performed for the purposes of increasing the vestibular depth,[52] gaining keratinized gingiva before crown preparation,[53] and root coverage.[54]

In a review discussing the principles of successful FGG, Sullivan and Atkins recognized three different stages of healing: plasmatic circulation, revascularization, and organic union.[55] Oliver et al recommended dividing the healing of FGG into initial, revascularization, and maturation phases (Table 14-4 and Fig 14-3).[56]

During the first 2 to 3 days, the FGG survived due to the plasmatic circulation, while anastomosis between FGG vessels and recipient site capillaries took place. A trend in reduction of the capillary vessels along with the increasing density of the CT was then observed in the following days.[56] In line with Sullivan and Atktins,[55] Oliver et al concluded that FGGs heal similarly to free skin grafts.

Lange and Bernimoulin analyzed the cytologic changes during the healing of a FGG, showing that the epithelialization is not affected by the wound margins but by the graft.[57] In particular, the reepithelialization process is guided by the basal layers of the FGG that remained intact, while, on the contrary, the healing of the palatal donor site occurred from the wound margins.[57]

Later on, further investigations were performed to evaluate whether the recipient bed, periosteum, or denuded bone could affect the healing of FGG. James and McFall concluded that a 1.5- to 2-fold increase in FGG shrinkage should be expected when the FGG is positioned over the periosteum.[58] On the other hand, an angiographic study reported that FGGs of thin or intermediate thickness had faster revascularization when positioned over a periosteal recipient bed, while thick FGGs sutured over denuded bone showed delayed revascularization and healing compared with an FGG placed over a periosteal recipient bed (25% vs 75% of revascularization after 7

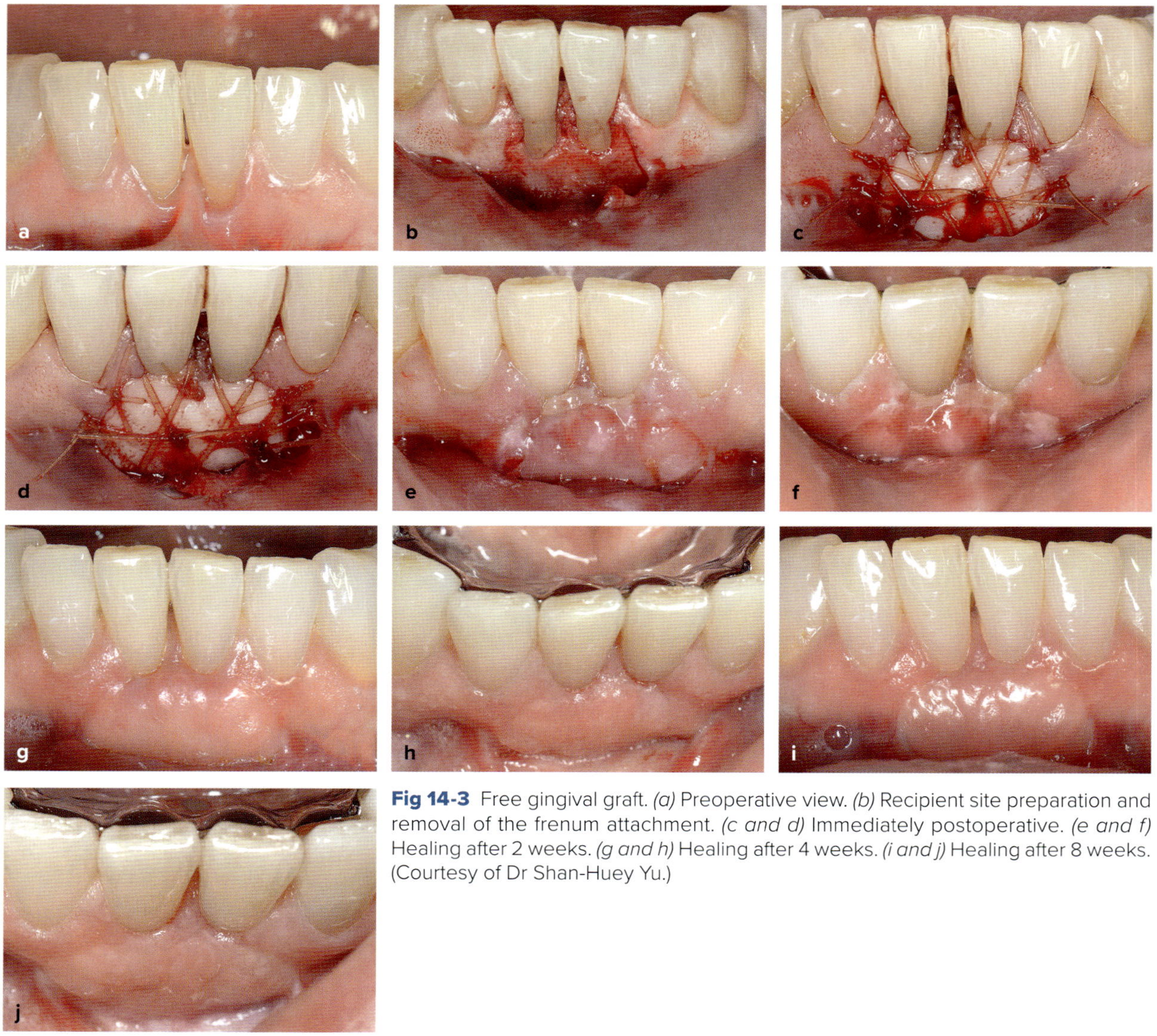

Fig 14-3 Free gingival graft. *(a)* Preoperative view. *(b)* Recipient site preparation and removal of the frenum attachment. *(c and d)* Immediately postoperative. *(e and f)* Healing after 2 weeks. *(g and h)* Healing after 4 weeks. *(i and j)* Healing after 8 weeks. (Courtesy of Dr Shan-Huey Yu.)

days, respectively). In addition, the shrinkage after 1 year was 30% for thick FGGs, 38% for intermediate thickness grafts, and 44% to 45% for thin or very thin FGGs.[59]

The shrinkage of FGG has been divided into primary and secondary contraction.[55] *Primary contraction* is strictly related to the elastic fibers and occurs 2 to 4 days after the surgery, while *secondary contraction* is due to the cicatrization of the tissue between the graft and the recipient bed and takes place 4 to 10 days following the procedure. The secondary contraction depends on the rigidity of the recipient bed and on the thickness of the graft's lamina propria: thicker FGGs undergo less secondary contraction.[55]

Nishimura showed that an FGG heals with LJE in the coronal half of the defect and new CT attachment at the apical half, while no cementum formation was observed. However, at most areas in which new CT attachment was seen, the periodontal fibers were not functionally oriented.[60]

The integration of FGG is a dynamic process that continues over the years, as demonstrated by the tendency of the gingival margin of the grafted site to migrate coronally. This phenomenon, which has been termed *creeping attachment*, may occur due to the progressive coronal movement of the attachment apparatus or to an "overhealing" process.[61] In addition, the increased thickness of

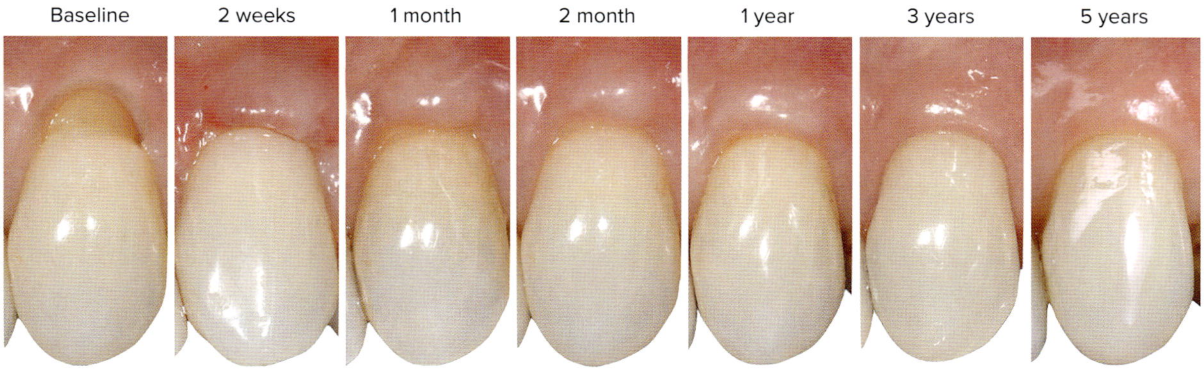

Fig 14-4 Coronally advanced flap in comparison with a CTG. Note the creeping attachment phenomenon that occurred over time until a complete root coverage was achieved.

the gingival tissue and the patient's oral hygiene may play a key role in favoring the creeping attachment phenomenon.[61] Bell et al observed an average creeping attachment of 0.89 ± 0.46 mm in 1 year.[62] Similarly, Agudio et al found that the gingival margin of sites previously treated with FGG tended to migrate coronally over time, while contralateral untreated sites exhibited a tendency to develop gingival recession or increase the recession depth.[63,64]

The esthetic outcome is considered one of the main disadvantages of this technique[65] because the grafted site may retain the appearance of the palatal soft tissue.[66,67]

Connective tissue graft

The early wound-healing events following a connective tissue graft (CTG) resemble those of an FGG. Despite the possibility of leaving a CTG partially exposed,[68] CTGs are mostly used underneath a flap to achieve healing by **primary intention**.

Guiha et al demonstrated that, similarly to FGG, the healing of a CTG is a combination of LJE and CT attachment, with no (or minimal) new bone or cementum formation.[69] Blood vessels in the CTG were observed at 7 days in both sides of the graft (superficial and deeper) originating from vessels from the periodontal plexus, supraperiosteal plexus, and the flap. The vascularization of the graft was completed at 14 days. The authors highlighted the importance of total coverage of the CTG and its intimate adaptation to the root surface in order to provide a blood supply to the graft. Indeed, areas of hematoma were observed between the CTG and the root when the CTG was not closely adapted with consequent impairment of blood vessels to penetrate the graft.[69]

McGuire et al conducted a series of human pilot studies aimed at investigating the clinical and histologic outcomes following the treatment of gingival recessions. In the first study,[70] it was confirmed that no histologic evidence of periodontal regeneration should be expected when a CTG is used, while enamel matrix derivative (EMD) was able to regenerate new cementum and organized PDL fibers. In another study, a group that received growth factors (ie, recombinant human platelet-derived growth factor-BB, β-tricalcium phosphate) showed cementum regeneration, PDL fibers functionally oriented and inserted into bundle bone, and cementum. Conversely, healing by repair with LJE was observed in the CTG group.[71]

Therefore, these studies demonstrated that gingival recession can be successfully treated with a regenerative approach. However, it is important to note that both studies achieved superior clinical outcomes with CTG alone.[71,72]

The phenomenon of creeping attachment has also been demonstrated for CTG (Fig 14-4). Harris reported an average creeping attachment of 0.8 mm at 6 months following a double pedicle flap combined with a CTG,[73] while Henderson et al did not observe additional root coverage gain using acellular dermal matrix.[74] It is believed that creeping attachment is an unpredictable process[75] that can be facilitated by the increased marginal thickness due to the addition of a graft[76] and by a strict postsurgical regimen where oral hygiene and brushing instruction are frequently reinforced.[77]

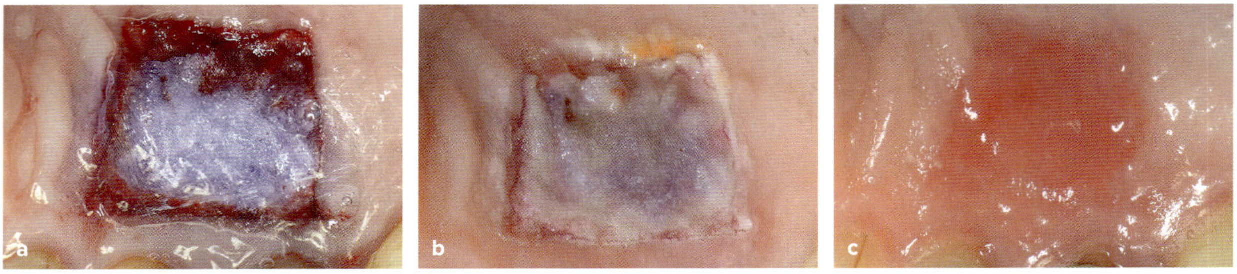

Fig 14-5 Palatal donor site following free gingival graft harvesting. *(a)* Immediate postoperative view where collagen sponge, cyanoacrylate, and palatal stent were applied. *(b)* Healing after 2 weeks. *(c)* Healing after 4 weeks. (Courtesy of Dr Shan-Huey Yu.)

EHI = 1	Complete flap closure without fibrin line at the palate
EHI = 2	Complete flap closure with fibrin line at the palate
EHI = 3	Complete flap closure with small fibrin clot(s) at the palate
EHI = 4	Incomplete flap closure with partial necrosis of the palatal tissue
EHI = 5	Incomplete flap closure with complete necrosis of the palatal tissue (more than 50% of the former flap is involved)

Fig 14-6 Early healing index (EHI) as proposed by Fickl et al.[86]

Palatal harvesting

FGG harvesting approaches involve the healing of the donor site by **secondary intention**. Consequently, attempts have been made to create techniques for obtaining CTG that allow healing by primary intention.[78,79]

Overall, these techniques (ie, envelope, parallel incisions, or trap-door) are thought to be associated with faster and less painful healing than FGG harvesting.[80,81] However, sloughing or necrosis of the primary flap during healing are common complications of these harvesting approaches[82,83] and may result in more prolonged patient discomfort.[84] Zucchelli et al demonstrated that, when the palatal wound is properly managed, there are no differences in postoperative morbidity between FGG and trap-door harvesting techniques.[83] In particular, a recent randomized clinical trial showed that adding an external layer of cyanoacrylate on a hemostatic sponge positioned over the palatal wound can highly minimize patient morbidity following FGG harvesting (Fig 14-5).[85]

The healing of the palatal donor site has also been evaluated in terms of complete epithelialization rate, color match, wound sensitivity, variation of feeding habits, and bleeding patterns.[80,86,87] In particular, by using a modified early healing index (EHI; Fig 14-6), Fickl et al showed that the single-incision technique is related to an improved healing compared to the trap-door harvesting technique.[86]

According to Ozcan et al, complete epithelialization is not achieved during the first week following FGG harvesting. On the contrary, it is obtained within 1 month regardless of the approach performed.[88] Soileau and Brannon concluded that 9 weeks (63 days) should be considered as the minimal healing time before reharvesting an FGG from the same donor site.[89]

BOX 14-2 Factors affecting patient morbidity and donor site epithelialization following FGG harvesting

Factors minimizing postoperative pain	• Graft thickness < 2 mm[90] • Graft length < 14 mm[85] • Protective material on the donor site: – Cyanoacrylate[85] – Growth factors: platelet-rich plasma,[91] platelet-rich fibrin,[92] platelet-rich fibrin + cyanoacrylate[88] – Ozone therapy[93] – Medicinal plant extracted[94] – Hyaluronic acid[95] – Diode laser[96]
Factors accelerating donor site epithelialization	• Nonsmoking patients[97] • Growth factors: platelet-rich plasma,[91] platelet-rich fibrin + cyanoacrylate[88] • Medicinal plant extracted[94] • Hyaluronic acid[95] • Ozone therapy[93] • Topical erythropoietin[98] • Aminoguanidine, an advanced glycation end-products inhibitor, and N-phenacylthiazolium bromide, a glycated cross-link breaker[99] • Topically applied antimicrobial agents[100]* • Chondroitin sulfate[101]*

*Animal study

Several attempts have been made to accelerate palatal wound healing following FGG and reduce patient discomfort (Box 14-2).[85,88,90–101] In particular, Delima et al demonstrated that prewounded FGG can positively affect the postoperative healing of the donor site.[102] They found that, after 2 weeks, none of the FGG sites and 40% of the prewounded FGG sites resulted in complete epithelialization and in a significantly lower number of bacteria species.[102]

GUIDED TISSUE REGENERATION

In the 1970s, several procedures (including SRP, modified Widman flap, interdental denudation, coronally positioned flap, free gingival grafts, bone graft) were claimed to be able to obtain periodontal regeneration.[103] However, these approaches resulted mostly in pocket depth reduction due to increased gingival recession and healing by repair (histologically characterized by LJE).[104,105]

Periodontal **regeneration** is histologically defined as regeneration of cementum, PDL, and alveolar bone on a root surface previously denuded by periodontal disease.[103]

The 2005 American Academy of Periodontology (AAP) position paper on periodontal regeneration recognized three procedures able to induce periodontal regeneration: *(1)* bone replacement graft, *(2)* guided tissue regeneration, and *(3)* biologics-based technique (eg, bone morphogenetic protein, EMD).[103] In the 2015 AAP Regeneration Workshop, laser therapy was also added among these approaches, despite limited clinical data.[106]

The concept of compartmentalization was introduced by Melcher, who suggested that four different cell types (ie, epithelial cells, gingival CT cells, PDL cells, and bone cells) compete for the colonization of the wound following periodontal surgeries.[107] The rationale of GTR is that if cells from the PDL and bone can populate the intrabony defect before epithelial and CT cells, periodontal regeneration is possible.

Starting from this theory, several approaches were developed based on the use of a barrier membrane to prevent epithelial cells from colonizing the defect. Nyman et al were the first to histologically demonstrate new attachment in humans by using a Millipore filter as a membrane. Three months after the surgery, the treated tooth was extracted and epithelium proliferating along

TABLE 14-5 EHI for assessing interproximal flap closure in the first 2 weeks following GTR, as proposed by Wachtel et al[111]

Early wound healing index	Flap closure	Interproximal area
EHI 1	Complete	No fibrin line at 2 weeks
EHI 2	Complete	Fine fibrin line at 2 weeks
EHI 3	Complete	Fibrin clot 1 week after the surgery
EHI 4	Incomplete	Partial necrosis of the interproximal tissue at 1 week
EHI 5	Incomplete	Complete necrosis of the interproximal tissue at 2 weeks

the barrier was observed, while new cementum and PDL were noted below the membrane.[108]

Different histologic studies demonstrated the efficacy of the use of barrier membranes in achieving periodontal tissue regeneration, showing newly formed PDL and new connective fibers oriented from the cementum to the alveolar bone.[109,110]

It has been suggested that the healing following periodontal surgery is similar to that after incisional wounds[103]; however, in the periodontium, the early adherence of the blood clot to the root surface may also provide a barrier against the apical epithelial and CT cell migration.[37] The fibrin clot between the flap margin and the root surface is progressively replaced by CT matrix. The disruption of this fibrin linkage may result in LJE instead of new CT attachment.[103] Indeed, as demonstrated by Wikesjö et al, the stability of the blood clot in the early healing plays a key role in regenerative periodontal surgery.[37]

Wachtel et al introduced an EHI for evaluating the flap closure in the interproximal space in the first 2 weeks following GTR (Table 14-5).[111] According to the authors, a microsurgical approach may increase the likelihood of achieving primary flap closure and interproximal soft tissue preservation.[111]

Microsurgical Approach

The benefits of using microsurgical approaches have been shown by several studies, demonstrating improved outcomes when compared with regular techniques.[112–114] In particular, Burkhardt and Lang showed a better graft vascularization in the microsurgical group, speculating that this approach was able to reduce the trauma and vessel injuries, thus accelerating wound healing.[113]

A microsurgical approach may also affect the shrinkage of the flap, which is a crucial factor in root-coverage procedures and in GTR.[112,113] In addition, the improved illumination and magnification of the surgical field, the atraumatic manipulation of the flap, together with a more precise membrane positioning, flap adaptation, and suturing, are the main benefits described by Cortellini and Tonetti.[112] Furthermore, postoperative pain seems to be reduced when a microsurgical technique is performed.[115] A recent meta-analysis also concluded that the outcomes of tunneling procedures for root-coverage purposes can be enhanced by using a microsurgical approach.[116]

Complications During Wound Healing

Surgical procedures are becoming more and more patient-centered, and thus pain management has become a key factor. Curtis et al evaluated the incidence and the severity of postoperative complications in 304 consecutive periodontal surgeries, measuring the pain using a verbal rating scale. The authors found that mucogingival surgery was related to the highest postoperative pain, followed by osseous surgery and soft tissue surgeries. Almost 95% of patients reported minimal or no postoperative complications. They also found that increased surgical time was related to higher perceived pain.[117] Vogel et al showed that ibuprofen was effective in delaying pain onset compared to placebo when the painkiller was prescribed immediately before surgery.[118] Lastly, it should be mentioned that anxiety, depression, stress, and well-being can affect the level of postsurgical pain, the need for painkillers, and the wound healing after periodontal treatment.[10]

Swelling is a possible postoperative complication resulting from an accumulation of fluid caused by altered capillarity permeability. According to Curtis et al, osseous surgery was three times more likely to cause swelling, bleeding, and infection than mucogingival surgery.[117] Postoperative swelling has also been related to the surgical time.[119]

Baab et al reported an average blood loss of 134 mL during periodontal surgery that increased in the mandibular posterior area, and that was affected by the duration of the surgery and the use of local anesthetic agents.[120] Hemostasis can be achieved by using a variety of measures including but not limited to local anesthetics with epinephrine[121]; applying pressure with a gauze over the wound; suturing the vessels with resorbable sutures; and using bone, electrosurgery, and hemostatic agents, among others.

According to Pack and Haber, the frequency of infection after periodontal surgery was 1%, regardless of the use of antibiotic prophylaxis.[122] Similar results were also found by Curtis et al.[117] Although not statistically significant, osseous surgery was the procedure most related to postoperative infection.[122] In line with previous investigations, Powell et al reported an incidence of infection of 2% following periodontal surgeries.[123]

Lastly, it should be noted that some procedures are more prone to develop specific complications. In particular, FGG has been related to patient morbidity, excessive palatal hemorrhage, palatal pain, failure in the graft union resulting in graft necrosis, delayed healing, exostoses, and unpleasant esthetic results.[124,125] On the other hand, frequent postoperative complications of GTR that may impair the outcomes include membrane exposure and infection, swelling, erythema, flap sloughing or perforation, and postoperative pain.[126] The introduction of minimally invasive techniques and biologic agents will allow the prevalence of some of these complications to be reduced.[127,128]

References

1. American Academy of Periodontology. Glossary of Periodontal Terms. American Academy of Periodontology, 2001.
2. Bosshardt DD, Sculean A. Does periodontal tissue regeneration really work? Periodontol 2000 2009;51:208–219.
3. Polimeni G, Xiropaidis AV, Wikesjö UM. Biology and principles of periodontal wound healing/regeneration. Periodontol 2000 2006;41:30–47.
4. Hämmerle CH, Giannobile WV, Working Group 1 of the European Workshop on Periodontology. Biology of soft tissue wound healing and regeneration—consensus report of Group 1 of the 10th European Workshop on Periodontology. J Clin Periodontol 2014;41(15 suppl):S1–S5.
5. Guo S, DiPietro LA. Factors affecting wound healing. J Dent Res 2010;89:219–229.
6. Sculean A, Gruber R, Bosshardt DD. Soft tissue wound healing around teeth and dental implants. J Clin Periodontol 2014; 15(41 suppl):S6–S22.
7. Neiva RF, Al-Shammari K, Nociti FH Jr, Soehren S, Wang HL. Effects of vitamin-B complex supplementation on periodontal wound healing. J Periodontol 2005;76:1084–1091.
8. Bashutski JD, Eber RM, Kinney JS, et al. The impact of vitamin D status on periodontal surgery outcomes. J Dent Res 2011;90:1007–1012.
9. Lau BY, Johnston BD, Fritz PC, Ward WE. Dietary strategies to optimize wound healing after periodontal and dental implant surgery: An evidence-based review. Open Dent J 2013;7:36–46.
10. Kloostra PW, Eber RM, Wang HL, Inglehart MR. Surgical versus non-surgical periodontal treatment: Psychosocial factors and treatment outcomes. J Periodontol 2006;77:1253–1260.
11. Tonetti MS, Pini-Prato G, Cortellini P. Effect of cigarette smoking on periodontal healing following GTR in infrabony defects. A preliminary retrospective study. J Clin Periodontol 1995;22:229–234.
12. Souza SL, Macedo GO, Tunes RS, et al. Subepithelial connective tissue graft for root coverage in smokers and non-smokers: A clinical and histologic controlled study in humans. J Periodontol 2008;79:1014–1021.
13. Chambrone L, Chambrone D, Pustiglioni FE, Chambrone LA, Lima LA. The influence of tobacco smoking on the outcomes achieved by root-coverage procedures: A systematic review. J Am Dent Assoc 2009;140:294–306.
14. Stahl SS, Weiner JM, Benjamin S, Yamada L. Soft tissue healing following curettage and root planing. J Periodontol 1971;42:678–684.
15. Waerhaug J. Healing of the dento-epithelial junction following subgingival plaque control. I. As observed in human biopsy material. J Periodontol 1978;49:1–8.
16. Caton JG, Zander HA. The attachment between tooth and gingival tissues after periodic root planing and soft tissue curettage. J Periodontol 1979;50:462–466.
17. Egelberg J. The topography and permeability of vessels at the dento-gingival junction in dogs. J Periodontal Res Suppl 1967;1:1–39.
18. Proye M, Caton J, Polson A. Initial healing of periodontal pockets after a single episode of root planing monitored by controlled probing forces. J Periodontol 1982;53:296–301.
19. Magnusson I, Runstad L, Nyman S, Lindhe J. A long junctional epithelium: A locus minoris resistentiae in plaque infection? J Clin Periodontol 1983;10:333–340.
20. Beaumont RH, O'Leary TJ, Kafrawy AH. Relative resistance of long junctional epithelial adhesions and connective tissue attachments to plaque-induced inflammation. J Periodontol 1984;55:213–223.
21. Orban B. Gingivectomy or flap operation? J Am Dent Assoc 1939;26:1276–1283.
22. Engler WO, Ramfjord SP, Hiniker JJ. Healing following simple gingivectomy. A tritiated thymidine radioautographic study. I. Epithelialization. J Periodontol 1966;37:298–308.
23. Ramfjord SP, Engler WO, Hiniker JJ. A radioautographic study of healing following simple gingivectomy. II. The connective tissue. J Periodontol 1966;37:179–189.

24. Stahl SS, Slavkin HC, Yamada L, Levine S. Speculations about gingival repair. J Periodontol 1972;43:395–402.
25. Listgarten M. Ultrastructure of the dento-gingival junction after gingivectomy. J Periodontal Res 1972;7:151–160.
26. Ramfjord S, Ash, M. Periodontology and Periodontics. Philadephia: Saunders, 1979.
27. Chambrone L, Chambrone LA, Tatakis DN, Costa Hanemann JA, Shibli JA, Nevins M. Wound healing of the laterally positioned flap: A histomorphometric assessment. Int J Periodontics Restorative Dent 2015;35:785–792.
28. Wilderman MN, Wentz FM. Repair of a dentogingival defect with a pedicle flap. J Periodontol 1965;36:218–231.
29. Caffesse RG, Kon S, Castelli WA, Nasjleti CE. Revascularization following the lateral sliding flap procedure. J Periodontol 1984;55:352–358.
30. Hiatt WH, Stallard RE, Butler ED, Badgett B. Repair following mucoperiosteal flap surgery with full gingival retention. J Periodontol 1968;39:11–16.
31. Cattermole AE, Wade AB. A comparison of the scalloped and linear incisions as used in the reverse bevel technique. J Clin Periodontol 1978;5:41–49.
32. Smith BA, Echeverri M, Caffesse RG. Mucoperiosteal flaps with and without removal of the pocket epithelium. J Periodontol 1987;58:78–85.
33. Wikesjö UM, Crigger M, Nilvéus R, Selvig KA. Early healing events at the dentin-connective tissue interface. Light and transmission electron microscopy observations. J Periodontol 1991;62:5–14.
34. Kon S, Novaes AB, Ruben MP, Goldman HM. Visualization of the microvascularization of the healing periodontal wound. IV. Mucogingival surgery: Full thickness flap. J Periodontol 1969;40:441–456.
35. Stahl SS, Froum SJ, Kushner L. Periodontal healing following open debridement flap procedures. II. Histologic observations. J Periodontol 1982;53:15–21.
36. Lee EJ, Meraw SJ, Oh TJ, Giannobile WV, Wang HL. Comparative histologic analysis of coronally advanced flap with and without collagen membrane for root coverage. J Periodontol 2002;73:779–788.
37. Wikesjö UM, Claffey N, Egelberg J. Periodontal repair in dogs. Effect of heparin treatment of the root surface. J Clin Periodontol 1991;18:60–64.
38. Wilderman MN, Wentz FM, Orban BJ. Histogenesis of repair after mucogingival surgery. J Periodontol 1960;31:283–299.
39. Staffileno H. Significant differences and advantages between the full thickness and split thickness flaps. J Periodontol 1974;45:421–425.
40. Pfeifer JS. The reaction of alveolar bone to flap procedures in man. Periodontics 1965;3:135–140.
41. Wood DL, Hoag PM, Donnenfeld OW, Rosenfeld LD. Alveolar crest reduction following full and partial thickness flaps. J Periodontol 1972;43:141–144.
42. Pfeifer JS, Heller R. Histologic evaluation of full and partial thickness lateral repositioned flaps: A pilot study. J Periodontol 1971;42:331–333.
43. Donnenfeld OW, Marks R, Glickman I. The apically repositioned flap: A clinical study. J Periodontol 1964;35:381–387.
44. Fickl S, Kebschull M, Schupbach P, Zuhr O, Schlagenhauf U, Hürzeler MB. Bone loss after full-thickness and partial-thickness flap elevation. J Clin Periodontol 2011;38:157–162.
45. Pfeifer JS. The growth of gingival tissues over denuded bone. J Periodontol 1965;34:10–16.
46. Costich ER, Ramfjord SP. Healing after partial denudation of the alveolar process. J Periodontol 1968;39:127–134.
47. Wilderman MN, Pennel BM, King K, Barron JM. Histogenesis of repair following osseous surgery. J Periodontol 1970;41:551–565.
48. Moghaddas H, Stahl SS. Alveolar bone remodeling following osseous surgery. A clinical study. J Periodontol 1980;51:376–381.
49. Selipsky H. Osseous surgery: How much need we compromise? Dent Clin North Am 1976;20:79–106.
50. Caton J, Nyman S. Histometric evaluation of periodontal surgery. III. The effect of bone resection on the connective tissue attachment level. J Periodontol 1981;52:405–409.
51. Björn H. Fri transplantation av gingiva propria [abstract]. In: Symposium i parodontologi. Sveriges Tandlaekarefoerbunds Tiding 1963;55:676–684.
52. Nabers JM. Free gingival grafts. Periodontics 1966;4:243–245.
53. Haggerty PC. The use of a free gingival graft to create a healthy environment for full crown preparation. Case history. Periodontics 1966;4:329–331.
54. Mlinek A, Smukler H, Buchner A. The use of free gingival grafts for the coverage of denuded roots. J Periodontol 1973;44:248–254.
55. Sullivan HC, Atkins JH. Free autogenous gingival grafts. I. Principles of successful grafting. Periodontics 1968;6:121–129.
56. Oliver RC, Loe H, Karring T. Microscopic evaluation of the healing and revascularization of free gingival grafts. J Periodontal Res 1968;3:84–95.
57. Lange DE, Bernimoulin JP. Exfoliative cytological studies in evaluation of free gingival graft healing. J Clin Periodontol 1974;1:89–96.
58. James WC, McFall WT Jr. Placement of free gingival grafts on denuded alveolar bone. Part I: Clinical evaluations. J Periodontol 1978;49:283–290.
59. Mörmann W, Schaer F, Firestone AR. The relationship between success of free gingival grafts and transplant thickness. Revascularization and shrinkage—A one year clinical study. J Per odontol 1981;52:74–80.
60. Nishimura K. Histologic evaluation of free gingival graft especially about the attachment between the graft and the exposed root. J Osaka Dent Univ 1981;15:1–10.
61. Matter J, Cimasoni G. Creeping attachment after free gingival grafts. J Periodontol 1976;47:574–579.
62. Bell LA, Valluzzo TA, Garnick JJ, Pennel BM. The presence of "creeping attachment" in human gingiva. J Periodontol 1978;49:513–517.
63. Agudio G, Nieri M, Rotundo R, Franceschi D, Cortellini P, Pini Prato GP. Periodontal conditions of sites treated with gingival-augmentation surgery compared to untreated contralateral homologous sites: A 10- to 27-year long-term study. J Periodontol 2009;80:1399–1405.
64. Agudio G, Cortellini P, Buti J, Pini Prato G. Periodontal conditions of sites treated with gingival augmentation surgery compared with untreated contralateral homologous sites: An 18- to 35-year long-term study. J Periodontol 2016;87:1371–1378.
65. Cairo F, Rotundo R, Miller PD, Pini Prato GP. Root coverage esthetic score: A system to evaluate the esthetic outcome of the treatment of gingival recession through evaluation of clinical cases. J Periodontol 2009;80:705–710.
66. Ellegaard B, Karring T, Loe H. The fate of vital and devitalized bone grafts in the healing of interradicular lesions. J Periodontal Res 1975;10:88–97.
67. Scheyer ET, Nevins ML, Neiva R, et al. Generation of site-appropriate tissue by a living cellular sheet in the treatment of mucogingival defects. J Periodontol 2014;85:e57–e64.
68. Byun HY, Oh TJ, Abuhussein HM, Yamashita J, Soehren SE, Wang HL. Significance of the epithelial collar on the subepithelial connective tissue graft. J Periodontol 2009;80:924–932.

69. Guiha R, el Khodeiry S, Mota L, Caffesse R. Histological evaluation of healing and revascularization of the subepithelial connective tissue graft. J Periodontol 2001;72:470–478.
70. McGuire MK, Cochran DL. Evaluation of human recession defects treated with coronally advanced flaps and either enamel matrix derivative or connective tissue. Part 2: Histological evaluation. J Periodontol 2003;74:1126–1135.
71. McGuire MK, Scheyer ET, Schupbach P. Growth factor-mediated treatment of recession defects: A randomized controlled trial and histologic and microcomputed tomography examination. J Periodontol 2009;80:550–564.
72. McGuire MK, Nunn M. Evaluation of human recession defects treated with coronally advanced flaps and either enamel matrix derivative or connective tissue. Part 1: Comparison of clinical parameters. J Periodontol 2003;74:1110–1125.
73. Harris RJ. Creeping attachment associated with the connective tissue with partial-thickness double pedicle graft. J Periodontol 1997;68:890–899.
74. Henderson RD, Greenwell H, Drisko C, et al. Predictable multiple site root coverage using an acellular dermal matrix allograft. J Periodontol 2001;72:571–582.
75. Matter J. Creeping attachment of free gingival grafts. A five-year follow-up study. J Periodontol 1980;51:681–685.
76. Rebele SF, Zuhr O, Schneider D, Jung RE, Hürzeler MB. Tunnel technique with connective tissue graft versus coronally advanced flap with enamel matrix derivative for root coverage: A RCT using 3D digital measuring methods. Part II. Volumetric studies on healing dynamics and gingival dimensions. J Clin Periodontol 2014;41:593–603.
77. Zucchelli G, Felice P, Mazzotti C, et al. 5-year outcomes after coverage of soft tissue dehiscence around single implants: A prospective cohort study. Eur J Oral Implantol 2018;11:215–224.
78. Edel A. Clinical evaluation of free connective tissue grafts used to increase the width of keratinised gingiva. J Clin Periodontol 1974;1:185–196.
79. Langer B, Langer L. Subepithelial connective tissue graft technique for root coverage. J Periodontol 1985;56:715–720.
80. Del Pizzo M, Modica F, Bethaz N, Priotto P, Romagnoli R. The connective tissue graft: A comparative clinical evaluation of wound healing at the palatal donor site. A preliminary study. J Clin Periodontol 2002;29:848–854.
81. Wessel JR, Tatakis DN. Patient outcomes following subepithelial connective tissue graft and free gingival graft procedures. J Periodontol 2008;79:425–430.
82. Jahnke PV, Sandifer JB, Gher ME, Gray JL, Richardson AC. Thick free gingival and connective tissue autografts for root coverage. J Periodontol 1993;64:315–322.
83. Zucchelli G, Mele M, Stefanini M, et al. Patient morbidity and root coverage outcome after subepithelial connective tissue and de-epithelialized grafts: A comparative randomized-controlled clinical trial. J Clin Periodontol 2010;37:728–738.
84. Maino GNE, Valles C, Santos A, Pascual A, Esquinas C, Nart J. Influence of suturing technique on wound healing and patient morbidity after connective tissue harvesting. A randomized clinical trial. J Clin Periodontol 2018;45:977–985.
85. Tavelli L, Ravidà A, Saleh MHA, et al. Pain perception following epithelialized gingival graft harvesting: A randomized clinical trial. Clin Oral Investig 2019;23:459–468.
86. Fickl S, Fischer KR, Jockel-Schneider Y, Stappert CF, Schlagenhauf U, Kebschull M. Early wound healing and patient morbidity after single-incision vs trap-door graft harvesting from the palate: A clinical study. Clin Oral Investig 2014;18:2213–2219.
87. Thoma DS, Sancho-Puchades M, Ettlin DA, Hämmerle CH, Jung RE. Impact of a collagen matrix on early healing, aesthetics and patient morbidity in oral mucosal wounds: A randomized study in humans. J Clin Periodontol 2012;39:157–165.
88. Ozcan M, Ucak O, Alkaya B, Keceli S, Seydaoglu G, Haytac MC. Effects of platelet-rich fibrin on palatal wound healing after free gingival graft harvesting: A comparative randomized controlled clinical trial. Int J Periodontics Restorative Dent 2017;37:e270–e278.
89. Soileau KM, Brannon RB. A histologic evaluation of various stages of palatal healing following subepithelial connective tissue grafting procedures: A comparison of eight cases. J Periodontol 2006;77:1267–1273.
90. Burkhardt R, Hämmerle CH, Lang NP, Research Group on Oral Soft Tissue Biology & Wound Healing. Self-reported pain perception of patients after mucosal graft harvesting in the palatal area. J Clin Periodontol 2015;42:281–287.
91. Bahammam MA. Effect of platelet-rich fibrin palatal bandage on pain scores and wound healing after free gingival graft: A randomized controlled clinical trial. Clin Oral Investig 2018;22:3179–3188.
92. Femminella B, Iaconi MC, Di Tullio M, et al. Clinical comparison of platelet-rich fibrin and a gelatin sponge in the management of palatal wounds after epithelialized free gingival graft harvest: A randomized clinical trial. J Periodontol 2016;87:103–113.
93. Tasdemir Z, Alkan BA, Albayrak H. Effects of ozone therapy on the early healing period of deepithelialized gingival grafts: A randomized placebo-controlled clinical trial. J Periodontol 2016;87:663–671.
94. Keceli HG, Aylikci BU, Koseoglu S, Dolgun A. Evaluation of palatal donor site haemostasis and wound healing after free gingival graft surgery. J Clin Periodontol 2015;42:582–589.
95. Yıldırım S, Özener HÖ, Doğan B, Kuru B. Effect of topically applied hyaluronic acid on pain and palatal epithelial wound healing: An examiner-masked, randomized, controlled clinical trial. J Periodontol 2018;89:36–45.
96. Ozcelik O, Seydaoglu G, Haytac CM. Diode laser for harvesting de-epithelialized palatal graft in the treatment of gingival recession defects: A randomized clinical trial. J Clin Periodontol 2016;43:63–71.
97. Silva CO, de Lima AF, Sallum AW, Tatakis DN. Coronally positioned flap for root coverage in smokers and non-smokers: Stability of outcomes between 6 months and 2 years. J Periodontol 2007;78:1702–1707.
98. Yaghobee S, Rouzmeh N, Aslroosta H, Mahmoodi S, Khorsand A, Kharrazifard MJ. Effect of topical erythropoietin (EPO) on palatal wound healing subsequent to free gingival grafting (FGG). Braz Oral Res 2018;32:e55.
99. Chang PC, Tsai SC, Jheng YH, Lin YF, Chen CC. Soft-tissue wound healing by anti-advanced glycation end-products agents. J Dent Res 2014;93:388–393.
100. Kozlovsky A, Artzi Z, Hirshberg A, Israeli-Tobias C, Reich L. Effect of local antimicrobial agents on excisional palatal wound healing: A clinical and histomorphometric study in rats. J Clin Periodontol 2007;34:164–171.
101. Zou XH, Foong WC, Cao T, Bay BH, Ouyang HW, Yip GW. Chondroitin sulfate in palatal wound healing. J Dent Res 2004;83:880–885.
102. Delima SL, Kumar PS, Tatakis DN. Bacterial community shifts during healing of palatal wounds: Comparison of two graft harvesting approaches. J Clin Periodontol 2016;43:271–278.
103. Position paper: Periodontal regeneration. J Periodontol 2005;76:1601–1622.

104. Caton J, Nyman S, Zander H. Histometric evaluation of periodontal surgery. II. Connective tissue attachment levels after four regenerative procedures. J Clin Periodontol 1980;7:224–231.
105. Caton J, Nyman S. Histometric evaluation of periodontal surgery. I. The modified Widman flap procedure. J Clin Periodontol 1980;7:212–223.
106. Kao RT, Nares S, Reynolds MA. Periodontal regeneration—Intrabony defects: A systematic review from the AAP Regeneration Workshop. J Periodontol 2015;86(2 suppl):S77–S104.
107. Melcher AH. On the repair potential of periodontal tissues. J Periodontol 1976;47:256–260.
108. Nyman S, Lindhe J, Karring T, Rylander H. New attachment following surgical treatment of human periodontal disease. J Clin Periodontol 1982;9:290–296.
109. Gottlow J, Nyman S, Karring T, Lindhe J. New attachment formation as the result of controlled tissue regeneration. J Clin Periodontol 1984;11:494–503.
110. Gottlow J, Nyman S, Lindhe J, Karring T, Wennström J. New attachment formation in the human periodontium by guided tissue regeneration. Case reports. J Clin Periodontol 1986;13:604–616.
111. Wachtel H, Schenk G, Böhm S, Weng D, Zuhr O, Hürzeler MB. Microsurgical access flap and enamel matrix derivative for the treatment of periodontal intrabony defects: A controlled clinical study. J Clin Periodontol 2003;30:496–504.
112. Cortellini P, Tonetti MS. Microsurgical approach to periodontal regeneration. Initial evaluation in a case cohort. J Periodontol 2001;72:559–569.
113. Burkhardt R, Lang NP. Coverage of localized gingival recessions: Comparison of micro- and macrosurgical techniques. J Clin Periodontol 2005;32:287–293.
114. Ucak O, Ozcan M, Seydaoglu G, Haytac MC. Microsurgical instruments in laterally moved, coronally advanced flap for Miller Class III isolated recession defects: A randomized controlled clinical trial. Int J Periodontics Restorative Dent 2017;37:109–115.
115. Nizam N, Bengisu O, Sönmez S. Micro- and macrosurgical techniques in the coverage of gingival recession using connective tissue graft: 2 years follow-up. J Esthet Restor Dent 2015;27:71–83.
116. Tavelli L, Barootchi S, Nguyen TVN, Tattan M, Ravidà A, Wang HL. Efficacy of tunnel technique in the treatment of localized and multiple gingival recessions: A systematic review and a meta-analysis. J Periodontol 2018;89:1075–1090.
117. Curtis JW Jr, McLain JB, Hutchinson RA. The incidence and severity of complications and pain following periodontal surgery. J Periodontol 1985;56:597–601.
118. Vogel RI, Desjardins PJ, Major KV. Comparison of presurgical and immediate postsurgical ibuprofen on postoperative periodontal pain. J Periodontol 1992;63:914–918.
119. Griffin TJ, Cheung WS, Zavras AI, Damoulis PD. Postoperative complications following gingival augmentation procedures. J Periodontol 2006;77:2070–2079.
120. Baab DA, Ammons WF Jr, Selipsky H. Blood loss during periodontal flap surgery. J Periodontol 1977;48:693–698.
121. Buckley JA, Ciancio SG, McMullen JA. Efficacy of epinephrine concentration in local anesthesia during periodontal surgery. J Periodontol 1984;55:653–657.
122. Pack PD, Haber J. The incidence of clinical infection after periodontal surgery. A retrospective study. J Periodontol 1983;54:441–443.
123. Powell CA, Mealey BL, Deas DE, McDonnell HT, Moritz AJ. Post-surgical infections: Prevalence associated with various periodontal surgical procedures. J Periodontol 2005;76:329–333.
124. Echeverria JJ, Montero M, Abad D, Gay C. Exostosis following a free gingival graft. J Clin Periodontol 2002;29:474–477.
125. Otero-Cagide FJ, Singer DL, Hoover JN. Exostosis associated with autogenous gingival grafts: A report of 9 cases. J Periodontol 1996;67:611–616.
126. Cortellini P, Tonetti MS. Focus on intrabony defects: Guided tissue regeneration. Periodontol 2000 2000;22:104–132.
127. Sanz M, Tonetti MS, Zabalegui I, et al. Treatment of intrabony defects with enamel matrix proteins or barrier membranes: Results from a multicenter practice-based clinical trial. J Periodontol 2004;75:726–733.
128. Cortellini P, Tonetti MS. Clinical concepts for regenerative therapy in intrabony defects. Periodontol 2000 2015;68:282–307.

15

ALVEOLAR RIDGE PRESERVATION

Fernando Suárez López del Amo, DDS, MS
Juan C. Rodríguez, DDS, MS

The alveolar process forms concurrently with the development and eruption of the dentition. As such, the morphologic features and the remodeling of this structure are directly related to the characteristics of the teeth. After tooth extraction, the bundle bone along with portions of the adjacent bony walls of the socket will resorb, resulting in significant structural changes. These changes are characterized by a series of local biologic events that typically result in a net loss of alveolar ridge volume. This phenomenon is initiated after tooth extraction and could continue for decades.[1,2] The dynamics and magnitude of these changes have been extensively investigated in animal models[3–6] as well as in humans.[7–9] As a public health concern, tooth loss has a detrimental impact on various aspects related to quality of life, including self-perception, facial esthetic changes, decreased ability to properly masticate, and alterations of normal speech. Several etiologies are known for tooth loss, ranging from periodontal disease to trauma or severe decay leading to unrestorability, making extractions one of the three most common procedures performed in dental offices.[10] This chapter reviews the events associated with dimensional changes to the hard and soft alveolar tissues postextraction, as well as the different therapeutic alternatives that can be used to minimize these changes.

Anatomical Characteristics

Both maxillary and mandibular bones are composed of several structures, namely the basal bone, the alveolar process, and the bundle bone (Fig 15-1). The **basal bone** constitutes the structural component of the maxilla and the mandible. This bone invariably forms together with the skeleton whether or not teeth are developed. Consequently, in cases of total tooth agenesis, the basal bone is the only portion of the jawbones that is formed. Many years after tooth extraction, this structure is often the only bone that remains following the resorption processes, although external stimuli from a removable prosthesis might cause a considerable portion of it to be lost.

DEFINITIONS AND TERMINOLOGY

Alveolar bone proper: Compact bone that composes the alveolus (tooth socket). Also known as the *lamina dura* or *cribriform plate*, the fibers of the periodontal ligament insert into it.[11]

Alveolar process: The compact and cancellous bony structure that contains tooth sockets that surrounds and supports the teeth.

Alveolus: The socket in the bone into which a tooth is attached by means of the periodontal ligament.[11]

Basal bone: The bone of the mandible and maxilla exclusive of the alveolar process.[11]

Bundle bone: A type of alveolar bone, so-called because of the "bundle" pattern caused by the continuation of the principal (Sharpey) fibers into it.[11]

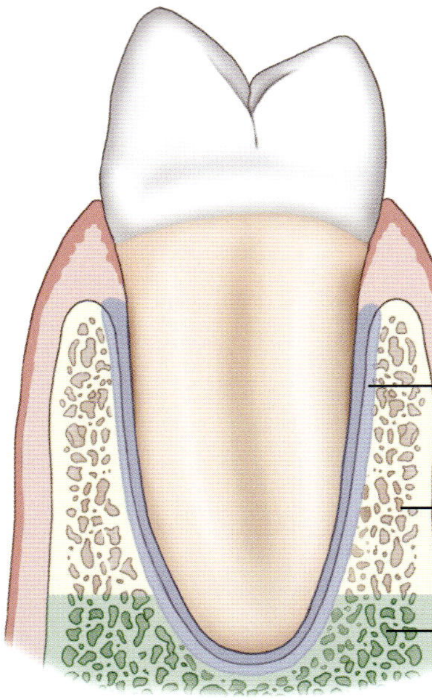

Fig 15-1 Anatomical structures surrounding the root.

The alveolar bone or **alveolar process**, on the other hand, is the bone that forms during the different stages of tooth development, at the end of which it surrounds the vast majority of the roots and houses what is called the **alveolus**. After tooth extraction, the alveolar bone is gradually resorbed until it is completely lost. Lastly, the **bundle bone** is the portion of the alveolar process in which the Sharpey fibers of the periodontal ligament insert. The bundle bone is a dense lamina that receives its vascularity from both alveolar bone and periodontal ligament vascular systems. This bone lines the alveolar socket, and it is completely resorbed after tooth extraction. In addition, this tooth-dependent structure appears to be the first bone to be resorbed after extraction.

Postextraction Socket Healing

The spontaneous healing of a socket leads to a cascade of events that ultimately result in the loss of both hard and soft tissues. These occur in immediate succession of one another as well as simultaneously. Many authors have studied this series of events,[7,8,12] which can be briefly summarized as follows:

1. The tooth is extracted.
2. The empty socket is filled with blood and a clot forms.
3. Inflammatory cells (polymorphonuclear and macrophages/monocytes) migrate into the clot and start to phagocytize elements of necrotic tissue, thereby initiating the process of wound cleansing.
4. Sprouts of newly formed blood vessels and mesenchymal cells enter the clot, and granulation tissue is formed.
5. The granulation tissue is gradually replaced with provisional connective tissue, and subsequently immature woven bone is formed.
6. The hard tissue walls of the socket (**alveolar bone proper**) are resorbed, and the socket wound becomes filled with woven bone.
7. In the later phases, the woven bone is remodeled into lamellar bone and marrow.

One of the first human studies conducted to histologically investigate the cascade of events associated with socket healing was published in 1960 by Amler et al (Table 15-1).[7]

In a similar landmark study evaluating the osteogenic potential of healing bone from extraction sockets, Evian et al focused their efforts in describing the progression that bone experiences after a tooth is lost from the moment of epithelial closure to 16 weeks later (Table 15-2).[8]

DIMENSIONAL TISSUE ALTERATIONS

When alveolar ridge preservation (ARP) is not performed after tooth extraction, the alveolus and surrounding bony structures often suffer from major dimensional changes characterized by a profound resorption process. These alterations occur in both hard and soft tissues and have been extensively studied in clinical and preclinical models.

Hard tissue

The dimensional changes occurring after tooth extraction are initiated by the resorption of the bundle bone. This structure lining of the extraction socket is composed of lamellar bone and presents with an average thickness of 0.2 to 0.4 mm.[13] As a tooth-dependent structure, the bundle bone is always gradually resorbed after tooth extraction, ultimately resulting in vertical and/or horizontal bone loss.

The thickness of the socket's bony walls—and more importantly, the facial bony wall—represents one of the

TABLE 15-1 Socket healing as described in 1960 by Amler et al[7]

Stage	Timing	Events
Blood clot	Immediately after extraction	• Fills up the socket space immediately after extraction. • Mainly composed of RBCs, WBCs, and precipitating fibrin.
Granulation tissue	2 to 3 days	• Characterized by RBCs, increase in WBCs, cells of the reticuloendothelial system, and cells associated with the creation of capillaries. • Metachromatic GS appears as well as glycoprotein and AP. • At day 7, the RBCs look fragmented and mix with well-organized fibrin. By this time, granulation tissue has replaced the blood clot.
Young connective tissue	4 to 20 days	• Seen at day 4, this is characterized by spindle-shaped cells and collagen fibers, disappearance of the granulation tissue (by day 20), and increase in vascularity. • Increase in the metachromatic GS, AP, and glycoprotein framework. • Osteogenic fibers and osteoblasts start to show.
Bone formation	7 to 25 days	• At day 7, uncalcified bone spicules are evident attached to old spicules as well as new ones. • Metachromatic GS as well as glycoprotein and AP are highly expressed at this point, especially in more mature areas. • At day 14, mineralization starts and is more evident at day 25.
Filling of socket with primary bone	20 to 38 days	• After day 20 and by day 38, two-thirds of the socket is filled by bone.
Epithelization	4 to 40 days	• At the day 4, epithelization starts at the edges of the socket. • At day 7, a high infiltration of mast cells into the epithelium is observed, which grows exponentially until day 14. It then becomes stable until day 40, when it peaks again. • Complete fusion of the epithelium is seen as early as day 24 but occurs most commonly after day 35.

RBCs, red blood cells; WBCs, white blood cells; GS, ground substance; AP, alkaline phosphatase.

TABLE 15-2 Socket healing as described in 1982 by Evian et al[8]

Timing	Characteristics
4 weeks	• Abundance of fibrous connective tissue • Islands of new bone within connective tissue surrounded by an osteoid seam • Layers of osteoblasts present external to this osteoid layer • High osteoblastic activity
6 weeks	• Increased bone content and elongated islands of new bone with a primitive trabecular network • Osteoid tissue surrounded by new bone • High osteoblastic activity
8 weeks	• Sheets and trabeculae of new bone appear to occupy a greater proportion of the tissue • Osteoid seam less pronounced with fewer osteoblasts present • Less connective tissue component largely surrounded by bone • Less osteoblastic activity than 4 to 6 weeks
10 weeks	• Trabeculae of interconnected bone with minimum osteoid surrounding bone • Greater bone volume than 8 weeks
12 weeks	• Similar to 10 weeks with well-formed trabeculae of bone surrounding a lightly staining and less cellular connective tissue • Very little osteoid tissue • Reduction of osteoblasts
16 weeks	• Masses of mature dense bony trabeculae • Connective tissue with fewer cellular elements • Blood vessel within connective tissue • Very little bone formation with apparent signs of remodeling • Osteoblasts still present in a few areas • Greater bone volume relative to connective tissue than 10 to 12 weeks

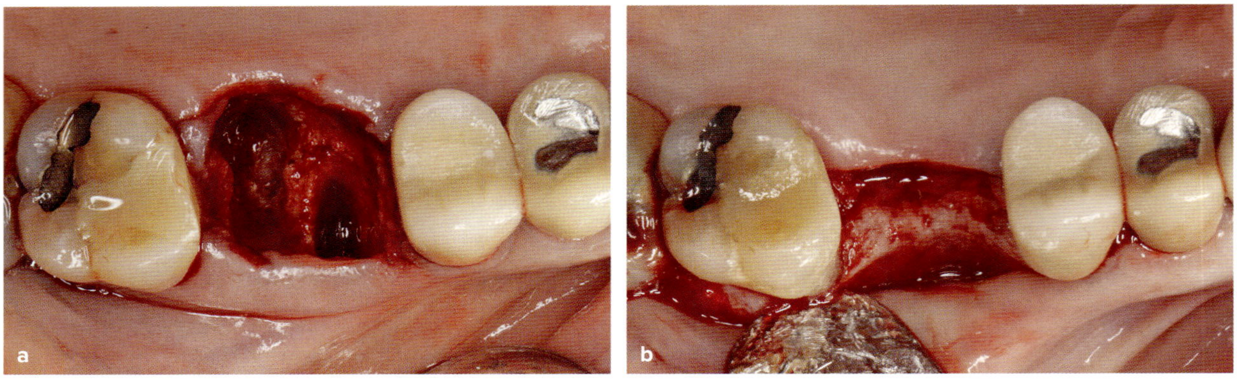

Fig 15-2 Ridge width reduction after extraction of maxillary molar. *(a)* Fresh extraction socket. *(b)* Postextraction changes 4 months later.

most determinant factors in the remodeling process occurring after tooth extraction. Multiple investigations have demonstrated that the facial socket bony wall in the anterior maxilla is less than 0.5 mm in 50% of cases and less than 1 mm in 90% of cases.[14,15] On the other hand, only 3% of sites presented with 2 mm of buccal bony wall.[14] Consequently, oftentimes in the anterior maxilla, the majority of the facial bone is composed of bundle bone, leading to a higher degree of resorption after extraction. The importance of the thickness of the buccal bone was confirmed in a study by Chappuis et al[16] demonstrating that at sites with facial bone of 1 mm or less, a vertical average of 7.5 mm corresponding to 62% of the bone height was lost after 8 weeks. In contrast, sites with greater than 1 mm of facial bone showed an average loss of 1.1 mm, corresponding to only 9% of the vertical bone present prior to extraction.[16] More recently, Tomasi et al confirmed the previous findings demonstrating that at sockets with 1 mm or less of buccal bone wall, the reduction in buccal volume was three times greater than sites with more than 1 mm of bone wall.[17]

With regard to the horizontal ridge reduction after extraction, it has been reported to occur up to 50% of the original width and was more significant at buccal than lingual sites and in the molar region[18] (Fig 15-2).

The differences in terms of ridge resorption (width and height) reported in the literature can be attributed to a variety of factors, including but not limited to bone wall thickness, tooth anatomy and location, surgical trauma, lack of functional stimuli, and genetics.[16] In addition, the dimensional alterations are greatly influenced by the different locations within the socket. As such, for single extraction sites with healthy adjacent dentition, the dimensional changes occur mostly at the central area, while the interproximal sites remain almost unchanged.[16] This was recently confirmed by a systematic review and meta-analysis reporting that mesial and distal sites did not experience substantial differences with or without ARP.[19]

Soft tissue

Interestingly, while the soft tissue represents a key component of the final esthetic outcomes of implant therapy, especially for the anterior maxilla, the investigations of the volumetric and morphologic changes—as well as their influence on the postextraction healing process—have not been as extensively investigated as they occur with the surrounding bony structures. Indeed, the soft tissue changes occurring after tooth extraction have received little attention. Nevertheless, a recent investigation focused on this topic.[20] After single-tooth extractions in 33 patients, an analysis of the soft tissue alterations was conducted every 2 weeks until a total of 8 weeks. Results indicated that for thin bone phenotypes, the facial tissue thickness increased sevenfold, whereas for thick bone phenotypes, the soft tissues remained unchanged. These results could be attributed to the quick resorption of the thin buccal wall after tooth extraction along with the rapid growth of the soft tissue inward and toward the socket. It is important to mention that more than 50% of these dimensional soft tissue changes occurred within the first 2 weeks, regardless of the phenotype.

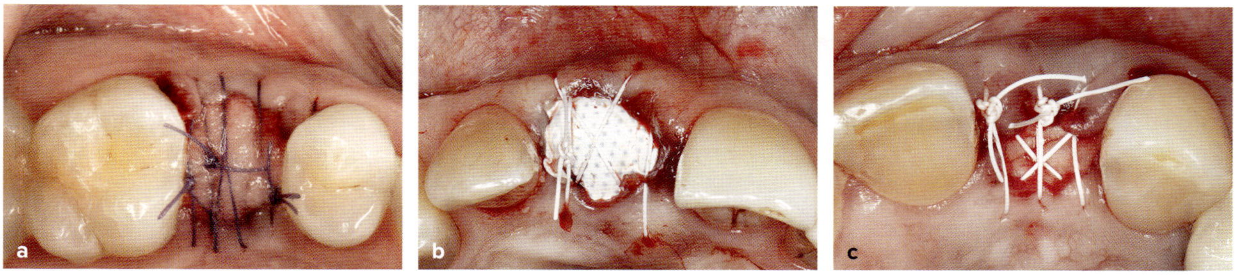

Fig 15-3 Alveolar ridge preservation. *(a)* Absorbable collagen sponge. *(b)* Nonabsorbable membrane. *(c)* Absorbable collagen membrane.

Management of the Extraction Socket

Once the tooth is extracted from its alveolus, multiple grafting materials and/or techniques can be employed (Fig 15-3). Postextraction grafting of the socket with different biomaterials has been demonstrated as effective in minimizing the dimensional changes.[19] However, the biologic remodeling process after extraction is inevitable.[21] In general terms, these techniques can be divided into the maintenance of the root (partially or totally), socket grafting, and immediate implant placement.[21]

Also, a number of variables have been studied affecting the degree of postextraction resorption. These variables include but are not limited to soft tissue manipulation (flap vs flapless), tissue phenotype, use of barrier membranes, number and integrity of bony walls, and type of grafting, among others. The following section focuses on the description of the treatment modalities most commonly used after tooth extraction.

ALVEOLAR RIDGE PRESERVATION

Bone formation in the alveolar socket is a naturally occurring event given the presence of the surrounding bony walls. However, the osteoclastic activity and the resulting resorption process of these bony walls[6,22] causes an undesired remodeling of the alveolar ridge that could possibly compromise or preclude the placement of dental implants in the adequate prosthetically driven position. In addition, loss of alveolar height and width could compromise the esthetic appearance of pontic areas or the stability of removable dentures. Consequently, the utilization of different ARP techniques has been extensively investigated, demonstrating to be an effective therapy diminishing the dimensional reduction of the alveolar ridge after tooth extraction.[19] The goals of ARP include the following[23]:

- To enable placement and stability of a dental implant
- To reduce loss of alveolar bone volume
- To reduce need for additional bone grafting procedures
- To enable the generated tissues to provide implant osseointegration
- To improve the esthetic outcome of the definitive prosthesis

ARP can be performed with a variety of grafting materials and barrier membranes. Recently, for the conduction of a systematic review and meta-analysis, Avila-Ortiz et al grouped these treatment modalities into nine different categories[19]:

1. Bovine bone particles plus socket sealing
2. Construct made of 90% bovine bone granules and 10% porcine collagen plus socket sealing
3. Corticocancellous porcine bone particles plus socket sealing
4. Allograft particles plus socket sealing
5. Alloplastic material with or without socket sealing
6. Autologous blood-derived products
7. Cell therapy
8. Recombinant bone morphogenetic protein 2
9. Socket sealing alone

Overall, multiple investigations have demonstrated the beneficial effect of ARP compared with spontaneous socket healing.[24–29] Recent systematic reviews and meta-analyses have demonstrated the clinical magnitude of this effect compared with tooth extraction alone to be approximately 2 mm for horizontal and midbuccal height, 1 mm for vertical midlingual height, 0.5 mm for mesial height, and 0.2 mm for distal height changes.[2,19] In addition, the utilization of particulate xenogenic or allogenic material in combination with absorbable collagen sponge or membrane resulted in superior outcomes with regard to horizontal ridge preservation.[2,19]

It is important to bear in mind that several factors, including the thickness of the buccal bone wall, play a very critical role in the postextraction remodeling process. Unfortunately, many of these factors remain commonly underreported in multitudes of investigations. Conversely, investigations evaluating the thickness of the buccal wall have demonstrated the critical effect of this structure with regard to the dimensional reduction.[16,17,19] Indeed, a recent study concluded that only sites with a thin phenotype could significantly benefit from ARP.[17]

ARP is one of the most researched subjects in periodontal and oral surgery literature. A vast amount of evidence, including clinical and preclinical studies as well as narrative and systematic reviews, has been published on this topic over the last decades.[5,9,17,18,21] The most current and comprehensive systematic review from the XIII European Workshop in Periodontology reviewed 22 randomized controlled trials that evaluated different ARP techniques compared to spontaneous socket healing.[19] This systematic review and meta-analysis focused into endpoints of interest that included clinical, radiographic, and patient-reported outcome measures. With regard to clinical outcomes, ARP demonstrated superiority in terms of horizontal, vertical, linear, and volumetric soft tissue changes. Implant-related outcomes revealed a reduced need for additional bone grafting at time of or prior to implant placement when ARP was previously performed. With regard to radiographic outcomes, most of the included investigations also reported superior outcomes for ARP compared with spontaneous socket healing. Lastly, patient-reported outcomes were only evaluated in two investigations, reporting no differences between ARP and the control group.

Multiple other systematic reviews and meta-analyses have also evaluated the effect of ARP.[30–33] Thus, although they presented with several differences, all of these investigations demonstrated the beneficial effect of ARP for attenuation of the dimensional reduction of the alveolar ridge.

IMMEDIATE IMPLANT PLACEMENT

The placement of dental implants into fresh extraction sockets was once believed to prevent bone resorption and help maintain the original architecture of the ridge. However, numerous investigations have refuted this concept, concluding that immediate implant placement does not prevent the resorption process occurring after tooth extraction,[34] and it may even promote a greater degree of bone remodeling.[35,36] On the other hand, ARP with or without immediate implant placement has been demonstrated as effective in attenuating the resorption process.[37] In this study, no statistically significant differences were observed when ARP was performed with or without simultaneous immediate implant placement. However, results from both of these groups were superior to spontaneous healing. As such, immediate implant placement is most commonly used in combination with guided bone regeneration and/or different techniques for ARP.

While the resorption process is diminished when immediate implant placement is performed in conjunction with ARP, some degree of bone resorption is still expected. In this sense, several investigations have reported midbuccal soft tissue recession and bone resorption with this treatment modality.[38,39] Therefore, it is imperative to perform proper case selection when performing immediate implant placement. Sockets with a thick intact buccal bone wall and thick gingival phenotype, a flapless approach, and immediate provisional restoration are associated with a reduced risk for developing midfacial recession.[38]

ALTERNATIVE TREATMENTS

While the utilization of different ARP techniques with or without immediate implant placement are the most commonly employed approaches for the management of the extraction socket, several other alternative therapies exist. Thus, investigations have evaluated the possibility of grafting over the buccal bone wall and underneath the soft tissue (known as *buccal plate augmentation* or *overbuilding*),[40,41] as well as the total or partial maintenance of the root.[42,43] Recently, the utilization of the socket shield technique has been gaining popularity. This approach consists of the maintenance of the buccal portion of the root, aiming at preservation of the periodontal ligament and bundle bone. Although successful outcomes up to 5 years have been reported, the use of this technique is not advisable until further research and higher level of evidence is available.[43]

Conclusions

A significant amount of evidence supported by numerous randomized controlled trials and systematic reviews have demonstrated that ARP represents an effective therapy to minimize the dimensional reduction that occurs after tooth extraction. These dimensional changes are influenced by a variety of factors, with the thickness of the surrounding bony walls playing one of the most critical roles. Finally, it is important to bear in mind that ARP minimizes the dimensional changes; however, it does not eliminate the bone resorption process.

References

1. Tan WL, Wong TL, Wong MC, Lang NP. A systematic review of post-extractional alveolar hard and soft tissue dimensional changes in humans. Clin Oral Implants Res 2012;23(5 suppl 5):1–21.
2. Avila-Ortiz G, Elangovan S, Kramer KW, Blanchette D, Dawson DV. Effect of alveolar ridge preservation after tooth extraction: A systematic review and meta-analysis. J Dent Res 2014;93:950–958.
3. Kuboki Y, Hashimoto F, Ishibashi K. Time-dependent changes of collagen crosslinks in the socket after tooth extraction in rabbits. J Dent Res 1988;67:944–948.
4. Devlin H, Hoyland J, Newall JF, Ayad S. Trabecular bone formation in the healing of the rodent molar tooth extraction socket. J Bone Miner Res 1997;12:2061–2067.
5. Cardaropoli G, Araújo M, Lindhe J. Dynamics of bone tissue formation in tooth extraction sites. An experimental study in dogs. J Clin Periodontol 2003;30:809–818.
6. Araújo MG, Lindhe J. Dimensional ridge alterations following tooth extraction. An experimental study in the dog. J Clin Periodontol 2005;32:212–218.
7. Amler MH, Johnson PL, Salman I. Histological and histochemical investigation of human alveolar socket healing in undisturbed extraction wounds. J Am Dent Assoc 1960;61:32–44.
8. Evian CI, Rosenberg ES, Coslet JG, Corn H. The osteogenic activity of bone removed from healing extraction sockets in humans. J Periodontol 1982;53:81–85.
9. Trombelli L, Farina R, Marzola A, Bozzi L, Liljenberg B, Lindhe J. Modeling and remodeling of human extraction sockets. J Clin Periodontol 2008;35:630–639.
10. Gilbert GH, Gordan VV, Korelitz JJ, et al. Provision of specific dental procedures by general dentists in the National Dental Practice-Based Research Network: Questionnaire findings. BMC Oral Health 2015;15:11.
11. American Academy of Periodontology. Glossary of Periodontal Terms. American Academy of Periodontology, 2001.
12. Amler MH. The time sequence of tissue regeneration in human extraction wounds. Oral Surg Oral Med Oral Pathol 1969;27:309–318.
13. Schroeder HE. Handbook of Microscopic Anatomy. Vol 5: The Periodontium. Berlin: Springer, 1986.
14. Huynh-Ba G, Pjetursson BE, Sanz M, et al. Analysis of the socket bone wall dimensions in the upper maxilla in relation to immediate implant placement. Clin Oral Implants Res 2010;21:37–42.
15. Januário AL, Duarte WR, Barriviera M, Mesti JC, Araújo MG, Lindhe J. Dimension of the facial bone wall in the anterior maxilla: A cone-beam computed tomography study. Clin Oral Implants Res 2011;22:1168–1171.
16. Chappuis V, Engel O, Reyes M, Shahim K, Nolte LP, Buser D. Ridge alterations post-extraction in the esthetic zone: A 3D analysis with CBCT. J Dent Res 2013;92(12 suppl):195S–201S.
17. Tomasi C, Donati M, Cecchinato D, Szathvary I, Corrà E, Lindhe J. Effect of socket grafting with deproteinized bone mineral: An RCT on dimensional alterations after 6 months. Clin Oral Implants Res 2018;29:435–442.
18. Araújo MG, Silva CO, Misawa M, Sukekava F. Alveolar socket healing: What can we learn? Periodontol 2000 2015;68:122–134.
19. Avila-Ortiz G, Chambrone L, Vignoletti F. Effect of alveolar ridge preservation interventions following tooth extraction: A systematic review and meta-analysis. J Clin Periodontol 2019;46(21 suppl):195–223.
20. Chappuis V, Engel O, Shahim K, Reyes M, Katsaros C, Buser D. Soft tissue alterations in esthetic postextraction sites: A 3-dimensional analysis. J Dent Res 2015;94(9 suppl):187S–193S.
21. Chappuis V, Araújo MG, Buser D. Clinical relevance of dimensional bone and soft tissue alterations post-extraction in esthetic sites. Periodontol 2000 2017;73:73–83.
22. Schropp L, Wenzel A, Kostopoulos L, Karring T. Bone healing and soft tissue contour changes following single-tooth extraction: A clinical and radiographic 12-month prospective study. Int J Periodontics Restorative Dent 2003;23:313–323.
23. Pagni G, Pellegrini G, Giannobile WV, Rasperini G. Postextraction alveolar ridge preservation: Biological basis and treatments. Int J Dent 2012;151030.
24. Aimetti M, Romano F, Griga FB, Godio L. Clinical and histologic healing of human extraction sockets filled with calcium sulfate. Int J Oral Maxillofac Implants 2009;24:902–909.
25. Barone A, Aldini NN, Fini M, Giardino R, Calvo Guirado JL, Covani U. Xenograft versus extraction alone for ridge preservation after tooth removal: A clinical and histomorphometric study. J Periodontol 2008;79:1370–1377.
26. Barone A, Orlando B, Cingano L, Marconcini S, Derchi G, Covani U. A randomized clinical trial to evaluate and compare implants placed in augmented versus non-augmented extraction sockets: 3-year results. J Periodontol 2012;83:836–846.
27. Camargo PM, Lekovic V, Weinlaender M, et al. Influence of bioactive glass on changes in alveolar process dimensions after exodontia. Oral Surg Oral Med Oral Pathol Oral Radiol Endod 2000;90:581–586.
28. Cardaropoli D, Tamagnone L, Roffredo A, Gaveglio L, Cardaropoli G. Socket preservation using bovine bone mineral and collagen membrane: A randomized controlled clinical trial with histologic analysis. Int J Periodontics Restorative Dent 2012;32:421–430.
29. Iasella JM, Greenwell H, Miller RL, et al. Ridge preservation with freeze-dried bone allograft and a collagen membrane compared to extraction alone for implant site development: A clinical and histologic study in humans. J Periodontol 2003;74:990–999.
30. Bassir SH, Alhareky M, Wangsrimongkol B, Jia Y, Karimbux N. Systematic review and meta-analysis of hard tissue outcomes of alveolar ridge preservation. Int J Oral Maxillofac Implants 2018;33:979–994.
31. Troiano G, Zhurakivska K, Lo Muzio L, Laino L, Cicciù M, Lo Russo L. Combination of bone graft and resorbable membrane for alveolar ridge preservation: A systematic review, meta-analysis, and trial sequential analysis. J Periodontol 2018;89:46–57.

32. Iocca O, Farcomeni A, Pardiñas Lopez S, Talib HS. Alveolar ridge preservation after tooth extraction: A Bayesian network meta-analysis of grafting materials efficacy on prevention of bone height and width reduction. J Clin Periodontol 2017;44:104–114.
33. MacBeth N, Trullenque-Eriksson A, Donos N, Mardas N. Hard and soft tissue changes following alveolar ridge preservation: A systematic review. Clin Oral Implants Res 2017;28:982–1004.
34. Araújo MG, Sukekava F, Wennström JL, Lindhe J. Ridge alterations following implant placement in fresh extraction sockets: An experimental study in the dog. J Clin Periodontol 2005;32:645–652.
35. Vignoletti F, Discepoli N, Müller A, de Sanctis M, Muñoz F, Sanz M. Bone modelling at fresh extraction sockets: Immediate implant placement versus spontaneous healing: An experimental study in the beagle dog. J Clin Periodontol 2012;39:91–97.
36. Discepoli N, Vignoletti F, Laino L, de Sanctis M, Muñoz F, Sanz M. Fresh extraction socket: Spontaneous healing vs immediate implant placement. Clin Oral Implants Res 2015;26:1250–1255.
37. Clementini M, Agostinelli A, Castelluzzo W, Cugnata F, Vignoletti F, De Sanctis M. The effect of immediate implant placement on alveolar ridge preservation compared to spontaneous healing after tooth extraction: Radiographic results of a randomized controlled clinical trial. J Clin Periodontol 2019;46:776–786.
38. Cosyn J, Hooghe N, De Bruyn H. A systematic review on the frequency of advanced recession following single immediate implant treatment. J Clin Periodontol 2012;39:582–589.
39. Vera C, De Kok IJ, Reinhold D, et al. Evaluation of buccal alveolar bone dimension of maxillary anterior and premolar teeth: A cone beam computed tomography investigation. Int J Oral Maxillofac Implants 2012;27:1514–1519.
40. Avila-Ortiz G, Rodriguez JC, Rudek I, Benavides E, Rios H, Wang HL. Effectiveness of three different alveolar ridge preservation techniques: A pilot randomized controlled trial. Int J Periodontics Restorative Dent 2014;34:509–521.
41. Caiazzo A, Brugnami F, Mehra P. Buccal plate augmentation: A new alternative to socket preservation. J Oral Maxillofac Surg 2010;68:2503–2506.
42. Filippi A, Pohl Y, von Arx T. Decoronation of an ankylosed tooth for preservation of alveolar bone prior to implant placement. Dent Traumatol 2001;17:93–95.
43. Baumer D, Zuhr O, Rebele S, Hürzeler M. Socket Shield Technique for immediate implant placement—Clinical, radiographic and volumetric data after 5 years. Clin Oral Implants Res 2017;28:1450–1458.

16

DENTAL IMPLANTS

Aaeshah Alkanderi, BMedSc, BDM, MS
Fernando Suárez López del Amo, DDS, MS

The dental implant has evolved tremendously over the past decades into a highly predictable treatment alternative to replace the missing dentition with excellent long-term outcomes. Professors Per-Ingvar Brånemark and André Schroeder were the pioneers of modern implant dentistry and performed the first preclinical and clinical studies.

Osseointegration

Osseointegration as a term was originally proposed by Brånemark et al.[2] Later, Albrektsson et al[3] redefined it as "a direct—on the light microscopic level—contact between living bone and implant." Zarb and Albrektsson[4] defined it as "a process whereby clinically asymptomatic rigid fixation of alloplastic materials is achieved and maintained in bone during functional loading." On the other hand, Schroeder et al[5,6] used the term *functional ankylosis* to demonstrate the rigid fixation of the dental **implant** to the jawbone and stated that "new bone is laid down directly upon the implant surface, provided that the rules for atraumatic implant placement are followed and the implant exhibits primary stability."

One of the most critical factors for successful implant osseointegration is *primary stability*. This phenomenon refers to the stability of the implant within the osteotomy at the time of placement. As peri-implant bone remodeling takes place, the primary mechanical stability is gradually replaced by secondary stability. The latter denotes new bone deposition around the implant; ie, the implant is **osseointegrated**.[7]

Implant versus Tooth

Although the peri-implant supporting tissues and the periodontium share similar clinical as well as histologic features, there are several differences between the attachment apparatus around teeth and dental implants. These are depicted in Table 16-1 and Fig 16-1.[8–18]

DEFINITIONS AND TERMINOLOGY

Implant abutment: That part of an implant system that connects the implant with a prosthesis or other device.[1]

Implant fixture: A synonym for an implant, especially an endosseous implant.[1]

Implant, oral: 1. An alloplastic material or device that is surgically placed into the oral tissue beneath the mucosal or periosteal layer or within the bone for functional, therapeutic, or esthetic purposes. 2. To insert a graft or alloplastic device into the oral hard or soft tissues for replacement of missing or damaged anatomical parts, or for stabilization of a periodontally compromised tooth or group of teeth.[1]

Implant surgery: Procedures concerned with the placement, uncovering, and removal of implants and the repair or modification of associated hard or soft tissues.[1]

Osseointegrated implant: A direct structural and functional connection between ordered, living bone and the surface of an immobile, load-bearing implant as detected on a light microscopic level.[1]

Osseointegration: A direct contact, on the light microscopic level, between living bone tissue and an implant.[1]

TABLE 16-1 Comparison between the attachment apparatus of teeth and implants

	Tooth	Implant
Attachment	Periodontium	Osseointegration
Epithelial attachment		
Origin[8]	Reduced enamel epithelium	Epithelial cells from oral mucosa
Epithelial attachment	Basal lamina and hemidesmosomes[8]	Basal lamina and hemidesmosomes[9]
Connective tissue attachment		
Fiber groups	Dentogingival, dentoperiosteal, alveolo-gingival, periosteo-gingival, interpapillary, circular or semicircular transgingival, and transseptal fibers[10]	Fibers extending from alveolar bone crest to the gingival margin[11]
Cellular composition[11]	Greater percentage of fibroblasts and smaller percentage of collagen and vasculature Mostly collagen fibers	Greater percentage of collagen and vascula-ture, and smaller percentage of fibroblasts Mostly collagen fibers
Vascularity[12]	Supraperiosteal blood vessels and vascular plexus of the PDL Richly vascular CT adjacent to root cementum	Supraperiosteal blood vessels only CT adjacent to implant surface is almost completely devoid of vasculature
Orientation of collagen fibers[11]	Collagen fibers insert into the cementum in a perpendicular direction	Fibers originate from periosteum to mucosal margin and run parallel to implant/abutment surface
Supracrestal attached tissues (biologic width)/peri-implant mucosa dimension		
Sulcus (mm)	0.69[13] 1.32[14]	0.2–0.5[15]
Junctional epithelium (mm)	0.97[13] 1.14[14]	Dog: 2–2.1[16]; 1.88[17] Human: 1.9[18]
CT (mm)	1.07[13] 0.77[14]	Dog: 1.3–1.8[16]; 1.05[17] Human: 1.7[18]

PDL, periodontal ligament; CT, connective tissue.

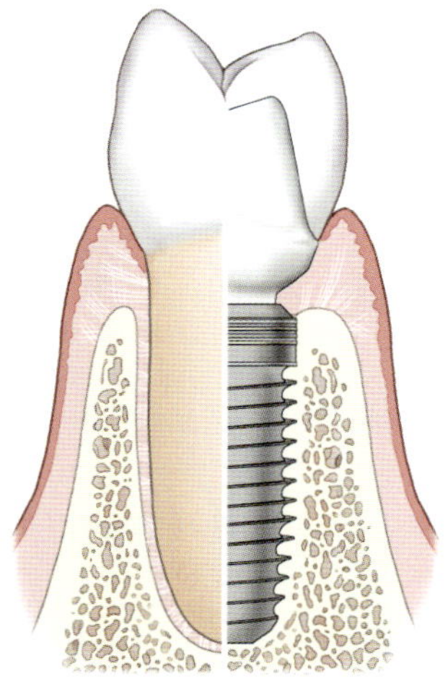

Fig 16-1 Comparison between tooth and implant.

Implant Design and Components

Implant design basically refers to the 3D structure of the dental implant. Factors such as material biocompatibility, the design itself, and surface topography, among others, have been shown to influence the process of osseointegration.[19] In particular, certain designs and surface modifications have been suggested to improve implant performance by obtaining better stability and providing more implant-to-bone surface area.

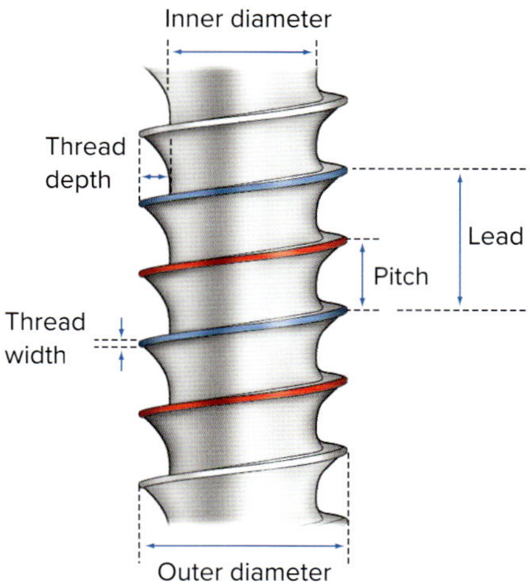

Fig 16-2 Example of threaded implant and macro design features.

TABLE 16-2 Effect of threads, pitch height, and thread pattern on BIC and marginal/crestal bone loss

Study	Model	Groups	Conclusion
Abrahamsson and Berglundh[22] (2006)	Beagle dogs	Both threaded but the test had additional microthreads coronally	Higher BIC in the coronal portion of the microthreaded group (81.8%) vs 72.8% for the control (no microthreads)
Lee et al[23] (2007)	Human	With vs without microthreads	Less MBL for the microthreaded group
Steigenga et al[24] (2004)	Rabbit tibia	Square vs V-shaped vs reverse buttress thread design	Greater BIC and reverse torque measurements for the square thread design
Chung et al[25] (2008)	Beagle dogs	0.5-mm vs 0.6-mm pitch height	0.6-mm pitch height showed more MBL

MBL, marginal bone loss.

IMPLANT BODY

The **implant fixture** or implant body denotes the segment that is meant to be surrounded by bone. Different implant systems present with a wide variety of designs, dimensions, surface characteristics, and more.

Threads

Implants can be classified into *(1)* threaded and *(2)* nonthreaded, cylindric, or press-fit designs. Threads are used to maximize initial bone-to-implant contact (BIC), improve primary stability, enlarge the implant surface area,[20] and favor dissipation of stress.[21] In the second half of the 1980s, the threaded solid screw type of dental implant started to become the preferred design (Fig 16-2). Threaded implants can be further classified based on the following:

- Thread pattern:
  - Standard V-thread
  - Square thread
  - Buttress thread
  - Reverse buttress thread
  - Spiral thread
- Number of threads:
  - Single thread
  - Double thread
  - Triple thread

Table 16-2 summarizes the effect of threads, pitch height, and thread pattern on BIC and marginal bone loss (MBL).[22–25]

In conclusion, the addition of threads and microthreads to an implant might provide a positive effect on BIC. A reduced thread pitch (distance from the center of the thread to the center of the next thread) may positively influence implant stability. Deeper threads might improve stabilization, especially in trabecular or cancellous bone.[26]

Morphology

The shape or morphology of the dental implant can determine the surface area available for stress distribution and influence the implant's initial stability. Implants can be classified based on different body shapes as tapered, parallel, and stepped.

Surface

The implant systems launched in the 1980s and 1990s included the machined Brånemark system[3] and rough titanium plasma sprayed (TPS) Straumann implants.[6] Currently used implant systems differ from the previously mentioned in microroughness and physiochemical

TABLE 16-3 Different levels of Sa along with examples of some of the most widely used implant systems[33]

Surface roughness (Sa)	Description	Examples of implant systems
0–0.4 µm	Smooth	Abutments, some experimental implants
0.5–1 µm	Minimally rough	Machined implants, Osseotite (Zimmer Biomet)
1–2 µm	Moderately rough	TiOblast (Astra Tech), SLA (Straumann), TiUnite (Nobel Biocare), most currently available implant systems
> 2 µm	Rough	TPS, hydroxyapatite-coated implants

SLA, sandblasted, large-grit acid-etched.

TABLE 16-4 Effect of implant diameter on survival rates

Study	Groups	Conclusions
Renouard and Nisand[34] (2006)	Narrow: < 3.5 mm Wide: ≥ 4.5 mm	Previous studies reported higher failure rates for wider diameter compared to standard diameter. Recent studies show comparable survival rates for both wide and standard diameter.
Ortega-Oller et al[35] (2014)	Narrow: < 3.3 mm Wider: ≥ 3.3 mm	Significantly lower survival rates (75%) for narrow implants vs wider implants (87%).

properties[27] achieved through implant surface modification. These modification methods can be applied either through additive (eg, titanium plasma spraying) or subtractive (eg, blasting, etching, or oxidation) processes. Overall, these modifications seem to positively influence the host-to-implant response[28] and might explain the higher implant survival rates. Experimental investigations show less robust bone response around smooth and minimally rough surfaces than their rougher counterparts.[29] Alterations in the surface composition of most of the widely marketed implant systems showed improvement in bone integration compared with their predecessors.[30] Nevertheless, more recent evidence suggested that implant surface roughness may accelerate the progression of peri-implantitis compared to machined surfaces.[31] In addition, certain surface characteristics can negatively affect the resolution of peri-implantitis.[32]

Implant surface roughness can be described in terms of Sa, which is a 3D parameter that examines the height of surface structure (Table 16-3).[29,33]

Width

Currently, there is no universal or widely accepted classification for implant width or diameter (Table 16-4).[34,35] However, several studies considered implant diameters ranging from 1.8 to 3.3 mm as *narrow* implants. Quek et al[36] proposed classifying implants based on their diameter into mini (< 2.9 mm), narrow (3.0–3.4 mm), regular (3.75–4 mm), and wide (5–6 mm).

Length

Currently, there is no universal definition regarding implant length However, different researchers defined *short* dental implants as 7 mm or shorter,[37] 8 mm or shorter,[34] or 10 mm or shorter[38] (Table 16-5).[34,39–44]

Crown-to-implant ratio

The crown-to-implant (C/I) ratio describes the relationship between the length of the implant restoration and the length of the fixture. With the increased use of short implants, it is common to observe higher C/I ratios (Table 16-6).[45–47]

CONNECTION

The Brånemark system was characterized by an external hexagon to facilitate implant insertion.[48] However, this design presented with some disadvantages due to its limited height, which could result in **abutment** screw loosening or fatigue fracture.[49,50] Hence, internal connections were introduced to reduce the incidence of these mechanical complications. A systematic review by Gracis et al[51] showed that the most frequent mechanical

TABLE 16-5 Influence of implant length

Study	Definitions	Conclusions
Renouard and Nisand[34] (2006)	Short: ≤ 8 mm	Previous studies reported higher failure rates for short implants. Recent studies show comparable survival rates for both short and long implants.
Telleman et al[39] (2011)	Short: < 10 mm	2-year survival rate was 93.1% for 5-mm implants, increasing slightly with longer implants, reaching 98.6% for 9.5-mm implants. A higher failure rate was observed in the maxilla.
Annibali et al[40] (2012)	Short: < 10 mm	99% survival rate and low incidence of biomechanical and biologic complications in the short term, regardless of implant location. Long-term studies are needed.
Monje et al[41,42] (2013, 2014)	Short: < 10 mm	The peak failure for short and standard implants occurred between 4 and 6 years and between 6 and 8 years of function, respectively. Implant length did not influence MBL.
Monje et al[43] (2013)	Short: 7–9 mm Extra-short: ≤ 6 mm	5-year failure rates were 1.61% and 2.92% for extra-short and short implants, respectively. The wider the implant, the higher the failure rate.
Ravidà et al[44] (2019)	Extra-short: ≤ 6 mm Long: ≥ 10 mm	Less MBL but greater prosthetic complications for extra-short implants compared with long implants during the first 3 years of function.

MBL, marginal bone loss.

TABLE 16-6 Systematic reviews on the influence of C/I ratio

Study	Conclusions
Blanes[45] (2009)	MBL seemed not to be affected by the C/I ratio. In addition, the C/I ratio does not influence the rate of technical complications.
Garaicoa-Pazmiño et al[46] (2014)	Within a range of 0.6:1 to 2.36:1 for C/I ratio, the higher the ratio, the less the MBL.
Ravidà et al[47] (2019)	No significant correlation between anatomical C/I ratios and survival rate, MBL, or prosthetic complications.

MBL, marginal bone loss.

complication related to abutments and single-implant reconstructions was screw loosening and that the rate was higher for external connections. This was followed by screw fracture, which was not reported for internal connection implants. Apart from these technical complications, implant-abutment connection appears to be a significant factor on MBL, with greater bone loss noted around implants with an external connection compared with their internal counterparts.[52,53] Another factor related to the implant connection is platform switching. *Platform switching* refers to the use of a smaller-diameter prosthetic component with a larger-diameter implant platform. Several clinical studies and systematic reviews reported less MBL around platform-switched compared to platform-matched implants.[54,55]

Protocols

During the early years of osseointegration, standard implant protocol was based on implant placement in healed ridges following at least 6 months from the time of tooth extraction and allowing 3 to 6 months of undisturbed healing following implant placement.[3,56] The advancements in implant design and surface modifications have made possible a faster osseointegration process, reducing the healing time. This change has allowed predictable outcomes in multiple clinical scenarios, including more challenging conditions such as immediate placement and immediate loading protocols.

TABLE 16-7 Timing of implant placement following tooth extraction

Type	Time line	Description/definition	Healing events
1	Same day	Immediate implant placement	NA
2	4–8 weeks	Early implant placement	Soft tissue healing
3	12–16 weeks	Early implant placement	Partial bone healing
4	> 6 months	Late implant placement	Complete bone healing

NA, not applicable.

TABLE 16-8 Characteristics of the different protocols for implant placement

Type	Indications	Advantages	Disadvantages
1	• Intact facial bone • Thick wall phenotype • Thick gingival phenotype • No acute infection • Adequate bone apical and palatal of the socket	• Reduced number of procedures • Reduced overall treatment time	• Socket morphology may complicate ideal implant positioning and primary stability • Hard and soft tissue remodeling may result in esthetic complications
2	When the previous conditions are not met	• Resolution of local pathology • Complete soft tissue coverage	• Socket morphology may complicate ideal implant positioning and primary stability • Increased treatment time
3	When primary stability cannot be achieved after 4 to 8 weeks	• Substantial bone fill • Mature soft tissues	• Increased treatment time • Varying amounts of resorption
4	• Preferable to avoid unless dealing with a growing patient or large apical bone lesions • Ridge preservation is recommended	• Completely healed ridge • Mature soft tissues	• Increased treatment time • Ridge alteration/ridge atrophy

TABLE 16-9 Implant loading protocols

Loading protocol	Time of prosthesis connection subsequent to implant placement
Immediate	Within 1 week
Early	Between 1 week and 2 months
Conventional	After 2 months

TIMING OF IMPLANT PLACEMENT

In 2004, Hämmerle et al[57] proposed a classification of the different timing options for implant placement. This was further modified by Chen and Buser[58] (Table 16-7). Today, this classification has been widely adopted. Advantages and disadvantages of each category are described in Table 16-8.

TIMING OF IMPLANT RESTORATION

Different loading protocols were described by Esposito et al[59] and later by Weber et al[60] (Table 16-9).

Immediate loading can also be further divided into functional and nonfunctional[61]:

TABLE 16-10 Randomized clinical trials on implant loading protocols and timing of placement.

Study	Timing of implant placement	Insertion torque (Ncm)	Loading protocol	Follow-up (m)	Papilla recession (mm)	Midfacial recession (mm) (mean ± SD)	Survival rate
De Rouck et al[63] (2009)	Type 1	35	INFL	12	0.31–0.44	0.41 ± 0.75*	96%
			CL		0.43–0.53	1.16 ± 0.66*	92%
Palattella et al[64] (2008)	Type 1	56	INFL	24	No significant difference based on Jemt papilla index	0.8 ± 0.7†	100%
	Type 2	74	INFL			0.6 ± 0.6†	100%
Den Hartog et al[65] (2011)	Types 3 and 4	≥ 45	INFL	18	0.27–0.41†	0.06 ± 0.42†	96.8%
			CL		0.19–0.35†	0.09 ± 0.34†	100%
Donati et al[66] (2008)	Types 3 and 4	≥ 20	IFL	12	0.21–0.43†	Not reported	98%
			CL		0.5–0.55†		100%

CL, conventional loading; IFL, immediate functional loading; INFL, immediate nonfunctional loading.
*Significant difference between groups.
†No significant difference between groups.

- Immediate functional loading: The prosthesis is in occlusion on the day of implant placement.
- Immediate nonfunctional loading, also known as *immediate restoration*[62]: The provisional restoration is cleared out of occlusion.

Table 16-10 demonstrates the effects of loading protocol and timing of implant placement on soft tissue parameters.[63–66]

With regard to MBL, Suárez et al[67] reported no differences with several loading protocols and various timings of implant placement. Similar findings were also reported by Benic et al.[68] Reduction of treatment time and faster comfort, esthetics, and function are the main advantages of immediate loading.[69]

GUIDED SURGERY

3D planning has gained popularity during the last years. Computer-guided and computer-navigated protocols have been used to transfer virtual digital planning to surgery through the use of different methods. Computer-guided implant surgery can be divided into dynamic and static computer-assisted guidance. The former includes surgical navigation, whereas the latter involves the use of a surgical guide, which can be either produced through stereolithography or manually in a laboratory.[70]

Some of the major advantages of guided surgery include the potential to reduce surgical time[71] and increased level of accuracy.[72,73] Accuracy can be assessed by measuring deviation in the *(1)* entry point, *(2)* apex, *(3)* long axis or angulation, and *(4)* height or depth. The corresponding values for static guides based on Van Assche et al[74] are 1 mm, 1.2 mm, 3.8 degrees, and 0.5 mm, respectively.

Sources of errors for a surgical guide include motion or metal artifact,[75] surgical guide production, and positioning and stabilization of the guide.[71]

Performance

SURVIVAL

Survival refers to the physical presence of the implant in the oral cavity. This measure of implant treatment outcomes was primarily employed in the 1990s and early 2000s. While still used today, other outcomes such as implant success and patient-centered outcomes are more valuable measures for evaluation of the implant treatment.

TABLE 16-11 Criteria defining implant success

Criteria	Success rate	Reference(s)
• No mobility or peri-implant radiolucency • < 0.2 mm annual bone loss following the first year in function	5 years: 85% 10 years: 80%	Albrektsson et al[76] (1986)
• Absence of subjective complaints, recurrent infection, mobility, or peri-implant radiolucency • Possibility for restoration	1 year: 98% 3 years: 96.2%	Buser et al[77] (1990) Buser et al[78] (1991)
• No mobility or peri-implant radiolucency • < 0.2 mm annual bone loss following the first year in function • No PD > 5 mm • No PD of 5 mm with BOP	10 years: 69.8% (73.2% when 6 mm was used as border-line for PD)	Karoussis et al[79] (2004)

PD, probing depth; BOP, bleeding on probing.

SUCCESS

Several definitions of success have been proposed over the years (Table 16-11).[76–79] Schnitman and Shulman[80] considered an implant as successful if less than 1 mm of mobility was detected, if the bone loss was no greater than one-third of the implant length, and if symptoms and/or infection were absent. In 1986, Albrektsson et al[76] proposed a new criterion to define implant success. MBL less than 1.5 mm was used as one of the factors to describe a successful implant therapy following the first year in function.[76] Currently, with the advancements in implant surface technology and the understanding of the factors associated with bone remodeling and with peri-implant diseases,[81] the definition of implant success proposed by Albrektsson et al[76] is considered outdated. Indeed, Galindo-Moreno et al[82] showed that implants that had MBL of 0.44 mm or greater during the first 6 months postloading tended to have 2 mm or more of MBL at 18 months. Another method for evaluating implant treatment is the use of patient-reported outcomes. Fortunately, this approach has gained popularity in the field of implant dentistry as shown in a recent systematic review.[83]

IMPLANT FAILURE

According to Romeo et al,[84] an implant is regarded as a failure if it had to be removed for any reason. However, the International Congress of Oral Implantologists Pisa Consensus Conference considered an implant a failure if it exhibits any of the following conditions: pain on function, mobility, radiographic bone loss greater than one-half of implant length, uncontrolled exudate, or it is no longer in the mouth.[85] Table 16-12 summarizes the failure rate of commonly used implant protocols.[86–91]

COMPLICATIONS

Dental implants can present with a variety of complications intra- or postoperatively. These complications can be divided into surgical, biologic, and technical or prosthetic. Peri-implantitis and MBL are further discussed in chapters 17 and 18.

Surgical complications include, but are not limited to, hemorrhage-related complications, neurosensory disturbance, adjacent tooth damage, and mandibular fracture.[92] Biologic complications include functional disturbances of the implant and are characterized by a biologic process involving the implant-supporting tissues, such as peri-implantitis and soft tissue complications.[86]

Technical or *prosthetic complication* is a collective term to describe mechanical damage of the implant or implant components and suprastructure.[93] Technical complications related to implant-supported single crowns[94] consist of (5-year cumulative incidence): abutment or screw loosening (8.8%), loss of retention (4.1%), veneer material fracture (3.5%), and implant fracture (0.18%). Regarding implant-supported fixed partial dentures, the most common technical complication is fracture of veneer material, followed by loss of the screw access hole restoration. The third most common is abutment or occlusal screw loosening.[95] Screw fracture and chipping or fracture of veneering material are the most common complications related to fixed implant prostheses for completely edentulous patients.[96] The most common implant mechanical complication in overdenture wearers is loss of retention, followed by the need for reline.[92]

TABLE 16-12 Estimated implant survival and failure rates

	Survival rate	Failure rate (per 100 implant-years)	Study
Implant-supported single crown	5 years: 96.8%	0.64	Jung et al[86] (2008)
Implant-supported FPD	5 years: 95.4% 10 years: 92.8%	0.94	Pjetursson et al[87] (2004)
Implant/tooth–supported FPD	5 years: 90.1% 10 years: 82.1%	2.09	Lang et al[88] (2004)
Immediate implant placement	4 years: 97.5%	0.62	Lang et al[89] (2012)
Implant placed in augmented sinus: lateral approach	3 years: 96.5%	1.19	Pjetursson et al[90] (2008)
Implant placed in augmented sinus: transalveolar approach	3 years: 92.8%	2.48	Tan et al[91] (2008)

FPD, fixed partial denture.

Positioning Guidelines

The position of the implant platform can be evaluated in three dimensions: mesiodistal, bucco/faciolingual, and apicocoronal. Inappropriate implant positioning can result in esthetic and functional complications. Ideal implant position should be restoratively driven and formulated on a case-by-case basis. However, general guidelines to optimize the clinical outcomes of implant therapy are presented in the following sections.

MESIODISTAL

Implant-tooth distance

- A minimum of 1.25 mm is recommended between the implant and adjacent teeth for proper osseointegration and to avoid damage to neighboring dentition.[97]
- With platform-switched implants, Vela et al[98] showed that this distance can be as short as 1 mm and still maintain the bone levels at the adjacent teeth.

Interimplant distance

- 1.04 mm of radiographic crestal bone loss was observed for machined implants with 3 mm or less interimplant distance. On the other hand, 0.45 mm was noted when this distance was greater than 3 mm. Lateral bone loss was even greater and ranged from 1.34 to 1.4 mm.[99]
- When platform-switched Biomet 3i implants (Zimmer Biomet) are placed less than 3 mm apart (mean = 2.23 mm), the peri-implant crestal bone peak was preserved in 64% of pairs.[100]

APICOCORONAL

Implant placement in an apicocoronal dimension can be assessed through different distances: implant shoulder to free gingival margin (FGM), implant shoulder to cemento-enamel junction (CEJ), or implant shoulder to alveolar crest.

- Implant-to-FGM:
  - Approximately 3 to 4 mm is required for an appropriate emergence profile.[101,102]
  - According to the International Team for Implantology (ITI) consensus meeting in 2000, the location of the implant shoulder needs to be approximately 2 mm apical to the midfacial gingiva of the planned restoration.[103]
- Implant-to-CEJ:
  - For a soft tissue–level implant, the implant shoulder needs to be located about 1 mm apical to the facial CEJ of the contralateral tooth in cases without recession.[104]
- Implant-to-alveolar crest:
  - For bone-level implants, greater bone remodeling was noted for subcrestal placement compared to epicrestal. However, no bone loss was found beyond the implant platform when placed subcrestally.[105]

- When considering immediate implant placement, the implant shoulder should be positioned apical to the midfacial bone crest because 0.5 to 1 mm of crestal bone resorption might be expected following extraction.[106]

BUCCOLINGUAL

- When facial bone thickness of 1.8 mm or greater following osteotomy preparation was present, bone loss decreased, and evidence of bone apposition was observed.[107]
- The correct implant position is when the implant shoulder is located about 1 mm palatal to the point of emergence at neighboring teeth. Implants placed too far palatally will result in ridge lap restorations, which are unhygienic and unesthetic.[104]
- Three times more recession was noted for immediate implants with buccal shoulder position compared to those with lingual shoulder location.[108]

Alternatives to Titanium

ZIRCONIA

Titanium dental implants have demonstrated excellent results and high levels of biocompatibility. Only a very low percentage of the population has been reported to experience allergy to titanium.[109] However, the high esthetic demands and the concerns about sensitivity to titanium have led to growing interest in ceramic as a material for dental implants. The first generation was made of aluminum oxide; however, these were withdrawn from the market and replaced by zirconium dioxide (zirconia) implants.

When compared with titanium, zirconia implants have shown low affinity to bacterial biofilm,[110] smaller inflammatory cell infiltrate,[111] and better soft tissue integration.[112] However, it seems that zirconia implants have generally higher early implant failure and are also more susceptible to fracture.[113]

References

1. American Academy of Periodontology. Glossary of Periodontal Terms. American Academy of Periodontology, 2001.
2. Brånemark PI, Breine U, Adell R, Hansson BO, Lindström J, Ohlsson Å. Intra-osseous anchorage of dental prostheses. I. Experimental studies. Scand J Plast Reconstr Surg 1969;3:81–100.
3. Albrektsson T, Brånemark PI, Hansson HA, Lindström J. Osseointegrated titanium implants: Requirements for ensuring a long-lasting, direct bone-to-implant anchorage in man. Acta Orthop Scand 1981;52:155–170.
4. Zarb GA, Albrektsson T. Osseointegration: A requiem for the periodontal ligament? Int J Periodontics Restor Dent 1991;11:88–91.
5. Schroeder A, Pohler O, Sutter, F. Tissue reaction to an implant of a titanium hollow cylinder with a titanium surface spray layer [in German]. SSO Schweiz Monatsschr Zahnheilkd 1976;86:713–727.
6. Schroeder A, van der Zypen E, Stich H, Sutter F. The reactions of bone, connective tissue, and epithelium to endosteal implants with titanium-sprayed surfaces. J Maxillofac Surg 1981;9:15–25.
7. Raghavendra S, Wood MC, Taylor TD. Early wound healing around endosseous implants: A review of the literature. Int J Oral Maxillofac Implants 2005;20:425–431.
8. Bosshardt DD, Lang NP. The junctional epithelium: From health to disease. J Dent Res 2005;84:9–20.
9. Lindhe J, Berglundh T. The interface between the mucosa and the implant. Periodontol 2000 1998;17:47–54.
10. Schroeder HE, Listgarten MA. The gingival tissues: The architecture of periodontal protection. Periodontol 2000 1997;13:91–120.
11. Berglundh T, Lindhe J, Ericsson I, Marinello CP, Liljenberg B, Thornsen P. The soft tissue barrier at implants and teeth. Clin Oral Implants Res 1991;2:81–90.
12. Berglundh T, Lindhe J, Jonsson K, Ericsson I. The topography of the vascular systems in the periodontal and peri-implant tissues in the dog. J Clin Periodontol 1994;21:189–193.
13. Gargiulo AW, Wentz FM, Orban B. Dimensions and relations of the dentogingival junction in humans. J Periodontol 1961;32:261–267.
14. Vacek JS, Gher ME, Assad DA, Richardson AC, Giambarresi LI. The dimensions of the human dentogingival junction. Int J Periodontics Restorative Dent 1994;14:154–165.
15. Glauser R, Schüpbach P, Gottlow J, Hämmerle CH. Periimplant soft tissue barrier at experimental one-piece mini-implants with different surface topography in humans: A light-microscopic overview and histometric analysis. Clin Implant Dent Relat Res 2005(1 suppl);7:S44–S51.
16. Berglundh T, Lindhe J. Dimension of the periimplant mucosa. Biological width revisited. J Clin Periodontol 1996;23:971–973.
17. Cochran DL, Hermann JS, Schenk RK, Higginbottom FL, Buser D. Biologic width around titanium implants. A histometric analysis of the implanto-gingival junction around unloaded and loaded nonsubmerged implants in the canine mandible. J Periodontol 1997;68:186–197.
18. Tomasi C, Tessarolo F, Caola I, Wennström J, Nollo G, Berglundh T. Morphogenesis of peri-implant mucosa revisited: An experimental study in humans. Clin Oral Implants Res 2014;25:997–1003.
19. Albrektsson T, Lekholm U. Osseointegration: Current state of the art. Dent Clin North Am 1989;33:537–554.
20. Ivanoff CJ, Gröndahl K, Sennerby L, Bergström C, Lekholm U. Influence of variations in implant diameters: A 3- to 5-year retrospective clinical report. Int J Oral Maxillofac Implants 1999;14:173–180.

21. Brunski JB. Biomaterials and biomechanics in dental implant design. Int J Oral Maxillofac Implants 1988;3:85–97.
22. Abrahamsson I, Berglundh T. Tissue characteristics at micro-threaded implants: An experimental study in dogs. Clin Implant Dent Relat Res 2006;8:107–113.
23. Lee DW, Choi YS, Park KH, Kim CS, Moon IS. Effect of microthread on the maintenance of marginal bone level: A 3-year prospective study. Clin Oral Implants Res 2007;18:465–470.
24. Steigenga J, Al-Shammari K, Misch C, Nociti FH Jr, Wang HL. Effects of implant thread geometry on percentage of osseointegration and resistance to reverse torque in the tibia of rabbits. J Periodontol 2004;75:1233–1241.
25. Chung SH, Heo SJ, Koak JY, et al. Effects of implant geometry and surface treatment on osseointegration after functional loading: A dog study. J Oral Rehabil 2008;35:229–236.
26. Abuhussein H, Pagni G, Rebaudi A, Wang HL. The effect of thread pattern upon implant osseointegration. Clin Oral Implants Res 2010;21:129–136.
27. Wennerberg A, Albrektsson T. On implant surfaces: A review of current knowledge and opinions. Int J Oral Maxillofac Implants 2010;25:63–74.
28. Coelho PG, Granjeiro JM, Romanos GE, et al. Basic research methods and current trends of dental implant surfaces. J Biomed Mater Res B Appl Biomater 2009;88:579–596.
29. Wennerberg A, Albrektsson T. Effects of titanium surface topography on bone integration: A systematic review. Clin Oral Implants Res 2009;20(4 suppl):172–184.
30. Lang NP, Jepsen S. Implant surfaces and design (Working Group 4). Clin Oral Implants Res 2009;20(4 suppl):228–231.
31. Carcuac O, Abrahamsson I, Albouy JP, Linder E, Larsson L, Berglundh T. Experimental periodontitis and peri-implantitis in dogs. Clin Oral Implants Res 2013;24:363–371.
32. Albouy JP, Abrahamsson I, Persson LG, Berglundh T. Implant surface characteristics influence the outcome of treatment of peri-implantitis: An experimental study in dogs. J Clin Periodontol 2011;38:58–64.
33. Albrektsson T, Wennerberg A. Oral implant surfaces: Part 1—Review focusing on topographic and chemical properties of different surfaces and in vivo responses to them. Int J Prosthodont 2004;17:536–543.
34. Renouard F, Nisand D. Impact of implant length and diameter on survival rates. Clin Oral Implants Res 2006;17(2 suppl):35–51.
35. Ortega-Oller I, Suárez F, Galindo-Moreno P, et al. The influence of implant diameter on its survival: A meta-analysis based on prospective clinical trials. J Periodontol 2014;85:569–580.
36. Quek CE, Tan KB, Nicholls JI. Load fatigue performance of a single-tooth implant abutment system: Effect of diameter. Int J Oral Maxillofac Implants 2006;21:929–936.
37. Friberg B, Gröndahl K, Lekholm U, Brånemark PI. Long-term follow-up of severely atrophic edentulous mandibles reconstructed with short Brånemark implants. Clin Implant Dent Relat Res 2000;2:184–189.
38. das Neves FD, Fones D, Bernardes SR, do Prado CJ, Neto AJ. Short implants: An analysis of longitudinal studies. Int J Oral Maxillofac Implants 2006;21:86–93.
39. Telleman G, Raghoebar GM, Vissink A, den Hartog L, Huddleston Slater JJ, Meijer HJ. A systematic review of the prognosis of short (< 10 mm) dental implants placed in the partially edentulous patient. J Clin Periodontol 2011;38:667–676.
40. Annibali S, Cristalli MP, Dell'Aquila D, Bignozzi I, La Monaca G, Pilloni A. Short dental implants: A systematic review. J Dent Res 2012;91:25–32.
41. Monje A, Chan HL, Fu JH, Suarez F, Galindo-Moreno P, Wang HL. Are short dental implants (< 10 mm) effective? A meta-analysis on prospective clinical trials. J Periodontol 2013;84:895–904.
42. Monje A, Suarez F, Galindo-Moreno P, García-Nogales A, Fu JH, Wang HL. A systematic review on marginal bone loss around short dental implants (<10 mm) for implant-supported fixed prostheses. Clin Oral Implants Res 2014;25:1119–1124.
43. Monje A, Fu JH, Chan HL, et al. Do implant length and width matter for short dental implants (< 10 mm)? A meta-analysis of prospective studies. J Periodontol 2013;84:1783–1791.
44. Ravidà A, Barootchi S, Askar H, Suárez-López del Amo F, Tavelli L, Wang HL. Long-term effectiveness of extra-short (≤ 6 mm) dental implants: A systematic review. Int J Oral Maxillofac Implants 2019;34:68–84.
45. Blanes RJ. To what extent does the crown-implant ratio affect the survival and complications of implant-supported reconstructions? A systematic review. Clin Oral Implants Res 2009;20(4 suppl):67–72.
46. Garaicoa-Pazmiño C, Suárez-López del Amo F, Monje A, et al. Influence of crown/implant ratio on marginal bone loss: A systematic review. J Periodontol 2014;85:1214–1221.
47. Ravidà A, Barootchi S, Alkanderi A, Tavelli L, Suárez-López del Amo F. The effect of crown-to-implant ratio on the clinical outcomes of dental implants: A systematic review. Int J Oral Maxillofac Implants 2019;34:1121–1131.
48. Brånemark PI, Zarb GA, Albrektsson T, Rosen H. Tissue-integrated prostheses. Osseointegration in clinical dentistry. Plast Reconstr Surg 1986;77:496–497.
49. Adell R, Eriksson B, Lekholm U, Brånemark PI, Jemt T. A long-term follow-up study of osseointegrated implants in the treatment of totally edentulous jaws. Int J Oral Maxillofac Implants 1990;5:347–359.
50. Jemt T, Laney WR, Harris D, Henry PJ, Krogh PH Jr, Polizzi G. Osseointegrated implants for single tooth replacement: A 1-year report from a multicenter prospective study. Int J Oral Maxillofac Implants 1991;6:29–35.
51. Gracis S, Michalakis K, Vigolo P, Vult von Steyern P, Zwahlen M, Sailer I. Internal vs external connections for abutments/reconstructions: A systematic review. Clin Oral Implants Res 2012;23(6 suppl):202–216.
52. Galindo-Moreno P, León-Cano A, Ortega-Oller I, et al. Prosthetic abutment height is a key factor in peri-implant marginal bone loss. J Dent Res 2014;93(7 suppl):80S–85S.
53. Peñarrocha-Diago MA, Flichy-Fernández AJ, Alonso-González R, Peñarrocha-Oltra D, Balaguer-Martínez J, Peñarrocha-Diago M. Influence of implant neck design and implant–abutment connection type on peri-implant health. Radiological study. Clin Oral Implants Res 2013;24:1192–1200.
54. Atieh MA, Ibrahim HM, Atieh AH. Platform switching for marginal bone preservation around dental implants: A systematic review and meta-analysis. J Periodontol 2010;81:1350–1366.
55. Annibali S, Bignozzi I, Cristalli MP, Graziani F, La Monaca G, Polimeni A. Peri-implant marginal bone level: A systematic review and meta-analysis of studies comparing platform switching versus conventionally restored implants. J Clin Periodontol 2012;39:1097–1113.
56. Adell R, Lekholm U, Rockler B, Brånemark PI. A 15-year study of osseointegrated implants in the treatment of the edentulous jaw. Int J Oral Surg 1981;10:387–416.
57. Hämmerle CH, Chen ST, Wilson TG Jr. Consensus statements and recommended clinical procedures regarding the placement of implants in extraction sockets. Int J Oral Maxillofac Implants 2004;19:26–28.

58. Chen B, Buser D. ITI Treatment Guide. Vol 1: Implant Placement in Post-Extraction Sites: Treatment Options. Berlin: Quintessence, 2009.
59. Esposito M, Grusovin MG, Willings M, Coulthard P, Worthington HV. The effectiveness of immediate, early, and conventional loading of dental implants: A Cochrane systematic review of randomized controlled clinical trials. Int J Oral Maxillofac Implants 2007;22:893–904.
60. Weber HP, Morton D, Gallucci GO, Roccuzzo M, Cordaro L, Grütter L. Consensus statements and recommended clinical procedures regarding loading protocols. Int J Oral Maxillofac Implants 2009;24:180–183.
61. Degidi M, Piattelli A. Immediate functional and non-functional loading of dental implants: A 2- to 60-month follow-up study of 646 titanium implants. J Periodontol 2003;74:225–241.
62. Morton D, Jaffin R, Weber HP. Immediate restoration and loading of dental implants: Clinical considerations and protocols. Int J Oral Maxillofac Implants 2004;19:103–108.
63. De Rouck T, Collys K, Wyn I, Cosyn J. Instant provisionalization of immediate single-tooth implants is essential to optimize esthetic treatment outcome. Clin Oral Implants Res 2009;20:566–570.
64. Palattella P, Torsello F, Cordaro L. Two-year prospective clinical comparison of immediate replacement vs immediate restoration of single tooth in the esthetic zone. Clin Oral Implants Res 2008;19:1148–1153.
65. den Hartog L, Raghoebar GM, Stellingsma K, Vissink A, Meijer HJ. Immediate non-occlusal loading of single implants in the aesthetic zone: A randomized clinical trial. J Clin Periodontol 2011;38:186–194.
66. Donati M, La Scala V, Billi M, Di Dino B, Torrisi P, Berglundh T. Immediate functional loading of implants in single tooth replacement: A prospective clinical multicenter study. Clin Oral Implants Res 2008;19:740–748.
67. Suárez F, Chan HL, Monje A, Galindo-Moreno P, Wang HL. Effect of the timing of restoration on implant marginal bone loss: A systematic review. J Periodontol 2013;84:159–169.
68. Benic GI, Mir-Mari J, Hämmerle F. Loading protocols for single-implant crowns: A systematic review and meta-analysis. Int J Oral Maxillofac Implants 2014;29:222–238.
69. Kinsel RP, Liss M. Retrospective analysis of 56 edentulous dental arches restored with 344 single-stage implants using an immediate loading fixed provisional protocol: Statistical predictors of implant failure. Int J Oral Maxillofac Implants 2007;22:823–830.
70. Jung RE, Schneider D, Ganeles J, et al. Computer technology applications in surgical implant dentistry: A systematic review. Int J Oral Maxillofac Implants 2009;24:92–109.
71. Arısan V, Karabuda CZ, Özdemir T. Implant surgery using bone- and mucosa-supported stereolithographic guides in totally edentulous jaws: Surgical and postoperative outcomes of computer-aided vs standard techniques. Clin Oral Implants Res 2010;21:980–988.
72. Vercruyssen M, Hultin M, Van Assche N, Svensson K, Naert I, Quirynen M. Guided surgery: Accuracy and efficacy. Periodontol 2000 2014;66:228–246.
73. Chen CK, Yuh DY, Huang RY, Fu E, Tsai CF, Chiang CY. Accuracy of implant placement with a navigation system, a laboratory guide, and freehand drilling. Int J Oral Maxillofac Implants 2018;33:1213–1218.
74. Van Assche N, Vercruyssen M, Coucke W, Teughels W, Jacobs R, Quirynen M. Accuracy of computer-aided implant placement. Clin Oral Implants Res 2012;23:112–123.
75. Dreiseidler T, Neugebauer J, Ritter L, et al. Accuracy of a newly developed integrated system for dental implant planning. Clin Oral Implants Res 2009;20:1191–1199.
76. Albrektsson T, Zarb G, Worthington P, Eriksson AR. The long-term efficacy of currently used dental implants: A review and proposed criteria of success. Int J Oral Maxillofac Implants 1986;1:11–5.
77. Buser D, Weber HP, Lang NP. Tissue integration of non-submerged implants. l-year results of a prospective study with 100 ITI hollow-cylinder and hollow-screw implants. Clin Oral Implants Res 1990;1:33–40.
78. Buser D, Weber HP, Brägger U, Balsiger C. Tissue integration of one-stage ITI implants: 3-year results of a longitudinal study with hollow-cylinder and hollow-screw implants. Int J Oral Maxillofac Implants 1991;6:405–412.
79. Karoussis IK, Brägger U, Salvi GE, Bürgin W, Lang NP. Effect of implant design on survival and success rates of titanium oral implants: A 10-year prospective cohort study of the ITI Dental Implant System. Clin Oral Implants Res 2004;15:8–17.
80. Schnitman PA, Shulman LB. Recommendations of the consensus development conference on dental implants. J Am Dent Assoc 1979;98:373–377.
81. Albrektsson T, Dahlin C, Jemt T, Sennerby L, Turri A, Wennerberg A. Is marginal bone loss around oral implants the result of a provoked foreign body reaction? Clin Implant Dent Relat Res 2014;16:155–165.
82. Galindo-Moreno P, León-Cano A, Ortega-Oller I, Monje A, O'Valle F, Catena A. Marginal bone loss as success criterion in implant dentistry: Beyond 2 mm. Clin Oral Implants Res 2015;26:e28–e34.
83. De Bruyn H, Raes S, Matthys C, Cosyn J. The current use of patient-centered/reported outcomes in implant dentistry: A systematic review. Clin Oral Implants Res 2015;26(11 suppl):45–56.
84. Romeo E, Lops D, Margutti E, Ghisolfi M, Chiapasco M, Vogel G. Long-term survival and success of oral implants in the treatment of full and partial arches: A 7-year prospective study with the ITI dental implant system. Int J Oral Maxillofac Implants 2004;19:247–259.
85. Misch CE, Perel ML, Wang HL, et al. Implant success, survival, and failure: The International Congress of Oral Implantologists (ICOI) Pisa Consensus Conference. Implant Dent 2008;17:5–15.
86. Jung RE, Pjetursson BE, Glauser R, Zembic A, Zwahlen M, Lang NP. A systematic review of the 5-year survival and complication rates of implant-supported single crowns. Clin Oral Implants Res 2008;19:119–130.
87. Pjetursson BE, Tan K, Lang NP, Brägger U, Egger M, Zwahlen M. A systematic review of the survival and complication rates of fixed partial dentures (FPDs) after an observation period of at least 5 years. Clin Oral Implants Res 2004;15:625–642.
88. Lang NP, Pjetursson BE, Tan K, Brägger U, Egger M, Zwahlen M. A systematic review of the survival and complication rates of fixed partial dentures (FPDs) after an observation period of at least 5 years. Clin Oral Implants Res 2004;15:643–653.
89. Lang NP, Pun L, Lau KY, Li KY, Wong MC. A systematic review on survival and success rates of implants placed immediately into fresh extraction sockets after at least 1 year. Clin Oral Implants Res 2012;23(5 suppl):39–66.
90. Pjetursson BE, Tan WC, Zwahlen M, Lang NP. A systematic review of the success of sinus floor elevation and survival of implants inserted in combination with sinus floor elevation. J Clin Periodontol 2008;35(8 suppl):216–240.
91. Tan WC, Lang NP, Zwahlen M, Pjetursson BE. A systematic review of the success of sinus floor elevation and survival of implants inserted in combination with sinus floor elevation Part II: Transalveolar technique. J Clin Periodontol 2008;35:241–254.

92. Goodacre CJ, Bernal G, Rungcharassaeng K, Kan JYK. Clinical complications with implants and implant prostheses. J Prosthet Dent 2003;90:121–132.
93. Berglundh T, Persson L, Klinge B. A systematic review of the incidence of biological and technical complications in implant dentistry reported in prospective longitudinal studies of at least 5 years. J Clin Periodontol 2002;29(3 suppl):197–212.
94. Jung RE, Zembic A, Pjetursson BE, Zwahlen M, Thoma DS. Systematic review of the survival rate and the incidence of biological, technical, and aesthetic complications of single crowns on implants reported in longitudinal studies with a mean follow-up of 5 years. Clin Oral Implants Res 2012;23(6 suppl):2–21.
95. Pjetursson BE, Thoma D, Jung R, Zwahlen M, Zembic A. A systematic review of the survival and complication rates of implant-supported fixed dental prostheses (FDPs) after a mean observation period of at least 5 years. Clin Oral Implants Res 2012;23(6 suppl):22–38.
96. Papaspyridakos P, Chen CJ, Chuang SK, Weber HP, Gallucci GO. A systematic review of biologic and technical complications with fixed implant rehabilitations for edentulous patients. Int J Oral Maxillofac Implants 2012;27:102–110.
97. Saadoun AP, LeGall M, Touati B. Selection and ideal tridimensional implant position for soft tissue aesthetics. Pract Periodontics Aesthetic Dent 1999;11:1063–1072.
98. Vela X, Méndez V, Rodríguez X, Segalá M, Tarnow DP. Crestal bone changes on platform-switched implants and adjacent teeth when the tooth-implant distance is less than 1.5 mm. Int J Periodontics Restorative Dent 2012;32:149–155.
99. Tarnow DP, Cho SC, Wallace SS. The effect of inter-implant distance on the height of inter-implant bone crest. J Periodontol 2000;71:546–549.
100. Rodríguez-Ciurana X, Vela-Nebot X, Segalà-Torres M, et al. The effect of interimplant distance on the height of the interimplant bone crest when using platform-switched implants. Int J Periodontics Restorative Dent 2009;29:141–151.
101. Kan JY, Rungcharassaeng K. Immediate placement and provisionalization of maxillary anterior single implants: A surgical and prosthodontic rationale. Pract Periodontics Aesthetic Dent 2000;12:817–824.
102. Kois JC, Kan JY. Predictable peri-implant gingival esthetics: Surgical and prosthodontic rationales. Pract Proced Aesthet Dent 2001;13:691-698.
103. Buser D, von Arx T. Surgical procedures in partially edentulous patients with ITI implants. Clin Oral Implants Res 2000;11(1 suppl):83–100.
104. Buser D, Martin W, Belser UC. Optimizing esthetics for implant restorations in the anterior maxilla: Anatomic and surgical considerations. Int J Oral Maxillofac Implants 2004;19(19 suppl):43–61.
105. Froum SJ, Cho SC, Suzuki T, Yu P, Corby P, Khouly I. Epicrestal and subcrestal placement of platform-switched implants: 18 month-result of a randomized, controlled, split-mouth, prospective clinical trial. Clin Oral Implants Res 2018;29:353–366.
106. Chen ST, Darby I. The relationship between facial bone wall defects and dimensional alterations of the ridge following flapless tooth extraction in the anterior maxilla. Clin Oral Implants Res 2017;28:931–937.
107. Spray JR, Black CG, Morris HF, Ochi S. The influence of bone thickness on facial marginal bone response: Stage 1 placement through stage 2 uncovering. Ann Periodontol 2000;5:119–128.
108. Evans CDJ, Chen ST. Esthetic outcomes of immediate implant placements. Clin Oral Implants Res 2008;19:73–80.
109. Sicilia A, Cuesta S, Coma G, et al. Titanium allergy in dental implant patients: A clinical study on 1500 consecutive patients. Clin Oral Implants Res 2008;19:823–835.
110. Rimondini L, Cerroni L, Carrassi A, Torriceni P. Bacterial colonization of zirconia ceramic surfaces: An in vitro and in vivo study. Int J Oral Maxillofac Implants 2002;17:793–798.
111. Liñares A, Grize L, Muñoz F, Pippenger BE, Dard M, Domken O. Histological assessment of hard and soft tissues surrounding a novel ceramic implant: A pilot study in the minipig. J Clin Periodontol 2016;43:538–546.
112. Kohal RJ, Weng D, Bächle M, Strub JR. Loaded custom-made zirconia and titanium implants show similar osseointegration: An animal experiment. J Periodontol 2004;75:1262–1268.
113. Cionca N, Hashim D, Mombelli A. Zirconia dental implants: Where are we now, and where are we heading? Periodontol 2000 2017;73:241–258.

17

MARGINAL BONE LOSS

Vahid Khoshkam, DDS, MS
Fernando Suárez López del Amo, DDS, MS

DEFINITIONS AND TERMINOLOGY

Bone resorption: Bone loss due to osteoclastic activity.[4]

Marginal: Pertaining to or connected with a margin or border.[4]

The stability of peri-implant hard and soft tissues is one of the most critical factors for the long-term success of implant therapy. Preclinical studies have demonstrated that following implant placement, a soft tissue seal of approximately 3 to 4 mm will form corresponding to the supracrestal attached tissues.[1–3] Alterations of the peri-implant bone level may jeopardize this soft tissue seal and consequently have a negative impact on the long-term outcomes of implant therapy.

The significance of **marginal** bone loss (MBL) around dental implants also draws specific attention given that its progression represents a contributing factor for peri-implantitis. Accordingly, eliminating or minimizing MBL is key in the prevention of peri-implantitis. This chapter is focused on the changes occurring at the bone level following implant placement and in the short term after prosthesis delivery. Aside from the concept of microbial biofilm–related peri-implantitis, surgical, prosthetic, and biomechanical factors are also known to be additional trigger mechanisms for MBL, with varying degrees of available evidence. Peri-implant diseases are comprehensively discussed in chapter 18.

Etiology

Early MBL is a well-documented process also referred to as *bone remodeling* or *physiologic bone loss* following implant placement and tends to occur mostly during the first year.[5] Understanding the etiologic factors to eliminate or minimize this bone loss is key for the long-term implant success and the prevention of peri-implantitis.[6]

As a measure for implant success, MBL has been historically reported to occur during the first year with an average bone loss not exceeding 1.5 mm, followed by a maximum of 0.2 mm annually.[5,7] More recently, it was determined that following implant healing, there should be no further bone loss beyond 2 mm.[8] However, with the understanding of the biologic processes of osseointegration and biologic width formation, the phenomenon of early MBL can indeed be eliminated or significantly minimized. Of importance, given the tremendous variability in terms of local and systemic factors, it is impossible to determine a threshold to differentiate between physiologic and pathologic MBL applicable to all implants and scenarios.

The factors affecting early MBL are numerous. Moreover, many of these factors are unequivocally interconnected (eg, position of the implant relative to the alveolar crest and location of the implant-abutment interface, biologic width formation and dimensions of the soft tissues). Investigated local factors that may contribute to MBL include but are not limited to the following:

- Location of the implant-abutment interface[9–11]
- Abutment characteristics[12–14]
- Implant-abutment connection[15,16]
- Implant size[17–22]
- Position of the implant relative to the alveolar crest[23–25]
- Position of the implant relative to adjacent dentition[26–28]
- Position of the implant relative to adjacent implants[26,29–31]
- Formation of supracrestal attached tissues[2,32–34]
- Peri-implant soft tissues[2,35]
- Occlusal forces[36,37]
- Insertion torque[38,39]
- Metal particle release[40–42]
- Timing of implant placement and implant loading[43–46]

Implant-Abutment Interface

LOCATION

Several preclinical and clinical studies have been conducted to investigate whether the interface between rough and smooth implant surfaces as well as the location of the microgap have a significant influence on peri-implant tissue formation during healing.[10,11,34,47] The key findings of these studies were as follows:

- The rough-smooth implant interface in addition to the location of the microgap have a significant effect on marginal bone level and remodeling.
- Marginal bone level changes around two-piece, nonsubmerged titanium implants were significantly influenced by possible movements between implants and abutments, but not by the size of the microgap (interface).
- The dimensional bone levels changes, or bone loss, occurring from the implant-abutment interface to the first bone-to-implant contact are usually consistent with the formation of supracrestal attached tissues or biologic width.
- The supracrestal attached tissues formed in one-piece implants are established early and maintained over time.

ABUTMENT CHARACTERISTICS

Properties

The lack of direct attachment between the abutment and the supracrestal tissues[1,2] may impact the formation and maintenance of the soft tissue seal around dental implants. Hence, the material selection for abutments is of critical importance.

To date, titanium has been the material of choice for most of the abutments used in implant dentistry. One drawback of titanium for this purpose has been the dark coloration of its surface. Consequently, in recent years, a tendency toward the investigation of other materials has emerged. In a study by Abrahamsson et al,[14] it was found that when compared with titanium, other materials such as gold alloy or ceramic (highly sintered Al_2O_3) resulted in lack of adequate attachment formation at the abutment level, demonstrating higher levels of MBL. Nevertheless, available evidence suggests that there is no significant difference in terms of MBL when comparing different abutment materials (aluminum, gold, titanium nitride, or zirconia) with titanium.[48]

A recent systematic review revealed that although both metallic and ceramic abutments rendered high survival rates for their prostheses, the ceramic abutments at both internal or external connections showed significantly higher rates of fracture compared with metallic abutments.[49]

For implant-supported single crowns, both metal and ceramic abutments with internal and external connections can be recommended based on the available evidence; however, for implant-supported fixed prostheses, metal abutments (titanium) with internal and external connections are recommended. Due to the lack of sufficient data, zirconia abutments cannot yet be recommended for multiple-unit implant-supported fixed prostheses, and their utility remains limited to single crowns.[50] Nevertheless, zirconia abutments have demonstrated a lower inflammatory response through decreased bleeding on probing values when compared with titanium abutments.[51,52]

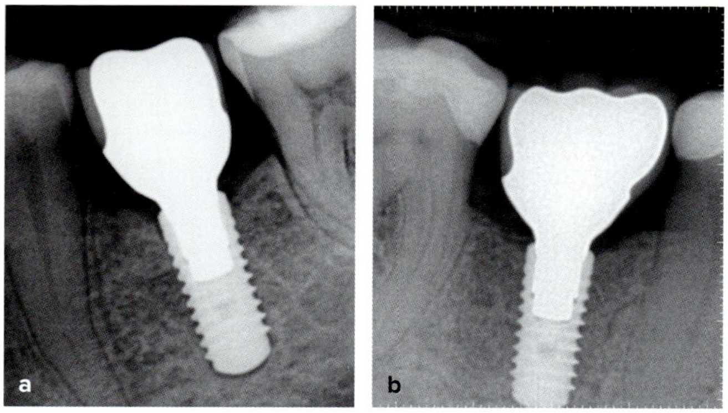

Fig 17-1 *(a and b)* Examples of platform-switched connections.

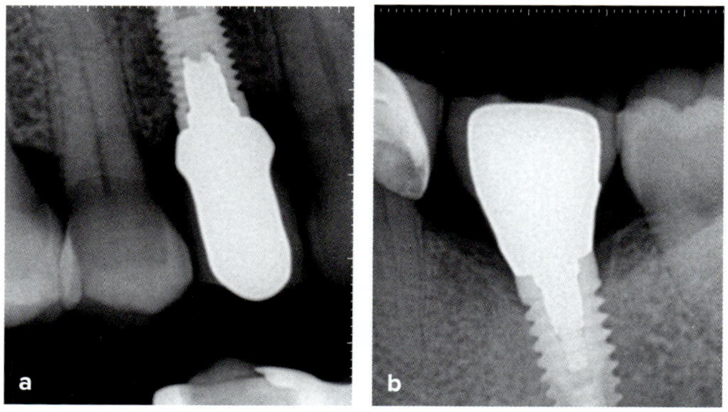

Fig 17-2 *(a and b)* Examples of platform-matched connections.

Size (platform switching)

The use of an abutment that is narrower than the width of the implant platform, known as *platform switching*, has been historically identified as a potential factor to reduce MBL around osseointegrated implants.[53] When the outer edge of the implant-abutment interface is horizontally repositioned inward and away from the outer edge of the implant platform, this allows the microgap to be further from the first bone-to-implant contact. It has been suggested that this may contribute to the creation of more space for tissue formation, further distancing the microgap from the alveolar crest and promoting a reduction in crestal bone loss.[12] Today, this concept has been adopted by many implant systems, although conflicting data has been reported with regard to its effectiveness on reduction of MBL.[13,54–56]

While a randomized controlled trial (RCT)[13] with 3 years of follow-up did not report any significant differences between the implants with platform-matched and platform-switched abutments in terms of marginal bone level alterations, others studies have reported superior results for platform switching.[12,55] This conflicting information could be due to the many other local and systemic factors playing a role in MBL as well as the differences in the methodologies of the studies. Indeed, a recent systematic review suggested that platform switching may have an indirect protective effect against bone loss.[57]

It is worth mentioning that in most of the comparative studies,[12,55,58] implants with narrower diameters and matched abutments were evaluated against wider fixtures with platform switching. Interestingly, in the study that reported no differences between platform switching and matched platforms, all the implants used had the same diameter.[13] The differences in the implant body design and geometry, implant surface characteristics, and the implant-abutment connection, among others, may also explain the conflicting data.[59]

In general, platform switching seems to be advantageous in terms of soft and hard tissue stability around osseointegrated implants[54] (Figs 17-1 and 17-2).

TABLE 17-1 Summary of studies with different implant-abutment connections

Authors	Follow-up time (m)	Implant system	Connection type	Marginal bone loss (mm)	Outcome
Arnhart et al[61] (2012)	36	Nobel active*	Conical	0.89 ± 1.65	External connection resulted in less bone loss
		Nobel active*	External	0.16 ± 1.06	
		Nobel replace*	Internal	0.85 ± 1.32	
Pozzi et al[62] (2014)	36	Nobel active*	Conical	0.67 ± 0.39	Significantly less bone loss with conical connection
		Nobel speedy groovy*	External	1.24 ± 0.47	
Esposito et al[16] (2016)	60	EZ Plus†	External	1.13	No significant difference was observed
		EZ Plus†	Internal	1.21	

*Nobel Biocare
†MegaGen

IMPLANT-ABUTMENT CONNECTION

Implant systems present with different morphologies and different implant-abutment interface geometries. A variety of connections between the implant and the abutment have been introduced. External connections consist of an external hexagon on the implant platform; internal connections comprise a variety of connection types (eg, internal hexagon, internal octagon, internal trilobe) in addition to conical internal connection or Morse taper, which has been considered as a separate category.[60] Implant-abutment connection has a critical role for the long-term success of the implant-prosthetic restoration because it plays a major role in both biologic and technical aspects. As such, several studies have investigated the impact of the connection type. Table 17-1 summarizes RCTs with at least 3 years of follow-up.[16,61,62]

Once again, the differences presented in the above-mentioned investigations may also be due to the vast amount of local and systemic factors affecting the stability of the peri-implant hard tissue. A recent systematic review[60] concluded that all different types of implant-abutment connections (ie, external, internal, and conical) can result in successful implant-prosthetic rehabilitation. However, results also showed that crestal bone levels are better maintained with internal types of connections. In general, internal conical connections seem to be more advantageous, presenting with reduced levels of MBL.

Implant Size

Since the introduction of dental implants, there has been a dramatic evolution in the geometry and the size of these fixtures, resulting in the use of narrower and shorter implants now compared with those used decades ago. One main reason is the improvement in the surface characteristics that have optimized the amount of bone-to-implant contact and the overall osseointegration process. As such, when the bone volume is not sufficient, the utility of shorter and/or narrower implants has been proposed as an alternative option to simplify the treatment procedures.

LENGTH

Over the years, there have been different definitions for *short implants*, such as 10 mm or less,[63,64] 8 mm or less,[65] or 6 mm or less.[19,66] Multiple studies have also documented and compared the amount of MBL between short and longer implants. Table 17-2 summarizes the major findings from some of these investigations with at least 3 years of follow-up.[18,67–71]

Today, the use of short implants represents a reliable alternative for the rehabilitation of edentulous patients, particularly in atrophic posterior mandibles where vertical ridge augmentation might pose more morbidity, expenses, and complications. In general, the survival rate of implants 6 mm or shorter is slightly lower than longer implants; however, the amount of MBL is comparable.

TABLE 17-2 Studies comparing implants with different lengths

Author	Study design and follow-up (m)	Implant features				Marginal bone loss ± SD (mm)
		Length (mm)	Survival rate (%)	Number and location	Implant type (surface)	
Romeo et al[69] (2014)	RCT (60)	10	100	21 mand 7 max	Straumann Tissue Level (SLA)	0.43 ± 0.34
		6	90	21 mand 5 max		0.24 ± 0.45
Felice et al[70] (2014)	RCT (60)	9.6	88	25 mand	Nanotite, Zimmer Biomet	2.34 ± 0.75
		6.6	80	27 mand		1.49 ± 0.40
Esposito et al[68] (2014)	RCT (36)	7, 8.5, 10	97	30 mand 38 max	EZ Plus	1.54 ± 0.44
		5	92	26 mand 34 max	Rescue, MegaGen	1.22 ± 0.49
Rossi et al[71] (2016)	RCT (60)	10	96.7	15 mand 15 max	Straumann Tissue Level (SLA)	0.14
		6	86.7	18 mand 12 max		0.18
Sahrmann et al[18] (2016)	RCT (36)	10	100	25 mand 15 max	Straumann Tissue Level (SLA)	0.33 ± 0.71
		6	98	31 mand 10 max		0.19 ± 0.62
Pohl et al[67] (2017)	RCT (36)	11, 13, 15	100	Max	Osseospeed, Astra Tech (TiOblast)	0.43 ± 0.58
		6	100			0.44 ± 0.56

SD, standard deviation; mand, mandible; max, maxilla; SLA, sandblasted, large-grit acid-etched.

It should be noted that the variability in the success of short implants might also be related to other factors, such as the specific type of implant or the loading protocols. A recent systematic review recommended splinting implants 6 mm or shorter to increase the survival rate.[22,72]

The efficacy of short implants as an alternative to sinus augmentation procedures has also been well documented.[67,68] Overall, short implants were found equivalent in terms of survival rate and MBL to longer implants placed in combination with sinus elevation after 3 years in function. However, studies with longer follow-up periods are necessary to confirm their utility as a standard approach to replace sinus floor elevation procedures.[67]

WIDTH

The definition of *narrow-diameter implant* has also been subjected to changes over the years. Nevertheless, a diameter of 3.5 mm or less has been generally considered as *narrow*.[73] One study[21] classified narrow-diameter implants in three different categories:

- Category 1: Diameter of less than 3.0 mm (also known as *mini implants*)
- Category 2: Diameter of 3.0 to 3.25 mm
- Category 3: Diameter of 3.3 to 3.5 mm

TABLE 17-3 Implant placement protocol and main findings

Authors	Study type	Characteristics	Main findings
Hermann et al[76] (2000)	Animal	One-piece and two-piece implants	For one-piece implants, the placement of the border between the rough and smooth surfaces 1 mm below the alveolar crest resulted in no bone loss beyond the smooth-rough interface.
Cochran et al[23] (2009)	Animal	Bone level with Morse taper connection and nonmatching abutment	Implants that were placed 1 mm below the alveolar crest in both submerged and nonsubmerged healing models showed significantly less bone loss compared with those placed at the crest level or 1 mm above the alveolar crest level.
Ercoli et al[24] (2017)	Human	Not defined	Subcrestal placement of the implants resulted in reduced odds of having implant threads exposed.
Froum et al[25] (2018)	Human	Platform-switched connection	No significant difference between the epicrestal and subcrestal implants in terms of marginal bone loss, and no bone loss beyond the implant-abutment junction detected in subcrestal group.

A recent systematic review[73] modified these categories as follows:

- Category 1: Implants with a diameter of less than 2.5 mm (mini implants). Their utility remains for highly atrophic edentulous jaws or for single non-load-bearing teeth in the anterior area.
- Category 2: Implants with a diameter of 2.5 mm to 3.3 mm, mostly used for single-tooth restorations in the anterior zone (eg, mandibular incisors or maxillary lateral incisors).
- Category 3: Implants with a diameter of 3.3 mm to 3.5 mm that may be used for all regions, including posterior single-tooth restorations.

Several other studies with medium-term follow-up have corroborated the aforementioned indications,[74,75] stating that category 3 implants may be used for all regions.

In a randomized clinical trial[74] with 3 years of follow-up, the performance of 3.3-mm titanium-zirconia implants was found to be no different than 4.1-mm titanium implants for the replacement of implant-supported single crowns in the anterior maxilla. No significant differences between the two groups in terms of changes in marginal bone level, changes in mucosa level, and the occurrence of complications were found. Another prospective clinical study[75] that investigated the effectiveness of 97 implants with 3-mm diameters for restoring single spaces in the anterior zone reported more than 1 mm of MBL for only 8.43% of the implants and a failure rate of 4.12% after 5 years.

Overall, it can be concluded that narrow-diameter implants should be considered as a possible treatment alternative with promising survival rates. However, long-term data are missing, and there is inconclusive evidence regarding the potential technical risks.[73]

Implant Positioning

RELATIVE TO THE ALVEOLAR CREST

The position of the implants relative to the alveolar crest (eg, supracrestal, equicrestal, or subcrestal) and its impact on MBL has been a topic of interest for many researchers.[23–25,76] Highlights from some of these studies are summarized in Table 17-3. In summary, all studies have confirmed that regardless of the implant type, subcrestal placement of the fixture (1 to 1.5 mm below the alveolar crest) will result in less bone remodeling beyond the implant platform, and consequently, less exposure of the implant threads. It should also be noted that in some cases, subcrestal placement of the implants is also necessary to achieve an ideal emergence profile and sufficient abutment height (Fig 17-3).

Overall, a strong body of evidence advocates for the subcrestal placement of implants. For one-piece

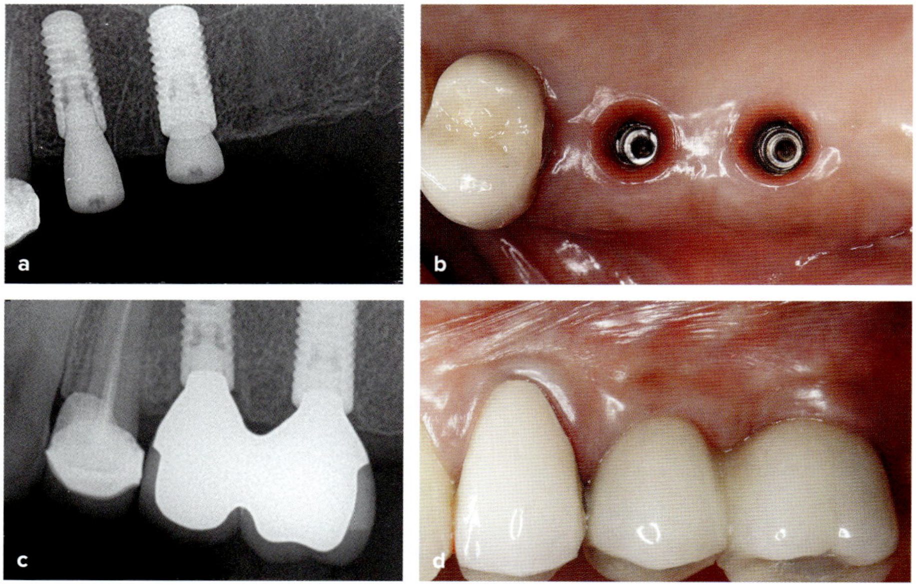

Fig 17-3 Subcrestal placement of the implants often reduces the possibility of marginal bone loss beyond the implant platform. *(a)* Radiograph at time of implant placement. *(b)* Clinical photograph before loading. *(c)* Radiograph at 1 year postloading. *(d)* Clinical photograph at 1 year postloading.

tissue-level implants, it is prudent to place 1 to 2 mm of the transmucosal part below the crest. For bone-level or two-piece implants, subcrestal placement may help prevent the implant threads from being exposed during the early healing phases. Although this subcrestal positioning may create further bone remodeling, it will likely help in maintaining full bony coverage of the rough surface.[77] Interestingly, one study has also documented osseointegration coronal to the implant-abutment interface for a specific two-part implant; however, this might be due to the surface characteristics of the investigated fixtures and abutments.[78]

RELATIVE TO ADJACENT DENTITION

The impact of the horizontal distance between implants and the adjacent dentition was initially investigated by Esposito et al.[79] The authors reported an increased level of MBL at the implant sites when the horizontal distance between the machine-surfaced Brånemark implants and the adjacent teeth was decreased. Thus, a minimum distance of 1.5 mm between the implant and the adjacent teeth, especially in the anterior maxilla, was proposed.[79] It should be noted that the MBL reported in this study was confined to the time between implant placement and crown delivery, and no further loss was observed during the subsequent follow-up period.

This hypothesis was later rejected by several studies[26,30,80–82] demonstrating at tooth/implant units, no statistically significant association between the horizontal distance and MBL. In addition, Vela et al[80] showed that with the use of platform-switched abutments, the placement of the implant 1 mm next to the adjacent tooth had no negative impact on MBL.

A recent radiographic study[81] examined the records of 180 patients with a total of 278 interproximal units. Various tooth-to-implant distances with corresponding marginal bone level changes were investigated and are presented in Table 17-4.

The proximity of the implant to the adjacent dentition might also have a negative impact on the soft tissue topography, jeopardizing the esthetic outcomes.[83] Gastaldo et al[83] suggested that when the distance between the implant and the adjacent tooth was less than 3 mm, there was an absence of complete papilla. Another study[84] suggested that the proximity of single implants in the anterior maxilla increases the odds ratio of having incomplete distal papilla. However, a recent systematic review[85] concluded that for single-crown implant-supported restorations, the height of the papilla between the implant and a tooth is predominantly determined by the clinical attachment level of the tooth.[86,87]

The information about the impact of the vertical distance of the implant platform relative to the adjacent dentition and MBL is scarce. While a prospective study[27] failed to find an association in 16 patients, a retrospective study[28] with 139 patients demonstrated that in the posterior area, for implants that were placed more than 3 mm

TABLE 17-4 Distance from implant to tooth and marginal bone loss levels*

Horizontal distance	Number of implants	Marginal bone level change at tooth (mm)	Marginal bone level change at implant (mm)
≤ 2 mm	59	0.33 ± 0.42	0.33 ± 0.60
≤ 3 mm	119	0.36 ± 0.57	0.34 ± 0.75
≤ 4 mm	85	0.41 ± 0.53	0.39 ± 0.73

*None of the values were statistically significant.

deeper than the cementoenamel junction of the adjacent tooth, the MBL in both mesial (mean difference of 0.57 mm) and distal (mean difference of 0.83 mm) sides was significantly higher than with shallower implants.

RELATIVE TO ADJACENT IMPLANTS

The effect of the interimplant horizontal distance on MBL was first shown by a cross-sectional study concluding that the lateral component of vertical bone loss to the first thread might result in the loss in crest height at sites with less than 3 mm of interimplant distance.[29] However, a longitudinal retrospective study[30] using the same type of implants (machine-surfaced Brånemark implants) failed to identify lateral bone loss as a significant factor for reduction of the interimplant bone level.

Moreover, experimental and preclinical studies[31,88–92] using platform-switched and internal conical implant-abutment connections investigated the effect of the horizontal interimplant distance on MBL and failed to report an association between these two parameters. Similarly, a recent systematic review[93] failed to define an optimal threshold for the horizontal interimplant distance based on the available evidence. The reason for this might also be that MBL is a multifactorial phenomenon with numerous factors responsible for bone remodeling, not only the horizontal interimplant distance. Nevertheless, a tendency for higher risk of incomplete interimplant mucosa fill was identified when implants are placed at a distance of less than 3 mm.[93] Therefore, in the anterior maxilla, it is recommended that two adjacent implants should have an interimplant bone distance of 3 to 4 mm in order to optimize papilla fill. In cases with interimplant distance of less than 3 mm in the anterior maxilla, a single implant with a cantilever could be considered.[86]

Biologic Factors

FORMATION OF SUPRACRESTAL ATTACHED TISSUES

Preclinical and human studies[2,32,33] have shown that once the implants are exposed to the oral cavity, a certain minimum dimension of soft tissue attachment will always form. As a result, if insufficient tissue is present to allow for the formation of the supracrestal attached tissues (formerly referred to as *biologic width*), **bone resorption** will occur. This attachment is composed of connective tissue and the junctional epithelium, which forms after 6 to 8 weeks of healing.[94] The junctional epithelium is separated from the crestal bone by a zone of connective tissue mainly composed of collagen fibers and matrix elements (85%), a small amount of fibroblasts (3%), and vasculature (5%).[2,95] The establishment of these supracrestal attached tissues always occurs independently of the implant design or surface characteristics (eg, one-piece or two-piece).[1,34] However, the implant design may influence the dimensions of this soft tissue attachment.[32]

Findings from human and preclinical studies are generally in agreement, demonstrating that the peri-implant mucosa is about 3 to 4 mm in height with a 2-mm epithelium.[95] Preclinical studies also showed that one-piece implants present with smaller supracrestal attached tissue dimensions than two-piece implants (Table 17-5).[2,32–34]

Cross-sectional studies have confirmed the aforementioned findings reporting that over time, tissue-level implants will undergo less MBL than bone-level implants.[96–98] However, due to limitations in prosthetic versatility and potential esthetic complications, one-piece implants are not widely used in daily practice. Another study[32] showed that for two-piece implants, the location of the interface (ie, microgap) played a role in the formation of biologic width regardless of the placement protocol (submerged or nonsubmerged; Figs 17-4 and 17-5).

TABLE 17-5 Supracrestal attached tissue (biologic width) dimensions

Study	Study type	Findings
Berglundh and Lindhe[2] (1996)	Animal (dogs)	• Junctional epithelium length between 2 to 2.1 mm • Connective tissue length between 1.3 mm and 1.8 mm • In sites with thin mucosa (≤ 2 mm), more MBL occurred compared to sites with thicker mucosa
Cochran et al[34] (1997)	Animal (dogs)	• Junctional epithelium length: 1.88 mm • Connective tissue length: 1.05 mm
Hermann et al[32] (2001)	Animal (dogs)	• Significantly more crestal bone loss around two-piece than one-piece implants • Biologic width dimensions were significantly smaller in one-piece implants than two-piece implants
Tomasi et al[33] (2014)	Human	• Peri-implant mucosa dimension: 3.6 mm • Epithelium: 1.9 mm • Connective tissue: 1.7 mm

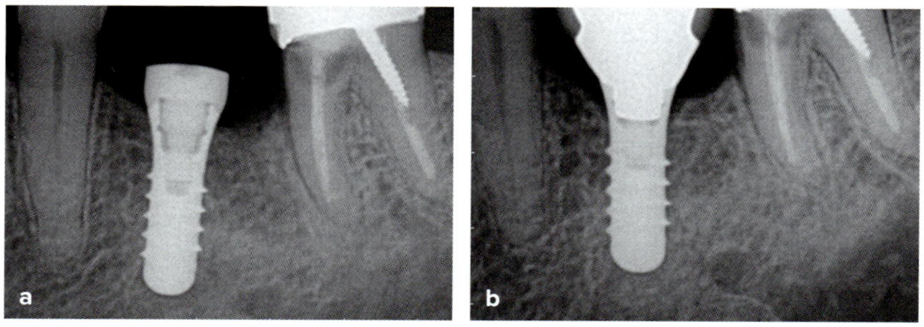

Fig 17-4 *(a)* Radiograph at time of implant placement. *(b)* Radiograph at 24 months post loading demonstrating the amount of bone loss that occurred possibly due to biologic width formation up to the level of the junction between the rough and smooth surfaces.

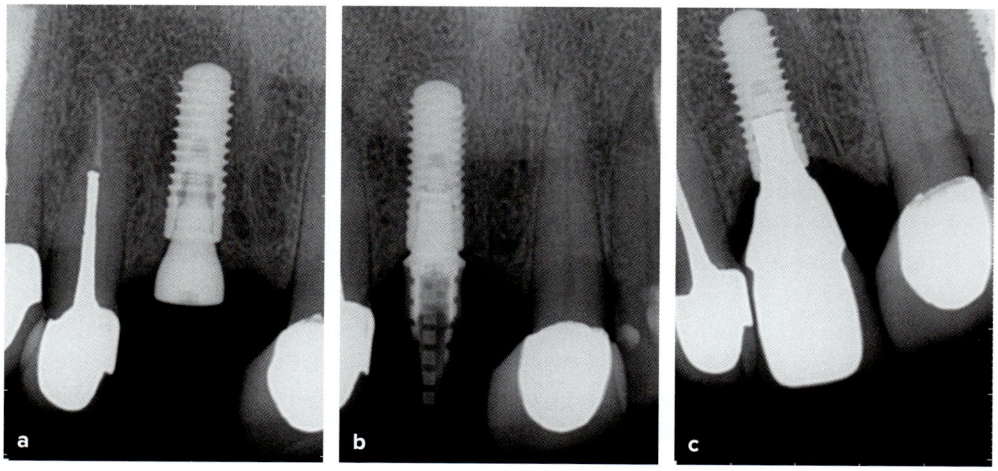

Fig 17-5 *(a)* Radiograph at time of implant placement. *(b)* Radiograph at loading time. *(c)* Radiograph 6 months after placement of the definitive restoration of the two-piece implant. Note the amount of bone loss possibly due to biologic width formation slightly beyond the implant platform.

PERI-IMPLANT SOFT TISSUES

In the evaluation of the factors relevant to MBL, the roles of the soft tissue height and thickness around osseointegrated implants have often been underestimated and misreported.[12,35]

More than two decades ago, in a preclinical study, Berglundh and Lindhe[2] demonstrated that at sites where the peri-implant mucosa was made thin prior to abutment placement (ie, ≤ 2 mm), wound healing consistently included MBL. This important finding showed that a certain minimum width of peri-implant mucosa is required, and that if necessary, bone resorption would take place to allow the formation of a stable soft tissue attachment.[2,34] In concordance with these findings, a recent systematic review[35] confirmed that implants with an initially thicker peri-implant soft tissue had less MBL. Moreover, this tissue thickness played a major role in minimizing bone loss when implants were placed supracrestally. This could also be because the location of the implant-abutment interface (microgap) influences the amount of initial MBL.[95]

Soft tissue augmentation procedures to increase the thickness of the peri-implant mucosa have been shown to be effective methods to reduce the negative effects of thin peri-implant mucosa.[99,100]

On the other hand, while the need for a minimum amount of keratinized mucosa to maintain peri-implant health still remains a controversial topic,[95] it appears that plaque control is facilitated in the presence of more than 2 mm of keratinized tissue.[100,101] To increase the zone of keratinized tissue around implants, the autogenous free gingival graft still remains as the gold standard. Statistically significant differences have been noted for marginal bone level changes in favor of this treatment modality versus other treatment alternatives.[99,100]

Mechanical Factors

OCCLUSAL FORCES

For decades, peri-implantitis and occlusal overload have been identified as the major etiologic factors responsible for late failures of dental implants.[37] While a cause-and-effect relationship between bacterial load and peri-implant bone loss has been identified,[87] it is impossible to quantify the stress and strain evoked at the implant-to-bone interface to measure occlusal overload in an animal or clinical setting.[102] Therefore, it is very challenging, if not impossible, to correlate occlusal loading to implant failure,[36] and at best, the role of occlusal overload as a risk indicator for peri-implantitis remains to be determined.[87] The studies aimed at evaluating occlusal overload have traditionally presented with several drawbacks. First, *occlusal overload* is often vaguely defined, and second, most of the studies in the literature refer to occlusal overload when forces do not really reach what has been defined as *true overload* (> 3,000 microstrain) as coined by Frost.[103] Due to this lack of proper definition, several other factors were studied as possible sources of occlusal overload on osseointegrated implants; however, no strong evidence was ever presented to substantiate a cause–effect relationship. For example, the presence of cantilevers was considered as a possible cause of MBL for decades. Later, a strong body of evidence rejected this hypothesis because the presence of a mesial or distal cantilever does not necessarily lead to MBL.[104–110]

It is unethical to conduct a trial on humans to investigate the role of occlusal overload on MBL. However, a strong body of preclinical evidence is present.[36,111–113] In addition, two systematic reviews[36,111] on animal studies concluded that based on the mucosal health, supraocclusal contacts acting in an uninflamed peri-implant environment did not have any negative impact on osseointegration and even resulted in greater bone density. In contrast, occlusal overload in the presence of inflammation significantly increased the plaque-induced bone resorption. In addition, occlusal overload can also lead to further mechanical complications.

INSERTION TORQUE

High insertion torque values are believed to be a reason for compression necrosis and early implant failures.[114] While several studies[38,39,115,116] have shown that high insertion torque does not lead to implant failure, other investigations found an association between high insertion torque and MBL.[38,39,117] In one prospective study,[38] 42 implants were placed with high insertion torque values in partially edentulous patients and were loaded after a healing period of 2 months (mean: 110.6 Ncm; range: 70.8–176 Ncm). Later, no negative effect of high insertion torque on MBL was detected. On the other hand, in an RCT,[39] implants that were placed with insertion torque values (ie, ≥ 50 Ncm) presented with significantly more MBL than the control group. It should be noted that the designs of the implants in the test and control groups were different.[39]

TABLE 17-6 Influence of insertion torque on marginal bone loss

Study	Follow-up (m)	Implant system	Number of implants	Insertion torque	Marginal bone loss (mm)	Outcome
Khayat et al[38] (2013)	12	Tapered Screw-Vent (Zimmer Biomet)	42	> 70 Ncm	0.72 ± 0.56	No significant difference with the implants placed at lower insertion torque
Barone et al[39] (2016)	12	CT (Intra-Lock)	58	≥ 50 Ncm	0.94 ± 0.50	Significantly more bone loss in the high insertion torque group

A longitudinal analysis of the latter showed that after 3 years, the mean MBL and facial soft tissue recession were significantly greater for the high insertion torque group (1.53 mm vs 1.03 mm).[39,116] It also appears that the implant design might play a major role in the association between high insertion torque and MBL (Table 17-6).[38,39]

Other Factors

METAL PARTICLES

The influence of metal particles and ions on the peri-implant tissues as a potential contributor to MBL and peri-implantitis has been investigated in several clinical, preclinical, and in vitro studies.[41] As such, titanium particles have been frequently observed around dental implants, especially when presenting with peri-implantitis.[41,118] While the biologic repercussions of these metal debris on the peri-implant hard and soft tissues remain to be further elucidated, multiple studies have investigated the detrimental effects of these particles/ions demonstrating phenomena such as osteolysis, modification of the peri-implant microbiome, inflammation, bone loss, epigenetic changes, DNA damage in oral epithelial cells, and more.[119–125] The most common pathways for titanium particle release[40–42] are as follows:

- During implant insertion due to friction
- Friction between the implant platform and abutment
- Wear during debridement, implantoplasty, or other decontamination methods
- Saliva, bacteria, and chemicals that can potentially dissolve the titanium oxide layer, resulting in corrosion cycles

A cross-sectional study also revealed greater levels of dissolved titanium in submucosal plaque samples around implants diagnosed with peri-implantitis compared with their healthy counterparts.[118]

Given the available evidence, it appears prudent to minimize the release of titanium debris to the peri-implant environment as much as possible. Several measures could be applied to reduce titanium particle release, including enhancement of the insertion procedures to avoid excessive friction, as well as precise and delicate maintenance protocols.[41] Additional research is necessary to further elucidate the possible causality between metal particle or ion release and MBL.

TIMING OF IMPLANT PLACEMENT AND IMPLANT LOADING

A variety of surgical and prosthetic protocols have been introduced in the field of oral implantology with satisfactory long-term survival rates.[126,127] The timing of implant placement has been defined by the duration of the healing period following tooth extraction before implant installation. In the same manner, implant loading protocols have been defined by the duration of the healing period following implant placement prior to the delivery of a provisional or definitive implant restoration.[45,128]

A recent systematic review[43] including 12 RCTs compared the outcomes of early, immediate, and delayed implant placement and concluded that there was no significant difference between the three protocols with regard to risk of implant failures. However, the immediate implant protocol presented significantly more MBL compared with the early implant placement protocol. These findings are in contrast with a previously published review[126] that reported more failures for the immediate implant placement group.

With regard to the impact of implant loading protocols upon MBL, the available evidence does not show a significant difference between the different protocols.[46] It should be noted that immediate implant placement in conjunction with immediate loading is a complex treatment, and several factors must be considered when choosing this treatment modality.[44,129]

Conclusion

While MBL may or may not be associated with peri-implantitis, peri-implantitis is always preceded or accompanied by MBL. Hence, the elimination or reduction of MBL represents one of the key factors in the prevention of peri-implantitis. Of paramount importance is the minimization of the early or so-called physiologic MBL, because higher levels of this process have been related with further bone loss. On the other hand, minimal MBL during the first months has been related to stable bone levels over time. Finally, multiple factors play a role in MBL, including a variety of local, systemic, surgical, and prosthetic factors.

References

1. Abrahamsson I, Berglundh T, Wennström J, Lindhe J. The peri-implant hard and soft tissues at different implant systems. A comparative study in the dog. Clin Oral Implants Res 1996;7:212–219.
2. Berglundh T, Lindhe J. Dimension of the periimplant mucosa. Biological width revisited. J Clin Periodontol 1996;23:971–973.
3. Galindo-Moreno P, Léon-Cano A, Ortega-Oller I, Monje A, O'Valle F, Catena A. Marginal bone loss as success criterion in implant dentistry: Beyond 2 mm. Clin Oral Implants Res 2015;26:e28–e34.
4. American Academy of Periodontology. Glossary of Periodontal Terms. American Academy of Periodontology, 2001.
5. Albrektsson T, Zarb G, Worthington P, Eriksson AR. The long-term efficacy of currently used dental implants: A review and proposed criteria of success. Int J Oral Maxillofac Implants 1986;1:11–25.
6. Albrektsson T, Chrcanovic B, Östman PO, Sennerby L. Initial and long-term crestal bone responses to modern dental implants. Periodontol 2000 2017;73:41–50.
7. Roos J, Sennerby L, Lekholm U, Jemt T, Gröndahl K, Albrektsson T. A qualitative and quantitative method for evaluating implant success: A 5-year retrospective analysis of the Brånemark implant. Int J Oral Maxillofac Implants 1997;12:504–514.
8. Renvert S, Persson GR, Pirih FQ, Camargo PM. Peri-implant health, peri-implant mucositis, and peri-implantitis: Case definitions and diagnostic considerations. J Clin Periodontol 2018;45(20 suppl):S278–S285.
9. Hermann JS, Schoolfield JD, Nummikoski PV, Buser D, Schenk RK, Cochran DL. Crestal bone changes around titanium implants: A methodologic study comparing linear radiographic with histometric measurements. Int J Oral Maxillofac Implants 2001;16:475–485.
10. Hermann JS, Schoolfield JD, Schenk RK, Buser D, Cochran DL. Influence of the size of the microgap on crestal bone changes around titanium implants. A histometric evaluation of unloaded nonsubmerged implants in the canine mandible. J Periodontol 2001;72:1372–1383.
11. Hermann JS, Cochran DL, Nummikoski PV, Buser D. Crestal bone changes around titanium implants. A radiographic evaluation of unloaded nonsubmerged and submerged implants in the canine mandible. J Periodontol 1997;68:1117–1130.
12. Canullo L, Fedele GR, Iannello G, Jepsen S. Platform switching and marginal bone-level alterations: The results of a randomized-controlled trial. Clin Oral Implants Res 2010;21:115–121.
13. Enkling N, Jöhren P, Katsoulis J, et al. Influence of platform switching on bone-level alterations: A three-year randomized clinical trial. J Dent Res 2013;92(12 suppl):139S–145S.
14. Abrahamsson I, Berglundh T, Glantz PO, Lindhe J. The mucosal attachment at different abutments. An experimental study in dogs. J Clin Periodontol 1998;25:721–727.
15. Galindo-Moreno P, Fernández-Jiménez A, O'Valle F, et al. Influence of the crown-implant connection on the preservation of peri-implant bone: A retrospective multifactorial analysis. Int J Oral Maxillofac Implants 2015;30:384–390.
16. Esposito M, Maghaireh H, Pistilli R, et al. Dental implants with internal versus external connections: 5-year post-loading results from a pragmatic multicenter randomised controlled trial. Eur J Oral Implantol 2016;9(1 suppl):129–141.
17. Monje A, Suarez F, Galindo-Moreno P, García-Nogales A, Fu JH, Wang HL. A systematic review on marginal bone loss around short dental implants (< 10 mm) for implant-supported fixed prostheses. Clin Oral Implants Res 2014;25:1119–1124.
18. Sahrmann P, Naenni N, Jung RE, et al. Success of 6-mm implants with single-tooth restorations: A 3-year randomized controlled clinical trial. J of Dent Res 2016;95:623–628.
19. Rossi F, Lang NP, Ricci E, Ferraioli L, Marchetti C, Botticelli D. Early loading of 6-mm-short implants with a moderately rough surface supporting single crowns: A prospective 5-year cohort study. Clin Oral Implants Res 2015;26:471–477.
20. Degidi M, Piattelli A, Iezzi G, Carinci F. Wide-diameter implants: Analysis of clinical outcome of 304 fixtures. J Periodontol 2007;78:52–58.
21. Klein MO, Schiegnitz E, Al-Nawas B. Systematic review on success of narrow-diameter dental implants. Int J Oral Maxillofac Implants 2014;29(suppl):43–54.
22. Papaspyridakos P, De Souza A, Vazouras K, Gholami H, Pagni S, Weber HP. Survival rates of short dental implants (≤6 mm) compared with implants longer than 6 mm in posterior jaw areas: A meta-analysis. Clin Oral Implants Res 2018;29(16 suppl):8–20.
23. Cochran DL, Bosshardt DD, Grize L, et al. Bone response to loaded implants with non-matching implant-abutment diameters in the canine mandible. J Periodontol 2009;80:609–617.
24. Ercoli C, Jammal G, Buyers M, et al. Influence of apico-coronal implant placement on post-surgical crestal bone loss in humans. J Periodontol 2017;88:762–770.
25. Froum SJ, Cho SC, Suzuki T, Yu P, Corby P, Khouly I. Epicrestal and subcrestal placement of platform-switched implants: 18 month-result of a randomized, controlled, split-mouth, prospective clinical trial. Clin Oral Implants Res 2018;29:353–366.
26. Chang M, Wennström JL. Bone alterations at implant-supported FDPs in relation to inter-unit distances: A 5-year radiographic study. Clin Oral Implants Res 2010;21:735–740.
27. Chang M, Wennström JL. Peri-implant soft tissue and bone crest alterations at fixed dental prostheses: A 3-year prospective study. Clini Oral Implants Res 2010;21:527–534.

28. Mailoa J, Fu JH, Chan HL, Khoshkam V, Li J, Wang HL. The effect of vertical implant position in relation to adjacent teeth on marginal bone loss in posterior arches: A retrospective study. Int J Oral Maxillofac Implants 2015;30:931–936.
29. Tarnow DP, Cho SC, Wallace SS. The effect of inter-implant distance on the height of inter-implant bone crest. J Periodontol 2000;71:546–549.
30. Cardaropoli G, Wennström JL, Lekholm U. Peri-implant bone alterations in relation to inter-unit distances. A 3-year retrospective study. Clinical Oral Implants Res 2003;14:430–436.
31. Koutouzis T, Neiva R, Lipton D, Lundgren T. The effect of inter-implant distance on peri-implant bone and soft tissue dimensional changes: A nonrandomized, prospective, 2-year follow-up study. Int J Oral Maxillofac Implants 2015;30:900–908.
32. Hermann JS, Buser D, Schenk RK, Schoolfield JD, Cochran DL. Biologic width around one- and two-piece titanium implants. Clin Oral Implants Res 2001;12:559–571.
33. Tomasi C, Tessarolo F, Caola I, Wennström J, Nollo G, Berglundh T. Morphogenesis of peri-implant mucosa revisited: An experimental study in humans. Clin Oral Implants Res 2014;25:997–1003.
34. Cochran DL, Hermann JS, Schenk RK, Higginbottom FL, Buser D. Biologic width around titanium implants. A histometric analysis of the implanto-gingival junction around unloaded and loaded nonsubmerged implants in the canine mandible. J Periodontol 1997;68:186–198.
35. Suárez-López Del Amo F, Lin GH, Monje A, Galindo-Moreno P, Wang HL. Influence of soft tissue thickness on peri-implant marginal bone loss: A systematic review and meta-analysis. J Periodontol 2016;87:690–699.
36. Naert I, Duyck J, Vandamme K. Occlusal overload and bone/implant loss. Clin Oral Implants Res 2012;23(6 suppl):95–107.
37. Esposito M, Hirsch JM, Lekholm U, Thomsen P. Biological factors contributing to failures of osseointegrated oral implants. (II). Etiopathogenesis. Eur J Oral Sci 1998;106:721–764.
38. Khayat PG, Arnal HM, Tourbah BI, Sennerby L. Clinical outcome of dental implants placed with high insertion torques (up to 176 Ncm). Clin Implant Dent Relat Res 2013;15:227–233.
39. Barone A, Alfonsi F, Derchi G, et al. The effect of insertion torque on the clinical outcome of single implants: A randomized clinical trial. Clin Implant Dent Relat Res 2016;18:588–600.
40. Fretwurst T, Nelson K, Tarnow DP, Wang HL, Giannobile WV. Is metal particle release associated with peri-implant bone destruction? An emerging concept. J Dent Res 2018;97:259–265.
41. Suárez-López Del Amo F, Garaicoa-Pazmiño C, Fretwurst T, Castilho RM, Squarize CH. Dental implants-associated release of titanium particles: A systematic review. Clin Oral Implants Res 2018 doi:10.1111/clr.13372.
42. Delgado-Ruiz R, Romanos G. Potential causes of titanium particle and ion release in implant dentistry: A systematic review. Int J Mol Sci 2018;19:3585.
43. Bassir SH, El Kholy K, Chen CY, Lee KH, Intini G. Outcome of early dental implant placement versus other dental implant placement protocols: A systematic review and meta-analysis. J Periodontol 2018;90:493–506.
44. Morton D, Gallucci G, Lin WS, et al. Group 2 ITI consensus report: Prosthodontics and implant dentistry. Clin Oral Implants Res 2018;29(16 suppl):215–223.
45. Gallucci GO, Hamilton A, Zhou W, Buser D, Chen S. Implant placement and loading protocols in partially edentulous patients: A systematic review. Clin Oral Implants Res 2018;29(16 suppl):106–134.
46. Suarez F, Chan HL, Monje A, Galindo-Moreno P, Wang HL. Effect of the timing of restoration on implant marginal bone loss: A systematic review. J Periodontol 2013;84:159–169.
47. Hartman GA, Cochran DL. Initial implant position determines the magnitude of crestal bone remodeling. J Periodontol 2004;75:572–577.
48. Sanz M, Klinge B, Alcoforado G, et al. Biological aspects: Summary and consensus statements of group 2. The 5th EAO Consensus Conference 2018. Clin Oral Implants Res 2018;29(18 suppl):152–156.
49. Pjetursson BE, Zarauz C, Strasding M, Sailer I, Zwahlen M, Zembic A. A systematic review of the influence of the implant-abutment connection on the clinical outcomes of ceramic and metal implant abutments supporting fixed implant reconstructions. Clin Oral Implants Res 2018;29(18 suppl):160–183.
50. Sailer I, Mühlemann S, Kohal RJ, et al. Reconstructive aspects: Summary and consensus statements of group 3. The 5th EAO Consensus Conference 2018. Clin Oral Implants Res 2018;29(18 suppl):237–242.
51. Sanz-Sánchez I, Sanz-Martín I, Carrillo de Albornoz A, Figuero E, Sanz M. Biological effect of the abutment material on the stability of peri-implant marginal bone levels: A systematic review and meta-analysis. Clin Oral Implants Res 2018;29(18 suppl):124–144.
52. Sanz-Martín I, Sanz-Sánchez I, Carrillo de Albornoz A, Figuero E, Sanz M. Effects of modified abutment characteristics on peri-implant soft tissue health: A systematic review and meta-analysis. Clin Oral Implants Res 2018;29:118–129.
53. Lazzara RJ, Porter SS. Platform switching: A new concept in implant dentistry for controlling postrestorative crestal bone levels. Int J Periodontics Restorative Dent 2006;26:9–17.
54. Canullo L, Caneva M, Tallarico M. Ten-year hard and soft tissue results of a pilot double-blinded randomized controlled trial on immediately loaded post-extractive implants using platform-switching concept. Clin Oral Implants Res 2017;28:1195–1203.
55. Fickl S, Zuhr O, Stein JM, Hurzeler MB. Peri-implant bone level around implants with platform-switched abutments. Int J Oral Maxillofac Implants 2010;25:577–581.
56. Vigolo P, Givani A. Platform-switched restorations on wide-diameter implants: A 5-year clinical prospective study. Int J Oral Maxillofac Implants 2009;24:103–109.
57. Hsu YT, Lin GH, Wang HL. Effects of platform-switching on peri-implant soft and hard tissue outcomes: A systematic Review and meta-analysis. Int J Oral Maxillofac Implants 2017;32:e9–e24.
58. Crespi R, Capparè P, Gherlone E. Radiographic evaluation of marginal bone levels around platform-switched and non-platform-switched implants used in an immediate loading protocol. Int J Oral Maxillofac Implants 2009;24:920–926.
59. Al-Nsour MM, Chan HL, Wang HL. Effect of the platform-switching technique on preservation of peri-implant marginal bone: A systematic review. Int J Oral Maxillofac Implants 2012;27:138–145.
60. Caricasulo R, Malchiodi L, Ghensi P, Fantozzi G, Cucchi A. The influence of implant-abutment connection to peri-implant bone loss: A systematic review and meta-analysis. Clin Implant Dent Relat Res 2018;20:653–664.
61. Arnhart C, Kielbassa AM, Martinez-de Fuentes R, et al. Comparison of variable-thread tapered implant designs to a standard tapered implant design after immediate loading. A 3-year multicentre randomised controlled trial. Eur J Oral Implantol 2012;5:123–136.
62. Pozzi A, Agliardi E, Tallarico M, Barlattani A. Clinical and radiological outcomes of two implants with different prosthetic interfaces and neck configurations: Randomized, controlled, split-mouth clinical trial. Clin Implant Dent Relat Res 2014;16:96–106.

63. Friberg B, Jemt T, Lekholm U. Early failures in 4,641 consecutively placed Brånemark dental implants: A study from stage 1 surgery to the connection of completed prostheses. Int J Oral Maxillofac Implants 1991;6:142–146.
64. Feldman S, Boitel N, Weng D, Kohles SS, Stach RM. Five-year survival distributions of short-length (10 mm or less) machined-surfaced and Osseotite implants. Clin Implant Dent Relat Res 2004;6:16–23.
65. Renouard F, Nisand D. Impact of implant length and diameter on survival rates. Clin Oral Implants Res 2006;17(2 suppl):35–51.
66. Rossi F, Ricci E, Marchetti C, Lang NP, Botticelli D. Early loading of single crowns supported by 6-mm-long implants with a moderately rough surface: A prospective 2-year follow-up cohort study. Clin Oral Implants Res 2010;21:937–943.
67. Pohl V, Thoma DS, Sporniak-Tutak K, et al. Short dental implants (6 mm) versus long dental implants (11–15 mm) in combination with sinus floor elevation procedures: 3-year results from a multicentre, randomized, controlled clinical trial. J Clin Periodontol 2017;44:438–445.
68. Esposito M, Pistilli R, Barausse C, Felice P. Three-year results from a randomised controlled trial comparing prostheses supported by 5-mm long implants or by longer implants in augmented bone in posterior atrophic edentulous jaws. Eur J Oral Implantol 2014;7:383–395.
69. Romeo E, Storelli S, Casano G, Scanferla M, Botticelli D. Six-mm versus 10-mm long implants in the rehabilitation of posterior edentulous jaws: A 5-year follow-up of a randomised controlled trial. Eur J Oral Implantol 2014;7:371–381.
70. Felice P, Cannizzaro G, Barausse C, Pistilli R, Esposito M. Short implants versus longer implants in vertically augmented posterior mandibles: A randomised controlled trial with 5-year after loading follow-up. Eur J Oral Implantol 2014;7:359–369.
71. Rossi F, Botticelli D, Cesaretti G, De Santis E, Storelli S, Lang NP. Use of short implants (6 mm) in a single-tooth replacement: A 5-year follow-up prospective randomized controlled multicenter clinical study. Clin Oral Implants Res 2016;27:458–464.
72. Jung RE, Al-Nawas B, Araujo M, et al. Group 1 ITI consensus report: The influence of implant length and design and medications on clinical and patient-reported outcomes. Clin Oral Implants Res 2018;29(16 suppl):69–77.
73. Schiegnitz E, Al-Nawas B. Narrow-diameter implants: A systematic review and meta-analysis. Clin Oral Implants Res 2018;29(16 suppl):21–40.
74. Ioannidis A, Gallucci GO, Jung RE, Borzangy S, Hämmerle CH, Benic GI. Titanium-zirconium narrow-diameter versus titanium regular-diameter implants for anterior and premolar single crowns: 3-year results of a randomized controlled clinical study. J Clin Periodontol 2015;42:1060–1070.
75. Galindo-Moreno P, Nilsson P, King P, et al. Clinical and radiographic evaluation of early loaded narrow-diameter implants: 5-year follow-up of a multicenter prospective clinical study. Clin Oral Implants Res 2017;28:1584–1591.
76. Hermann JS, Buser D, Schenk RK, Cochran DL. Crestal bone changes around titanium implants. A histometric evaluation of unloaded non-submerged and submerged implants in the canine mandible. J Periodontol 2000;71:1412–1424.
77. Jung RE, Jones AA, Higginbottom FL, et al. The influence of non-matching implant and abutment diameters on radiographic crestal bone levels in dogs. J Periodontol 2008;79:260–270.
78. Welander M, Abrahamsson I, Berglundh T. Subcrestal placement of two-part implants. Clin Oral Implants Res 2009;20:226–231.
79. Esposito M, Ekestubbe A, Gröndahl K. Radiological evaluation of marginal bone loss at tooth surfaces facing single Brånemark implants. Clinical Oral Implants Res 1993;4:151–157.
80. Vela X, Mendez V, Rodriguez X, Segalá M, Tarnow DP. Crestal bone changes on platform-switched implants and adjacent teeth when the tooth-implant distance is less than 1.5 mm. Int J Periodontics Restorative Dent 2012;32:149–155.
81. Cecchinato D, Marino M, Toia M, Cecchinato F, Lindhe J. Bone loss at implants and teeth in the same inter-proximal unit: A radiographic study. Clin Oral Implants Res 2018;29:375–380.
82. Al Amri MD. Influence of interimplant distance on the crestal bone height around dental implants: A systematic review and meta-analysis. J Prosthet Dent 2016;115:278–282.
83. Gastaldo JF, Cury PR, Sendyk WR. Effect of the vertical and horizontal distances between adjacent implants and between a tooth and an implant on the incidence of interproximal papilla. J Periodontol 2004;75:1242–1246.
84. Cosyn J, Sabzevar MM, De Bruyn H. Predictors of inter-proximal and midfacial recession following single implant treatment in the anterior maxilla: A multivariate analysis. J Clin Periodontol 2012;39:895–903.
85. Roccuzzo M, Roccuzzo A, Ramanuskaite A. Papilla height in relation to the distance between bone crest and interproximal contact point at single-tooth implants: A systematic review. Clin Oral Implants Res 2018;29(15 suppl):50–61.
86. Jung RE, Heitz-Mayfield L, Schwarz F, Groups of the 2nd Osteology Foundation Consensus Meeting. Evidence-based knowledge on the aesthetics and maintenance of peri-implant soft tissues: Osteology Foundation Consensus Report Part 3—Aesthetics of peri-implant soft tissues. Clin Oral Implants Res 2018;29(15 suppl):14–17.
87. Berglundh T, Armitage G, Araujo MG, et al. Peri-implant diseases and conditions: Consensus report of workgroup 4 of the 2017 World Workshop on the Classification of Periodontal and Peri-implant Diseases and Conditions. J Clin Periodontol 2018;45(20 suppl):S286–S291.
88. Elian N, Bloom M, Dard M, Cho SC, Trushkowsky RD, Tarnow D. Radiological and micro-computed tomography analysis of the bone at dental implants inserted 2, 3 and 4 mm apart in a minipig model with platform switching incorporated. Clin Oral Implants Res 2014;25:e22–e29.
89. Novaes AB Jr, de Oliveira RR, Muglia VA, Papalexiou V, Taba M. The effects of interimplant distances on papilla formation and crestal resorption in implants with a Morse cone connection and a platform switch: A histomorphometric study in dogs. J Periodontol 2006;77:1839–1849.
90. de Oliveira RR, Novaes AB Jr, Papalexiou V, Muglia VA, Taba M Jr. Influence of interimplant distance on papilla formation and bone resorption: A clinical-radiographic study in dogs. J Oral Implantol 2006;32:218–227.
91. Papalexiou V, Novaes AB Jr, Ribeiro RF, Muglia V, Oliveira RR. Influence of the interimplant distance on crestal bone resorption and bone density: A histomorphometric study in dogs. J Periodontol 2006;77:614–621.
92. Novaes AB Jr, Papalexiou V, Muglia V, Taba M Jr. Influence of interimplant distance on gingival papilla formation and bone resorption: Clinical-radiographic study in dogs. Int J Oral Maxillofac Implants 2006;21:45–51.
93. Ramanauskaite A, Roccuzzo A, Schwarz F. A systematic review on the influence of the horizontal distance between two adjacent implants inserted in the anterior maxilla on the inter-implant mucosa fill. Clin Oral Implants Res 2018;29(15 suppl):62–70.
94. Berglundh T, Abrahamsson I, Welander M, Lang NP, Lindhe J. Morphogenesis of the peri-implant mucosa: An experimental study in dogs. Clin Oral Implant Res 2007;18:1–8.
95. Araujo MG, Lindhe J. Peri-implant health. J Clin Periodontol 2018;45(20 suppl):S230–S236.

96. Derks J, Håkansson J, Wennström JL, Tomasi C, Larsson M, Berglundh T. Effectiveness of implant therapy analyzed in a Swedish population: Early and late implant loss. J Dent Res 2015;94(3 suppl):44S–51S.
97. Derks J, Schaller D, Håkansson J, Wennström JL, Tomasi C, Berglundh T. Effectiveness of implant therapy analyzed in a Swedish population: Prevalence of peri-implantitis. J Dent Res 2016;95:43–49.
98. Tarnow DP. Increasing prevalence of peri-implantitis: How will we manage? J Dent Res 2016;95:7–8.
99. Thoma DS, Naenni N, Figuero E, et al. Effects of soft tissue augmentation procedures on peri-implant health or disease: A systematic review and meta-analysis. Clin Oral Implants Res 2018;29(15 suppl):32–49.
100. Giannobile WV, Jung RE, Schwarz F, Groups of the 2nd Osteology Foundation Consensus Meeting. Evidence-based knowledge on the aesthetics and maintenance of peri-implant soft tissues: Osteology Foundation Consensus Report Part 1—Effects of soft tissue augmentation procedures on the maintenance of peri-implant soft tissue health. Clin Oral Implants Res 2018;29(15 suppl):7–10.
101. Monje A, Blasi G. Significance of keratinized mucosa/gingiva on peri-implant and adjacent periodontal conditions in erratic maintenance compliers. J Periodontol 2018;90:445–453.
102. Mellal A, Wiskott HW, Botsis J, Scherrer SS, Belser UC. Stimulating effect of implant loading on surrounding bone. Comparison of three numerical models and validation by in vivo data. Clin Oral Implants Res 2004;15:239–248.
103. Frost HM. A 2003 update of bone physiology and Wolff's Law for clinicians. Angle Orthod 2004;74:3–15.
104. Romeo E, Tomasi C, Finini I, Casentini P, Lops D. Implant-supported fixed cantilever prosthesis in partially edentulous jaws: A cohort prospective study. Clin Oral Implants Res 2009;20:1278–1285.
105. Romeo E, Lops D, Margutti E, Ghisolfi M, Chiapasco M, Vogel G. Implant-supported fixed cantilever prostheses in partially edentulous arches. A seven-year prospective study. Clin Oral Implants Res 2003;14:303–311.
106. Aglietta M, Siciliano VI, Zwahlen M, et al. A systematic review of the survival and complication rates of implant supported fixed dental prostheses with cantilever extensions after an observation period of at least 5 years. Clini Oral Implants Res 2009;20:441–451.
107. Aglietta M, Iorio Siciliano V, Blasi A, et al. Clinical and radiographic changes at implants supporting single-unit crowns (SCs) and fixed dental prostheses (FDPs) with one cantilever extension. A retrospective study. Clin Oral Implants Res 2012;23:550–555.
108. Storelli S, Del Fabbro M, Scanferla M, Palandrani G, Romeo E. Implant-supported cantilevered fixed dental rehabilitations in fully edentulous patients: Systematic review of the literature. Part II. Clin Oral Implants Res 2018;29(18 suppl):275–294.
109. Storelli S, Del Fabbro M, Scanferla M, Palandrani G, Romeo E. Implant supported cantilevered fixed dental rehabilitations in partially edentulous patients: Systematic review of the literature. Part I. Clin Oral Implants Res 2018;29(18 suppl):253–274.
110. Hammerle CHF, Cordaro L, Alccayhuaman KAA, et al. Biomechanical aspects: Summary and consensus statements of group 4. The 5th EAO Consensus Conference 2018. Clin Oral Implants Res 2018;29(18 suppl):326–331.
111. Chambrone L, Chambrone LA, Lima LA. Effects of occlusal overload on peri-implant tissue health: A systematic review of animal-model studies. J Periodontol 2010;81:1367–1378.
112. Kozlovsky A, Tal H, Laufer BZ, et al. Impact of implant overloading on the peri-implant bone in inflamed and non-inflamed peri-implant mucosa. Clin Oral Implant Res 2007;18:601–610.
113. Hürzeler MB, Quiñones CR, Kohal RJ, et al. Changes in peri-implant tissues subjected to orthodontic forces and ligature breakdown in monkeys. J Periodontol 1998;69:396–404.
114. Bashutski JD, D'Silva NJ, Wang HL. Implant compression necrosis: Current understanding and case report. J Periodontol 2009;80:700–704.
115. Grandi T, Garuti G, Guazzi P, Tarabini L, Forabosco A. Survival and success rates of immediately and early loaded implants: 12-month results from a multicentric randomized clinical study. J Oral Implantol 2012;38:239–249.
116. Marconcini S, Giammarinaro E, Toti P, Alfonsi F, Covani U, Barone A. Longitudinal analysis on the effect of insertion torque on delayed single implants: A 3-year randomized clinical study. Clin Implant Dent Relat Res 2018;20:322–332.
117. Li H, Liang Y, Zheng Q. Meta-analysis of correlations between marginal bone resorption and high insertion torque of dental implants. Int J Oral Maxillofac Implants 2015;30:767–772.
118. Safioti LM, Kotsakis GA, Pozhitkov AE, Chung WO, Daubert DM. Increased levels of dissolved titanium are associated with peri-implantitis: A cross-sectional study. J Periodontol 2017;88:436–442.
119. Daubert D, Pozhitkov A, McLean J, Kotsakis G. Titanium as a modifier of the peri-implant microbiome structure. Clin Implant Dent Relat Res 2018;20:945–953.
120. Pettersson M, Kelk P, Belibasakis GN, Bylund D, Molin Thorén M, Johansson A. Titanium ions form particles that activate and execute interleukin-1β release from lipopolysaccharide-primed macrophages. J Periodontal Res 2017;52:21–32.
121. Samelko L, Landgraeber S, McAllister K, Jacobs J, Hallab NJ. Cobalt alloy implant debris induces inflammation and bone loss primarily through danger signaling, not TLR4 activation: Implications for DAMP-ening implant related inflammation. PLoS One 2016;11:e0160141.
122. Souza JGS, Costa Oliveira BE, Bertolini M, et al. Titanium particles and ions favor dysbiosis in oral biofilms. J Periodontal Res 2020;55:258–266.
123. Suárez-López Del Amo F, Rudek I, Wagner VP, et al. Titanium activates the DNA damage response pathway in oral epithelial cells: A pilot study. Int J Oral Maxillofac Implants 2017;32:1413–1420.
124. Wang X, Li Y, Feng Y, Cheng H, Li D. Macrophage polarization in aseptic bone resorption around dental implants induced by Ti particles in a murine model. J Periodontal Res 2019;54:329–338.
125. Magone K, Luckenbill D, Goswami T. Metal ions as inflammatory initiators of osteolysis. Arch Orthop Trauma Surg 2015;135:683–695.
126. Esposito M, Grusovin MG, Polyzos IP, Felice P, Worthington HV. Timing of implant placement after tooth extraction: Immediate, immediate-delayed or delayed implants? A Cochrane systematic review. Eur J Oral Implantol 2010;3:189–205.
127. Esposito M, Grusovin MG, Coulthard P, Worthington HV. Different loading strategies of dental implants: A Cochrane systematic review of randomised controlled clinical trials. Eur J Oral Implantol 2008;1:259–276.
128. Hämmerle CH, Chen ST, Wilson TG Jr. Consensus statements and recommended clinical procedures regarding the placement of implants in extraction sockets. Int J Oral Maxillofac Implants 2004;19 suppl:26–28.
129. Huynh-Ba G, Oates TW, Williams MAH. Immediate loading vs early/conventional loading of immediately placed implants in partially edentulous patients from the patients' perspective: A systematic review. Clin Oral Implants Res 2018;29(16 suppl):255–269.

18

PERI-IMPLANT DISEASES

Alberto Monje, DDS, MS, PhD

Dental implants have been readily embraced by clinicians and researchers owing to their outstanding restorative properties and long-term success and survival rates. As such, over the last few decades, we have witnessed a significant increase in the number of implants placed every year as well as an increasing number of implant systems and models on the market. However, this explosive growth was disproportionally faster than the related clinical and scientific evidence. This has also resulted in an increasing prevalence of peri-implant diseases and a lack of predictable treatment protocols.

DEFINITIONS AND TERMINOLOGY

Peri-implant mucositis: Inflammatory lesion of the soft tissues surrounding an endosseous implant in the absence of loss of supporting bone or continuing marginal bone loss.[1]

Peri-implantitis: Pathologic condition occurring in tissues around dental implants, characterized by inflammation in the peri-implant mucosa and progressive loss of supporting bone.[2]

Diagnosis

The following considerations for diagnosis are based on the consensus report of workgroup 4 of the 2017 World Workshop on the Classification of Periodontal and Peri-implant Diseases and Conditions.[3]

- Health
  - Absence of clinical signs of inflammation
  - Absence of bleeding and/or suppuration on gentle probing (0.15 Ncm)
  - No increase in probing depth (PD) compared to previous examinations
  - Absence of bone loss beyond crestal bone level changes resulting from initial bone remodeling
- **Peri-implant mucositis**
  - Presence of bleeding and/or suppuration on gentle probing (0.15 Ncm)
  - Absence of bone loss beyond crestal bone level changes resulting from initial bone remodeling
- **Peri-implantitis**
  - Presence of bleeding and/or suppuration on gentle probing (0.15 Ncm)
  - PDs of 6 mm or more (Fig 18-1)
  - Bone loss 3 mm or greater apical to the most coronal portion of the intraosseous part of the implant

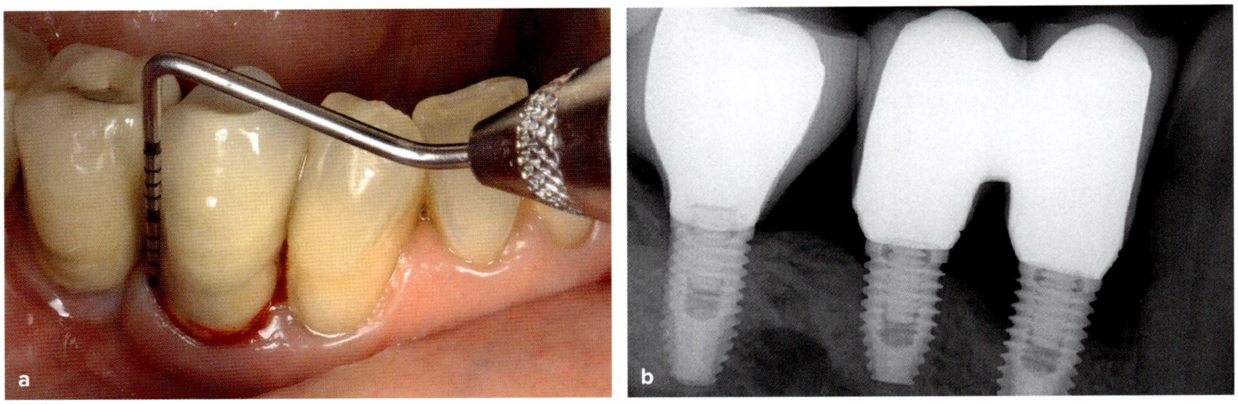

Fig 18-1 Example of peri-implantitis based on the presence of signs of inflammation with progressive bone loss beyond the physiologic bone remodeling. *(a)* Profuse bleeding on probing. *(b)* Radiographic bone loss.

The following are key considerations for the diagnosis and monitoring of peri-implant conditions:

- Probing around dental implants is not detrimental for the peri-implant tissue sealing.[4]
- Clinical parameters have shown to be accurate in diagnosing and monitoring peri-implant conditions.[5–9]
- Bleeding on peri-implant probing (BOP) does not seem to be very sensitive for peri-implant tissue breakdown; however, it is correlated with PD greater than 4 mm.[10]
- In smokers, BOP is less sensitive for tissue breakdown.
- Suppuration is not consistent in every peri-implantitis site (10% to 20% at the implant level).[11]
- The diagnosis should be made on a longitudinal basis; ie, a baseline radiograph should always be obtained at the time of definitive prosthesis delivery to monitor peri-implant bone loss.[2]
- Plastic probes might be helpful around restorations with difficult access (eg, overcontoured).
- If needed, the prosthesis should be removed for a more accurate diagnosis.
- The final diagnosis should be made by combining the clinical and radiographic features.
- The use of CBCT for the diagnosis of peri-implantitis may offer several advantages, including the assessment of lingual and buccal bone.

Prevalence

The prevalence of peri-implant diseases remains as a subject of controversy due to the heterogeneous case definitions used. Peri-implant mucositis is frequently observed (50% to 70%), while peri-implantitis is less common. Based on epidemiologic data, it could be stated that the prevalence of peri-implantitis at the patient level is overestimated roughly 2 times compared to the prevalence at implant level. Also, both peri-implant mucositis and peri-implantitis are site-specific phenomena (Table 18-1).[12–15]

Etiology

Peri-implant diseases are biofilm-mediated conditions occurring in susceptible patients. Mucositis is characterized by its reversibility at a biomarker level at 3 weeks and longer at a clinical level.[16] Peri-implantitis, like periodontitis, is an irreversible condition that includes peri-implant bone loss. In addition, a multitude of local and systemic factors are related to mucositis and peri-implantitis.

Risk Factors and Risk Indicators

PERI-IMPLANT MUCOSITIS

Given the reversibility of mucositis, data linking risk factors is scarce. Hence, most of the evidence is limited to retrospective and cross-sectional studies. According to the 2017 World Workshop on the Classification of Periodontal and Peri-implant Diseases and Conditions, biofilm accumulation, smoking, and radiation therapy have all been considered as risk factors or indicators for peri-implant mucositis.[1] Other potential risk factors have been suggested, including diabetes, lack of keratinized mucosa (KM), and presence of excess cement; however, further investigations and more evidence are required for

TABLE 18-1 Prevalence of peri-implant diseases

Systematic review	Prevalence (patient level)	
	Peri-implant mucositis	Peri-implantitis
Derks and Tomasi[12] (2015)	19%–65%	1%–47%
Monje et al[13] (2016)	40%–44%	13%–37%
Lee et al[14] (2017)	47%	20%
Rakic et al[15] (2018)	–	13%

–, not reported.

these factors. Lastly, other aspects such as the materials and surface characteristics of the restorative components, along with the design of the prosthesis, may also influence the occurrence of inflammation in the peri-implant tissues.

PERI-IMPLANTITIS

As occurs with the onset and progression of periodontitis, each individual has a different susceptibility to an inflammatory response around implants. Certain conditions may increase susceptibility, making an individual more prone to develop peri-implant diseases.

Risk factors

History of periodontitis. History of periodontitis has been regarded as the most determinant risk factor for the development of peri-implantitis. Karoussis et al showed that the 10-year incidence of peri-implantitis in patients with no history of periodontitis was 6% (at the implant level) compared to 29% in individuals with history of periodontitis.[17] Similarly, Roccuzzo et al followed 101 patients with dental implants after they were categorized as *(1)* not periodontally compromised, *(2)* moderately compromised, and *(3)* severely compromised.[18,19] The authors reported that both the frequency of implant sites demonstrating PDs of 6 mm or more and bone loss 3 mm or more differed significantly between groups: PD 6 mm or greater was 2% for group 1, 16% for group 2, and 27% for group 3; bone loss 3 mm or more was 5% for group 1, 11% for group 2, and 15% for group 3. Another investigation by Costa et al assessed the incidence of peri-implantitis over 5 years in individuals initially diagnosed with mucositis. In this study, patients with a history of periodontitis at the final examination were 9 times more likely to develop peri-implantitis when compared with individuals without periodontitis.[20]

Lack of regular peri-implant maintenance therapy and poor plaque control. There is also strong evidence linking peri-implant diseases with irregular compliance with supportive peri-implant maintenance therapy (PIMT). In a comparative 12-month study, it was found that PIMT every 4 months potentially reduces the risk of developing peri-implantitis (3.7% vs 22.7%) at the patient level.[21] Ferreira et al observed an 8.5% incidence of peri-implantitis at the implant level for patients attending maintenance appointments at least twice per year (≤ 6 months). The incidence was slightly higher at 9.3% for those who adhered to recall intervals once per year (> 6 months).[22] Monje et al also demonstrated that compliance with PIMT was associated with an 86% fewer incidence rate of peri-implantitis.[23] Rokn et al showed that, without a regular maintenance program, one out of five patients would experience peri-implantitis (though this was less frequent in tissue-level implants).[24] Lastly, a systematic review by Monje et al found that PIMT every 5 to 6 months was effective in minimizing the frequency of peri-implantitis.[13]

Tobacco smoking. According to the 2017 World Workshop, limited and conflicting evidence exists regarding the link between tobacco smoking and peri-implantitis.[2] Nevertheless, the effect of nicotine and tobacco byproducts at cellular and vascular levels seem to indicate that tobacco smoking should be cautiously examined as it might be linked with peri-implant diseases. As such, a practice-based cross-sectional study identified that smokers had an odds ratio of 3.8 for developing peri-implant mucositis and an odds ratio of 31.6 for peri-implantitis.[25] Likewise, a 9- to 14-year follow-up study demonstrated that smokers presented an odds ratio for developing

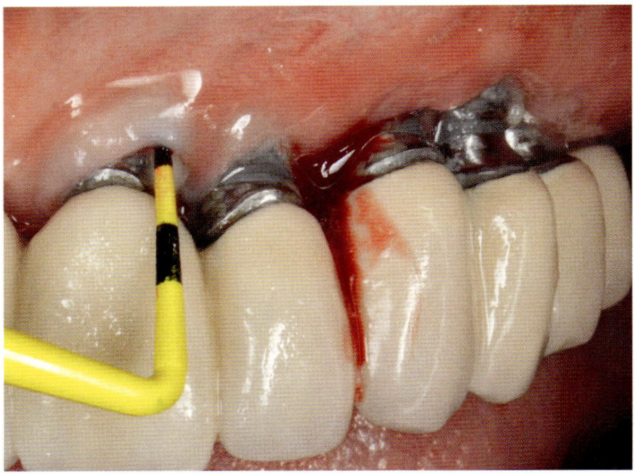

Fig 18-2 Keratinized mucosa plays a pivotal role in the development of peri-implantitis in those with erratic compliance to maintenance.

peri-implantitis of 7.7 compared to nonsmokers (odds ratio of 1) and to former smokers (odds ratio of 0.52).[26] In contrast, other reports demonstrated that smoking did not represent a risk factor for peri-implantitis as other confounding variables studied reached greater significance.[27,28]

Diabetes mellitus. Limited and inconclusive data are reported in the literature to link diabetes mellitus and peri-implant diseases.[2] However, a recent systematic review based on 12 studies detected that the risk of peri-implantitis was approximately 50% higher in diabetic patients than in nondiabetic patients (risk ratio = 1.46). Importantly, among nonsmokers, those with hyperglycemia had 3.39-fold higher risk for peri-implantitis compared to those with normoglycemia.[29]

Risk indicators

Aside from the previously mentioned factors, there is some limited evidence linking several other conditions to peri-implantitis. These include residual submucosal cement, lack of peri-implant keratinized tissue, and incorrect implant positioning.[2]

Residual cement. Residual cement has been associated with peri-implant diseases due to the inflammatory reaction originated by the cement itself and for the inherent roughness that might facilitate further biofilm accumulation. As such, in a landmark retrospective case analysis, 81% of peri-implantitis cases occurred in the presence of residual cement. Interestingly, it was also observed that after the cement was mechanically removed, 74% of these cases healed without further intervention.[30]

Lack of attached keratinized mucosa. The significance of KM on peri-implant conditions has been a subject of controversy for decades. Recent meta-analytic literature based on seven cross-sectional and four longitudinal human studies showed statistically significant differences in plaque index and modified plaque index, modified gingival index, mucosal recession, and attachment loss, all favoring implants with a wide band of KM.[31] Moreover, it has been demonstrated that KM plays a pivotal role in the development of peri-implantitis in those with erratic compliance to maintenance[32] (Fig 18-2). Contrarily, Wennström et al showed that the presence of KM might be negligible in individuals with adequate personal and professionally administered oral hygiene.[33]

Malpositioned implants. Numerous local predisposing (iatrogenic) factors have been shown to influence the onset of peri-implant diseases by hindering adequate oral hygiene measures (Table 18-2[34–37] and Figs 18-3 and 18-4).

Areas of future research

In addition to the multiple local and systemic conditions demonstrated to play a role in the development and progression of peri-implantitis, several other factors have been recognized that require additional research to further investigate the potential influence on this inflammatory disease. These factors include the following:

- Keratinized mucosa
- Excess cement
- Genetic factors
- Systemic conditions other than diabetes
- Occlusal overload
- Iatrogenic factors
- Titanium particles

Histopathologic Characteristics and Progression Pattern

HISTOPATHOLOGIC CHARACTERISTICS

Peri-implantitis and periodontitis lesions share some common characteristics. As such, similar to periodontitis, the lesions at peri-implantitis sites are also dominated by plasma cells and lymphocytes,[38–40] but they are

TABLE 18-2 Surgical and prosthetic predisposing factors for peri-implantitis

Local predisposing factor	Considerations
Prosthetic predisposing factors	• In single crowns, the emergence should always be reachable to clean, minimizing convex profiles (< 30 degrees)[34] (Fig 18-3). • In fixed hybrid prostheses, the prosthetic abutment or implant neck (tissue-level implants) should be exposed for better self-cleanability.[35]
Surgical predisposing factors (implant position)	• Implants positioned too buccally with thinner buccal bone often experience further bone loss after physiologic bone remodeling[36] (Fig 18-4). • Implants positioned too buccally often lack keratinized mucosa. • Implants positioned too lingually are often difficult to clean. • Implants positioned too mesially or distally often lead to greater interproximal bone loss and more plaque accumulation. • Insufficient thickness (< 1.5 mm) at the buccal aspect of dental implants during placement is associated with physiological bone loss of approximately 4 mm.[37] • Buccal bone thickness < 1.5 mm is associated with more rapid progression of peri-implantitis.[37]

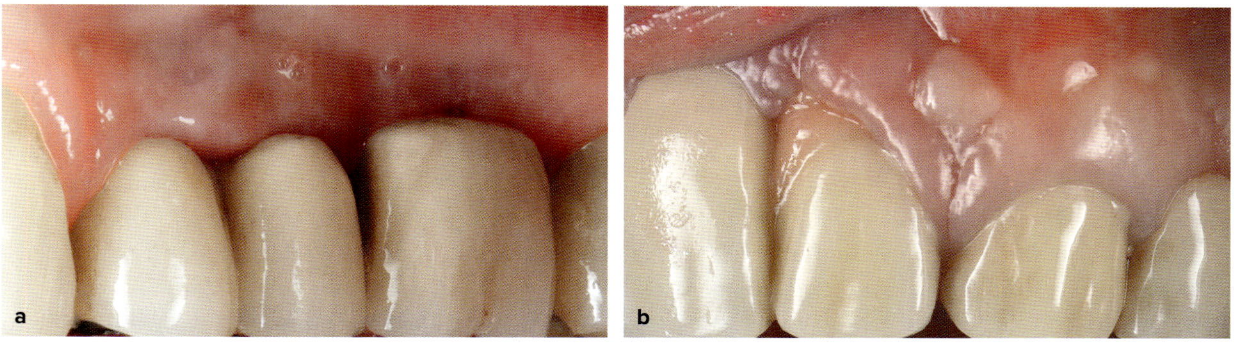

Fig 18-3 *(a and b)* Inadequate prosthesis designs often do not permit or significantly interfere with proper home oral hygiene measures.

characterized by a larger proportion of polymorphonuclear leukocytes and macrophages[41,42] (Fig 18-5). On the other hand, the size of a peri-implantitis lesion is more than twice as large as periodontitis sites (3.5 mm^2 vs 1.5 mm^2).[43] Also, peri-implantitis features a higher density of vascular structures outside and lateral to the cell infiltrate.[43] When compared with peri-implant mucositis, the lesions at peri-implantitis sites harbor more neutrophil granulocytes and larger proportions of B cells (CD19+).[44]

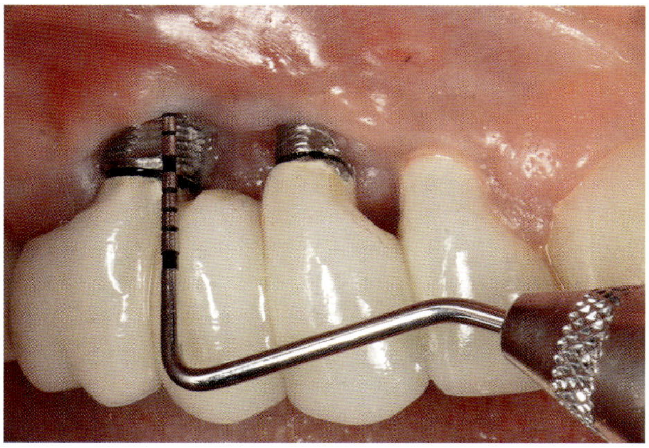

Fig 18-4 Implants placed too buccally often experience greater recession and bone loss.

ONSET AND PROGRESSION

Peri-implantitis presents with a nonlinear, accelerating pattern of bone loss.[45] These lesions are usually more aggressive and present with more rapid progression than periodontitis. The onset of peri-implantitis usually occurs within 3 years of function.[46]

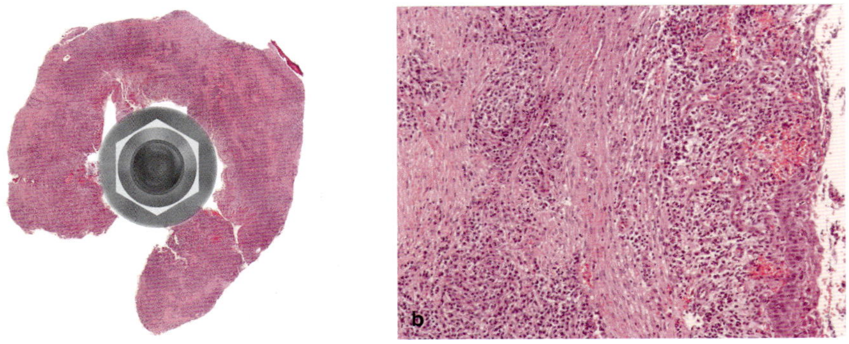

a b

Fig 18-5 *(a and b)* Peri-implant lesions are dominated by plasma cells and characterized by larger proportions of polymorphonuclear leukocytes and macrophages. (Courtesy of Prof Pablo Galindo-Moreno and Prof Francisco O'Valle-Ravassa.)

Prognosis

MUCOSITIS

Like gingivitis, peri-implant mucositis has shown to be reversible after mechanical treatment with or without adjunctive antimicrobial agents. Hence, the prognosis is favorable.

PERI-IMPLANTITIS

The management and prognosis of peri-implantitis are generally less predictable. Depending on the severity, extension, and morphology of the defect, peri-implantitis lesions can be managed very differently. The prognosis is linked to the patient's risk profile, the modification of the local predisposing factors, and the treatment approach.

Treatment

THERAPEUTIC CRITERIA FOR SUCCESS

- PD ≤ 5 mm
- Lack of BOP (excluding isolated areas as consequence of trauma)
- Lack of suppuration
- Arrestment of progressive bone loss

PREREQUISITES FOR TREATMENT

There are several aspects that can influence the outcomes of the treatment of peri-implant diseases. It is paramount to identify these factors before treatment can begin, and some factors may even require separate treatment or management during or before the treatment of the implant lesion itself. Examples include the following:

- Removal of local contributing factors (eg, prosthesis design)
- Conditioning of the soft tissues (eg, augment the band of KM; Fig 18-6)
- Modifying the patient's risk profile (eg, smoking, inadequate habits, oral hygiene education)
- Ascertainment of postoperative maintenance compliance

MUCOSITIS

The treatment of mucositis includes the utilization of a wide variety of instruments and adjunctive methods (Table 18-3). In general, the therapeutic outcome of peri-implant mucositis can be improved by using locally delivered antibiotics as an adjunct to mechanical debridement. However, the use of locally delivered agents alone is not effective. The adjunctive use of systemic antibiotics for the treatment of mucositis is yet to be elucidated.

PERI-IMPLANTITIS

Three main alternatives have been proposed for the treatment of peri-implantitis. Table 18-4 presents a summary of the most commonly employed techniques. The aim for the treatment of peri-implantitis is complete disease resolution, including lack of BOP, PD less than 5 mm, and no further loss of support (Fig 18-7).

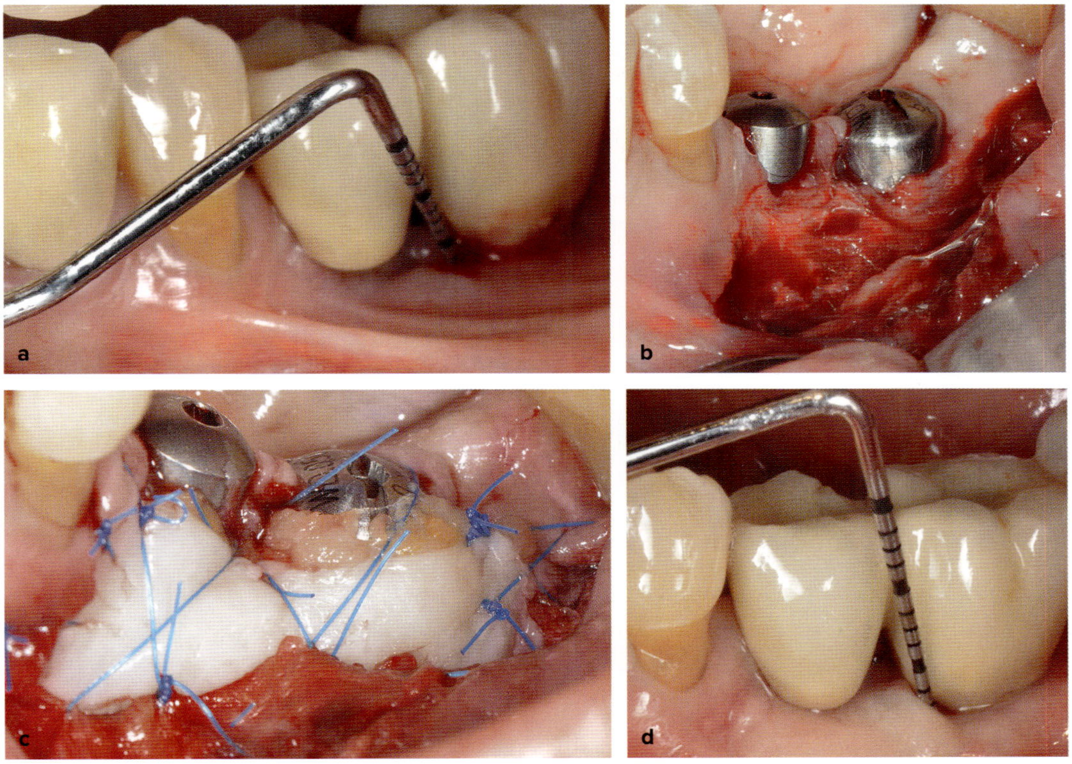

Fig 18-6 Clinical presentation of implants with signs of peri-implant inflammation. The KM will be augmented. *(a)* Profuse bleeding on gentle probing. *(b)* Partial-thickness flap. *(c)* Placement of thick free gingival graft. *(d)* Lack of BOP and increased band of KM.

TABLE 18-3 Treatment alternatives for peri-implant mucositis

Instrument	Types/materials	Description
Curette	Steel	High external hardness
	Titanium-coated	Similar hardness to implants
	Polytetrafluoroethylene	Weaker properties
	Carbon fiber	Softer than the implant surface
	Plastic	Flexible but fragile
Ultrasonic	Coated with polyetheretherketone (PEEK)	Stainless steel core to protect the instrument
Locally delivered agents	Antiseptics (chlorhexidine)	Subgingival irrigation of 0.06% to 0.12% as adjunct to mechanical debridement
	Antibiotics	Tetracycline fibers or doxycycline gel
Systemic antibiotics	Antibiotics	Amoxicillin, amoxicillin + metronidazole, or azithromycin

TABLE 18-4 Main treatment modalities for peri-implantitis

Therapeutic option	Advantages	Disadvantages
Nonsurgical debridement	• Minimal recession • Minimal postoperative discomfort	• Inefficient surface detoxification • Less predictable
Resective treatment with or without implantoplasty	• Pocket reduction or elimination • Surface modification	• Further loss of hard and soft tissues • Resection of KM
Reconstructive treatment	• Increased support • Pocket reduction	• Indication sensitive to defect containment • Preferable submerged healing

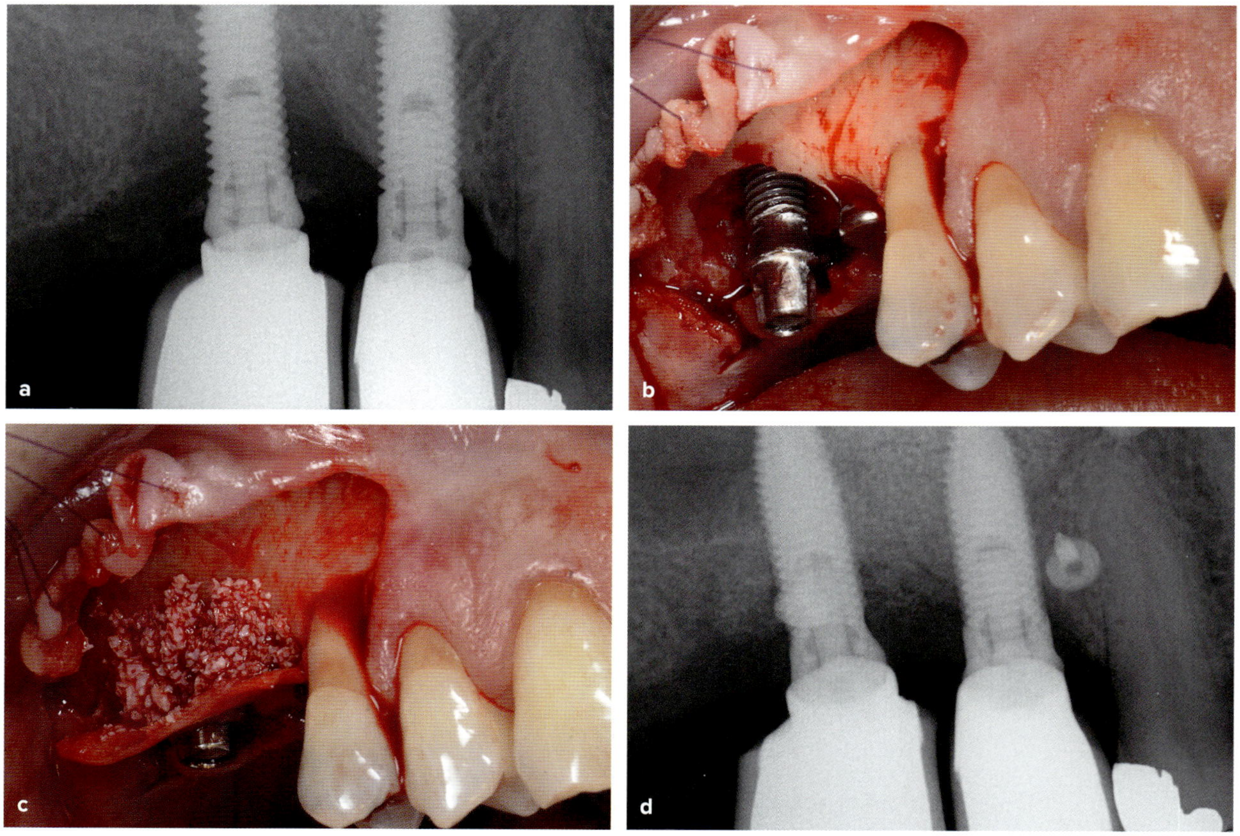

Fig 18-7 Peri-implantitis. *(a)* Periapical radiograph. *(b)* Flap after debridement of the peri-implant lesion. *(c)* Bone grafting with a 50-50 mix of autogenous bone and anorganic bovine bone. *(d)* Radiograph at 12-month follow up.

Peri-implant defect morphology

Defect severity and morphology also contribute to the decision-making process for the treatment of peri-implantitis. As such, the more contained the defect, the greater the repair capability. Two major defect types and five subtypes have been described by Schwarz and colleagues, as follows[47]:

TABLE 18-5 Treatment outcomes for peri-implantitis

Study	Method	Intervention	Main findings
Chambrone et al[49] (2018)	Surgical/nonsurgical	Photodynamic therapy	Photodynamic therapy may provide similar clinical improvements to conventional periodontal therapy for periodontitis and peri-implantitis.
Lin et al[50] (2018)	Surgical/nonsurgical	Lasers	Laser therapy in combination with surgical/nonsurgical therapy provides minimal clinical benefit in the treatment of peri-implant diseases.
Suárez-López del Amo et al[51] (2016)	Nonsurgical	Mechanical	Nonsurgical treatment is effective for peri-implant mucositis, while modest and unpredictable outcomes are expected for peri-implantitis lesions.
Schwarz et al[52] (2015)	Surgical/nonsurgical	Adjunctive measures	Mechanical debridement is effective for the treatment of peri-implant mucositis. Also, adjunctive measures may improve the efficacy of conventional nonsurgical therapy for peri-implantitis.
Khoshkam et al[53] (2016)	Surgical	Reconstructive	Regenerative treatment of peri-implantitis resulted in a mean radiographic defect fill of 2.41 mm after a minimum healing time of 36 months.
Schwarz et al[54] (2016)	Nonsurgical	Air polishing	Glycine powder air polishing is effective for the treatment of mucositis. Also, it may improve the efficacy of nonsurgical treatment of peri-implantitis.
Heitz-Mayfield and Mombelli[55] (2014)	Nonsurgical/surgical	Adjunctive measures	Favorable short-term outcomes are often reported. However, lack of disease resolution and progression or recurrence of disease as well as implant loss are also reported.
Chan et al[56] (2014)	Surgical	Adjunctive measures	The use of grafting materials and barrier membranes provided the greater reduction in probing depth and bone fill. However, there is a lack of high-quality comparative studies.
Khoshkam et al[57] (2013)	Surgical	Regenerative	Great variability has been reported in outcomes mainly attributed to patient factors, defect morphology, and the reconstructive methods used.

- Class I: Vertical component defect
  - Class Ia: Dehiscence-type defect
  - Class Ib: Two-wall defect
  - Class Ic: Three-wall defect
  - Class Id: Lack of buccal and oral bone plates
  - Class Ie: Circumferential defect
- Class II: Horizontal component defect

A modification from this classification on morphology and severity has been more recently proposed by Monje et al[48]:

- Class I: Intraosseous defect
  - Class Ia: Buccal dehiscence
  - Class Ib: Two- or three-wall defect
  - Class Ic: Circumferential defect
- Class II: Supracrestal/horizontal defect
- Class III: Combined defect
  - Class IIIa: Buccal dehiscence + horizontal bone loss
  - Class IIIb: Two- or three-wall defect + horizontal bone loss
  - Class IIIc: Circumferential defect + horizontal bone loss

In addition, peri-implantitis severity was classified as follows[48]:

- Grade S (slight): 3 to 4 mm or < 25% of the implant length

- Grade M (moderate): 4 to 5 mm or 25% to 50% of the implant length
- Grade A (advanced): > 6 mm or >50% of the implant length

Therapeutic outcomes

The outcomes of peri-implantitis treatment have been investigated after the employment of many different therapeutic approaches. Table 18-5 summarizes some of these investigations.[49–57]

Conclusion

The following conclusions can be obtained based on the currently available evidence. First, nonsurgical therapy should always precede surgical therapy; however, it is less predictable compared with surgical regenerative or resective approaches. Second, reconstructive therapy is plausible and effective as it may offer benefits regarding clinical attachment level gain and PD reduction. Nevertheless, resective therapy is also effective, although it is often accompanied by further loss of support. Third, the use of adjunctive measures such as lasers seems to be beneficial in certain scenarios. Last, the adherence to frequent supportive peri-implant maintenance therapy is crucial to prevent disease recurrence.

References

1. Heitz-Mayfield LJA, Salvi GE. Peri-implant mucositis. J Periodontol 2018;89(1 suppl):S257–S266.
2. Schwarz F, Derks J, Monje A, Wang HL. Peri-implantitis. J Periodontol 2018;89(1 suppl):S267–S290.
3. Berglundh T, Armitage G, Araujo MG, et al. Peri-implant diseases and conditions: Consensus report of workgroup 4 of the 2017 World Workshop on the Classification of Periodontal and Peri-implant Diseases and Conditions. J Clin Periodontol 2018;45(20 suppl):S286–S291.
4. Etter TH, Håkanson I, Lang NP, Trejo PM, Caffesse RG. Healing after standardized clinical probing of the perlimplant soft tissue seal: A histomorphometric study in dogs. Clin Oral Implants Res 2002;13:571–580.
5. Monje A, Insua A, Rakic M, Nart J, Moyano-Cuevas JL, Wang HL. Estimation of the diagnostic accuracy of clinical parameters for monitoring peri-implantitis progression: An experimental canine study. J Periodontol 2018;89:1442–1451.
6. Monje A, Caballé-Serrano J, Nart J, Peñarrocha D, Wang HL, Rakic M. Diagnostic accuracy of clinical parameters to monitor peri-implant conditions: A matched case-control study. J Periodontol 2018;89:407–417.
7. Fransson C, Tomasi C, Pikner SS, et al. Severity and pattern of peri-implantitis-associated bone loss. J Clin Periodontol 2010;37:442–448.
8. Fransson C, Wennström J, Tomasi C, Berglundh T. Extent of peri-implantitis-associated bone loss. J Clin Periodontol 2009;36:357–363.
9. Fransson C, Wennström J, Berglundh T. Clinical characteristics at implants with a history of progressive bone loss. Clin Oral Implants Res 2008;19:142–147.
10. Farina R, Filippi M, Brazzioli J, Tomasi C, Trombelli L. Bleeding on probing around dental implants: A retrospective study of associated factors. J Clin Periodontol 2017;44:115–122.
11. Ramanauskaite A, Becker K, Schwarz F. Clinical characteristics of peri-implant mucositis and peri-implantitis. Clin Oral Implants Res 2018;29:551–556.
12. Derks J, Tomasi C. Peri-implant health and disease. A systematic review of current epidemiology. J Clin Periodontol 2015;42(16 suppl):S158–S171.
13. Monje A, Aranda L, Diaz KT, et al. Impact of maintenance therapy for the prevention of peri-implant diseases: A systematic review and meta-analysis. J Dent Res 2016;95:372–379.
14. Lee CT, Huang YW, Zhu L, Weltman R. Prevalences of peri-implantitis and peri-implant mucositis: Systematic review and meta-analysis. J Dent 2017;62:1–12.
15. Rakic M, Galindo-Moreno P, Monje A, et al. How frequent does peri-implantitis occur? A systematic review and meta-analysis. Clin Oral Investig 2018;22:1805–1816.
16. Salvi GE, Aglietta M, Eick S, Sculean A, Lang NP, Ramseier CA. Reversibility of experimental peri-implant mucositis compared with experimental gingivitis in humans. Clin Oral Implants Res 2012;23:182–190.
17. Karoussis IK, Salvi GE, Heitz-Mayfield LJ, Brägger U, Hämmerle CH, Lang NP. Long-term implant prognosis in patients with and without a history of chronic periodontitis: A 10-year prospective cohort study of the ITI Dental Implant System. Clin Oral Implants Res 2003;14:329–339.
18. Roccuzzo M, Bonino F, Aglietta M, Dalmasso P. Ten-year results of a three arms prospective cohort study on implants in periodontally compromised patients. Part 2: Clinical results. Clin Oral Implants Res 2012;23:389–395.
19. Roccuzzo M, De Angelis N, Bonino L, Aglietta M. Ten-year results of a three-arm prospective cohort study on implants in periodontally compromised patients. Part 1: Implant loss and radiographic bone loss. Clin Oral Implants Res 2010;21:490–496.
20. Costa FO, Takenaka-Martinez S, Cota LO, Ferreira SD, Silva GL, Costa JE. Peri-implant disease in subjects with and without preventive maintenance: A 5-year follow-up. J Clin Periodontol 2012;39:173–181.
21. Aguirre-Zorzano LA, Vallejo-Aisa FJ, Estefanía-Fresco R. Supportive periodontal therapy and periodontal biotype as prognostic factors in implants placed in patients with a history of periodontitis. Med Oral Patol Oral Cir Bucal 2013;18:e786–e792.
22. Ferreira SD, Silva GL, Cortelli JR, Costa JE, Costa FO. Prevalence and risk variables for peri-implant disease in Brazilian subjects. J Clin Periodontol 2006;33:929–935.
23. Monje A, Wang HL, Nart J. Association of preventive maintenance therapy compliance and peri-implant diseases: A cross-sectional study. J Periodontol 2017;88:1030–1041.
24. Rokn A, Aslroosta H, Akbari S, Najafi H, Zayeri F, Hashemi K. Prevalence of peri-implantitis in patients not participating in well-designed supportive periodontal treatments: A cross-sectional study. Clin Oral implants Res 2017;28:314–319.

25. Rinke S, Ohl S, Ziebolz D, Lange K, Eickholz P. Prevalence of periimplant disease in partially edentulous patients: A practice-based cross-sectional study. Clin Oral Implants Res 2011;22:826–833.
26. Roos-Jansåker AM, Lindahl C, Renvert H, Renvert S. Nine- to fourteen-year follow-up of implant treatment. Part II: Presence of peri-implant lesions. J Clin Periodontol 2006;33:290–295.
27. Renvert S, Aghazadeh A, Hallström H, Persson GR. Factors related to peri-implantitis: A retrospective study. Clin Oral Implants Res 2014;25:522–529.
28. Marrone A, Lasserre J, Bercy P, Brecx MC. Prevalence and risk factors for peri-implant disease in Belgian adults. Clin Oral Implants Res 2013;24:934–940.
29. Monje A, Catena A, Borgnakke WS. Association between diabetes mellitus/hyperglycaemia and peri-implant diseases: Systematic review and meta-analysis. J Clin Periodontol 2017;44:636–648.
30. Wilson TG Jr. The positive relationship between excess cement and peri-implant disease: A prospective clinical endoscopic study. J Periodontol 2009;80:1388–1392.
31. Lin GH, Chan HL, Wang HL. The significance of keratinized mucosa on implant health: A systematic review. J Periodontol 2013;84:1755–1767.
32. Monje A, Blasi G. Significance of keratinized mucosa/gingiva on peri-implant and adjacent periodontal conditions in erratic maintenance compliers. J Periodontol 2019;90:445–453.
33. Wennström JL, Bengazi F, Lekholm U. The influence of the masticatory mucosa on the peri-implant soft tissue condition. Clin Oral Implants Res 1994;5:1–8.
34. Katafuchi M, Weinstein BF, Leroux BG, Chen YW, Daubert DM. Restoration contour is a risk indicator for peri-implantitis: A cross-sectional radiographic analysis. J Clin Periodontol 2018;45:225–232.
35. Serino G, Ström C. Peri-implantitis in partially edentulous patients: Association with inadequate plaque control. Clin Oral Implants Res 2009;20:169–174.
36. Spray JR, Black CG, Morris HF, Ochi S. The influence of bone thickness on facial marginal bone response: Stage 1 placement through stage 2 uncovering. Ann Periodontol 2000;5:119–128.
37. Monje A, Chappuis V, Monje F, et al. The critical peri-implant buccal bone wall thickness revisited: An experimental study in the beagle dog. Int J Oral Maxillofac Implants 2019;34:1328–1336.
38. Sanz M, Alandez J, Lazaro P, Calvo JL, Quirynen M, van Steenberghe D. Histo-pathologic characteristics of peri-implant soft tissues in Brånemark implants with 2 distinct clinical and radiological patterns. Clin Oral Implants Res 1991;2:128–134.
39. Bullon P, Fioroni M, Goteri G, Rubini C, Battino M. Immunohistochemical analysis of soft tissues in implants with healthy and peri-implantitis condition, and aggressive periodontitis. Clin Oral Implants Res 2004;15:553–559.
40. Cornelini R, Artese L, Rubini C, et al. Vascular endothelial growth factor and microvessel density around healthy and failing dental implants. Int J Oral Maxillofac Implants 2001;16:389–393.
41. Berglundh T, Zitzmann NU, Donati M. Are peri-implantitis lesions different from periodontitis lesions? J Clin Periodontol 2011;38(11 suppl):188–202.
42. Berglundh T, Gislason O, Lekholm U, Sennerby L, Lindhe J. Histopathological observations of human periimplantitis lesions. J Clin Periodontol 2004;31:341–347.
43. Carcuac O, Berglundh T. Composition of human peri-implantitis and periodontitis lesions. J Dent Res 2014;93:1083–1088.
44. Gualini F, Berglundh T. Immunohistochemical characteristics of inflammatory lesions at implants. J Clin Periodontol 2003;30:14–18.
45. Papantonopoulos G, Gogos C, Housos E, Bountis T, Loos BG. Peri-implantitis: A complex condition with non-linear characteristics. J Clin Periodontol 2015;42:789–798.
46. Derks J, Schaller D, Håkansson J, Wennström JL, Tomasi C, Berglundh T. Peri-implantitis—Onset and pattern of progression. J Clin Periodontol 2016;43:383–388.
47. Schwarz F, Herten M, Sager M, Bieling K, Sculean A, Becker J. Comparison of naturally occurring and ligature-induced peri-implantitis bone defects in humans and dogs. Clin Oral Implants Res 2007;18:161–170.
48. Monje A, Pons R, Insua A, Nart J, Wang H-L, Schwarz F. Morphology and severity of peri-implantitis bone defects. Clin Implant Dent Relat Res 2019;21:635–643.
49. Chambrone L, Wang HL, Romanos GE. Antimicrobial photodynamic therapy for the treatment of periodontitis and peri-implantitis: An American Academy of Periodontology best evidence review. J Periodontol 2018;89:783–803.
50. Lin GH, Suárez López del Amo F, Wang HL. Laser therapy for treatment of peri-implant mucositis and peri-implantitis: An American Academy of Periodontology best evidence review. J Periodontol 2018;89:766–782.
51. Suárez-López del Amo F, Yu SH, Wang HL. Non-surgical therapy for peri-implant diseases: A systematic review. J Oral Maxillofac Res 2016;7:e13.
52. Schwarz F, Schmucker A, Becker J. Efficacy of alternative or adjunctive measures to conventional treatment of peri-implant mucositis and peri-implantitis: A systematic review and meta-analysis. Int J Implant Dent 2015;1:22.
53. Khoshkam V, Suárez-López del Amo F, Monje A, Lin GH, Chan HL, Wang HL. Long-term radiographic and clinical outcomes of regenerative approach for treating peri-implantitis: A systematic review and meta-analysis. Int J Oral Maxillofac Implants 2016;31:1303–1310.
54. Schwarz F, Becker K, Bastendorf KD, et al. Recommendations on the clinical application of air polishing for the management of peri-implant mucositis and peri-implantitis. Quintessence Int 2016;47:293–296.
55. Heitz-Mayfield LJ, Mombelli A. The therapy of peri-implantitis: A systematic review. Int J Oral Maxillofac Implants 2014;29(suppl):325–345.
56. Chan HL, Lin GH, Suarez F, MacEachern M, Wang HL. Surgical management of peri-implantitis: A systematic review and meta-analysis of treatment outcomes. J Periodontol 2014;85:1027–1041.
57. Khoshkam V, Chan HL, Lin GH, et al. Reconstructive procedures for treating peri-implantitis: A systematic review. J Dent Res 2013;92:131S–138S.

19

HORIZONTAL BONE AUGMENTATION

Vahid Khoshkam, DDS, MS
Fernando Suárez López del Amo, DDS, MS

DEFINITIONS AND TERMINOLOGY

Membrane tack: A metal device used to stabilize a membrane by fixating it to the alveolar bone providing for stability.[3]

Particulate graft: A type of mineralized bone biomaterial (allogenic, xenogenic, or autogenous in nature) that has been processed or milled to include small particles of either cortical or cancellous or both types of bone, used for regenerative procedures.[3]

Ridge expansion: A surgical procedure, which increases the horizontal dimension of a narrow edentulous ridge in preparation for implant placement.[3]

Ridge split: A surgical procedure involving the use of one or more corticotomies in order to mobilize one or more bony segments for purposes of expanding an atrophic edentulous ridge in a faciolingual dimension. Typically, dental implants and/or bone graft materials are placed between the bony segments.[3]

A multitude of investigations have demonstrated that with adequate treatment planning and properly executed surgical procedures, implant-supported restorations can result in high survival and success rates. Similarly, numerous factors have been identified that are critical for the long-term stability of dental implants. In this sense, the detrimental effects of limited or compromised bone quantity have been investigated.[1,2] These studies demonstrated that the presence of adequate bone volume surrounding the intraosseous part of the implant is paramount for satisfactory long-term outcomes.

Currently, it is widely accepted that the correct positioning of dental implants is dictated by a prosthetically driven location. However, this prosthetically dictated 3D position can often differ from the area with the most abundant bone volume. In addition, trauma, tooth extraction, pathology, infections, and periodontitis, among others, will often result in insufficient or inadequate bone volume for implant placement. Consequently, procedures aiming at regenerating or increasing the preexisting bone topography have become increasingly popular over the last decades. This chapter focuses on horizontal bone deficiencies with emphasis on proper identification and classification systems, as well as the most current and commonly employed techniques and materials for horizontal bone augmentation.

Classifications

Over the last decades, several classifications have attempted to describe the different types of ridge deficiencies. A classic study in 1983 by Seibert[4,5] was the first to categorize these hard and soft tissue deficiencies into three groups as follows:

- Class I: Buccolingual loss of tissue with normal apicocoronal ridge height
- Class II: Apicocoronal loss of tissue with normal buccolingual ridge width
- Class III: Combination defects (ie, loss of height and width; Fig 19-1)

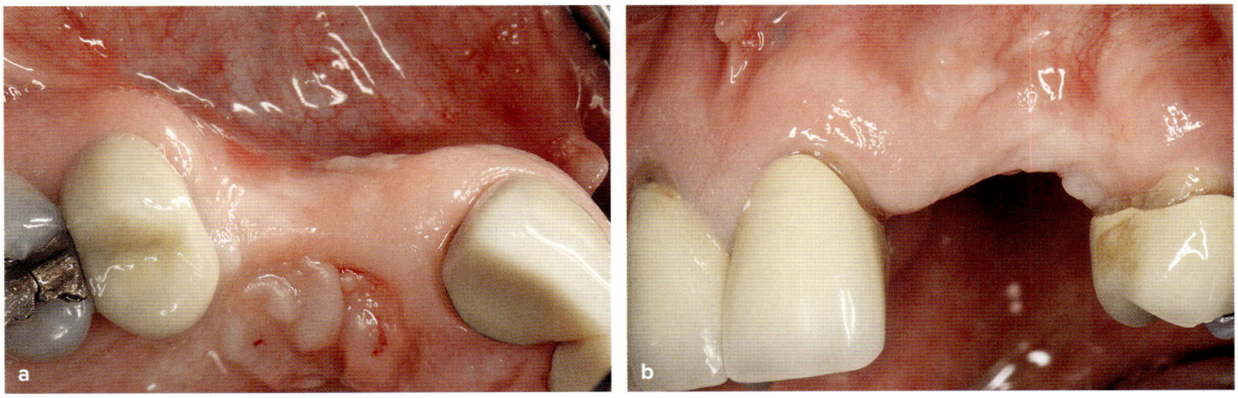

Fig 19-1 Example of Class III defect. *(a)* Horizontal deficiency. *(b)* Vertical deficiency.

Later on, Allen et al also described three different types of soft and hard tissue ridge defects: groups A, B, and C, for apicocoronal, buccolingual, and combination loss of tissue, respectively. In addition, these categories were further divided into mild, medium, and severe when defects were less than 3 mm, 3 to 6 mm, and greater than 6 mm, respectively.[6] Lekholm and Zarb[7] as well as Misch and Judy[8] also described different classifications for hard tissue defects ranging from ample bone volume to extremely resorbed ridges. Years later, in 2002, these classifications were modified by Wang and Al-Shammari[9] in an attempt to address some of the limitations previously encountered. This classification included three broad categories with the use of simpler terminology, referring to Seibert's Class I, II, and III defects as horizontal (H), vertical (V), and combination (C) defects, respectively. Each category was further subdivided into small (s, ≤ 3 mm), medium (m, 4 to 6 mm), and large (l, ≥ 7 mm). Lastly, a recent review[10] classified the horizontal defects based on prosthetically driven diagnostic protocols proposing also surgical alternatives. This classification included the following classes:

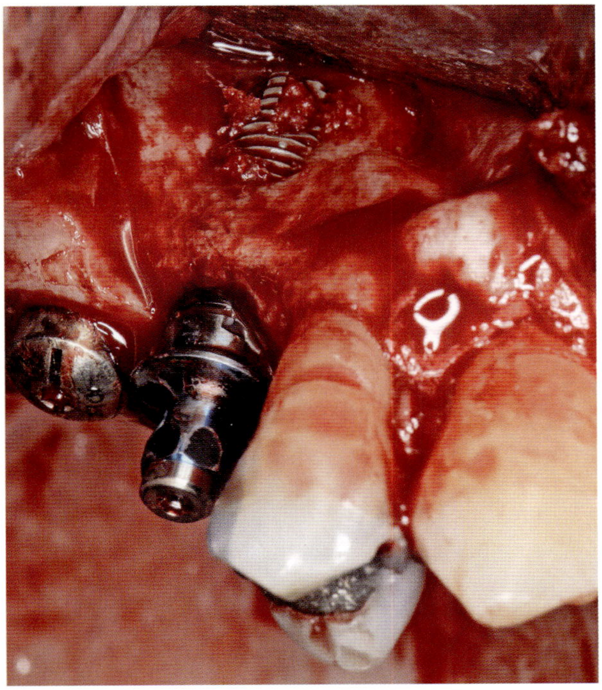

Fig 19-2 Class 2 defect.

1. Class 1: Favorable site for implant placement allowing for more than 1.5 to 2 mm of bone surrounding the fixture. There is no need for bone augmentation, although soft tissue grafting may be indicated to improve ridge contour.
2. Class 2: Moderate horizontal defect that allows for proper prosthetically driven implant positioning. However, simultaneous bone augmentation is required due to the presence of fenestration, dehiscence, and/or thin bony walls which could potentially compromise the long-term outcomes (Fig 19-2). Guided bone regeneration (GBR) is often used for these type of defects. Also, implants with a smaller diameter and/or the use of osteotomes could be considered. Similar to Class 1 defects, soft tissue augmentation can be performed in combination with the bone regenerative procedure.
3. Class 3: Significant horizontal deficiency precluding the placement of implants in the ideal position. Horizontal bone augmentation is indicated prior to implant placement. Many techniques and grafting materials can be used for the augmentative proce-

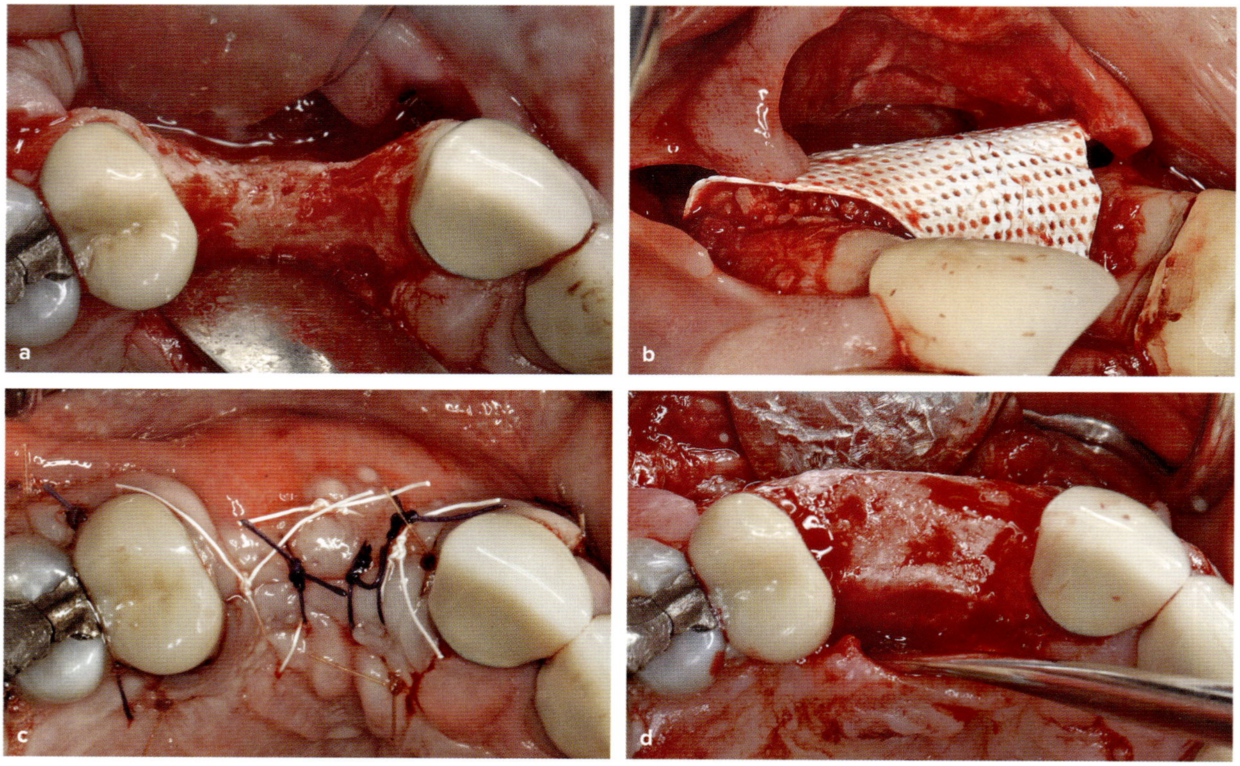

Fig 19-3 Vertical and horizonal bone augmentation procedure. *(a)* Bone atrophy. *(b)* Particulate bone allograft covered by stabilized nonabsorbable membrane. *(c)* Primary closure. *(d)* Reentry after 6 months.

dure. In addition, the use of diagnostic templates is recommended to ensure the augmentation of the future area for implant placement.

4. Class 4: Combined horizontal and vertical defect. In addition to the bone augmentation procedure, the use of pink porcelain could be considered.

Principles for Successful Bone Augmentation

The performance of successful bone augmentation procedures relies on a variety of principles that are applicable to both GBR and guided tissue regeneration (GTR) alike. These principles apply to almost all types of bone augmentation procedures regardless of the specific technique chosen. Moreover, while the selection of appropriate grafting materials and barrier membranes is critical to obtain successful outcomes, the use of adequate surgical protocols and proper flap manipulation are key for bone augmentation procedures. Similarly, proper case selection plays a critical role in bone regeneration.

In 2006, Wang and Boyapati reviewed the basic principles for bone regeneration and created the acronym *PASS* to emphasize the key components of these augmentative procedures. These principles included **p**rimary wound closure, **a**ngiogenesis, **s**tability, and **s**pace creation/maintenance[11] (Fig 19-3). *Primary wound closure* refers to the complete tension-free coverage of the surgical site that should be achieved and maintained during the entire healing process. Angiogenesis and adequate blood supply are fundamental for any regenerative procedure. Stability applies to different components of the surgical site, including the membrane, the blood clot, bone grafting material, and the dental implants. This stability should also be maintained over time. Lastly, space creation is necessary for the migration and proliferation of bone-forming cells while excluding unwanted cell populations from the regeneration site. Once again, the space created should also be maintained over time to allow for the slow process of bone formation.

Surgical Techniques

A large body of evidence suggests that surgical procedures for horizontal bone augmentation are highly predictable interventions, reporting high implant survival rates of 87% to 95% for fixtures placed simultaneously and 99% to 100% for implants placed following a staged approach.[12–14] A recent systematic review assessing horizontal ridge augmentation further confirmed that these procedures result in high survival and success rates (> 95%) for implants placed in augmented bone.[13]

Several strategies have been proposed to horizontally increase the alveolar bone, including but not limited to GBR,[15–18] block grafting,[19–21] and **ridge splitting/expansion**.[22–24] Although these three different treatment modalities can result in satisfactory outcomes, they present with significant differences with regard to indications, potential complications, morbidity, and resorption rate.[25]

GUIDED BONE REGENERATION

GBR is arguably the most researched and widely used treatment modality for horizontal bone augmentation.[25,26] Originally, this procedure was adapted by Nyman following the concept of GTR.[27] The biologic principle of GBR also depends on the use of barrier membranes to mechanically prevent the soft tissues from migrating into the osseous defect, allowing the cells with osteogenic potential to colonize the wound or defect. Membranes are also responsible for creating and maintaining the space for future bone augmentation. Thus, these barriers play a key role in GBR.

GBR can be performed alone or in combination with several other regenerative procedures. A recent systematic review[17] introduced a therapeutically oriented classification system for GBR describing three different types. *GBR I* was defined as the use of membranes and **particulate bone graft**. Next, the application of block grafts with an overlying membrane and particulate fillers was defined as *GBR II*. Lastly, the use of cortical bone blocks tented over a defect preserving particulate fillers was described as *GBR III*. As demonstrated by this review, GBR can be performed with a great variety of techniques and grafting materials as well as in combination with other regenerative approaches (eg, block grafts). Nevertheless, GBR procedures are most commonly performed with the sole use of bone grafts and barrier membranes. Hence, these two components represent some of the most critical aspects to be taken into consideration.

Barrier membranes

A variety of barrier membranes, including absorbable and nonabsorbable types, have been used for horizontal bone augmentation. These facilitate the most basic principle of GBR by creating new space for regeneration while excluding soft tissue infiltration. Barrier membranes physically separate the bone site or defect from the adjacent soft tissues. This newly formed space should be maintained over prolonged periods of time to allow for blood vessels and osteogenic cells to populate the area (Fig 19-4).

In general, absorbable membranes have been most widely used for horizontal augmentation, especially for the correction of small defects. These bioabsorbable barriers have several advantages, such as ease of handling and decreased complication rate compared with their nonabsorbable counterparts. In addition, if membrane exposures occur, these are usually relatively easy to manage with adequate disinfection. Absorbable membranes are classified into *natural* (xenogeneic collagen type I or III) that resorb by enzymatic degradation, or *synthetic*, made of polymers that resorb by hydrolysis[25,26] (Box 19-1). Their degradation rate, which depends on many factors (eg, membrane composition, pH, temperature, polymer crystallization degree, cross-linking) is variable, and it may interfere with the wound healing and bone regenerative outcomes.[28] Absorbable membranes usually lack sufficient rigidity to maintain space in noncontained bony defects, so they are most frequently used in combination with different bone grafting particles, serving as a scaffold that prevents the membrane from collapsing into the bone defect.[29] In order to achieve a greater degree of stability, absorbable membranes are frequently stabilized by screws, tacks, pins, and/or sutures[30] (Fig 19-5). Similarly, these barriers can be used in multiple layers to prolong their effectiveness.

The inability to preserve the barrier function for a prolonged period of time has been described as one of the major limitations of absorbable membranes.[25] However, studies have repeatedly shown success with these membranes. Interestingly, a recent preclinical study evaluated the healing after GBR in surgically created noncontained defects with bioabsorbable membranes and xenogeneic particulate grafting. Results revealed that from 4 to 14 days, there was a transition from coagulum and inflamed connective tissue to noninflamed connective tissue and small quantities of woven bone with remaining xenogeneic particles.[26] These findings demonstrate that in the presence of wound stability and adequate healing, the barrier function of absorbable membranes may not be needed for a long period of time.

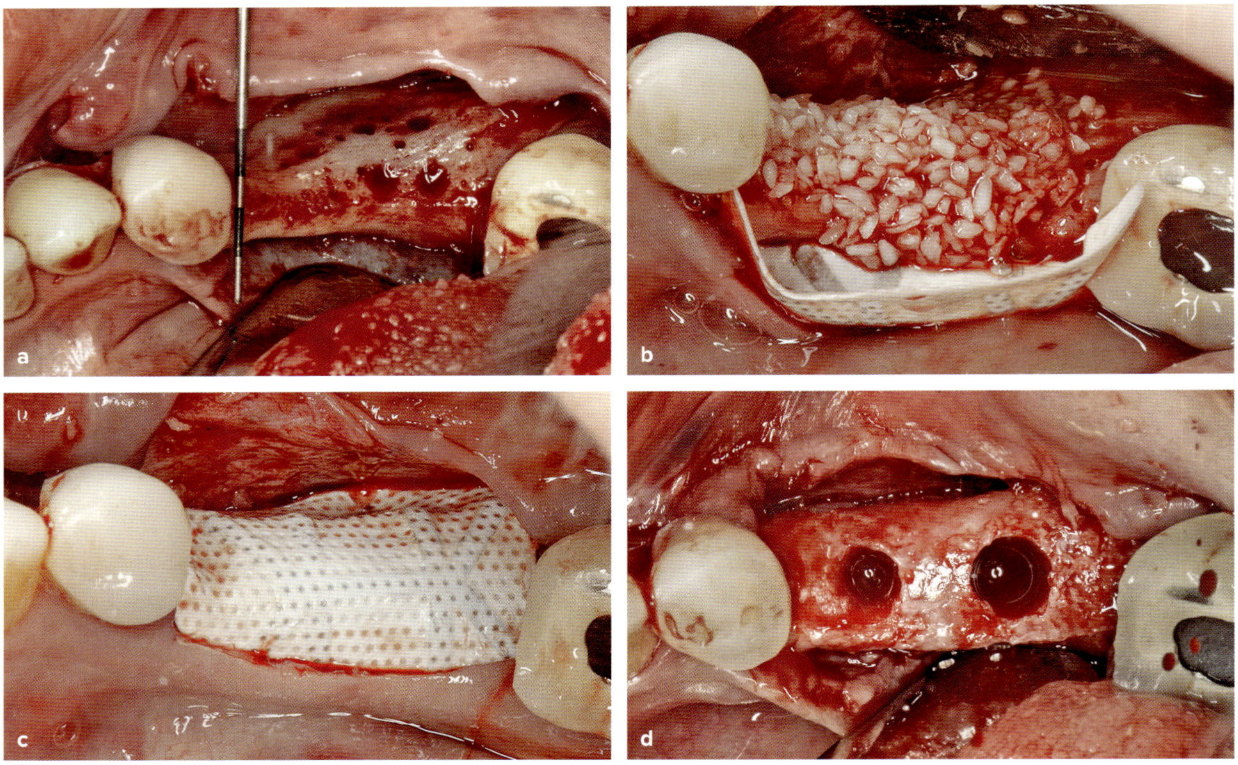

Fig 19-4 GBR. *(a)* Intraoperative view demonstrating ridge deficiency. *(b)* Grafting material. *(c)* Membrane adaptation. *(d)* Reentry after 6 months.

BOX 19-1 Different types of barrier membranes utilized in guided bone regeneration*

Nonabsorbable	Absorbable	
	Natural origin	Synthetic origin
• Expanded PTFE • Dense PTFE • Titanium mesh	• Native collagen • Cross-linked collagen • Freeze-dried fascia lata • Freeze-dried dura mater	• Polyglactin • Polyurethane • Polylactic acid • Polyglycolic acid • Polylactic acid/polyglycolic acid copolymers • Polyethylene glycol

PTFE, polytetrafluoroethylene.
*Adapted from Benic and Hämmerle.[25]

As mentioned previously, one of the main drawbacks of absorbable membranes is the lack of sufficient rigidity or space-making properties, often resulting in collapse into the bone defect. Consequently, the newly created space for bone formation can be compromised. Therefore, the use of a scaffold with particulate or block bone grafting materials is mandatory for both lateral and vertical bone augmentation procedures.[28]

The use of bioabsorbable membranes for horizontal bone augmentation has traditionally been proposed for smaller defects requiring limited bone augmentation.[10] Nevertheless, with the use of appropriate grafting techniques and materials providing tension-free primary wound closure and membrane fixation, Urban et al repeatedly demonstrated excellent clinical results with the use of absorbable membranes.[31–33] Results from these investigations demonstrated an average of 5 to 6 mm of lateral ridge augmentation with up to 10 mm of bone gain.

Nonabsorbable membranes or titanium meshes have also been frequently used in GBR.[25,34–36] These barriers in

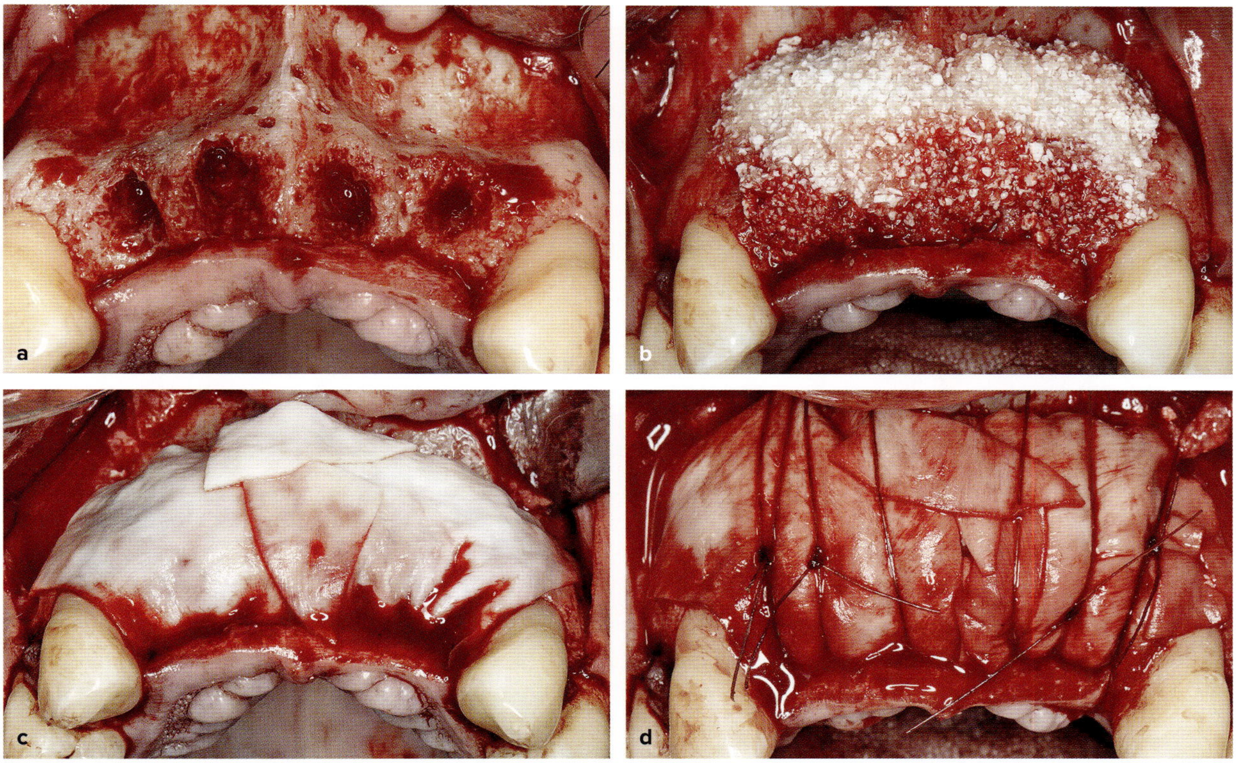

Fig 19-5 GBR with absorbable membrane. *(a)* Intraoperative view prior to grafting. *(b)* Particulate bone grafting. *(c)* Absorbable membranes over grafted area. *(d)* Stabilization of grafting material and membranes through periosteal sutures. (Courtesy of Dr Prashan Shanthakumar.)

general have been associated with a higher risk of early exposure and complications; therefore, their clinical usage has been typically limited to more advanced augmentative procedures requiring major bone reconstruction and/or vertical regeneration (Fig 19-6). Nevertheless, nonabsorbable membranes possess benefits such as sufficient rigidity that enables the maintenance of space for longer periods of time, usually until the membrane is removed. This superior stiffness compared to absorbable membranes typically results in significant bone augmentation if the basic principles of GBR are accomplished and complications do not arise.

Bone grafting materials

Bone grafting materials can be divided into four main groups based on their origin: autografts (same individual), allografts (same species, different individual), xenografts (different species), and alloplasts (synthetic; Table 19-1). See the "Bone Grafting Materials" section in chapter 11 and the "Grafting Alternatives" section in chapter 20 for more detailed information on each type. Currently, allografts, xenografts, and alloplasts are being produced with different forms and characteristics such as particles, block, moldable, and more. Bone graft substitutes for GBR need to meet the following criteria[25,37–39]:

- Biocompatibility
- Osteoconductivity
- Biodegradability
- Sufficient mechanical support for the membrane to create space for the newly formed bone
- Potential to be replaced with native bone

However, there is controversial information regarding the slow resorption rate of xenogeneic bone particles.[40,41] On the other hand, this slow resorption rate may be advantageous in some clinical scenarios to obtain long-term volumetric stability.[42–45]

Autogenous bone is arguably the best grafting material for bone augmentation due to its osteogenic, osteoinductive, and osteoconductive potential. Nevertheless, the patient's morbidity, limited availability, and (in some cases) unpredictable graft resorption represent important limitations of autogenous grafts.[46–48] Consequently,

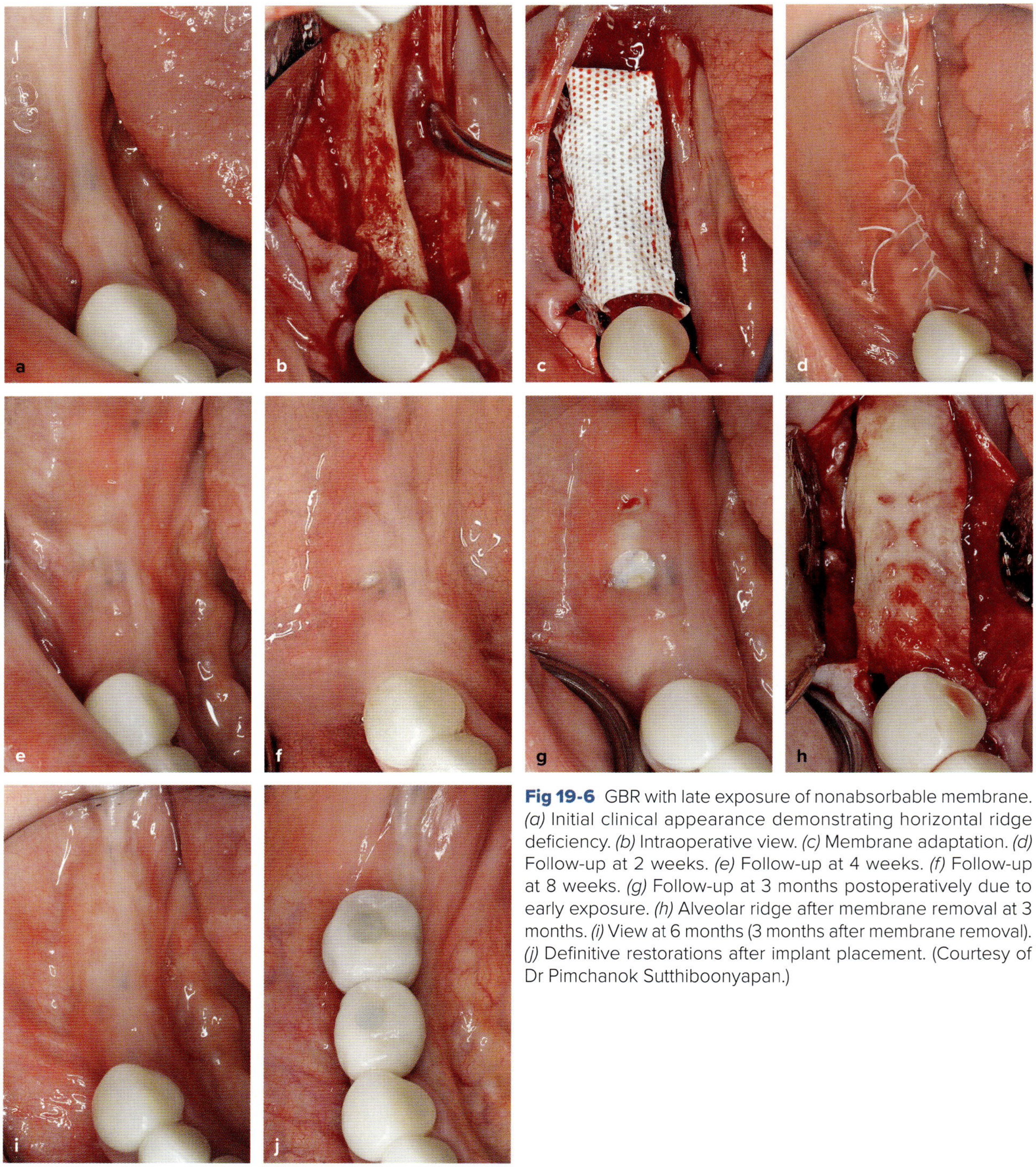

Fig 19-6 GBR with late exposure of nonabsorbable membrane. *(a)* Initial clinical appearance demonstrating horizontal ridge deficiency. *(b)* Intraoperative view. *(c)* Membrane adaptation. *(d)* Follow-up at 2 weeks. *(e)* Follow-up at 4 weeks. *(f)* Follow-up at 8 weeks. *(g)* Follow-up at 3 months postoperatively due to early exposure. *(h)* Alveolar ridge after membrane removal at 3 months. *(i)* View at 6 months (3 months after membrane removal). *(j)* Definitive restorations after implant placement. (Courtesy of Dr Pimchanok Sutthiboonyapan.)

TABLE 19-1 Bone grafting materials*

Grafting material	Source	Examples
Autograft	Same individual	• Intraoral (eg, mandibular ramus) • Extraoral (eg, iliac crest)
Allograft	Different individual, same species	• Freeze-dried bone • Demineralized freeze-dried bone
Xenograft	Different species	• Bovine • Equine • Porcine
Alloplast	Synthetically produced	• Tricalcium phosphate • Hydroxyapatite • Calcium phosphate cement • Calcium sulfate • Bioactive glass

*Adapted from Benic and Hämmerle.[25]

alternative grafting substitutes have been introduced as adjuncts or replacements for autogenous bone.[25,49] As an example, the combination of xenogeneic anorganic bovine bone mineral and autogenous particulate bone has been frequently employed with favorable clinical outcomes.[31,33] Similarly, the use of particulate bone allograft alone or in combination with autogenous bone has also been investigated.[50] It should be noted that most of the procedures for harvesting autogenous bone are technique sensitive and require significant surgical skills and experience.

Several investigations have shown successful results with prolonged periods of investigation after GBR.[49,51–53] Overall, the results obtained after correction of horizontal defects have been demonstrated to be relatively stable in the long term, providing high survival rates for the osseointegrated implants placed simultaneously or in a second stage.

Also, the available evidence suggests that GBR is a predictable treatment modality with both simultaneous or staged implant placement procedures. It is also less invasive than other techniques for horizontal bone augmentation, providing excellent outcomes with less morbidity and shorter treatment time in cases of simultaneous implant placement.[13]

BLOCK GRAFTING

Block grafts for horizontal ridge augmentation can be obtained from a variety of sources; however, autogenous bone blocks remain as the most widely studied and used source for this type of augmentation[14,54] (Fig 19-7). Similarly, block grafting with the adjunctive use of particulate bone grafts and membranes is a frequently used alternative. While bone blocks can be used for multiple scenarios, they are most typically applied for the correction of advanced ridge deficiencies and for the treatment of completely edentulous arches.[10]

With regard to the outcomes after horizontal ridge augmentation, multiple investigations have reported favorable results with the use of intraoral and extraoral autogenous block grafts.[49,55] A recent systematic review and meta-analysis by Elnayef et al demonstrated an overall mean gain at the time of regeneration of 4.18 ± 0.56 mm with the use of block grafts, compared to 3.61 ± 0.27 mm for GBR. Nevertheless, 6 months later, the estimated mean resorption was 0.75 ± 0.59 mm and 1.22 ± 0.28 mm for the block graft and GBR, respectively. Overall, both techniques presented with an estimated net bone gain of 2.86 ± 0.23 mm at the final evaluation.[56] The results from this investigation once again demonstrated block grafting and GBR as predictable and reliable techniques for horizontal ridge augmentation. It is important to mention that these results could have been influenced by the use of xenogeneic particulate grafting material as well as barrier membranes in combination with block grafting. Similarly, relatively short periods of investigation were analyzed, which could have also favored the outcomes of this approach. Lastly, implant survival rates after analyzing a total sample of 725 implants were 97% to 100%. On the other hand, the use of block grafting and, more specifically, autogenous bone blocks, also presents with

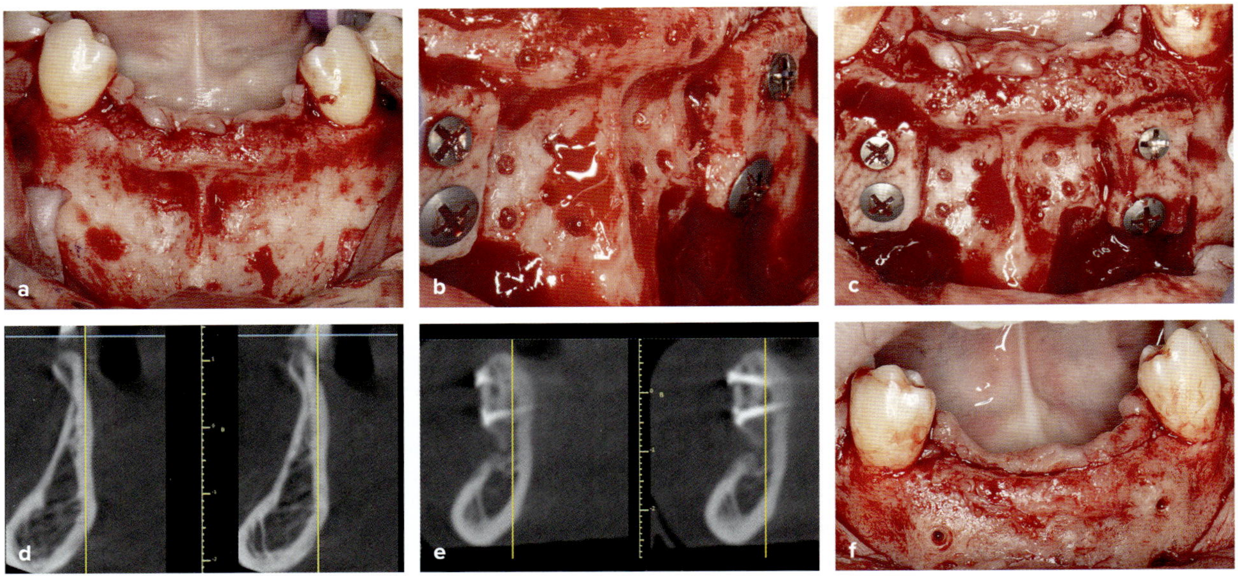

Fig 19-7 Symphysis bone block graft. *(a)* Intraoperative view demonstrating horizontal ridge deficiency. *(b)* Detailed view of stabilization and contact between block and recipient site. *(c)* Symphysis bone blocks stabilized in position for future implant placement. *(d)* Preoperative view. *(e)* Postoperative view. *(f)* Reentry after 6 months. (Courtesy of Dr Aaeshah Alkanderi.)

several disadvantages or limitations, including increased morbidity and surgical time, limited availability, and—in some scenarios—unpredictable graft resorption.

RIDGE SPLIT

Since the development of the technique during the 1990s, ridge or crest splitting techniques have been used as an alternative or in combination with GBR.[22,23] Through the use of different surgical instruments and devices, this procedure involves the longitudinal separation of the alveolar ridge and immediate placement of dental implants in between both cortical walls. This technique is also known as *ridge expansion* due to the separation of both cortical bony walls to augment the ridge.

Ridge splitting has been demonstrated as a predictable technique with a 95% to 97% implant survival rate. With regard to horizontal bone gain, a recent systematic review showed a mean gain of 3.2 mm for studies using ridge split with a full-thickness flap approach.[57] Although uncommon, the most prevalent complication was fracture of the buccal wall, followed by postoperative ridge resorption.[57]

Overall, ridge splitting has been demonstrated as a predictable alternative to GBR. However, due to the reduced indications and the potential for complications, the use of this technique remains limited.

TISSUE EXPANSION

In addition to the frequently used techniques for horizontal bone augmentation described previously, several other alternatives have been investigated to facilitate the reconstruction of ridge deficiencies and/or the placement of dental implants. In this sense, the use of a reshapable hydrogel for tissue expansion prior to the augmentative procedure has recently gained popularity.[58] Soft tissue expanders have been utilized as preaugmentation devices aiming at reducing complications by creating a larger amount of soft tissues.[59,60]

An animal investigation demonstrated successful expansion of the oral mucosa with 8.13 mm and 6.44 mm of linear oral mucosa gain for first and second insertion of the hydrogels, respectively.[61] Similarly, pilot human investigations have shown successful preliminary outcomes with 483.8 ± 251.7 mm^3 of mean soft tissue increase.[62]

Overall, this technique could significantly minimize the necessity for periosteal incisions, flap manipulation, and advancement during augmentative procedures, therefore reducing the potential for complications. While promising results have been shown so far, soft tissue expanders have been mainly investigated in preclinical trials, and their use in clinical practice is not advisable until further and larger clinical trials are conducted.

References

1. Spray JR, Black CG, Morris HF, Ochi S. The influence of bone thickness on facial marginal bone response: Stage 1 placement through stage 2 uncovering. Ann Periodontol 2000;5:119–128.
2. Grunder U, Gracis S, Capelli M. Influence of the 3-D bone-to-implant relationship on esthetics. Int J Periodontics Restorative Dent 2005;25:113–119.
3. American Academy of Periodontology. Glossary of Periodontal Terms. American Academy of Periodontology, 2001.
4. Seibert JS. Reconstruction of deformed, partially edentulous ridges, using full thickness onlay grafts. Part II. Prosthetic/periodontal interrelationships. Compend Contin Educ Dent 1983;4:549–562.
5. Seibert JS. Reconstruction of deformed, partially edentulous ridges, using full thickness onlay grafts. Part I. Technique and wound healing. Compend Contin Educ Dent 1983;4:437–453.
6. Allen EP, Gainza CS, Farthing GG, Newbold DA. Improved technique for localized ridge augmentation. A report of 21 cases. J Periodontol 1985;56:195–199.
7. Lekholm U, Zarb GA. Patient selection and preparation. In: Brånemark PI, Zarb GA, Albrektsson T (eds). Tissue-Integrated Prostheses: Osseointegration in Clinical Dentistry. Chicago: Quintessence, 1985:199–209.
8. Misch CE, Judy KW. Classification of partially edentulous arches for implant dentistry. Int J Oral Implantol 1987;4:7–13.
9. Wang HL, Al-Shammari K. HVC ridge deficiency classification: A therapeutically oriented classification. Int J Periodontics Restorative Dent 2002;22:335–343.
10. Chiapasco M, Casentini P. Horizontal bone-augmentation procedures in implant dentistry: Prosthetically guided regeneration. Periodontol 2000 2018;77:213–240.
11. Wang HL, Boyapati L. "PASS" principles for predictable bone regeneration. Implant Dent 2006;15:8–17.
12. Donos N, Mardas N, Chadha V. Clinical outcomes of implants following lateral bone augmentation: Systematic assessment of available options (barrier membranes, bone grafts, split osteotomy). J Clin Periodontol 2008;35(8 suppl):173–202.
13. Sanz-Sánchez I, Ortiz-Vigón A, Sanz-Martin I, Figuero E, Sanz M. Effectiveness of lateral bone augmentation on the alveolar crest dimension: A systematic review and meta-analysis. J Dent Res 2015;94(9 suppl):128S–142S.
14. Kuchler U, von Arx T. Horizontal ridge augmentation in conjunction with or prior to implant placement in the anterior maxilla: A systematic review. Int J Oral Maxillofac Implants 2014;(29 suppl):14–24.
15. Buser D, Dula K, Hirt HP, Schenk RK. Lateral ridge augmentation using autografts and barrier membranes: A clinical study with 40 partially edentulous patients. J Oral Maxillofac Surg 1996;54:420–432.
16. Hämmerle CH, Jung RE, Feloutzis A. A systematic review of the survival of implants in bone sites augmented with barrier membranes (guided bone regeneration) in partially edentulous patients. J Clin Periodontol 2002;29(3 suppl):226–231.
17. Khojasteh A, Kheiri L, Motamedian SR, Khoshkam V. Guided bone regeneration for the reconstruction of alveolar bone defects. Ann Maxillofac Surg 2017;7:263–277.
18. Dahlin C, Sennerby L, Lekholm U, Linde A, Nyman S. Generation of new bone around titanium implants using a membrane technique: An experimental study in rabbits. Int J Oral Maxillofac Implants 1989;4:19–25.
19. Misch CM, Misch CE. The repair of localized severe ridge defects for implant placement using mandibular bone grafts. Implant Dent 1995;4:261–267.
20. Verdugo F, Simonian K, D'Addona A, Pontón J, Nowzari H. Human bone repair after mandibular symphysis block harvesting: A clinical and tomographic study. J Periodontol 2010;81:702–709.
21. Monje A, Pikos MA, Chan HL, et al. On the feasibility of utilizing allogeneic bone blocks for atrophic maxillary augmentation. Biomed Res Int 2014;2014:814578.
22. Simion M, Baldoni M, Zaffe D. Jawbone enlargement using immediate implant placement associated with a split-crest technique and guided tissue regeneration. Int J Periodontics Restorative Dent 1992;12:462–473.
23. Vercellotti T. Piezoelectric surgery in implantology: A case report: A new piezoelectric ridge expansion technique. Int J Periodontics Restorative Dent 2000;20:358–365.
24. Chiapasco M, Ferrini F, Casentini P, Accardi S, Zaniboni M. Dental implants placed in expanded narrow edentulous ridges with the Extension Crest device. A 1–3-year multicenter follow-up study. Clin Oral Implants Res 2006;17:265–272.
25. Benic GI, Hämmerle CH. Horizontal bone augmentation by means of guided bone regeneration. Periodontol 2000 2014;66:13–40.
26. Sanz M, Ferrantino L, Vignoletti F, de Sanctis M, Berglundh T. Guided bone regeneration of non-contained mandibular buccal bone defects using deproteinized bovine bone mineral and a collagen membrane: An experimental in vivo investigation. Clin Oral Implants Res 2017;28:1466–1476.
27. Nyman S. Bone regeneration using the principle of guided tissue regeneration. J Clin Periodontol 1991;18:494–498.
28. Sanz M, Vignoletti F. Key aspects on the use of bone substitutes for bone regeneration of edentulous ridges. Dent Mater 2015;31:640–647.
29. Schenk RK, Buser D, Hardwick WR, Dahlin C. Healing pattern of bone regeneration in membrane-protected defects: A histologic study in the canine mandible. Int J Oral Maxillofac Implants 1994;9:13–29.
30. Urban IA, Lozada JL, Wessing B, Suarez-López del Amo F, Wang HL. Vertical bone grafting and periosteal vertical mattress suture for the fixation of resorbable membranes and stabilization of particulate grafts in horizontal guided bone regeneration to achieve more predictable results: A technical report. Int J Periodontics Restorative Dent 2016;36:153–159.
31. Urban IA, Nagursky H, Lozada JL. Horizontal ridge augmentation with a resorbable membrane and particulated autogenous bone with or without anorganic bovine bone-derived mineral: A prospective case series in 22 patients. Int J Oral Maxillofac Implants 2011;26:404–414.
32. Urban IA, Lozada JL, Jovanovic SA, Nagy K. Horizontal guided bone regeneration in the posterior maxilla using recombinant human platelet-derived growth factor: A case report. Int J Periodontics Restorative Dent 2013;33:421–425.
33. Urban IA, Nagursky H, Lozada JL, Nagy K. Horizontal ridge augmentation with a collagen membrane and a combination of particulated autogenous bone and anorganic bovine bone-derived mineral: A prospective case series in 25 patients. Int J Periodontics Restorative Dent 2013;33:299–307.
34. Buser D, Ingimarsson S, Dula K, Lussi A, Hirt HP, Belser UC. Long-term stability of osseointegrated implants in augmented bone: A 5-year prospective study in partially edentulous patients. Int J Periodontics Restorative Dent 2002;22:109–117.

35. Simion M, Jovanovic SA, Trisi P, Scarano A, Piattelli A. Vertical ridge augmentation around dental implants using a membrane technique and autogenous bone or allografts in humans. Int J Periodontics Restorative Dent 1998;18:8–23.
36. Chiapasco M, Abati S, Romeo E, Vogel G. Clinical outcome of autogenous bone blocks or guided bone regeneration with e-PTFE membranes for the reconstruction of narrow edentulous ridges. Clin Oral Implants Res 1999;10:278–288.
37. Jensen SS, Aaboe M, Pinholt EM, Hjørting-Hansen E, Melsen F, Ruyter IE. Tissue reaction and material characteristics of four bone substitutes. Int J Oral Maxillofac Implants 1996;11:55–66.
38. Fugazzotto PA. GBR using bovine bone matrix and resorbable and nonresorbable membranes. Part 2: Clinical results. Int J Periodontics Restorative Dent 2003;23:599–605.
39. Fugazzotto PA. GBR using bovine bone matrix and resorbable and nonresorbable membranes. Part 1: Histologic results. Int J Periodontics Restorative Dent 2003;23:361–369.
40. Berglundh T, Lindhe J. Healing around implants placed in bone defects treated with Bio-Oss. An experimental study in the dog. Clin Oral Implants Res 1997;8:117–124.
41. Mordenfeld A, Hallman M, Lindskog S. Tissue reactions to subperiosteal onlays of demineralized xenogenous dentin blocks in rats. Dent Traumatol 2011;27:446–451.
42. Chappuis V, Rahman L, Buser R, Janner SFM, Belser UC, Buser D. Effectiveness of contour augmentation with guided bone regeneration: 10-year results. J Dent Res 2018;97:266–274.
43. Jensen SS, Bosshardt DD, Gruber R, Buser D. Long-term stability of contour augmentation in the esthetic zone: Histologic and histomorphometric evaluation of 12 human biopsies 14 to 80 months after augmentation. J Periodontol 2014;85:1549–1556.
44. Buser D, Chappuis V, Kuchler U, et al. Long-term stability of early implant placement with contour augmentation. J Dent Res 2013;92(13 suppl):176S–182S.
45. Buser D, Chappuis V, Bornstein MM, Wittneben JG, Frei M, Belser UC. Long-term stability of contour augmentation with early implant placement following single tooth extraction in the esthetic zone: A prospective, cross-sectional study in 41 patients with a 5- to 9-year follow-up. J Periodontol 2013;84:1517–1527.
46. Cordaro L, Torsello F, Miuccio MT, di Torresanto VM, Eliopoulos D. Mandibular bone harvesting for alveolar reconstruction and implant placement: Subjective and objective cross-sectional evaluation of donor and recipient site up to 4 years. Clin Oral Implants Res 2011;22:1320–1326.
47. Nkenke E, Schultze-Mosgau S, Radespiel-Tröger M, Kloss F, Neukam FW. Morbidity of harvesting of chin grafts: A prospective study. Clin Oral Implants Res 2001;12:495–502.
48. von Arx T, Häfliger J, Chappuis V. Neurosensory disturbances following bone harvesting in the symphysis: A prospective clinical study. Clin Oral Implants Res 2005;16:432–439.
49. Cordaro L, Torsello F, Morcavallo S, di Torresanto VM. Effect of bovine bone and collagen membranes on healing of mandibular bone blocks: A prospective randomized controlled study. Clin Oral Implants Res 2011;22:1145–1150.
50. Caldwell GR, Mills MP, Finlayson R, Mealey BL. Lateral alveolar ridge augmentation using tenting screws, acellular dermal matrix, and freeze-dried bone allograft alone or with particulate autogenous bone. Int J Periodontics Restorative Dent 2015;35:75–83.
51. Jung RE, Glauser R, Schärer P, Hämmerle CH, Sailer HF, Weber FE. Effect of rhBMP-2 on guided bone regeneration in humans. Clin Oral Implants Res 2003;14:556–568.
52. Schneider D, Weber FE, Grunder U, Andreoni C, Burkhardt R, Jung RE. A randomized controlled clinical multicenter trial comparing the clinical and histological performance of a new, modified polylactide-co-glycolide acid membrane to an expanded polytetrafluorethylene membrane in guided bone regeneration procedures. Clin Oral Implants Res 2014;25:150–158.
53. Naenni N, Schneider D, Jung RE, Hüsler J, Hämmerle CHF, Thoma DS. Randomized clinical study assessing two membranes for guided bone regeneration of peri-implant bone defects: Clinical and histological outcomes at 6 months. Clin Oral Implants Res 2017;28:1309–1317.
54. Milinkovic I, Cordaro L. Are there specific indications for the different alveolar bone augmentation procedures for implant placement? A systematic review. Int J Oral Maxillofac Surg 2014;43:606–625.
55. Castagna L, Polido WD, Soares LG, Tinoco EM. Tomographic evaluation of iliac crest bone grafting and the use of immediate temporary implants to the atrophic maxilla. Int J Oral Maxillofac Surg 2013;42:1067–1072.
56. Elnayef B, Porta C, Suárez-López Del Amo F, Mordini L, Gargallo-Albiol J, Hernandez-Alfaro F. The fate of lateral ridge augmentation: A systematic review and meta-analysis. Int J Oral Maxillofac Implants 2018;33:622–635.
57. Elnayef B, Monje A, Lin GH, et al. Alveolar ridge split on horizontal bone augmentation: A systematic review. Int J Oral Maxillofac Implants 2015;30:596–606.
58. Asa'ad F, Rasperini G, Pagni G, Rios HF, Gianni AB. Pre-augmentation soft tissue expansion: An overview. Clin Oral Implants Res 2016;27:505–522.
59. Kaner D, Friedmann A. Soft tissue expansion with self-filling osmotic tissue expanders before vertical ridge augmentation: A proof of principle study. J Clin Periodontol 2011;38:95–101.
60. Mertens C, Thiele O, Engel M, Seeberger R, Hoffmann J, Freier K. The use of self-inflating soft tissue expanders prior to bone augmentation of atrophied alveolar ridges. Clin Implant Dent Relat Res 2015;17:44–51.
61. Garner J, Davidson DD, Barwinska D, et al. Reshapable hydrogel tissue expander for ridge augmentation: Results of a series of successive insertions at the same intraoral site. J Periodontol 2019;90:718–727.
62. Asa'ad F, Bellucci G, Ferrantino L, Trisciuoglio D, Taschieri S, Del Fabbro M. Preaugmentation soft tissue expansion: A report of four pilot cases. Case Rep Dent 2018;2018:3162617.

20

VERTICAL BONE AUGMENTATION

Arash Khojasteh, DDS, MS, PhD

Bone **atrophies** are frequently observed in the maxilla and mandible due to multiple different etiologies (eg, trauma, congenital deformities, periodontitis). Among these, the healing process of an extraction socket represents one of the most common reasons for deficient bone volume. This remodeling process often results in quantitative and qualitative alterations of the alveolar ridge.[1] In this sense, the 3D alveolar bone resorption causes vertical and horizontal deficiencies. To date, numerous techniques and grafting materials have been used for the reconstruction of the arches; among them, vertical bone augmentation remains as one of the most challenging approaches. In addition, vertical defects are often observed in combination with horizontal deficiencies.

This chapter summarizes the most commonly used techniques for vertical bone augmentation. The different techniques introduced to overcome vertically deficient ridges can be classified into three main approaches: *(1)* augmentative techniques, *(2)* anatomical repositioning of vital structures such as inferior alveolar nerve repositioning or sinus floor augmentation, and *(3)* **distraction osteogenesis** (DO). Augmentative techniques represent some of the most commonly performed approaches, and these may be subdivided into onlay and inlay techniques, as well as guided bone regeneration (GBR). In addition, augmentative techniques can be performed with a multitude of different grafting materials.

Determining Factors

Multiple factors play a role in the successful outcome of vertical bone augmentation procedures. These factors can be grouped into patient-related, operator-related, and surgical-related factors (Fig 20-1). Patient-related factors include the characteristics of the donor and recipient sites, as well as the local and systemic conditions. Operator-related factors include the surgical expertise, along with the selection of the technique and grafting material. Finally, surgical-related factors include proper manipulation of hard and soft tissues. Among all these factors, patient-related variables such as the morphologic

DEFINITIONS AND TERMINOLOGY

Atrophy: Diminution in size of a cell, organ, tissue, or part.[2]

Block graft: An autogenous or allogeneic bone graft in a block form used for augmentation of deficient bony ridges.[2]

Distraction osteogenesis: A vertical and volumetric bone augmentation procedure where new bone formation is created between two bony segments mobilized over time. It involves surgical access to the bone, separation of bony segments (either vertically or horizontally), and attachment and activation of distractors to bony segments that are being mobilized over time.[2]

Fixation screw: A mechanical device used to stabilize block grafts, membranes, and other devices by fixation to the alveolar bone.[2]

Titanium mesh: A nonocclusive barrier used in ridge augmentation procedures to provide space maintenance and graft containment.[2]

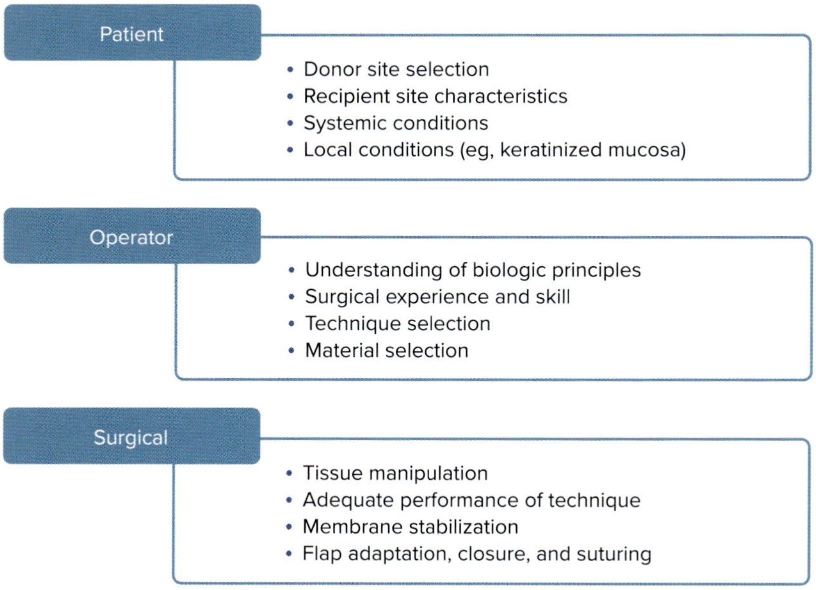

Fig 20-1 Determining factors in vertical bone augmentation.

characteristics of the recipient bone should be considered as essential elements in vertical bone augmentation.

A morphologic classification proposed by Tinti and Parma-Benfenati divided the jaw defects into vertical, horizontal, and combined defects.[3] In addition, Khojasteh et al[4] presented their classification based on the importance of the vertical bony walls and the width of the recipient site. When the recipient site has 2, 1, or 0 vertical walls, it is considered as class A, class B, or class C, respectively. The second feature considered in the current classification is the width of the base of the defect, which is divided into three groups: more than 5 mm, between 3 and 5 mm, and less than 3 mm for groups I, II, and III, respectively. Another potential factor affecting bone regeneration is the length of the edentulous span (ie, number of missing teeth), which can alter the surface area of a defect, ultimately influencing the degree of vascularization. Various studies have demarcated this factor by using terms such as *localized* or *extensive* ridge augmentation, although these have not been explicitly defined. Localized defects seem to pertain to areas missing a range of one to six teeth,[5,6] while extensive augmentations often indicate a fully edentulous jaw.[7]

Grafting Alternatives

Vertical bone augmentation can be performed with a great variety of different grafting materials and barrier membranes. Some of the most commonly used materials are autogenous bone blocks, xenografts, allografts, and sometimes biologic agents. These materials are also often used together, mostly with nonabsorbable membranes due to more rigid and longer lasting space maintenance capabilities compared with absorbable membranes. The following section summarizes some of the most commonly employed grafting materials for vertical bone augmentation. (See also the "Bone Grafting Materials" section in chapter 11.)

AUTOGENOUS

Autogenous bone can be harvested from intra- and extraoral donor sites. Although they were commonly used decades ago, extraoral donor sites have been decreasing in popularity in the periodontal field. The potential to use intraoral sites and the availability of allografting and xenografting materials have significantly reduced the need for extraoral harvesting. Nevertheless, these techniques are still commonly used in other fields. Autogenous grafts can be used as a block or in particulate form.

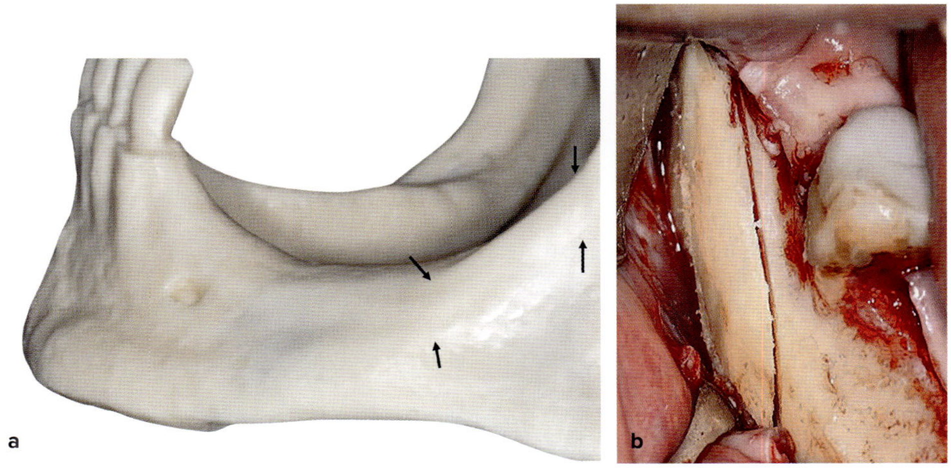

Fig 20-2 Mandibular lateral ramus. *(a)* Lateral ramus cortical bone. *(b)* Sulcular incision with distal crestal extension to harvest the block graft.

Extraoral donor sites

Extraoral sites were mainly used for the treatment of extensively atrophied ridges. Sources include the anterior and posterior iliac crest, calvaria, and anterior tibia bone. These grafts served as a nonvascularized free piece of corticocancellous bone for onlay or inlay techniques. Secondary bone resorption, increased patient morbidity, and limited availability remain as the main challenges in autogenous **block grafting**. In particular, the anterior iliac crest showed a resorption rate ranging between 20% to 92% after 10 years of follow-up.[8] In addition, significant postoperative complications could arise from these techniques, including but not limited to pain, iliac fractures, gate disturbances, hematoma, herniation of abdominal contents, vascular injury, nerve injury, unsightly contour defects along the iliac crest, and growth disturbances at young ages.[9] Today, extraoral bone harvesting is not used in the field of periodontics, although it is widely employed for other oral and maxillofacial purposes.

Intraoral donor sites

Although they have been decreasing in popularity in recent years due to the use of alternative grafting materials (eg, allografts, xenografts), intraoral donor sites remain widely used in the periodontal field. Areas for harvesting include the anterior palate, maxillary tuberosity, symphysis, and ramus. The anterior palate and the maxillary tuberosity are very rarely used as donor sites in periodontics.

Lateral ramus. The lateral mandibular surface area is the most popular source, providing blocks for bone augmentation. The external oblique ridge distal to the mandibular second molar represents the main anatomical area of this donor site (Fig 20-2). However, buccal shelf block grafts can also often provide sufficient bone to reconstruct alveolar defects of two to three teeth long (Fig 20-3). Horizontal and vertical defects up to 3 to 4 mm can be augmented with this donor site.[10] The dimensions of ramus cortical bone blocks are usually 4 mm (thickness) × 15 to 45 mm (length) × 10 to 15 mm (height), depending on the regional anatomy. The average buccal cortical plate thickness in dentate mandibles was 0.13 to 2.76 mm, whereas in edentulous posterior mandibles, it was 0.32 to 2.52 mm.[11] The bone is also primarily cortical in nature.[12]

As observed with blocks obtained from the symphysis area, the mandibular ramus also presents with resorption during the healing time. As such, 6 months after the regenerative procedure, a mean decrease of 23.5% and 42% has been reported for lateral and vertical augmentation, respectively.[13] The lateral ramus cortical bone can also be used in different forms (Fig 20-4).

Symphysis bone. Cortical or corticocancellous block grafts up to 4 cm in size can be harvested from the mandibular symphysis area. The mandibular symphysis as a donor site has been documented to provide sufficient bone to reconstruct alveolar ridge defects of about 15 mm in horizontal and up to 4 mm in vertical dimensions, usually covering edentulous spaces up to three teeth.[14] The bone block harvested from this site is usually 10 mm (height) × 15 to 17 mm (width) × 6 mm (thickness).[15] In general, the symphysis can provide over 50% larger graft volume in comparison to the lateral ramus region.[16] The typical symphysis corticocancellous graft consists of 65%

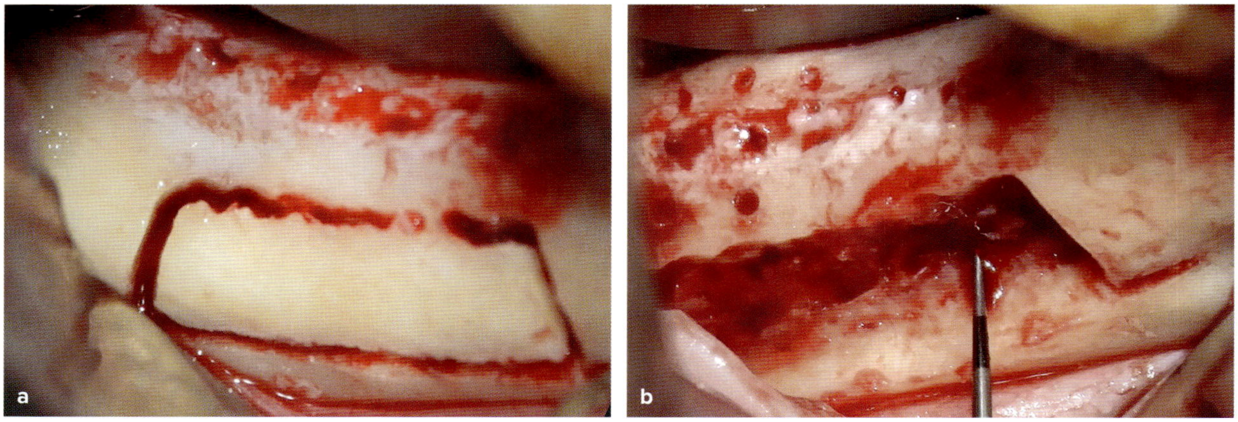

Fig 20-3 Buccal shelf as donor site. *(a)* Outline before harvesting. *(b)* Recipient bed after retrieval of bone block.

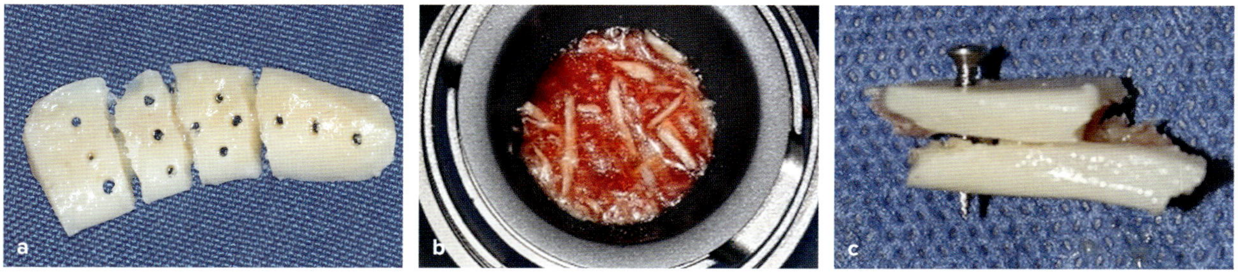

Fig 20-4 Lateral ramus cortical bone. *(a)* Bone graft sectioned and divided into four pieces of thin cortical plate. *(b)* Milled cortical particulate. *(c)* Double layer fixed with microscrew.

cortical and 36% cancellous bone.[15] There are three basic approaches to access the mandibular symphysis for bone graft harvesting: *(1)* sulcular, *(2)* attached gingiva, or *(3)* vestibular. For years, it was suggested that at least 5 mm of bone should be maintained below the teeth apices, around the mandibular inferior border, and bilaterally anterior to both mental foramina. When a large bone block is to be harvested, it is recommended to avoid the anterior-most portion of the symphysis, the mental protuberance. If necessary, two blocks from each side can be harvested, leaving a 3-mm midline connection to maintain support for the chin profile.[17] Although widely accepted and used for decades, with the 5-mm safety zone recommendation, the content of the mandibular incisive canal was endangered in 57% of the cases. There is also a risk of causing damage to the neurovascular bundles of the anterior dentition. Consequently, to minimize the risks related with this technique, Pommer et al more recently recommended a distance of 8 mm between the upper border of the harvesting site and the apices and limiting the depth of the block to 4 mm.[18]

XENOGRAFT

Xenografts are mostly obtained from bovine, porcine, or equine species. Deproteinized bovine bone mineral (DBBM) is considered one of the best suited substitutes for autogenous bone. DBBM is widely used in combination with autografts, and it is available in block and particulate forms. In a dog study, onlay grafted xenoblocks placed with the tunneling approach demonstrated 47% new bone formation in the posterior mandible.[19] In human trials, xenoblocks have been most often used with inlay techniques for posterior mandibular rehabilitation. The results showed success rates similar to autogenous bone (mean height gain = 5.48 mm).[20] A mixture of autogenous particulate bone and DBBM particulate in combination with GBR techniques has also been commonly used to treat vertical bone defects.[21]

ALLOGRAFT

Freeze-dried bone allograft (FDBA) and demineralized freeze-dried bone allograft (DFDBA) either in block or particulate forms have been used in numerous investigations. A case series with the use of particulate DFDBA and nonabsorbable membranes revealed a 4.1-mm increase in height in the posterior mandible.[22] Differences in vertical bone gain were not statistically significant when particulate FDBA or DBBM have been used in a mixture with autogenous particulate bone.[23]

BIOLOGIC AGENTS

Biologic agents stimulate a series of events including differentiation, migration, and proliferation. As an example, the migration of stem cells to the defect site or the ingrowth of new vessels creates a more favorable environment for bone regeneration. In periodontal therapy, and more specifically in vertical bone augmentation, a variety of biologic agents have been used.

Bone morphogenetic proteins

Recombinant human bone morphogenetic protein 2 (rhBMP-2) and rhBMP-7 have been reported as having regenerative potential in human and animal models. RhBMP-2 in combination with an absorbable collagen sponge (ACS) is the most commonly used recombinant protein in human bone regeneration studies.[24]

Although some clinical reports have been conducted for the reconstruction of large human critical defects such as alveolar clefts or mandibular continuity defects,[25] the lack of reliable data for the application in vertical bone augmentation as a sole agent in human models prevents the general use of rhBMP-2 with GBR methods. Nevertheless, Misch et al used a composite graft consisting of rhBMP-2/ACS and particulate mineralized bone allograft with **titanium mesh** in 15 patients. The average vertical bone gain was 8.53 mm.[26]

Platelet derivatives

Platelet-rich plasma (PRP), platelet rich in growth factor (PRGF), and platelet-rich fibrin (PRF) represent the three main categories of platelet-derived factors that have been used in regenerative medicine. Platelets play a fundamental role in hemostasis and are a natural source of growth factors, such as platelet-derived growth factor (PDGF), transforming growth factor β (TGF-β), insulinlike growth factor (IGF), and vascular endothelial growth factors (VEGF).[27]

Platelet derivatives in combination with different types of bone substitutes have shown positive effects on bone healing (eg, socket healing, sinus augmentation). However, these derivates have not demonstrated a significant benefit in vertical bone regeneration.[28] The use of PRF has also been investigated as a barrier membrane aiming at reducing graft resorption and promoting graft maturation. In this sense, the dimensional changes of intraoral block grafts covered with PRF and an absorbable membrane have been reported to be minimal.[29]

Cells

The use of embryonic stem cells is surrounded by ethical concerns. In addition, due to uncontrolled proliferation and differentiation rates, their use is not yet recommended in periodontics. On the other hand, adult mesenchymal stem cells (MSCs) derived from bone marrow aspirates have been frequently used as a cell source in bone tissue engineering. As such, MSCs showed promising results in posterior maxillary sinus augmentation.[30] Also, adipose tissue containing MSCs in a ratio of 1:2,000 (five times higher than bone marrow) represents an interesting source in plastic and reconstructive surgeries.[31] Farré-Guasch et al[32] isolated adipose-derived stem cells from the buccal fat pad and concluded that these cells have a similar phenotype to adipose-derived stem cells from the abdominal subcutaneous adipose tissue. Stem cells derived from the buccal fat pad in conjunction with iliac bone blocks showed an increase in the amount of new bone formation and a decrease in secondary bone resorption in extensively atrophic arches.[33] Also, buccal fat pad–derived cells, cultured over DBBM and protected with titanium mesh, showed 164.91 ± 3.74 mm^2 of new bone surface after horizontal and vertical defect reconstruction in the posterior mandible.[34]

Augmentation Techniques

Vertical augmentation of the atrophied arches has been extensively investigated by the use of different techniques including but not limited to GBR, blocks, and DO. Alternatively, the transposing of a vital anatomical structure (eg, inferior alveolar nerve lateralization) or different types of implants (eg, zygomatic) have also been studied. The following section focuses on the use of different augmentation techniques for vertical bone reconstruction.

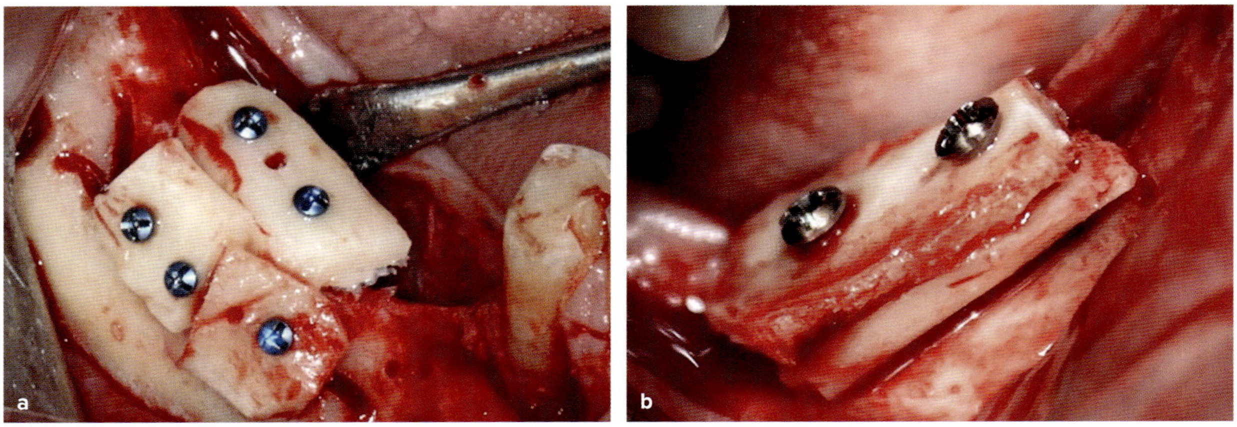

Fig 20-5 Onlay block grafting. *(a)* Multiple blocks obtained from the lateral ramus to treat a combination of horizontal and vertical defect in the posterior mandible. *(b)* Double-layered lateral ramus blocks for the treatment of a posterior mandibular vertical defect.

ONLAY GRAFTING

The use of onlay grafting techniques follows the same biologic principles as any other regenerative procedure. Among these principles, adequate primary stability is paramount, and it can be achieved through **fixation screws** or dental implants[35] (Fig 20-5). During the healing period, the grafted bone will be gradually replaced with new bone, and this process significantly depends on the revascularization from the recipient site.[24] Therefore, perforation of the recipient bed is also recommended to enhance angiogenesis and provide the regeneration site with osteogenic cells.[36]

For many years, autogenous blocks were considered as the gold standard for regeneration of atrophic arches. The different properties of this particular source of bone present with no comparison among all the different grafting materials. However, autogenous bone blocks also present with two main disadvantages: donor site morbidity and limited availability.[37] Hence, commercial allogeneic or xenogeneic blocks have been developed as alternatives.

Successful clinical application of these allogeneic or xenogeneic blocks has been reported in the literature[38–40]; however, further studies are required to histologically demonstrate new regenerated bone. Based on a retrospective study by Schwartz-Arad et al focused on the surgical success of intraoral autogenous onlay blocks for alveolar ridge augmentation, the average vertical gain was approximately 5.6 mm from the base of the vertical defect to the top of the onlay block. In addition, this study found no relationship between complications or failure rates and the type of bone source, the length of recipient site, or the recipient site area.[41] A recent systematic review on human trials reported vertical bone gain and complication rate to be 3.46 mm and 23.9%, respectively.[21]

During the last decades, different modifications to conventional augmentative methods have also been investigated. As such, onlay block bone grafting has been adapted by merging it with various concepts of GBR.[42] For instance, after fixing the block bone to the recipient site, DBBM or FBDA have been applied to fill the gap. An absorbable or nonabsorbable membrane is then used to cover the surgical site.

GUIDED BONE REGENERATION

One well-documented and highly successful procedure for augmenting the height and width of the atrophic arches is GBR by the application of cell occlusive membranes, which mechanically exclude nonosteogenic cell populations from the surrounding soft tissues.[43]

GBR can be further classified into three categories based on the materials and techniques: Type I is the use of space-maintaining membranes with particulate fillers, type II represents the application of bone blocks and particulate fillers with an overlying membranes, and type III is a cortical bone block tenting over a defect preserving particulate fillers.[44]

GBR type I

GBR type I refers to the use of either absorbable or nonabsorbable membranes over different kinds of bone substitutes alone or in conjunction with particulate autogenous bone. With regard to the clinical outcomes of this technique, one study reported a mean vertical defect fill of 5.63 mm in the group reconstructed with DBBM and polyethylene glycol hydrogel membrane and 4.25 mm with the use of DBBM plus collagen membrane.[45] A retrospective study reported 8.6 mm of vertical gain after the use of ramus bone, bovine bone particles, and PDGF.[46] When comparing expanded and dense polytetrafluoroethylene (ePTFE and dPTFE) membranes used in combination with a mix of autogenous and allograft bone, results demonstrated a mean vertical defect fill of 4.91 mm and 5.49 mm for ePTFE and dPTFE, respectively.[47] Nemcovsky and Artzi used GBR type I with absorbable membranes and reported 75.2% to 88.8% reduced defect height in the reconstruction of vertical defects larger than 3 mm and smaller than 7 mm.[48] Last, when compared with uncovered sites, the use of a membrane showed better results in the amount of bone gain in vertical defects.[49]

GBR type II

Type II refers to the application of bone blocks and particulate fillers with an overlying membrane. This technique is considered a modification of onlay bone grafting. The aim for the additional use of particulate bone substitutes is to compensate for the frequent resorption of the blocks. As such, these types of augmentative techniques usually employ xenogeneic or allogeneic bone with a barrier membrane. The most frequently used barriers for these procedures are absorbable collagen membranes. On the other hand, the bone blocks can be harvested from symphysis, ramus, retromolar area, or tuberosity.

With regard to the outcomes of implant therapy after the use of ramus and symphysis block grafts in combination with particulate autogenous bone and collagen membrane, an average marginal bone loss of 0.7 mm was observed after 12 months.[50] Similarly, Barone and Covani[51] used iliac block grafts and porcine bone particles in anterior and posterior maxillary defects smaller than 5 mm and showed a mean bone loss of 0.05 mm. Boronat et al chose intraoral blocks and particulate bone for similar defects, resulting in 0.64 mm mean bone loss after the first year of loading.[52]

GBR type III

In this technique, a thin cortical bone block from an intraoral donor site is used over a recipient bed to create a secured healing space for particulate bone. The key of this regenerative technique is exploiting the space created under the cortical bone block for protection of the particulate graft[53] (Fig 20-6). In fact, the thin cortical bone in this condition acts as an osteogenic membrane that provides a roof for a protected healing space. Also, it eliminates the pressure from the soft tissues to the particulate graft.[54] This augmentative technique is also considered as a modification of GBR and onlay bone grafting.

Khojasteh et al[55] reported both vertical and horizontal bone gain with the use of this technique. In this study, bone blocks were obtained from the ramus, chin, and tuberosity, in addition to allograft bone blocks. The authors also reported a 2.1% implant failure rate.[55] GBR type III has also been referred to in the literature as *osteogenic GBR* and *cortical autogenous tenting*. Lateral ramus and chin cortical bone are often used for this technique.

INLAY GRAFTING

A horizontal osteotomy with interposition of bone in the form of a sandwich, also known as *inlay*, was described in 1966 by Barros-Saint-Pasteur.[56] In this technique, the transposed segment can be fixed with miniscrews or miniplates, considering the crestal bone level of adjacent teeth and the available interarch space as the vertical limit for the mobilization of the osteotomized segment. Bone graft (block or particulate) fills the gap (Fig 20-7), which will eventually be replaced by new bone after the healing period.

Felice et al showed similar results with different types of bone blocks, suggesting the preferable use of heterologous blocks to avoid invasive procedures for harvesting autogenous bone.[20] Also, comparable results were found when using inlay bone grafting versus onlay xenografts with titanium mesh in vertical augmentation of the anterior maxilla.[57] Finally, similar volumetric changes were found when comparing onlay autogenous bone versus inlay xenogeneic grafts in the posterior mandible, reporting a vertical gain of 7.4 mm and 6.0 mm for the former and the latter, respectively.[58]

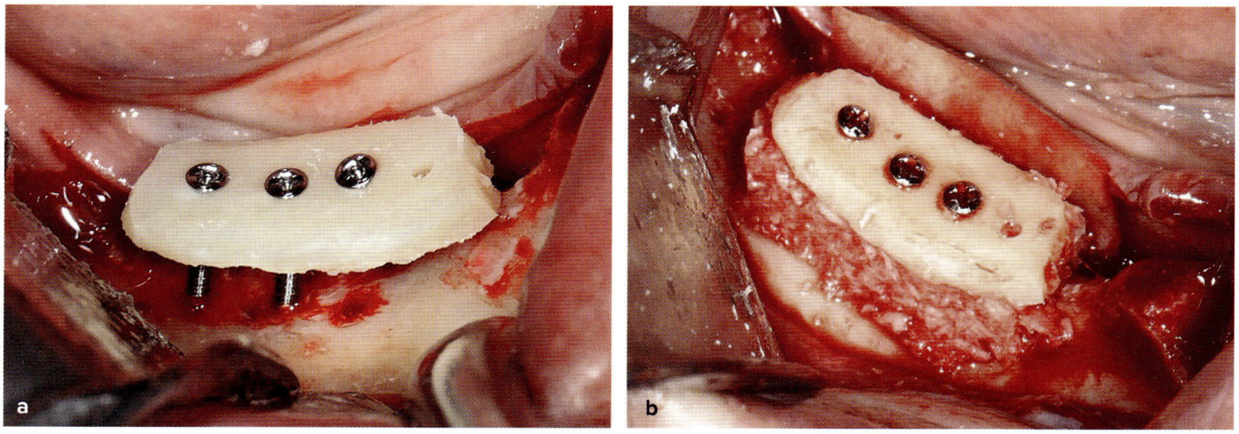

Fig 20-6 GBR type III. *(a)* Ramus block tented over the vertical defect in the posterior mandible. *(b)* Filling the space created by a mixture of autogenous particulate bone and bovine bone mineral.

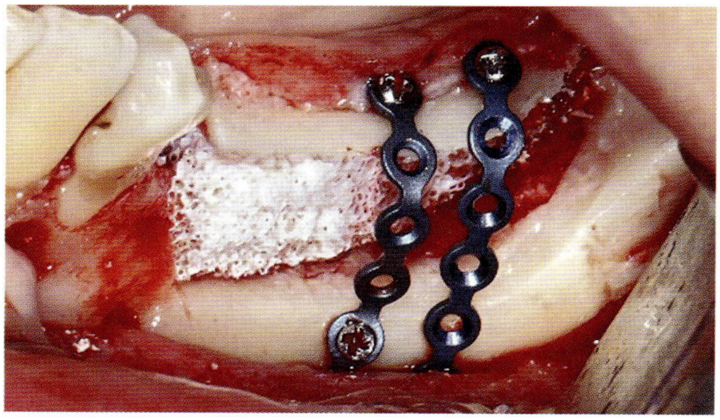

Fig 20-7 Example of the inlay technique.

Distraction Osteogenesis

DO, while first developed to correct deformities of the limbs,[59] is now a potential technique for vertical augmentation of atrophic ridges.[60] The biologic phenomenon occurring during DO allows for soft tissue expansion as well as bone regeneration. Therefore, more attached gingiva would be available with DO than with other augmentative procedures.[61] The basic principles involved in DO include a latency period of 7 days for initial postsurgical soft tissue wound healing, a distraction phase during which the two pieces of bone undergo gradual incremental separation at a rate of 1 mm per day, and a consolidation phase that allows bone regeneration in the created space.[60]

In an atrophic posterior mandible, DO is indicated for edentulous spans of three or more missing teeth when the vertical defect is more than 4 mm and a minimum of 6 to 7 mm of bone is available above the inferior alveolar nerve.[62]

A relatively large amount of vertical bone gain has been reported using this technique.[63] Nevertheless, sometimes a secondary augmentation is needed to increase bone width despite considerable vertical bone gain. DO has limited use for augmentation of the atrophic posterior mandible due to its disadvantages.[62] The most common complication with this technique is lingual inclination of the bone segment.[64] Other complications include relapse, tooth injury, nerve injury, distractor device failure, distraction chamber infection, fractures of distracted or basal bone, hypertrophic scarring, premature or delayed consolidation and fibrous nonunion, temporomandibular joint injury, and soft tissue dehiscences.[65]

Healing

Inflammation is the first phase of bone repair. Following the inflammatory phase, the endogenous stem and progenitor cells are recruited from local and distant sources to the site of injury. Immediately following the stabilization of bone substitutes in a protected healing space, macrophages also reach to the site. Dynamic changes to M2 macrophage cells are crucial following implantation of a biocompatible substitute in bone grafting procedures.[66] M2 macrophages produce a number of osteogenic growth factors, such as BMP-2, TGF-β, and osteopontin.[67] Hence, macrophages might be considered as responsible for guiding the bone healing process. A delicate flap elevation leaves the subgingival periosteum intact, and this can prevent high-speed epithelial cells from entering the wound. The periosteum is equivalent to a physical barrier that effectively prevents other soft tissues from invading, and it is also conducive to the supplement of bone cells.[68] Maintenance of a space under the periosteum as well as the stability of the grafted material are pivotal for successful bone regeneration.

Bone formation begins at week 2, and ostoclastic activity has been shown to be present between weeks 5 to 8 after cortical bone grafting. Histologic experiments revealed intramembranous bone formation without the presence of the cartilaginous tissue within or around the grafted tissue.[69] Perforating holes in the recipient bone (regional acceleratory phenomenon) can accelerate the migration of endogenous osteoprogenitors or bone marrow–derived MSCs.[70]

Complications

Vertical bone augmentation procedures have traditionally been related to higher complication rates than horizontal augmentation or guided tissue regeneration. While the biologic principles for bone regeneration are the same regardless of the specific characteristics of the defect, the higher level of complications could be related to the complexity of the procedures. In this sense, vertical bone augmentation often requires more technique-sensitive protocols. Also, the complication rate is influenced by the type of procedure, with a 47.3% complication rate for DO, 12.1% for GBR, and 23.9% for the use of bone blocks.[21] In a systematic review and meta-analysis,[21] the most commonly observed complication in the included investigations was graft and membrane exposure, with or without infection. Other complications included temporary paresthesia, additional grafting required, incomplete integration of the graft, and mandibular fracture, among others.

References

1. Araújo MG, Wennström JL, Lindhe J. Modeling of the buccal and lingual bone walls of fresh extraction sites following implant installation. Clin Oral Implants Res 2006;17:606–614.
2. American Academy of Periodontology. Glossary of Periodontal Terms. American Academy of Periodontology, 2001.
3. Tinti C, Parma-Benfenati S. Clinical classification of bone defects concerning the placement of dental implants. Int J Periodontics Restorative Dent 2003;23:147–155.
4. Khojasteh A, Morad G, Behnia H. Clinical importance of recipient site characteristics for vertical ridge augmentation: A systematic review of literature and proposal of a classification. J Oral Implantol 2013;39:386–398.
5. Jensen SS, Terheyden H. Bone augmentation procedures in localized defects in the alveolar ridge: Clinical results with different bone grafts and bone-substitute materials. Int J Oral Maxillofac Implants 2009;24(suppl):218–236.
6. Proussaefs P, Lozada J. Use of titanium mesh for staged localized alveolar ridge augmentation: Clinical and histologic-histomorphometric evaluation. J Oral Implantol 2006;32:237–247.
7. Iizuka T, Smolka W, Hallermann W, Mericske-Stern R. Extensive augmentation of the alveolar ridge using autogenous calvarial split bone grafts for dental rehabilitation. Clin Oral Implants Res 2004;15:607–615.
8. Baker RD, Terry BC, Davis WH, Connole PW. Long-term results of alveolar ridge augmentation. J Oral Surg 1979;37:486–489.
9. Bauer TW, Muschler GF. Bone graft materials. An overview of the basic science. Clin Orthop Relat Res 2000;(371):10–27.
10. Pikos MA. Block autografts for localized ridge augmentation: Part I. The posterior maxilla. Implant Dent 1999;8:279–285.
11. Leong DJ, Li J, Moreno I, Wang HL. Distance between external cortical bone and mandibular canal for harvesting ramus graft: A human cadaver study. J Periodontol 2010;81:239–243.
12. Misch CM. Use of the mandibular ramus as a donor site for onlay bone grafting. J Oral Implantol 2000;26:42–49.
13. Cordaro L, Amadé DS, Cordaro M. Clinical results of alveolar ridge augmentation with mandibular block bone grafts in partially edentulous patients prior to implant placement. Clin Oral Implants Res 2002;13:103–111.
14. Pikos MA. Mandibular block autografts for alveolar ridge augmentation. Atlas Oral Maxillofac Surg Clin North Am 2005;13:91–107.
15. Neiva RF, Gapski R, Wang HL. Morphometric analysis of implant-related anatomy in Caucasian skulls. J Periodontol 2004;75:1061–1067.
16. Misch CM. Comparison of intraoral donor sites for onlay grafting prior to implant placement. Int J Oral Maxillofac Implants 1997;12:767–776.
17. Toscano N, Shumaker N, Holtzclaw D. The art of block grafting: A review of the surgical protocol for reconstruction of alveolar ridge deficiency. J Implant Adv Clin Dent 2010;2:45–66.

18. Pommer B, Tepper G, Gahleitner A, Zechner W, Watzek G. New safety margins for chin bone harvesting based on the course of the mandibular incisive canal in CT. Clin Oral Implants Res 2008;19:1312–1316.
19. Xuan F, Lee CU, Son JS, Fang Y, Jeong SM, Choi BH. Vertical ridge augmentation using xenogenous bone blocks: A comparison between the flap and tunneling procedures. J Oral Maxillofac Surg 2014;72:1660–1670.
20. Felice P, Barausse C, Barone A, et al. Interpositional augmentation technique in the treatment of posterior mandibular atrophies: A retrospective study comparing 129 autogenous and heterologous bone blocks with 2 to 7 years follow-up. Int J Periodontics Restorative Dent 2017;37:469–480.
21. Urban IA, Montero E, Monje A, Sanz-Sánchez I. Effectiveness of vertical ridge augmentation interventions. A systematic review and meta-analysis. J Clin Periodontol 2019;46(21 suppl):319–339.
22. Fontana F, Santoro F, Maiorana C, Iezzi G, Piattelli A, Simion M. Clinical and histologic evaluation of allogeneic bone matrix versus autogenous bone chips associated with titanium-reinforced e-PTFE membrane for vertical ridge augmentation: A prospective pilot study. Int J Oral Maxillofac Implants 2008;23:1003–1012.
23. Chavda S, Levin L. Human studies of vertical and horizontal alveolar ridge augmentation comparing different types of bone graft materials: A systematic review. J Oral Implantol 2018;44:74–84.
24. Khojasteh A, Behnia H, Naghdi N, Esmaeelinejad M, Alikhassy Z, Stevens M. Effects of different growth factors and carriers on bone regeneration: A systematic review. Oral Surg Oral Med Oral Pathol Oral Radiol 2013;116:e405–e423.
25. Herford AS, Boyne PJ. Reconstruction of mandibular continuity defects with bone morphogenetic protein-2 (rhBMP-2). J Oral Maxillofac Surg 2008;66:616–624.
26. Misch CM, Jensen OT, Pikos MA, Malmquist JP. Vertical bone augmentation using recombinant bone morphogenetic protein, mineralized bone allograft, and titanium mesh: A retrospective cone beam computed tomography study. Int J Oral Maxillofac Implants 2015;30:202–207.
27. Anitua E, Andia I, Ardanza B, Nurden P, Nurden AT. Autologous platelets as a source of proteins for healing and tissue regeneration. Thromb Haemost 2004;91:4–15.
28. Plachokova AS, Nikolidakis D, Mulder J, Jansen JA, Creugers NH. Effect of platelet-rich plasma on bone regeneration in dentistry: A systematic review. Clin Oral Implants Res 2008;19:539–545.
29. Pripatnanont P, Thanakone P, Leepong N. Dimensional change and microstructure of intraoral bone block grafts covered with platelet-rich fibrin and a barrier membrane in ridge augmentation: A pilot investigation. Int J Periodontics Restorative Dent 2017;37:693–703.
30. Shayesteh YS, Khojasteh A, Soleimani M, Alikhasi M, Khoshzaban A, Ahmadbeigi N. Sinus augmentation using human mesenchymal stem cells loaded into a beta-tricalcium phosphate/hydroxyapatite scaffold. Oral Surg Oral Med Oral Pathol Oral Radiol Endod 2008;106:203–209.
31. Fraser JK, Wulur I, Alfonso Z, Hedrick MH. Fat tissue: An underappreciated source of stem cells for biotechnology. Trends Biotechnol 2006;24:150–154.
32. Farré-Guasch E, Martí-Pagè C, Hernádez-Alfaro F, Klein-Nulend J, Casals N. Buccal fat pad, an oral access source of human adipose stem cells with potential for osteochondral tissue engineering: An in vitro study. Tissue Eng Part C Methods 2010;16:1083–1094.
33. Khojasteh A, Sadeghi N. Application of buccal fat pad-derived stem cells in combination with autogenous iliac bone graft in the treatment of maxillomandibular atrophy: A preliminary human study. Int J Oral Maxillofac Surg 2016;45:864–871.
34. Khojasteh A, Hosseinpour S, Rezai Rad M, Alikhasi M, Zadeh HH. Buccal fat pad-derived stem cells with anorganic bovine bone mineral scaffold for augmentation of atrophic posterior mandible: An exploratory prospective clinical study. Clin Implant Dent Relat Res 2019;21:292–300.
35. Ozkan Y, Ozcan M, Varol A, Akoglu B, Ucankale M, Basa S. Resonance frequency analysis assessment of implant stability in labial onlay grafted posterior mandibles: A pilot clinical study. Int J Oral Maxillofac Implants 2007;22:235–242.
36. Pikos MA. Block autografts for localized ridge augmentation: Part II. The posterior mandible. Implant Dent 2000;9:67–75.
37. Scheerlinck LM, Muradin MS, van der Bilt A, Meijer GJ, Koole R, Van Cann EM. Donor site complications in bone grafting: Comparison of iliac crest, calvarial, and mandibular ramus bone. Int J Oral Maxillofac Implants 2013;28:222–227.
38. Araújo PP, Oliveira KP, Montenegro SC, Carreiro AF, Silva JS, Germano AR. Block allograft for reconstruction of alveolar bone ridge in implantology: A systematic review. Implant Dent 2013;22:304–308.
39. Waasdorp J, Reynolds MA. Allogeneic bone onlay grafts for alveolar ridge augmentation: A systematic review. Int J Oral Maxillofac Implants 2010;25:525–531.
40. Simion M, Rocchietta I, Dellavia C. Three-dimensional ridge augmentation with xenograft and recombinant human platelet-derived growth factor-BB in humans: Report of two cases. Int J Periodontics Restorative Dent 2007;27:109–115.
41. Schwartz-Arad D, Levin L, Sigal L. Surgical success of intraoral autogenous block onlay bone grafting for alveolar ridge augmentation. Implant Dent 2005;14:131–138.
42. von Arx T, Buser D. Horizontal ridge augmentation using autogenous block grafts and the guided bone regeneration technique with collagen membranes: A clinical study with 42 patients. Clin Oral Implants Res 2006;17:359–366.
43. Hammerle CH, Jung RE, Yaman D, Lang NP. Ridge augmentation by applying bioresorbable membranes and deproteinized bovine bone mineral: A report of twelve consecutive cases. Clin Oral Implants Res 2008;19:19–25.
44. Khojasteh A, Kheiri L, Motamedian SR, Khoshkam V. Guided bone regeneration for the reconstruction of alveolar bone defects. Ann Maxillofac Surg 2017;7:263–277.
45. Jung RE, Hälg GA, Thoma DS, Hämmerle CH. A randomized, controlled clinical trial to evaluate a new membrane for guided bone regeneration around dental implants. Clin Oral Implants Res 2009;20:162–168.
46. Funato A, Ishikawa T, Kitajima H, Yamada M, Moroi H. A novel combined surgical approach to vertical alveolar ridge augmentation with titanium mesh, resorbable membrane, and rhPDGF-BB: A retrospective consecutive case series. Int J Periodontics Restorative Dent 2013;33:437–445.
47. Ronda M, Rebaudi A, Torelli L, Stacchi C. Expanded vs dense polytetrafluoroethylene membranes in vertical ridge augmentation around dental implants: A prospective randomized controlled clinical trial. Clin Oral Implants Res 2014;25:859–866.
48. Nemcovsky CE, Artzi Z. Comparative study of buccal dehiscence defects in immediate, delayed, and late maxillary implant placement with collagen membranes: Clinical healing between placement and second-stage surgery. J Periodontol 2002;73:754–761.

49. Khojasteh A, Soheilifar S, Mohajerani H, Nowzari H. The effectiveness of barrier membranes on bone regeneration in localized bony defects: A systematic review. Int J Oral Maxillofac Implants 2013;28:1076–1089.
50. Peñarrocha-Oltra D, Aloy-Prósper A, Cervera-Ballester J, Peñarrocha-Diago M, Canullo L, Peñarrocha-Diago M. Implant treatment in atrophic posterior mandibles: Vertical regeneration with block bone grafts versus implants with 5.5-mm intrabony length. Int J Oral Maxillofac Implants 2014;29:659–666.
51. Barone A, Covani U. Maxillary alveolar ridge reconstruction with nonvascularized autogenous block bone: Clinical results. J Oral Maxillofac Surg 2007;65:2039–2046.
52. Boronat A, Carrillo C, Penarrocha M, Pennarocha M. Dental implants placed simultaneously with bone grafts in horizontal defects: A clinical retrospective study with 37 patients. Int J Oral Maxillofac Implants 2010;25:189–196.
53. Khoury F, Khoury C. Mandibular bone block grafts: Diagnosis, instrumentation, harvesting technique and surgical procedures. In: Khoury F, Antoun H, Missika P (eds). Bone Augmentation in Oral Implantology. London: Quintessence, 2007:169–183.
54. Khojasteh A, Hassani A, Motamedian SR, Saadat S, Alikhasi M. Cortical bone augmentation versus nerve lateralization for treatment of atrophic posterior mandible: A retrospective study and review of literature. Clin Implant Dent Relat Res 2016;18:342–359.
55. Khojasteh A, Behnia H, Shayesteh YS, Morad G, Alikhasi M. Localized bone augmentation with cortical bone blocks tented over different particulate bone substitutes: A retrospective study. Int J Oral Maxillofac Implants 2012;27:1481–1493.
56. Barros-Saint-Pasteur J. Plastic restoration of the alveolar crest of the mandible [in Spanish]. Acta Odontol Venez 1966;4:3–21.
57. Mounir M, Mounir S, Abou-Elfetouh A, Shaker MA. Assessment of vertical ridge augmentation in anterior aesthetic zone using onlay xenografts with titanium mesh versus the inlay bone grafting technique: A randomized clinical trial. Int J Oral Maxillofac Surg 2017;46:1458–1465.
58. Barone A, Toti P, Menchini-Fabris GB, Felice P, Marchionni S, Covani U. Early volumetric changes after vertical augmentation of the atrophic posterior mandible with interpositional block graft versus onlay bone graft: A retrospective radiological study. J Craniomaxillofac Surg 2017;45:1438–1447.
59. Codivilla A. On the means of lengthening, in the lower limbs, the muscles and tissues which are shortened through deformity. Clin Orthop Relat Res 1994:4–9.
60. McAllister BS, Haghighat K. Bone augmentation techniques. J Periodontol 2007;78:377–396.
61. Artzi Z, Tal H, Moses O, Kozlovsky A. Mucosal considerations for osseointegrated implants. J Prosthet Dent 1993;70:427–432.
62. Laster Z, Rachmiel A, Jensen OT. Alveolar width distraction osteogenesis for early implant placement. J Oral Maxillofac Surg 2005;63:1724–1730.
63. Bianchi A, Felice P, Lizio G, Marchetti C. Alveolar distraction osteogenesis versus inlay bone grafting in posterior mandibular atrophy: A prospective study. Oral Surg Oral Med Oral Pathol Oral Radiol Endod 2008;105:282–292.
64. Rocchietta I, Fontana F, Simion M. Clinical outcomes of vertical bone augmentation to enable dental implant placement: A systematic review. J Clin Periodontol 2008;35(8 suppl):203–215.
65. Chiapasco M, Casentini P, Zaniboni M. Bone augmentation procedures in implant dentistry. Int J Oral Maxillofac Implants 2009;24 suppl:237–259.
66. Sinder BP, Pettit AR, McCauley LK. Macrophages: Their emerging roles in bone. J Bone Miner Res 2015;30:2140–2149.
67. Champagne CM, Takebe J, Offenbacher S, Cooper LF. Macrophage cell lines produce osteoinductive signals that include bone morphogenetic protein-2. Bone 2002;30:26–31.
68. Dhaliwal K, Kunchur R, Farhadieh R. Review of the cellular and biological principles of distraction osteogenesis: An in vivo bioreactor tissue engineering model. J Plast Reconstr Aesthet Surg 2016;69:e19–e26.
69. Martinez-de la Cruz G, Yamauchi K, Odajima K, Kataoka Y, Nogami S, Takahashi T. Histologic and histomorphometric evaluation of the bone regeneration following cortical bone repositioning in a rabbit mandible. Clin Implant Dent Relat Res 2019;21:613–620.
70. Greenstein G, Greenstein B, Cavallaro J, Tarnow D. The role of bone decortication in enhancing the results of guided bone regeneration: A literature review. J Periodontol 2009;80:175–189.

21

SINUS AUGMENTATION

Basel Elnayef, DDS, MS, PhD
Carlos Garaicoa-Pazmiño, DDS, MS

DEFINITIONS AND TERMINOLOGY

Maxillary antrum: The air cavity in the body of the maxilla, lined with respiratory epithelium, that normally lies superior to the roots of the premolars and molars and generally extends from the canine or premolar region posterior to the molar or tuberosity region. It communicates with the middle meatus of the nose. Also known as *antrum of Highmore*.[7]

Osteotome: A surgical tool used to create or modify osteotomies for future implant placement in which the bone quality (compaction of local bone) and bone quantity (ridge expansion) can be improved. Can also be used in a sinus elevation procedure.[7]

Sinus: A cavity or hollow space in a bone or other tissue, such as the air-filled paranasal sinuses or the venous cavernous sinus in the cranium.[7]

Tooth loss unequivocally leads to a modification of the alveolar bone architecture, with dimensional changes affecting both height and width.[1] This bone remodeling process commences earlier and progresses further in posterior regions than in anterior and premolar sites.[2] As such, the augmentation of bone volume is often indicated in the posterior maxilla due to the presence of a reduced alveolar process. This decrease in available bone is mainly attributed to two phenomena: remodeling process after extraction and sinus pneumatization.

The elevation of the maxillary sinus membrane is an extensively investigated technique originally developed to increase the bone height for implant placement in the posterior maxilla. This sinus elevation technique was first described by Tatum during an implant conference in 1976[3,4]; however, Boyne and James[5] created the first publication in 1980 followed by Tatum[6] himself in 1986. This chapter reviews the current state of sinus augmentation procedures as well as the factors known to influence the outcomes of these techniques.

Anatomy of the Maxillary Sinus

The maxillary **sinus** is a pneumatic pyramid-shaped cavity located in the body of the maxillary bone. It is limited by anatomical landmarks as depicted in Table 21-1. This cavity is covered by the sinus membrane (also called the *Schneiderian membrane*), a thin mucosa of pseudostratified cubic epithelium with ciliated epithelial and mucosecretory cells. The ciliated epithelium transports fluids such as mucus to the nasal cavity, acting as an important defense mechanism of the sinus cavity.[8]

The maxillary sinus is connected with the nasal cavity through the ostium. This foramen is located on the highest part of medial wall, and it is necessary for drainage. Although uncommon, if this channel is collapsed by excessive packing of biomaterial during sinus grafting, the drainage to the nasal cavity will be compromised.[9]

The maxillary sinus represents the largest of the paranasal sinuses, with average dimensions of 15 to 32 mm in width (transverse), 23 to 52 mm in

TABLE 21-1 Borders of the maxillary sinus

Border	Anatomical landmark
Medial wall	Lateral nasal wall
Superior wall	Orbital bone
Anterior/buccal wall	Canine fossa
Posterior/pterygomaxillary wall	Zygomatic fossa
Apex	Zygomatic process of the maxilla

height (cephalocaudal), and 25 and 43 in length (anteroposterior).[10] Nonetheless, variations in size and shape can occur, including bilateral asymmetry within the same individual.[4] The sinus has an estimated volume of approximately 12 to 15 cm^3 after pneumatization is complete during adolescence[3] (Fig 21-1).

Multiples studies[11–14] have attempted to classify the maxillary sinus. Cawood and Howell classified the maxilla into six categories from dentate jaw (Class I) to depressed ridge (Class VI) based on the severity of ridge resorption.[12] In addition, Wang and Katranji described the ABC classification and provided treatment recommendations for each clinical scenario.[11] Newly introduced classification systems have used advanced radiographic imaging for presurgical assessment and to aid clinicians in the selection of surgical approaches.[15,16] Chan et al defined three categories to describe the mediolateral dimension of sinuses (narrow: < 8 mm; average: 8 to 10 mm; wide: > 10 mm) and proposed a new classification.[16] The edentulous sites were further classified as severely, moderately, or slightly deficient when the residual height was less than 4 mm, 4 to 7 mm, and 7 to 10 mm, respectively. Furthermore, Niu et al divided the sinus into five categories: narrow tapered, tapering, ovoid, square, and irregular.[15] For the first four types, subtypes are classified into three categories: without recess, with buccal sinus recess, and with palatonasal recess. Conversely, subtypes of irregularly shaped sinuses are classified into three categories: tooth protruding into sinus floor, irregular floor, and septa/exostosis on sinus floor.

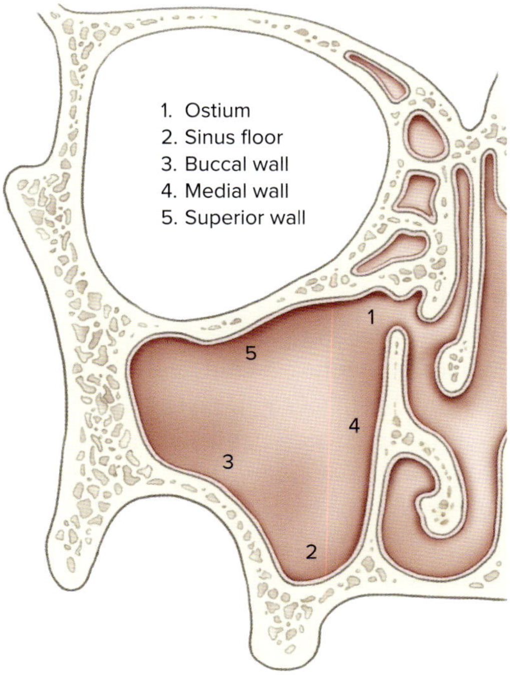

Fig 21-1 Frontal view of maxillary sinus.

SINUS MEMBRANE

The maxillary antral mucosa is thinner and less vascular than the nasal mucosa.[17] According to Pommer et al,[18] the sinus membrane is able to support a force of 7.3 N/mm^2 before a performation occurs. Additionally, the authors noted that it can be stretched to 132.6% and 124.7% of its original size in one- and two-dimensional elongation.

A recent systematic review reported a mean thickness of 1.17 mm with a range from 0.89 mm to 1.44 mm.[19] Interestingly, it was shown that 3D radiography overestimates the membrane thickness (1.33 mm) compared to histologic analysis (0.48 mm). Ultimately, different factors such as periodontitis, smoking, and gingival phenotype may influence the thickness of the membrane.[20–22]

SEPTUM

A *maxillary septum* is a thin cortical bone that divides the sinus cavity vertically or horizontally. In 1910, Underwood described these anatomical variations of the sinus cavity, and consequently, septa are sometimes referred to as *Underwood's septa*.[23] Different imaging techniques can assist in the identification of these anatomical structures; however, conventional panoramic radiographs often lead to inadequate diagnosis. Hence, 3D techniques such as CBCT are recommended to properly identify the presence of septa and anticipate potential challenges during the augmentation procedure.

Origin

Depending on the time of development, septa can be classified as primary or secondary. Primary septa are considered congenital, arising during development of the maxilla. On the other hand, secondary septa appear after sinus pneumatization and bone resorption.[24]

Extension

Regarding the extension of the septum, these can be classified as total or partial. A *total septum* is defined as a thin cortical bone that completely separates the sinus cavity into two individual compartments. This type is very uncommon with a 0.3% prevalence.[25] On the other hand, *partial* or *incomplete septa* are those extending into the sinus cavity without completely dividing it into different compartments. Moreover, the presence of septa might be associated with the degree of bone atrophy and dentate/edentulous alveolar ridge segments. Kim et al noted a prevalence of septa in 31.7% patients with an edentulous/atrophic maxilla, compared to 22.6% in denate/nonatrophic individuals.[26]

Size

Rancitelli et al conducted a detailed anatomical study of the maxillary septa.[27] The authors reported the median heights of primary and secondary septa to be 5.5 mm and 3.4 mm, respectively. Additionally, the median heights of anterior, medium, and posterior septa were 7.02 mm, 7.13 mm, and 4.38 mm, respectively. Similarly, Pommer et al reported a mean septal height of 7.5 mm.[25] Interestingly, Kim et al measured the mean height of septa in a lateral-medial perspective and reported values of 1.63 mm, 3.55 mm, and 5.46 mm in the lateral, middle, and medial areas, respectively.[26]

Prevalence

The prevalence of septa ranges from 7.1% to 58.3% according to a systematic review by Pommer et al.[25] This study reported the presence of septa in 28.4% of the 8,923 sinuses investigated. Septa were located in premolar, molar, and retromolar regions at rates of 24.4%, 54.6%, and 21.0%, respectively. The orientation of the septa was transverse in 87.6% of the cases, sagittal in 11.1% of cases, and horizontal in 1.3% of cases. These results are in concordance with the investigation by Park et al.[28] Among 400 maxillary sinuses, septa were present in 37% of the patients, and 22.5% were located in the anterior, 45.9% in the middle, and 31.5% in the posterior region.

The presence of septa is often associated with greater difficulty in performing sinus augmentation procedures and an increased risk of surgical complications (eg, membrane perforation).[29] As such, the presence of septa often defines the shape of the window during lateral approaches.

VASCULARIZATION

The vascularization of the sinus is mainly derived from two branches of the maxillary artery: the infraorbital artery and the posterior superior alveolar artery. The intraosseous anastomosis of the dental branch of the posterior superior alveolar artery (alveolar antral artery) and the infraorbital artery are located in the lateral antral wall.[30]

During a lateral window osteotomy procedure, the blood vessels of the lateral antral bony wall can be damaged. Severing any of these vascular structures can cause a hemorrhage, leading to poor visualization and consequential perforation of the sinus membrane. Different investigations have shown that this vessel is located at a distance between 16 mm and 19 mm from the alveolar ridge crest[31,32] (Fig 21-2). Furthermore, this distance is reduced to an average of 11.25 mm in first molar areas of an atrophic maxilla.[33] The mean diameter of these arteries is approximately 1.5 mm, and the bony canal harboring intraosseous anastomosis can be detected in 47% to 55% of cases through computed tomography.[31,33,34]

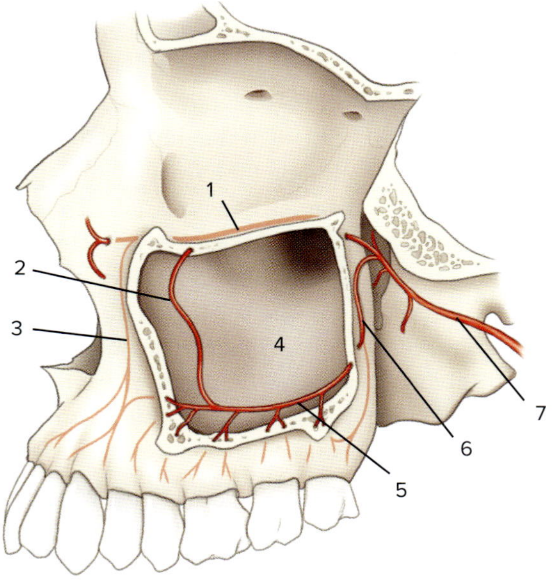

1. Infraorbital artery
2. Middle superior alveolar artery
3. Anterior superior alveolar artery
4. Maxillary sinus
5. Intraosseous branch of posterior superior alveolar artery
6. Posterior superior alveolar artery
7. Maxillary artery

Fig 21-2 Vascularization of the maxillary sinus.

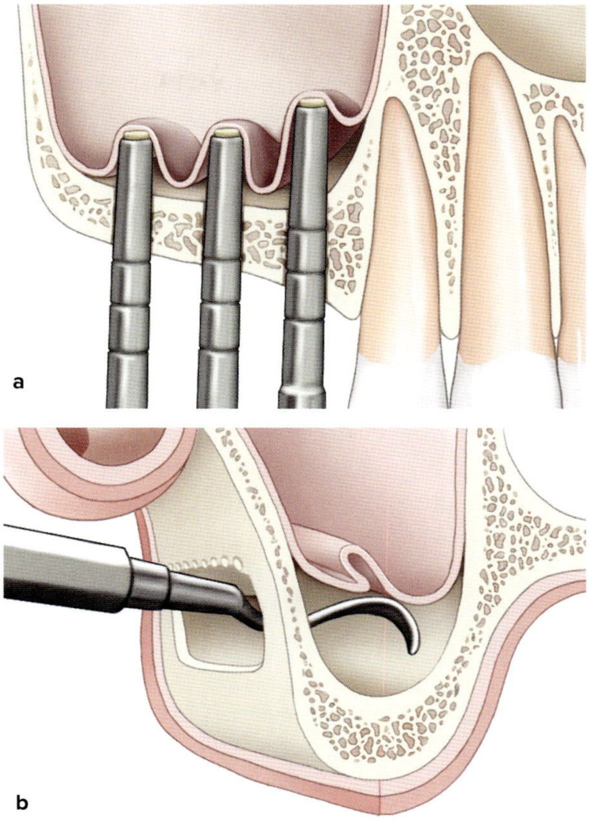

Fig 21-3 *(a)* Crestal approach. *(b)* Lateral approach.

Techniques

Several techniques have been described for the elevation of the sinus membrane.[35–38] However, two main approaches have been widely employed and investigated: the lateral window and the crestal approaches (Fig 21-3). As previously mentioned, Tatum[6] and Boyne and James[5] introduced the lateral window technique. The transalveolar or crestal approach was initially described by Summers, and it was indicated as a ridge expansion technique.[38] Both techniques have shown high survival rates similar to implants placed in the nongrafted posterior maxilla.[39]

CRESTAL APPROACH

The elevation of the sinus floor through a transcrestal approach is usually indicated when a residual bone height of 5 to 8 mm is present.[40,41] **Osteotome**-mediated sinus floor elevation is most suitable for placement of single implants, but it can also be used for multiple implants. The osteotome technique is considered less invasive and often requires less operative time.

Various studies have reported a high survival rate for implants placed with this technique by means of different variations (eg, graftless, collagen sponge, allografts, autografts, deproteinized bovine bone mineral [DBBM], tricalcium phosphate, bioactive glass).[42–46] However, the need to graft the space created after sinus augmentation osteotomes remains controversial. The most frequent intraoperative complication is perforation of the membrane, with an incidence of 3.8%.[46] In addition, crestal sinus augmentation as well as the employment of short implants at sites with less than 4 mm of residual bone height have reported lower implant survival rates compared with those sites with 5 mm or more.[44,47]

LATERAL WINDOW

This technique involves a crestal incision followed by full-thickness flap elevation to expose the lateral wall of the sinus and subsequently create a window that provides access to the interior of this anatomical structure. This approach will expose the sinus membrane and allow it to be reflected and elevated with different instruments.

As a result, a surgically created space is available for the placement of biomaterials into the sinus cavity and/or for osteotomies to be created without perforating the sinus membrane. The survival rate of implants placed in grafted sinuses with the lateral approach is comparable to those implants installed in pristine bone in the nongrafted posterior maxilla.[48] Wallace and Froum concluded that the following three factors were found to be related to implant survival: *(1)* machined implants versus rough implants (84.0% and 91.6%, respectively), *(2)* iliac block grafts versus particulate grafts (83.3% and 92.3%, respectively), and *(3)* membrane versus no membrane over lateral window (93.6% and 88.7%, respectively).[49] The lateral window sinus augmentation can also be performed with a variety of modifications with regard to grafting materials, barrier membranes, and implant placement protocols.

Grafting Materials

Different types of grafting materials have been used in sinus augmentation procedures. These materials include autografts, allografts (eg, freeze-dried or demineralized freeze-dried bone allografts [FDBA or DFDBA]), xenografts (eg, DBBM), alloplasts (eg, β-tricalcium phosphate [β-TCP]), growth factors (eg, bone morphogenetic proteins [BMPs], platelet-derived growth factor [PDGF], platelet-rich plasma [PRP]), and combinations of these. Clinical and in vitro investigations have failed to identify the most appropriate biomaterial to be used as a bone substitute, alone or in combination with other bone grafts.[50–53] These investigations demonstrate that a variety of materials can be used, reporting successful bone formation and high implant survival rates.[54–56] Nevertheless, the osteogenic potential depends on more than just the type of materials; the morphology and extension of the sinus cavity also play an important role in the final outcomes. It is paramount to bear in mind that the sinus cavity is a well-contained site, favoring clot stabilization and undisturbed bone formation; hence, the utilization of multiple different grafting materials tends to produce favorable outcomes.

NO GRAFTING MATERIAL

For decades, different grafting materials such as autografts, allografts, xenografts, and alloplasts have been used alone or in combination to achieve de novo bone formation. However, it has also been demonstrated that bone formation can occur with a graftless procedure. In 2004, Lundgren et al described the sinus augmentation by lateral approach without any graft material.[57] This technique requires there to be sufficient residual bone to achieve primary stability, allowing the implants to serve as tenting devices, elevating the sinus membrane and maintaining this elevation.

A systematic review by Shi et al reported a cumulative survival rate of implants after sinus floor elevation without grafting material of 97.3% compared to 95.89% for the grafted sites.[45] With regard to bone gain, a recent study by Fouad et al compared a xenograft group with the graftless technique.[58] Bone gain in the xenograft group ranged from 7.2 to 9.7 mm with a mean of 8.59 mm, whereas in the graftless group, bone gain ranged from 4.05 to 5.7 mm with a mean of 4.85 mm. This study demonstrated that although both represent reliable techniques, sinuses grafted with xenograft displayed a better potential for bone height gain and higher bone density compared with graftless sinuses.

Maintaining the space created after elevation of the sinus membrane is necessary for a successful outcome for this procedure. Therefore, the risk of implant perforation and membrane collapse during healing has led to the creation of space-maintaining devices. Nevertheless, the use of these devices is very technique sensitive and requires a second procedure for removal.[59,60] Overall, graftless approaches have shown sufficient bone gain, mean implant survival rates of 97.9%, and histologic evidence of vital bone formation up to 38.7%.[61–63]

AUTOGENOUS BONE

Different studies using autogenous bone grafts have shown moderate to high success associated with implant survival rates between 75% and 95%.[64–66] In a meta-analysis by Corbella et al, the authors reported a mean new bone volume of 37.5% with 54.4% of connective tissue after sinus augmentation using autogenous bone alone.[67]

In 2002, Hallman et al conducted a clinical and histologic evaluation using three groups: autogenous particulate bone from the mandibular ramus, bovine hydroxyapatite with membrane coverage, and an 80:20 mixture of bovine hydroxyapatite and autogenous bone.[68] After 6 to 9 months of healing, the mean bone-to-implant contact was 34.6%, with a total bone area of 37.7% within the sinuses grafted with autogenous bone. Ultimately, the histomorphometric analysis showed no differences between the three groups, indicating that autogenous bone graft can be substituted with bovine hydroxyapatite to 80% or 100% when used for maxillary sinus floor augmentation.

Autogenous bone is often combined with other bone substitutes (eg, allografts, xenografts, alloplasts) to reduce patient morbidity. Among studies using β-TCP, the newly formed bone and the residual bone material ranged from 31.8% to 44.2% and 16.5% to 33.8%, respectively.[69–71] The autogenous bone mixed with bovine bone showed mean percentages of 30.5% of new bone volume, 25.0% of residual biomaterial, and 47.7% of connective tissue.[67]

XENOGRAFT

Xenografts are obtained from species other than human (eg, bovine, porcine, equine), and these biomaterials are osteoconductive, serving as a scaffold for new bone formation. With the use of bovine-derived xenografts alone, Choi et al reported values of 26.6% to 33.1% for new bone formation, 31.6% to 27.3% for residual grafting material, and 39.6% to 41.8% for fibrous connective tissue among 59 sinuses after 6 months of healing.[72] Similarly, Martinez et al obtained 34.9% of new bone volume and 34.8% of residual material.[73]

When using xenograft alone or xenograft and autogenous bone for sinus augmentation, the relationship between implant survival and vital bone formation has been a topic of discussion. Froum et al could not establish a relationship because of the high overall implant survival rates.[74] On the other hand, a study by Hallman et al reported implant survival rates for sinuses grafted with particulate ramus autograft, a 20:80 autogenous/xenograft composite, and 100% xenograft to be 82.4%, 94.4%, and 96%, respectively.[68] Studies using porcine-derived xenograft for sinus augmentation have also shown results comparable to bovine bone.[75–77]

Nonbone substitutes and growth factors like PDGF, platelet-rich fibrin (PRF), PRP, or stem cells are usually combined with xenograft bone materials to promote osteoinduction. For example, Froum et al combined PDGF with a xenograft material for sinus augmentation and found a greater amount of vital bone formation after 4 to 5 months when compared to xenograft alone.[78]

ALLOGRAFT

Allogeneic bone grafts (eg, FDBA, DFDBA) have also been used for sinus augmentation. A comparison between DFDBA and FDBA revealed that FDBA resulted in significantly more new bone formation over time than DFDBA.[67] Kolerman et al reported values of 29.1% for new bone, 51.9% for connective tissue, and 19.0% of residual bone 9 months after sinus augmentation with FDBA alone.[79]

La Monaca et al performed a comparative histologic and histomorphometric study of six different biomaterials: *(1)* mineralized solvent-dehydrated bone allograft (also known as *mineralized cancellous bone allograft* or MCBA), *(2)* FDBA, *(3)* anorganic bovine bone (ABB), *(4)* equine-derived bone (EB), *(5)* synthetic micro-macroporous biphasic calcium-phosphate block consisting of 30% hydroxyapatite and 70% β-TCP (HA/β-TCP 30:70), and *(6)* bioapatite and collagen (BC). The histologic examination showed that all biomaterials were in close contact with newly formed bone.[80] The histomorphometric results revealed 20.1% of newly formed bone for MCBA, 32.1% for FDBA, 16.1% for ABB, 22.8% for EB, 20.3% for HA/β-TCP 30:70, and 21.4% for BC. Hence, the authors concluded that all six tested biomaterials showed good biocompatibility and osteoconductive properties when used in sinus augmentation procedures.

ALLOPLASTS

Alloplastic materials such as biphasic calcium phosphate (BCP), including α-TCP, β-TCP, and bioactive glass, have shown almost equal efficacy in sinus floor augmentation procedures compared with autogenous bone both clinically and histologically.[69–71,81–84] Histomorphometrically, alloplastic materials revealed values of 26% to 31% for new bone formation, 20% to 31% for residual grafting material, and 40% to 47% for connective tissue.[67]

SUMMARY

A recent systematic review by Starch-Jensen et al concluded that maxillary sinus floor augmentation is a highly predictable and successful surgical procedure to enhance the vertical alveolar bone height before or in conjunction with implant placement.[85] Table 21-2 summarizes total percentages of new bone formation, residual biomaterial, and connective tissue from histomorphometric studies reviewed by Corbella et al.[67] This comparative review did not find a significant advantage favoring any of the analyzed bone materials; however, it emphasized that the selection should be based on the clinician's judgment as well as the main purpose of the surgical procedure.

TABLE 21-2 Percentages of new bone volume, residual biomaterial, and connective tissue with different bone materials used in sinus augmentation procedures*

Bone material	Healing time (m)	New bone volume (%)		Residual biomaterial (%)		Connective tissue (%)	
		Mean	SD	Mean	SD	Mean	SD
AB alone	2–9	37.5	8.6	13.3	3.7	54.4	5.0
AB + β-TCP	3–10	28.3	8.9	25.2	5.9	40.8	8.3
AB + BB	3–84	30.5	11.2	25.0	11.4	47.7	10.3
AB + other substitutes	2–10	31.9	10.1	13.5	7.8	52.5	11.9
HA alone	3–12	31.0	4.9	31.5	5.7	42.4	5.5
HA + β-TCP	5–12	26.3	8.1	25.8	8.0	47.9	8.4
β-TCP alone	3–9	30.8	8.8	20.6	7.1	45.9	6.0
BB alone	3–20	28.0	6.8	29.4	7.1	42.4	7.7
BB + nonbone materials	3–9	14.1	4.2	30.1	5.9	48.1	4.5
AG	3–9	25.4	10.0	20.1	9.8	40.5	7.5

SD, standard deviation; AB, autogenous bone; BB, bovine bone; AG, allograft.

*Adapted from Corbella et al.[67]

Barrier Membranes

The application of a barrier membrane over the lateral sinus window has been used in an attempt to promote a higher degree and more rapid vital bone formation. It can also provide advantages such as containment of the bone graft and prevention of connective tissue migration inside the sinus.

The use of barrier membranes has led to more favorable implant survival rates.[86,87] These findings were confirmed in a meta-analysis of three comparative studies performed by Wallace and Froum. The authors concluded that the use of barrier membranes during lateral sinus augmentation increases the implant survival rate (93.6% vs 88.7%) compared with nonmembrane sites.[49]

With regard to histomorphometric outcomes, Barone et al revealed that when using a collagen membrane, newly formed bone was 30.7% of the total volume, the average percentage of connective tissue was 50.6%, and residual graft percentage was 18.4%.[88] On the other hand, data regarding the nonmembrane group showed that the percentage of newly formed bone was 28.1%, the mean percentage of connective tissues was 59.3%, and residual graft particles were 12.6%. A systematic review evaluating 37 studies also demonstrated that the use of a barrier membrane did not have an effect on the amount of vital bone formation after sinus augmentation.[89]

From these studies, it can be concluded that the use of a membrane over the lateral wall does not significantly influence the healing process. However, the membrane can also provide other advantages such as containment of the grafting material and prevention of soft tissue ingrowth, thus creating a positive effect on implant survival rate.

Implant Placement Protocol

Dental implants can be placed simultaneously when there is sufficient bone height for primary stability, or in a second procedure when bone remodeling of the graft has already occurred. The two-stage procedure is indicated when primary stability cannot be achieved, and it is usually performed for residual bone heights of less than 4 mm. The disadvantages of the two-stage protocol are the

BOX 21-1 Potential complications in lateral window technique

Intraoperative	Early postoperative	Late postoperative
• Membrane perforation • Hemorrhage • Obstruction of the ostium • Damage to adjacent dentition	• Hemorrhage • Wound dehiscence • Infection • Exposure of barrier membrane • Dental implant failure	• Graft loss • Implant loss or failure • Oroantral fistula • Migration of dental implants into the maxillary sinus • Chronic sinus disease • Chronic infection

need for a second procedure and increased overall time before restoration. Both residual bone height and primary stability are considered key factors when determining if simultaneous implant placement can be performed.

A single-stage protocol is recommended when the alveolar bone height is 5 mm or greater.[90] Available evidence suggests that with a single-stage approach, it is possible to achieve similar results as with the two-stage approach, with the advantages of shortening the healing period and avoiding another surgical intervention.[91] However, the authors concluded that for patients with residual bone height between 1 to 3 mm, there is a higher risk for implant failures when performing a single-stage procedure.

Complications

For decades, sinus augmentation procedures have been demonstrated as a highly successful surgical technique.[49] Nevertheless, complications may arise at different points. The different complications associated with lateral window sinus floor elevation are summarized in Box 21-1. For the osteotome technique, other complications have been described, including membrane perforation, vertigo, implant failure, and infection.[78,80–82] As such, it is paramount to use CBCT imaging for analysis of the sinus anatomy. This information can help clinicians to prevent possible complications.

Among these complications, the most frequent is the perforation of the sinus membrane, with a prevalence of 11% to 56%.[92] Cho et al found a correlation between the prevalence of perforations and the angle formed by the intersection of medial and lateral sinus walls.[93] The majority of perforations occurred when the membrane is being reflected in regions where the lateral and medial walls of the sinus are at an angle of less than 30 degrees (37.5%) or between 31 and 60 degrees (28.6%), whereas no perforations (0%) occured at the walls with angles greater than 61 degrees. In addition, the presence of anatomical variations within the maxillary sinus, such as septa, have been reported to increase the risk of sinus membrane perforation during the elevation procedure.[3] Also, the thickness of the sinus membrane has been related to the risk of perforation, where thinner (< 1-mm) or thicker (≥ 2-mm) membranes presented with higher risks for this intraoperative complication.[94] This study reported sinus membrane thicknesses between 1 and 1.5 mm to have the lowest incidence of perforations.

BOX 21-2 Size of sinus membrane perforations[96]

Small	≤ 5 mm
Medium	5–10 mm
Large	≥ 10 mm

With regard to the treatment of sinus membrane perforations, different approaches have been described.[92,95] The size of the perforated area should be carefully evaluated during sinus augmentation procedures (Box 21-2).[96]

If a perforation is smaller than 5 mm, a collagen plug or sponge could help to temporarily seal the perforation, allowing for successful graft and clot stabilization. Perforations larger than 5 mm can be covered with an absorbable membrane that serves as a barrier between the sinus and the grafting material. For extensive perforations (> 10 mm), the use of large absorbable membranes extending over the lateral wall might need stabilization by tacks or suturing.[97] On the other hand, for unmanageable perforations, aborting the procedure is highly recommended.

Perforations of the sinus membrane seem not to influence the final treatment outcome[96]; however, a higher prevalence of sinusitis has been reported.[29] Smokers also generally exhibit a greater predisposition for complications.[98] As such, a systematic review concluded that smoking seems to be associated with increased risk of wound dehiscence and infection after maxillary sinus floor augmentation.[97]

The second most common complication associated with this procedure is bleeding. The hemorrhage from the posterior superior alveolar artery may prolong the surgical time; increase the risk of perforation; and cause sinus mucosa swelling, accumulation of blood into the sinus cavity, and displacement of the grafting material due to the pressure. In case of damage to the artery, different techniques to control the bleeding can be performed, including but not limited to pressure, administering anesthesia with vasoconstrictor, antifibrinolytics, surgical wax, electrocautery, suturing of the damaged vessel, compressing the bone surrounding the artery, and a combination of these techniques. In addition, the use advanced radiographic imaging (eg, CBCT) and piezoelectric instruments are recommended to minimize the risk of intraoperative bleeding.

References

1. Schropp L, Wenzel A, Kostopoulos L, Karring T. Bone healing and soft tissue contour changes following single-tooth extraction: A clinical and radiographic 12-month prospective study. Int J Periodontics Restorative Dent 2003;23:313–323.
2. Ulm CW, Solar P, Gsellmann B, Matejka M, Watzek G. The edentulous maxillary alveolar process in the region of the maxillary sinus—A study of physical dimension. Int J Oral Maxillofac Surg 1995;24:279–282.
3. Chanavaz M. Maxillary sinus: Anatomy, physiology, surgery, and bone grafting related to implantology: Eleven years of surgical experience (1979–1990). J Oral Implantol 1990;16:199–209.
4. van den Bergh JP, ten Bruggenkate CM, Disch FJ, Tuinzing DB. Anatomical aspects of sinus floor elevations. Clin Oral Implants Res 2000;11:256–265.
5. Boyne PJ, James RA. Grafting of the maxillary sinus floor with autogenous marrow and bone. J Oral Surg 1980;38:613–616.
6. Tatum H, Jr. Maxillary and sinus implant reconstructions. Dent Clin North Am 1986;30:207–229.
7. American Academy of Periodontology. Glossary of Periodontal Terms. American Academy of Periodontology, 2001.
8. Griffa A, Berrone M, Boffano P, Viterbo S, Berrone S. Mucociliary function during maxillary sinus floor elevation. J Craniofac Surg 2010;21:1500–1502.
9. Asai S, Shimizu Y, Ooya K. Maxillary sinus augmentation model in rabbits: Effect of occluded nasal ostium on new bone formation. Clin Oral Implants Res 2002;13:405–409.
10. Ekizoglu O, Inci E, Hocaoglu E, Sayin I, Kayhan FT, Can IO. The use of maxillary sinus dimensions in gender determination: A thin-slice multidetector computed tomography assisted morphometric study. J Craniofac Surg 2014;25:957–960.
11. Wang HL, Katranji A. ABC sinus augmentation classification. Int J Periodontics Restorative Dent 2008;28:383–389.
12. Cawood JI, Howell RA. A classification of the edentulous jaws. Int J Oral Maxillofac Surg 1988;17:232–236.
13. Simion M, Fontana F, Rasperini G, Maiorana C. Long-term evaluation of osseointegrated implants placed in sites augmented with sinus floor elevation associated with vertical ridge augmentation: A retrospective study of 38 consecutive implants with 1- to 7-year follow-up. Int J Periodontics Restorative Dent 2004;24:208–221.
14. Misch CE, Judy KW. Classification of partially edentulous arches for implant dentistry. Int J Oral Implantol 1987;4:7–13.
15. Niu L, Wang J, Yu H, Qiu L. New classification of maxillary sinus contours and its relation to sinus floor elevation surgery. Clin Implant Dent Relat Res 2018;20:493–500.
16. Chan HL, Suarez F, Monje A, Benavides E, Wang HL. Evaluation of maxillary sinus width on cone-beam computed tomography for sinus augmentation and new sinus classification based on sinus width. Clin Oral Implants Res 2014;25:647–652.
17. May M, Sobol SM, Korzec K. The location of the maxillary os and its importance to the endoscopic sinus surgeon. Laryngoscope 1990;100:1037–1042.
18. Pommer B, Unger E, Sütö D, Hack N, Watzek G. Mechanical properties of the Schneiderian membrane in vitro. Clin Oral Implants Res 2009;20:633–637.
19. Monje A, Diaz KT, Aranda L, Insua A, Garcia-Nogales A, Wang HL. Schneiderian membrane thickness and clinical implications for sinus augmentation: A systematic review and meta-regression analyses. J Periodontol 2016;87:888–899.
20. Janner SF, Caversaccio MD, Dubach P, Sendi P, Buser D, Bornstein MM. Characteristics and dimensions of the Schneiderian membrane: A radiographic analysis using cone beam computed tomography in patients referred for dental implant surgery in the posterior maxilla. Clin Oral Implants Res 2011;22:1446–1453.
21. Engström H, Chamberlain D, Kiger R, Egelberg J. Radiographic evaluation of the effect of initial periodontal therapy on thickness of the maxillary sinus mucosa. J Periodontol 1988;59:604–608.
22. Aimetti M, Massei G, Morra M, Cardesi E, Romano F. Correlation between gingival phenotype and Schneiderian membrane thickness. Int J Oral Maxillofac Implants 2008;23:1128–1132.
23. Underwood AS. An inquiry into the anatomy and pathology of the maxillary sinus. J Anat Physiol 1910;44:354–369.
24. Krennmair G, Ulm CW, Lugmayr H, Solar P. The incidence, location, and height of maxillary sinus septa in the edentulous and dentate maxilla. J Oral Maxillofac Surg 1999;57:667–671.
25. Pommer B, Ulm C, Lorenzoni M, Palmer R, Watzek G, Zechner W. Prevalence, location and morphology of maxillary sinus septa: Systematic review and meta-analysis. J Clin Periodontol 2012;39:769–773.
26. Kim MJ, Jung UW, Kim CS, et al. Maxillary sinus septa: Prevalence, height, location, and morphology. A reformatted computed tomography scan analysis. J Periodontol 2006;77:903–908.
27. Rancitelli D, Borgonovo AE, Cicciù M, et al. Maxillary sinus septa and anatomic correlation with the Schneiderian membrane. J Craniofac Surg 2015;26:1394–1398.
28. Park YB, Jeon HS, Shim JS, Lee KW, Moon HS. Analysis of the anatomy of the maxillary sinus septum using 3-dimensional computed tomography. J Oral Maxillofac Surg 2011;69:1070–1078.
29. Hernández-Alfaro F, Torradeflot MM, Marti C. Prevalence and management of Schneiderian membrane perforations during sinus-lift procedures. Clin Oral Implants Res 2008;19:91–98.

30. Rosano G, Taschieri S, Gaudy JF, Del Fabbro M. Maxillary sinus vascularization: A cadaveric study. J Craniofac Surg 2009;20:940–943.
31. Solar P, Geyerhofer U, Traxler H, Windisch A, Ulm C, Watzek G. Blood supply to the maxillary sinus relevant to sinus floor elevation procedures. Clin Oral Implants Res 1999;10:34–44.
32. Elian N, Wallace S, Cho SC, Jalbout ZN, Froum S. Distribution of the maxillary artery as it relates to sinus floor augmentation. Int J Oral Maxillofac Implants 2005;20:784–787.
33. Rosano G, Taschieri S, Gaudy JF, Weinstein T, Del Fabbro M. Maxillary sinus vascular anatomy and its relation to sinus lift surgery. Clin Oral Implants Res 2011;22:711–715.
34. Mardinger O, Abba M, Hirshberg A, Schwartz-Arad D. Prevalence, diameter and course of the maxillary intraosseous vascular canal with relation to sinus augmentation procedure: A radiographic study. Int J Oral Maxillofac Surg 2007;36:735–738.
35. Berengo M, Sivolella S, Majzoub Z, Cordioli G. Endoscopic evaluation of the bone-added osteotome sinus floor elevation procedure. Int J Oral Maxillofac Surg 2004;33:189–194.
36. Kfir E, Kfir V, Mijiritsky E, Rafaeloff R, Kaluski E. Minimally invasive antral membrane balloon elevation followed by maxillary bone augmentation and implant fixation. J Oral Implantol 2006;32:26–33.
37. Nkenke E, Schlegel A, Schultze-Mosgau S, Neukam FW, Wiltfang J. The endoscopically controlled osteotome sinus floor elevation: A preliminary prospective study. Int J Oral Maxillofac Implants 2002;17:557–566.
38. Summers RB. A new concept in maxillary implant surgery: The osteotome technique. Compendium 1994;15:152–156.
39. Starch-Jensen T, Schou S. Maxillary sinus membrane elevation with simultaneous installation of implants without the use of a graft material: A systematic review. Implant Dent 2017;26:621–633.
40. Pjetursson BE, Lang NP. Sinus floor elevation utilizing the transalveolar approach. Periodontol 2000 2014;66:59–71.
41. Zitzmann NU, Schärer P. Sinus elevation procedures in the resorbed posterior maxilla. Comparison of the crestal and lateral approaches. Oral Surg Oral Med Oral Pathol Oral Radiol Endod 1998;85:8–17.
42. French D, Nadji N, Shariati B, Hatzimanolakis P, Larjava H. Survival and success rates of dental implants placed using osteotome sinus floor elevation without added bone grafting: A retrospective study with a follow-up of up to 10 years. Int J Periodontics Restorative Dent 2016;36(suppl):s89–s97.
43. Nedir R, Nurdin N, Vazquez L, Abi Najm S, Bischof M. Osteotome sinus floor elevation without grafting: A 10-year prospective study. Clin Implant Dent Relat Res 2016;18:609–617.
44. Rosen PS, Summers R, Mellado JR, et al. The bone-added osteotome sinus floor elevation technique: Multicenter retrospective report of consecutively treated patients. Int J Oral Maxillofac Implants 1999;14:853–858.
45. Shi JY, Gu YX, Zhuang LF, Lai HC. Survival of implants using the osteotome technique with or without grafting in the posterior maxilla: A systematic review. Int J Oral Maxillofac Implants 2016;31:1077–1088.
46. Tan WC, Lang NP, Zwahlen M, Pjetursson BE. A systematic review of the success of sinus floor elevation and survival of implants inserted in combination with sinus floor elevation. Part II: Transalveolar technique. J Clin Periodontol 2008;35:241–254.
47. Pjetursson BE, Rast C, Brägger U, Schmidlin K, Swahlen M, Lang NP. Maxillary sinus floor elevation using the (transalveolar) osteotome technique with or without grafting material. Part I: Implant survival and patients' perception. Clin Oral Implants Res 2009;20:667–676.
48. Del Fabbro M, Testori T, Francetti L, Weinstein R. Systematic review of survival rates for implants placed in the grafted maxillary sinus. Int J Periodontics Restorative Dent 2004;24:565–577.
49. Wallace SS, Froum SJ. Effect of maxillary sinus augmentation on the survival of endosseous dental implants. A systematic review. Ann Periodontol 2003;8:328–343.
50. Kühl S, Brochhausen C, Götz H, et al. The influence of bone substitute materials on the bone volume after maxillary sinus augmentation: A microcomputerized tomography study. Clin Oral Investig 2013;17:543–551.
51. Kühl S, Götz H, Brochhausen C, et al. The influence of substitute materials on bone density after maxillary sinus augmentation: A microcomputed tomography study. Int J Oral Maxillofac Implants 2012;27:1541–1546.
52. Torres J, Tamimi F, Martinez PP, et al. Effect of platelet-rich plasma on sinus lifting: A randomized-controlled clinical trial. J Clin Periodontol 2009;36:677–687.
53. de Melo WM, de Oliveira FS, Marcantonio E Jr, Beloti MM, de Oliveira PT, Rosa AL. Autogenous bone combined with anorganic bovine bone for maxillary sinus augmentation: Analysis of the osteogenic potential of cells derived from the donor and the grafted sites. Clin Oral Implants Res 2014;25:603–609.
54. Krennmair S, Weinländer M, Malek M, Forstner T, Krennmair G, Stimmelmayr M. Clinical outcome of implants placed in staged maxillary sinus augmentation using bovine bone mineral mixed with autogenous bone at three different ratios: A 5-year prospective follow-up study. Int J Oral Maxillofac Implants 2018;33:1351–1361.
55. Maddalone M, Mirabelli L, Venino PM, Karanxha L, Porcaro G, Del Fabbro M. Long-term stability of autologous bone graft of intraoral origin after lateral sinus floor elevation with simultaneous implant placement. Clin Implant Dent Relat Res 2018;20:713–721.
56. Menezes JD, Pereira RDS, Bonardi JP, Griza GL, Okamoto R, Hochuli-Vieira E. Bioactive glass added to autogenous bone graft in maxillary sinus augmentation: A prospective histomorphometric, immunohistochemical, and bone graft resorption assessment. J Appl Oral Sci 2018;26:e20170296.
57. Lundgren S, Andersson S, Gualini F, Sennerby L. Bone reformation with sinus membrane elevation: A new surgical technique for maxillary sinus floor augmentation. Clin Implant Dent Relat Res 2004;6:165–173.
58. Fouad W, Osman A, Atef M, Hakam M. Guided maxillary sinus floor elevation using deproteinized bovine bone versus graftless Schneiderian membrane elevation with simultaneous implant placement: Randomized clinical trial. Clin Implant Dent Relat Res 2018;20:424–433.
59. Johansson LA, Isaksson S, Adolfsson E, Lindh C, Sennerby L. Bone regeneration using a hollow hydroxyapatite space-maintaining device for maxillary sinus floor augmentation: A clinical pilot study. Clin Implant Dent Relat Res 2012;14:575–584.
60. Schweikert M, Botticelli D, de Oliveira JA, Scala A, Salata LA, Lang NP. Use of a titanium device in lateral sinus floor elevation: An experimental study in monkeys. Clin Oral Implants Res 2012;23:100–105.
61. Borges FL, Dias RO, Piattelli A, et al. Simultaneous sinus membrane elevation and dental implant placement without bone graft: A 6-month follow-up study. J Periodontol 2011;82:403–412.
62. Moon JW, Sohn DS, Heo JU, Shin HI, Jung JK. New bone formation in the maxillary sinus using peripheral venous blood alone. J Oral Maxillofac Surg 2011;69:2357–2367.
63. Duan DH, Fu JH, Qi W, Du Y, Pan J, Wang HL. Graft-free maxillary sinus floor elevation: A systematic review and meta-analysis. J Periodontol 2017;88:550–564.

64. Johansson B, Wannfors K, Ekenbäck J, Smedberg JI, Hirsch J. Implants and sinus-inlay bone grafts in a 1-stage procedure on severely atrophied maxillae: Surgical aspects of a 3-year follow-up study. Int J Oral Maxillofac Implants 1999;14:811–818.
65. Keller EE, Tolman DE, Eckert SE. Maxillary antral-nasal inlay autogenous bone graft reconstruction of compromised maxilla: A 12-year retrospective study. Int J Oral Maxillofac Implants 1999;14:707–721.
66. Khoury F. Augmentation of the sinus floor with mandibular bone block and simultaneous implantation: A 6-year clinical investigation. Int J Oral Maxillofac Implants 1999;14:557–564.
67. Corbella S, Taschieri S, Weinstein R, Del Fabbro M. Histomorphometric outcomes after lateral sinus floor elevation procedure: A systematic review of the literature and meta-analysis. Clin Oral Implants Res 2016;27:1106–1122.
68. Hallman M, Sennerby L, Lundgren S. A clinical and histologic evaluation of implant integration in the posterior maxilla after sinus floor augmentation with autogenous bone, bovine hydroxyapatite, or a 20:80 mixture. Int J Oral Maxillofac Implants 2002;17:635–643.
69. Boeck-Neto RJ, Gabrielli MF, Shibli JA, Marcantonio E, Lia RC, Marcantonio EJ. Histomorphometric evaluation of human sinus floor augmentation healing responses to placement of calcium phosphate or Ricinus communis polymer associated with autogenous bone. Clin Implant Dent Relat Res 2005;7:181–188.
70. Stavropoulos A, Becker J, Capsius B, Açil Y, Wagner W, Terheyden H. Histological evaluation of maxillary sinus floor augmentation with recombinant human growth and differentiation factor-5-coated beta-tricalcium phosphate: Results of a multicenter randomized clinical trial. J Clin Periodontol 2011;38:966–974.
71. Simunek A, Kopecka D, Somanathan RV, Pilathadka S, Brazda T. Deproteinized bovine bone versus beta-tricalcium phosphate in sinus augmentation surgery: A comparative histologic and histomorphometric study. Int J Oral Maxillofac Implants 2008;23:935–942.
72. Choi SY, Jang YJ, Choi JY, Jeong JH, Kwon TG. Histomorphometric analysis of sinus augmentation using bovine bone mineral with two different resorbable membranes. Clin Oral Implants Res 2013;24(suppl A100):68–74.
73. Martinez A, Franco J, Saiz E, Guitian F. Maxillary sinus floor augmentation on humans: Packing simulations and 8 months histomorphometric comparative study of anorganic bone matrix and beta-tricalcium phosphate particles as grafting materials. Mater Sci Eng C Mater Biol Appl 2010;30:763–769.
74. Froum SJ, Tarnow DP, Wallace SS, Rohrer MD, Cho SC. Sinus floor elevation using anorganic bovine bone matrix (OsteoGraf/N) with and without autogenous bone: A clinical, histologic, radiographic, and histomorphometric analysis–Part 2 of an ongoing prospective study. Int J Periodontics Restorative Dent 1998;18:528–543.
75. Barone A, Ricci M, Covani U, Nannmark U, Azarmehr I, Calvo-Guirado JL. Maxillary sinus augmentation using prehydrated corticocancellous porcine bone: Hystomorphometric evaluation after 6 months. Clin Implant Dent Relat Res 2012;14:373–379.
76. Iezzi G, Degidi M, Piattelli A, et al. Comparative histological results of different biomaterials used in sinus augmentation procedures: A human study at 6 months. Clin Oral Implants Res 2012;23:1369–1376.
77. Scarano A, Piattelli A, Perrotti V, Manzon L, Iezzi G. Maxillary sinus augmentation in humans using cortical porcine bone: A histological and histomorphometrical evaluation after 4 and 6 months. Clin Implant Dent Relat Res 2011;13:13–18.
78. Froum SJ, Wallace S, Cho SC, et al. A histomorphometric comparison of Bio-Oss alone versus Bio-Oss and platelet-derived growth factor for sinus augmentation: A postsurgical assessment. Int J Periodontics Restorative Dent 2013;33:269–279.
79. Kolerman R, Tal H, Moses O. Histomorphometric analysis of newly formed bone after maxillary sinus floor augmentation using ground cortical bone allograft and internal collagen membrane. J Periodontol 2008;79:2104–2111.
80. La Monaca G, Iezzi G, Cristalli MP, Pranno N, Sfasciotti GL, Vozza I. Comparative histological and histomorphometric results of six biomaterials used in two-stage maxillary sinus augmentation model after 6-month healing. Biomed Res Int 2018;2018:9430989.
81. Jensen SS, Gruber R, Buser D, Bosshardt DD. Osteoclast-like cells on deproteinized bovine bone mineral and biphasic calcium phosphate: Light and transmission electron microscopical observations. Clin Oral Implants Res 2015;26:859–864.
82. Wagner W, Wiltfang J, Pistner H, et al. Bone formation with a biphasic calcium phosphate combined with fibrin sealant in maxillary sinus floor elevation for delayed dental implant. Clin Oral Implants Res 2012;23:1112–1117.
83. Turunen T, Peltola J, Yli-Urpo A, Happonen RP. Bioactive glass granules as a bone adjunctive material in maxillary sinus floor augmentation. Clin Oral Implants Res 2004;15:135–141.
84. Stiller M, Kluk E, Bohner M, Lopez-Heredia MA, Müller-Mai C, Knabe C. Performance of beta-tricalcium phosphate granules and putty, bone grafting materials after bilateral sinus floor augmentation in humans. Biomaterials 2014;35:3154–3163.
85. Starch-Jensen T, Aludden H, Hallman M, Dahlin C, Christensen AE, Mordenfeld A. A systematic review and meta-analysis of long-term studies (five or more years) assessing maxillary sinus floor augmentation. Int J Oral Maxillofac Surg 2018;47:103–116.
86. Tarnow DP, Wallace SS, Froum SJ, Rohrer MD, Cho SC. Histologic and clinical comparison of bilateral sinus floor elevations with and without barrier membrane placement in 12 patients: Part 3 of an ongoing prospective study. Int J Periodontics Restorative Dent 2000;20:117–125.
87. Tawil G, Mawla M. Sinus floor elevation using a bovine bone mineral (Bio-Oss) with or without the concomitant use of a bilayered collagen barrier (Bio-Gide): A clinical report of immediate and delayed implant placement. Int J Oral Maxillofac Implants 2001;16:713–721.
88. Barone A, Ricci M, Grassi RF, Nannmark U, Quaranta A, Covani U. A 6-month histological analysis on maxillary sinus augmentation with and without use of collagen membranes over the osteotomy window: Randomized clinical trial. Clin Oral Implants Res 2013;24:1–6.
89. Suárez-López Del Amo F, Ortega-Oller I, Catena A, et al. Effect of barrier membranes on the outcomes of maxillary sinus floor augmentation: A meta-analysis of histomorphometric outcomes. Int J Oral Maxillofac Implants 2015;30:607–618.
90. Rios HF, Avila G, Galindo P, Bratu E, Wang HL. The influence of remaining alveolar bone upon lateral window sinus augmentation implant survival. Implant Dent 2009;18:402–412.
91. Felice P, Pistilli R, Piattelli M, Soardi E, Barausse C, Esposito M. 1-stage versus 2-stage lateral sinus lift procedures: 1-year post-loading results of a multicentre randomised controlled trial. Eur J Oral Implantol 2014;7:65–75.
92. Testori T, Wallace SS, Del Fabbro M, et al. Repair of large sinus membrane perforations using stabilized collagen barrier membranes: Surgical techniques with histologic and radiographic evidence of success. Int J Periodontics Restorative Dent 2008;28:9–17.

93. Cho SC, Wallace SS, Froum SJ, Tarnow DP. Influence of anatomy on Schneiderian membrane perforations during sinus elevation surgery: Three-dimensional analysis. Pract Proced Aesthet Dent 2001;13:160–163.
94. Lin YH, Yang YC, Wen SC, Wang HL. The influence of sinus membrane thickness upon membrane perforation during lateral window sinus augmentation. Clin Oral Implants Res 2016;27:612–617.
95. Proussaefs P, Lozada J, Kim J, Rohrer MD. Repair of the perforated sinus membrane with a resorbable collagen membrane: A human study. Int J Oral Maxillofac Implants 2004;19:413–420.
96. de Almeida Ferreira CE, Martinelli CB, Novaes AB Jr, et al. Effect of maxillary sinus membrane perforation on implant survival rate: A retrospective study. Int J Oral Maxillofac Implants 2017;32:401–407.
97. Ghasemi S, Fotouhi A, Moslemi N, Chinipardaz Z, Kolahi J, Paknejad M. Intra- and postoperative complications of lateral maxillary sinus augmentation in smokers vs nonsmokers: A systematic review and meta-analysis. Int J Oral Maxillofac Implants 2017;32:759–767.
98. Levin L, Herzberg R, Dolev E, Schwartz-Arad D. Smoking and complications of onlay bone grafts and sinus lift operations. Int J Oral Maxillofac Implants 2004;19:369–373.

22

MUCOGINGIVAL THERAPY

Fernando Suárez López del Amo, DDS, MS
Vahid Khoshkam, DDS, MS

DEFINITIONS AND TERMINOLOGY

Creeping attachment: The postoperative migration of the gingival marginal tissue in a coronal direction, partially or completely covering a previously denuded root.[1]

Gingival recession: Location of the gingival margin apical to the cemento-enamel junction.[2]

Mucogingival deformity: A departure from the normal dimension and morphology of, and/or interrelationship between gingiva and alveolar mucosa; the abnormality may be associated with a deformity of the underlying bone.[2]

Mucogingival surgery: A surgical procedure indicated to correct or enhance the thickness or amount of, or change the position of, mucogingival tissue.[2]

Periodontal plastic surgery: Procedures used to reshape the tissues around the teeth or implants to prevent or correct anatomical, developmental, traumatic, or plaque-induced defects of the gingiva, alveolar mucosa, or bone.[2]

Soft tissue graft: An autogenous or allogenic graft of masticatory mucosa and/or connective tissue completely or partially detached from its original site and placed in a prepared recipient bed.[2]

Mucogingival therapy is a general term that encompasses all the procedures aimed at correcting **mucogingival deformities** around teeth and dental implants. Although they present with subtle differences, several other terms have also been proposed to define the procedures directed at the prevention and correction of soft tissue deformities, including **mucogingival surgery** and **periodontal plastic surgery**. Operations under these categories include but are not limited to root coverage, crown lengthening, gingival augmentation, pocket reduction, frenulum removal, procedures to increase vestibular depth, ridge reconstruction, increase in keratinized mucosa, and correction of soft tissue deformities around dental implants. This chapter focuses on reviewing **gingival recession** (GR) defects with the multiple ramifications and considerations pertinent to their diagnosis, etiology, treatment, and influencing variables.

Gingival Recession

PREVALENCE

It is estimated that 23.8 million people in the United States (22.5%) above the age of 29 years present with at least one tooth surface with 3 mm or more of GR.[4] The extent, prevalence, and severity of these mucogingival deformities increase with age.[4–7] In fact, by the age of 50, more than 90% of individuals present with GR,[5] and by the age of 60, approximately 90% and 40% of Americans present with at least one site with recession of 1 mm or more and 3 mm or more, respectively.[4] Overall, investigations have found a prevalence ranging from 30% to 100% depending on the age group.[5–7] In addition, this condition affects a large part of the population regardless of the level of oral hygiene[5–7] (Fig 22-1).

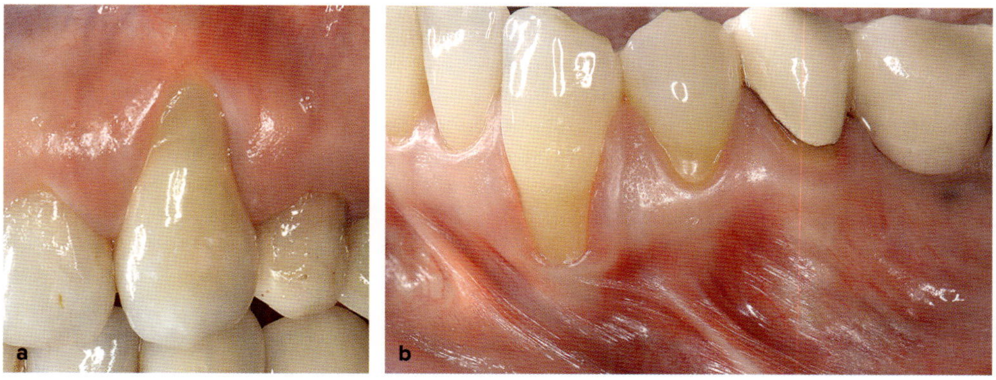

Fig 22-1 *(a and b)* Examples of gingival recession defects.

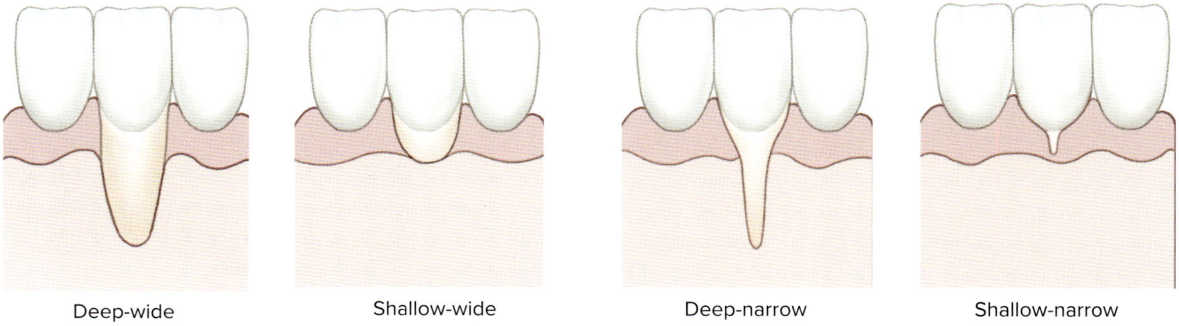

Fig 22-2 Classification proposed by Sullivan and Atkins[12] in 1968.

ETIOLOGY

Many different factors can be correlated with the incidence and progression of GR defects. Moreover, several of these factors or conditions can often play a role simultaneously on a particular mucogingival deformity. The proper diagnosis and identification of the etiologic and contributing factors is paramount for the performance of a successful therapy and the long-term maintenance of the outcomes.

Hall[8] described a series of predisposing and precipitating factors. Predisposing factors include inadequate attached gingiva, high frenulum attachment, tooth malposition, and osseous dehiscence. Precipitating factors include traumatic tooth brushing, laceration, recurrent inflammation, and iatrogenic factors.[8] In addition, several other reports have associated GRs with other factors, including but not limited to lack of keratinized tissue (KT), thin phenotype, smoking, frequent tooth brushing, presence of oral piercing, gingival inflammation, and biofilm accumulation.[7,9–11]

CLASSIFICATIONS

Several classifications for GR defects have been described (Fig 22-2 and Tables 22-1 and 22-2).[12–14] These methods for organization and classification allow for better communication among professionals and for other purposes such as research and estimating therapeutic outcomes. Miller's classification in 1985 remains as one of the most widely accepted and used worldwide.[13] However, the 2017 World Workshop on the Classification of Periodontal and Peri-implant Diseases and Conditions emphasized the utilization of a modern treatment-oriented classification by Cairo et al, which overcomes many of the limitations of previous systems.[14]

TABLE 22-1 Classification proposed by Miller[13] in 1985

Class	Depiction	Description
I	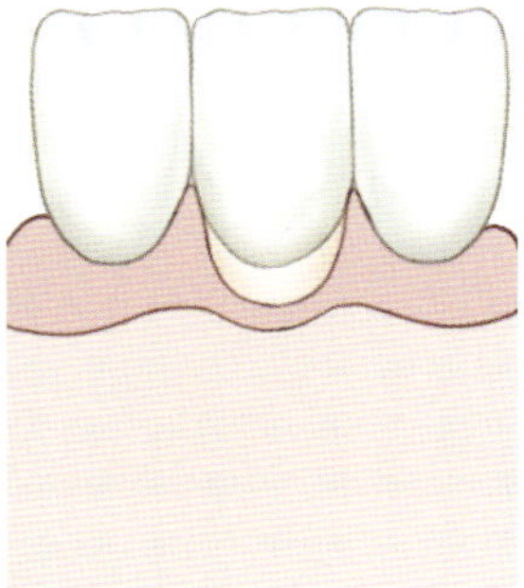	• Recession does not extend to MGJ • No attachment loss (bone or soft tissue) interproximally • 100% root coverage anticipated
II	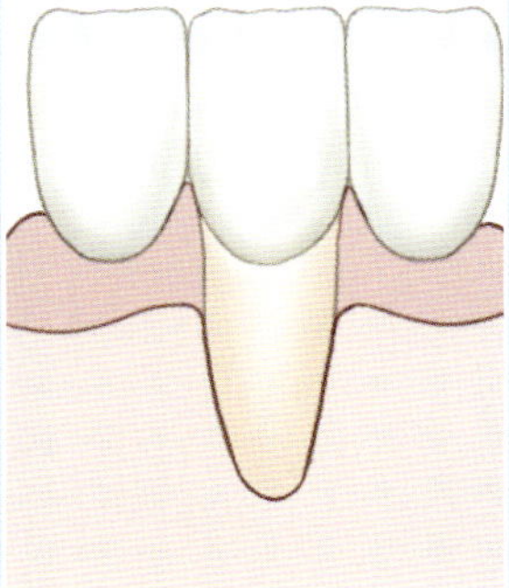	• Recession extends to or beyond MGJ • No attachment loss (bone or soft tissue) interproximally • 100% root coverage anticipated
III	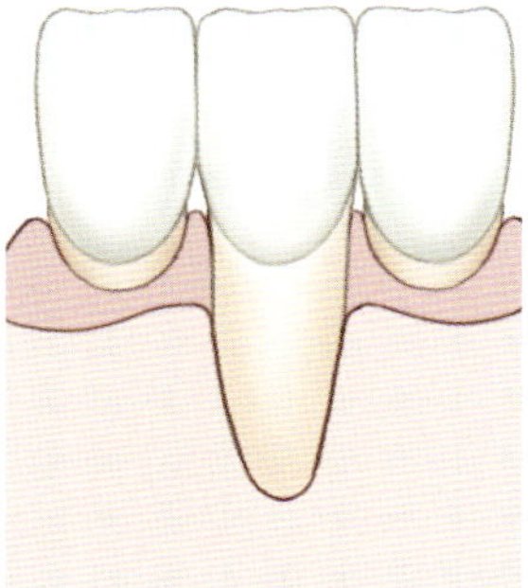	• Recession extends to or beyond MGJ • Bone or soft tissue loss present interproximally or malpositioned teeth • Partial root coverage anticipated
IV	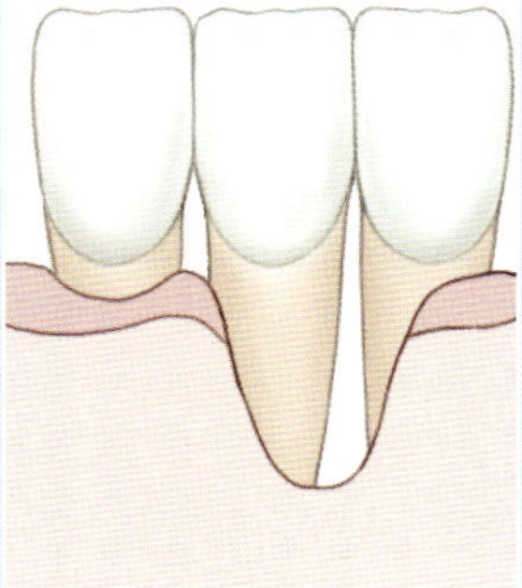	• Recession extends to or beyond MGJ • Bone or soft tissue loss present interproximally and/or severely malpositioned teeth • Root coverage cannot be anticipated

MGJ, mucogingival junction.

TABLE 22-2 Classification proposed by Cairo et al[14] in 2011

Class	Depiction	Description
RT1	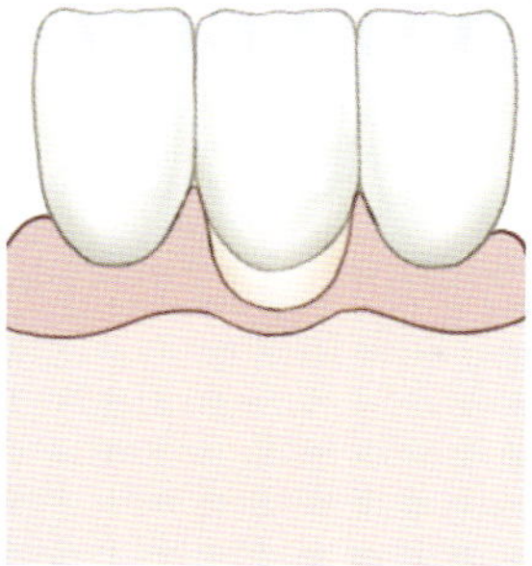	• No interproximal attachment loss • Not detectable interproximal CEJ
RT2	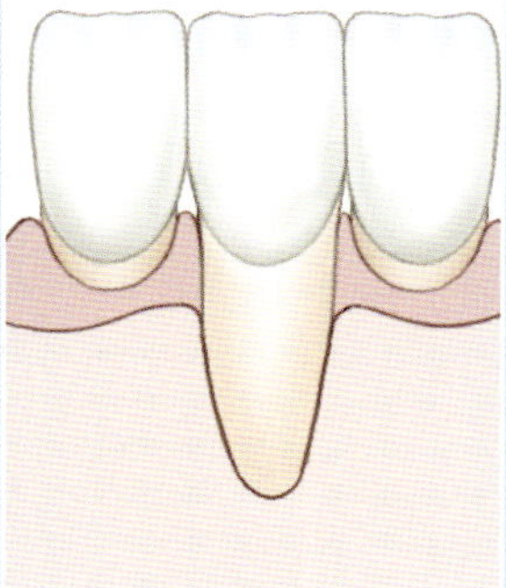	• Loss of interproximal attachment • Interproximal attachment loss ≤ buccal attachment loss
RT3	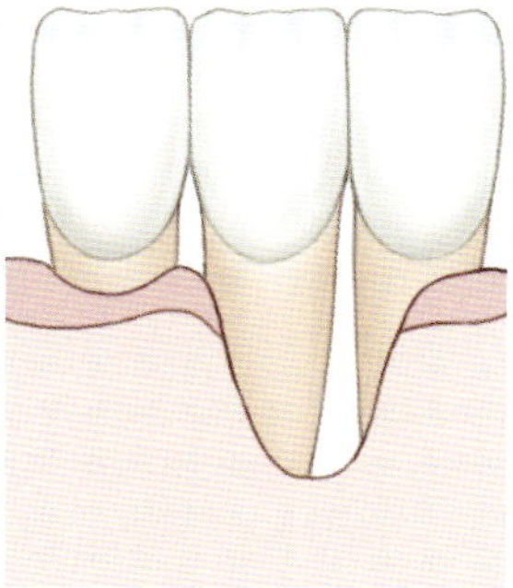	• Loss of interproximal attachment • Interproximal attachment loss > buccal attachment loss

RT, recession type; CEJ, cementoenamel juction.

Treatment

THERAPEUTIC OBJECTIVES

As described by the American Academy of Periodontology, there are two major objectives for mucogingival therapy[15]:

1. To maintain the dentition or its replacement in health, with adequate function and proper esthetics. This may include restoring the anatomical form and function.
2. To reduce the risk of progressive recession.

Consequently, the success of mucogingival therapy could be evaluated by a variety of different parameters, including the following (Fig 22-3):

- Root coverage
- Increase in clinical attachment level
- Reduction in probing depth
- Increase in tissue thickness
- Increase in KT
- Esthetic outcomes
- Facilitation of plaque control
- Increase in vestibular depth
- Elimination of frenulum
- Decrease in sensitivity
- Prevention of further recession

TECHNIQUES

Multiple techniques and grafting materials are currently available to treat mucogingival deformities and GR defects.

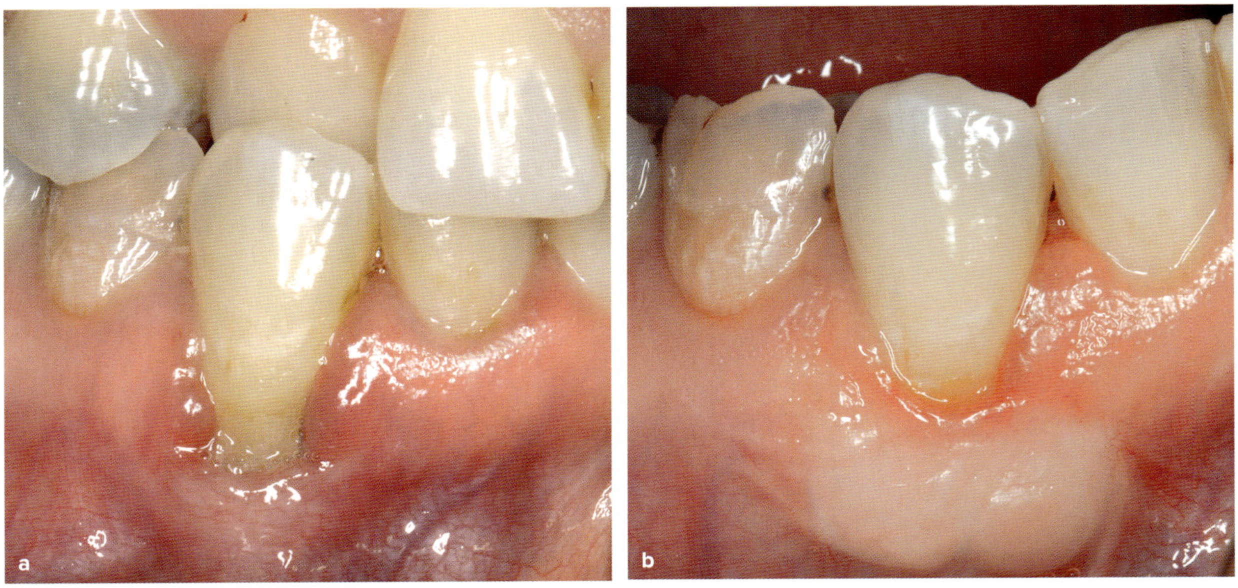

Fig 22-3 Mucogingival therapy. *(a)* Preoperative view. *(b)* Free gingival graft after 12 months.

These include but are not limited to guided tissue regeneration,[16] subepithelial connective tissue graft (CTG),[17] free gingival graft,[18] autogenous soft tissue graft substitutes,[19–21] coronally advanced flap,[22,23] laterally positioned flap,[24,25] double pedicle technique,[26] semilunar pedicle flap,[27] oblique rotated flap,[28] tunnel technique (intrasulcular or vestibular access),[29] and biologic agents.[30,31] Moreover, modifications of these techniques and combinations of different approaches have also been proposed. Today, the use of a subepithelial CTG with a coronally advanced flap is considered the best and most predictable procedure for root coverage.[32] Similarly, autogenous gingival grafts have demonstrated superior outcomes for non-root-coverage procedures.[33]

As described previously, the treatment of GRs encompasses a wide variety of techniques and grafting materials. It is important to bear in mind that in most circumstances, several different approaches could be successfully employed. However, depending on the specific clinical scenario and the patient's preferences, some approaches may be more suitable than others. Similarly, certain techniques and grafting materials have been more extensively investigated with regard to their efficacy and long-term outcomes. On the other hand, regardless of the technique chosen, properly executed surgical procedures with adequate flap design and precise surgical skills are critical for achieving satisfactory results.

Several guidelines and decision trees have been proposed to assist in the selection process for **soft tissue grafting**. For example, Leong and Wang suggested a series of considerations that guide clinicians toward the recommended therapeutic approach.[34] Later, the American Academy of Periodontology Regeneration Workshop published several practical applications for periodontal soft tissue grafting procedures. This report proposed a series of diagrams and decision trees to help identify an adequate treatment alternative for several different possible scenarios.[35] Ultimately, the selection of a specific approach should be based on a combination of patient preferences, the amount of tissue required, the indication(s) for the procedure, the personal preference and surgical expertise of the operator, as well as the evidence as reported in the literature.

OUTCOMES

Untreated gingival recessions

Untreated GRs in patients with good oral hygiene are likely to continue progressing over time. A recent systematic review and meta-analysis by Chambrone and Tatakis concluded that 78.1% of recession defects continued progressing during a follow-up period of at least 2 years.[36] The authors also found limited evidence suggesting that the presence of KT and/or greater KT width would decrease the likelihood of new or further increase in GR. In addition, limited evidence was found suggesting that GR does not lead to tooth loss. Similarly, Serino et al showed that in individuals with good oral hygiene, GR was a common finding that often increased over time.[7] The

TABLE 22-3 Mean defect coverage[38]

Technique	Mean defect coverage (%)
Laterally positioned flap	67
Free gingival graft	
Thick	69
Thin	41
Connective tissue graft	84
Free gingival graft + coronally positioned flap	61
Coronally positioned flap	78
Guided tissue regeneration	
Nonabsorbable membrane	73
Absorbable membrane	72
Acellular dermal matrix	86
Enamel matrix derivative + coronally positioned flap	86

results from these investigations are in concordance with a long-term study by Agudio et al reporting the outcomes of treated and untreated sites after 18 to 35 years.[37] In this study, 83% of sites treated with free gingival grafts showed a reduction in GR, whereas 48% of the untreated contralateral sites demonstrated an increase in GR.

Treated gingival recessions

The results of the different procedures pertaining to periodontal plastic surgery are influenced by a multitude of patient-, surgical-, and site-related factors. When evaluating the mean defect coverage, Greenwell et al reported on the different percentages depending on the technique used[38] (Table 22-3). It is important to mention that the differences in terms of study designs and evaluation periods may have played a key role in the reported outcomes.

The field of periodontal plastic surgery has continued evolving since its conception in terms of understanding the biologic principles and healing events, the development of additional techniques, as well as newer grafting materials. Hence, since the publication of the previously mentioned findings from the American Academy of Periodontology in 2005, it would not be overoptimistic to expect an overall improvement in the outcomes for most of the procedures evaluated. In this sense, Chambrone and Pini Prato reported on the evolution of different techniques for root coverage, including subepithelial CTG-based procedures and coronally advanced flap alone or in combination with acellular dermal matrix or enamel matrix derivative.[39] In this investigation, the authors evaluated randomized controlled trials treating nonsmoking patients with Miller Class I and II GR defects. The results showed an overall improvement over the last decades in terms of mean root coverage for most of the techniques investigated. In addition, the outcomes from 75 randomized controlled trials published between 1993 and 2017 showed an overall mean root coverage of 83.34% ± 12.46%, with a range of 41.8% to 99.3%. Today, there is substantial evidence that procedures involving CTGs provide the best outcomes with regard to mean root coverage, complete root coverage, and increase in the zone of KT.[40]

Creeping attachment

Creeping attachment is defined as the postoperative migration of the gingival marginal tissue in a coronal direction, partially or completely covering a previously denuded root.[1] In 1980, Matter reported an average of 0.89 mm of creeping attachment with free gingival grafts. This phenomenon occurred mostly within the first year with no significant changes occurring afterwards.[1] Later, in

TABLE 22-4 Long-term outcomes in the treatment of GR defects

Study	Follow-up	Study design	Miller Class	Outcomes (%)	
				MRC	CRC
Pini Prato et al[42] (1996)	4 years	FGG + CAF	–	72.3	–
		GTR-NAM + CAF		73.1	–
Harris[21] (2004)	4 years	SCTG + CAF or DPF	I and II	97	–
		ADM + CAF		65.8	–
Leknes et al[43] (2005)	6 years	CAF	I and II	–	9.1
		GTR-AM + CAF		–	18.2
Spahr et al[44] (2005)	2 years	Placebo + CAF	I and II	67	23
		EMD + CAF		84	53
Nickles et al[45] (2010)	10 years	SCTG + envelope flap	I and II	–	14.3*
		GTR-AM + CAF		–	0†
Moslemi et al[46] (2011)	5 years	SCTG + CAF	I and II	39.8	13.3
		ADM + CAF		54.6	20
McGuire et al[30] (2012)	10 years	SCTG + CAF	I and II	89.8 ± 22.7	77.8
		EMD + CAF		83.3 ± 21.7	55.6
Rosetti et al[47] (2013)	30 months	GTR-AM-DFDBA + CAF	I and II	87	–
		SCTG + CAF		95.5	–
Pini Prato et al[48] (2018)	20 years	SCTG + CAF	I	77.62	47.62
			III	58.18	20.83

*Relative root coverage of 43.7 ± 41.7 was also reported.

†Relative root coverage of 1.9 ± 36.4 was also reported.

FGG, free gingival graft; CAF, coronally advanced flap; GTR, guided tissue regeneration; NAM, nonabsorbable membrane; –, not reported; MRC, mean root coverage; SCTG, subepithelial connective tissue graft; DPF, double pedicle flap; ADM, acellular dermal matrix; AM, absorbable membrane; CRC, complete root coverage; EMD, enamel matrix derivative; DFDBA, demineralized freeze-dried bone allograft.

1997, Harris demonstrated a mean creeping attachment of 0.8 mm occurring in 95% of the defects after CTG with double pedicle graft.[41] Since then, multiple investigations have corroborated the outcomes reported by Matter and Harris. Also, it should be noted that although creeping attachment was observed with substitute materials, this phenomenon is more commonly present with the techniques involving soft tissue autografts.

Long-term outcomes

While the majority of the literature on mucogingival therapy reports on short- to medium-term outcomes (ie, 6 to 12 months), several investigations have shown long-term results with prolonged investigation periods. Table 22-4 summarizes the outcomes of some of these investigations with more than 12 months of follow-up.[21,30,42–48] Overall, the results obtained after correction of GR defects have been shown to be stable in the long term, especially after the use of techniques involving soft tissue autografts.[37,48]

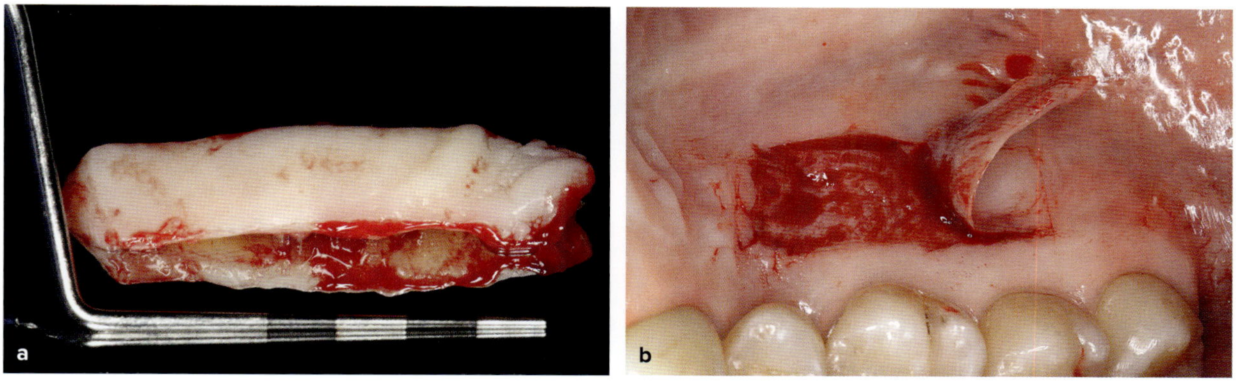

Fig 22-4 *(a and b)* Free gingival graft.

Grafting Materials

AUTOGENOUS GRAFTS

Several anatomical locations can be used as donor sites for harvesting autogenous soft tissue grafts. These locations include mainly the anterior and posterior palate, the maxillary tuberosity, and edentulous ridges. All of these possible donor sites provide grafts with distinct histologic compositions and morphologies. Today, the palate remains the most widely used source for autogenous grafts. The preferable area of the palate for harvesting autogenous connective tissue is located between the second molar and the lateral incisor region. Several aspects are taken into consideration for this statement:

- *Location of the greater palatine foramen:* Located primarily at the level of the third molar, it can also be found in between the second and third molars, and less commonly at the level of the second molar.[49] The greater palatine foramen is located at an average distance of 15.9 ± 1.5 mm from the maxillary midline and 3.0 ± 1.2 mm from the alveolar ridge.[50]
- *Thickness of the palatal tissue:* Several investigations have evaluated the thickness of the palate, concluding that canine and premolar areas are the most appropriate donor sites. Mean palatal thicknesses varied at different locations from 2.0 to 3.7 mm, increasing in thickness from the canine to the second molar area with the exception of the first molar region.[51] Studer et al found very similar results with thicknesses ranging from 1.5 to 4.0 mm.[52] In this study, the canine to premolar region was also found to be ideal for harvesting autogenous grafts, with the thinnest area around the first molar site.

With regard to the thickness of the harvested tissue, Soehren et al reported that the mean thickness of palatal epithelium was 0.34 mm, with a range from 0.1 to 0.6 mm.[53] Therefore, in order to ensure the presence of connective tissue, it is recommended to have a minimum thickness of 0.75 to 1.25 mm for the harvested graft.[33] This consideration is especially important when retrieving a free gingival graft (Fig 22-4).

Multiple techniques have been described for obtaining CTGs from the palate. Overall, these can be divided into approaches that result in healing by primary or secondary intention. While healing by primary intention has traditionally been related to reduced postoperative pain, a recent investigation demonstrated no differences when comparing primary intention healing or deepithelialized gingival grafts.[54] In addition, the connective tissue obtained by free or deepithelialized gingival grafts is primarily composed of lamina propria with large amounts of fibrous connective tissue, as well as less fatty and glandular tissue[55] than grafts obtained by traditional techniques for primary intention healing. While acknowledging the importance of these anatomical studies, the harvesting area should be tailored to each individual depending on the specific anatomy of the donor site and the surgical needs.

Last, with regard to the positioning of the graft, the orientation of the connective tissue has been proven not to influence the outcomes of periodontal plastic surgery

TABLE 22-5 Critical factors in mucogingival therapy

Parameter	Study	Main outcomes
Tissue thickness	Baldi et al[65] (1999)	Direct relationship between flap thickness and recession reduction. > 0.8 mm associated with complete root coverage. ≤ 0.8 mm associated with partial root coverage.
Treatment of root surface	Pini Prato et al[66] (1999)	No differences between polishing and root planing of the exposed root surfaces.
Flap tension	Pini Prato et al[67] (2000)	Minimal tension is compatible with favorable outcomes. The higher the tension, the lower the recession reduction.
Postsurgical position of the gingival margin	Pini Prato et al[68] (2005)	The more coronal the level of the gingival margin after suturing, the greater the probability of achieving complete root coverage.
Interdental papilla	Saletta et al[69] (2001)	Root coverage is not significantly influenced by papilla dimensions. Complete root coverage is significantly correlated with lower height of adjacent papilla.

procedures.[56,57] Similarly, acellular dermal matrix can be successfully used in combination with a coronally positioned flap regardless of the orientation of the graft.[58]

ALTERNATIVES TO AUTOGENOUS GRAFTS

Procedures involving autogenous gingival grafts have been repeatedly reported as the best and most predictable operations. However, due to the disadvantages associated with these procedures—namely patient morbidity and limited availability—numerous alternatives to autogenous grafts have been developed.[59–61] These alternative materials have also been extensively studied, often resulting in less favorable outcomes than autogenous grafts.[21,30] Nevertheless, they provide significant advantages, such as reduced patient morbidity and unlimited availability. In addition, the use of certain biologics, such as enamel matrix derivative, could provide other advantages, such as enhanced healing potential and the formation of a new attachment that more closely resembles the original architecture of the periodontium.

Modifying Factors

The outcomes of periodontal plastic surgery can be significantly influenced by a variety of patient-, surgical-, and site-related factors. The comprehensive understanding of these factors and conditions is critical for achieving successful results.

SMOKING

The detrimental effect of smoking on the periodontal tissues has been extensively investigated and is reported in more detail in chapter 4. With regard to periodontal plastic surgery, it has been shown that both smokers and nonsmokers can achieve statistically significant improvements in GR and clinical attachment level.[62,63] However, a systematic review concluded that smoking may negatively influence clinical attachment level gain and reduction in GR.[62] Similarly, smoking was shown to alter the donor site healing after free gingival graft by reducing immediate bleeding and delaying epithelialization. Also, although without significant differences, smokers experienced greater reduction in dimensional changes.[64]

CRITICAL FACTORS IN MUCOGINGIVAL THERAPY

A series of investigations conducted by Pini Prato and collaborators evaluated the influence of five different parameters on the outcomes of surgical procedures aimed at the correction of GR defects (Table 22-5).[65–69] It should be noted that these parameters were all evaluated in different studies with coronally advanced flaps. Variables evaluated included tissue thickness,[65] treatment of root surface,[66] flap tension,[67] postsurgical position of the gingival margin,[68] and interdental papilla.[69]

NONCARIOUS CERVICAL LESIONS

Noncarious cervical lesions, or *cervical wear*, are defined as the loss of tooth substance at the cementoenamal junction due to reasons other than caries.[3] These lesions present in a variety of forms and most often are related to an excessive or traumatic tooth brushing habit. Depending on the location and extension, noncarious cervical lesions can involve the crown, the root surface, or both. When the lesion involves the root, it is often associated with GR.

With regard to GR defects and mucogingival therapy, noncarious cervical lesions can cause the disappearance of the cementoenamal junction, leading to uncertainty regarding which corrective approach should be taken. Consequently, in 2011, Zucchelli et al proposed a series of recommendations for the treatment of GRs affected with these cervical lesions. The authors recommend five treatment modalities with the combination of restorative and mucogingival therapy.[70] Results from this investigation demonstrated favorable esthetic outcomes for the majority of the cases. Nevertheless, a long-term evaluation of GR defects treated with coronally advanced flap plus subepithelial CTG concluded that teeth presenting with noncarious cervical lesions are more likely to develop recession recurrence.[48] On the other hand, Agudio et al in 2016 demonstrated that gingival augmentation by means of free gingival graft may prevent the development and/or progression of noncarious cervical lesions.[37]

Mucosal Recession Around Dental Implants

Investigations have demonstrated that 38% to 57% of implants have 1 mm of recession or more on the facial/lingual aspects, depending on the characteristics of the adjacent soft tissues.[71] By means of coronally advanced flap and CTG, Zucchelli et al successfully treated soft tissue dehiscences around dental implants with a mean coverage of 96.3% and complete coverage achieved in 75% of the cases.[72] Hence, although the treatment of these soft tissue recession defects around dental implants have been proven successful,[72] currently the evidence is still limited. Case reports, case series, and descriptions of different techniques have been developed for the treatment of these recession defects.[72–74] Nonetheless, there is a lack of well-designed randomized controlled trials evaluating and comparing the efficacy of the different approaches. Moreover, the factors determining the long-term stability of the peri-implant soft tissues are complex and influenced by a multitude of variables, including patient-related and implant-related factors, anatomical variations, and material–host interactions.

Recently, several classifications have been proposed for the diagnosis, prognosis, and appropriate treatment selection of soft tissue dehiscences around dental implants.[75,76]

References

1. Matter J. Creeping attachment of free gingival grafts. A five-year follow-up study. J Periodontol 1980;51:681–685.
2. American Academy of Periodontology. Glossary of Periodontal Terms. American Academy of Periodontology, 2001.
3. Bartlett DW, Shah P. A critical review of non-carious cervical (wear) lesions and the role of abfraction, erosion, and abrasion. J Dent Res 2006;85:306–312.
4. Albandar JM, Kingman A. Gingival recession, gingival bleeding, and dental calculus in adults 30 years of age and older in the United States, 1988-1994. J Periodontol 1999;70:30–43.
5. Löe H, Anerud A, Boysen H. The natural history of periodontal disease in man: Prevalence, severity, and extent of gingival recession. J Periodontol 1992;63:489–495.
6. Gorman WJ. Prevalence and etiology of gingival recession. J Periodontol 1967;38:316–322.
7. Serino G, Wennström JL, Lindhe J, Eneroth L. The prevalence and distribution of gingival recession in subjects with a high standard of oral hygiene. J Clin Periodontol 1994;21:57–63.
8. Hall WB. Present status of soft tissue grafting. J Periodontol 1977;48:587–597.
9. Chrysanthakopoulos NA. Gingival recession: Prevalence and risk indicators among young Greek adults. J Clin Exp Dent 2014;6:e243–e249.
10. Jati AS, Furquim LZ, Consolaro A. Gingival recession: Its causes and types, and the importance of orthodontic treatment. Dental Press J Orthod 2016;21:18–29.
11. Wennström JL. Status of the art in mucogingival surgery. Schweiz Monatsschr Zahnmed (1984) 1985;95:343–352.
12. Sullivan HC, Atkins JH. Free autogenous gingival grafts. 3. Utilization of grafts in the treatment of gingival recession. Periodontics 1968;6:152–160.
13. Miller PD Jr. A classification of marginal tissue recession. Int J Periodontics Restorative Dent 1985;5:8–13.
14. Cairo F, Nieri M, Cincinelli S, Mervelt J, Pagliaro U. The interproximal clinical attachment level to classify gingival recessions and predict root coverage outcomes: An explorative and reliability study. J Clin Periodontol 2011;38:661–666.
15. American Academy of Periodontology. Parameter on mucogingival conditions. J Periodontol 2000;71(5S suppl):861–862.
16. Pini Prato G, Tinti C, Vincenzi G, Magnani C, Cortellini P, Clauser C. Guided tissue regeneration versus mucogingival surgery in the treatment of human buccal gingival recession. J Periodontol 1992;63:919–928.
17. Langer B, Langer L. Subepithelial connective tissue graft technique for root coverage. J Periodontol 1985;56:715–720.
18. Nabers JM. Free gingival grafts. Periodontics 1966;4:243–245.

19. Barros RR, Novaes AB, Grisi MF, Souza SL, Taba MJ, Palioto DB. A 6-month comparative clinical study of a conventional and a new surgical approach for root coverage with acellular dermal matrix. J Periodontol 2004;75:1350–1356.
20. Sanz M, Lorenzo R, Aranda JJ, Martin C, Orsini M. Clinical evaluation of a new collagen matrix (Mucograft prototype) to enhance the width of keratinized tissue in patients with fixed prosthetic restorations: A randomized prospective clinical trial. J Clin Periodontol 2009;36:868–876.
21. Harris RJ. A short-term and long-term comparison of root coverage with an acellular dermal matrix and a subepithelial graft. J Periodontol 2004;75:734–743.
22. Bernimoulin JP, Lüscher B, Mühlemann HR. Coronally repositioned periodontal flap. Clinical evaluation after one year. J Clin Periodontol 1975;2:1–13.
23. De Sanctis M, Zucchelli G. Coronally advanced flap: A modified surgical approach for isolated recession-type defects: Three-year results. J Clin Periodontol 2007;34:262–268.
24. Grupe HE. Modified technique for the sliding flap operation. J Periodontol 1966;37:491–495.
25. Grupe HE, Warren RF. Repair of gingival defect by a sliding flap operation. J Periodontol 1956;27:92–95.
26. Harris RJ. The connective tissue and partial thickness double pedicle graft: A predictable method of obtaining root coverage. J Periodontol 1992;63:477–486.
27. Tarnow DP. Semilunar coronally repositioned flap. J Clin Periodontol 1986;13:182–185.
28. Guinard EA, Caffesse RG. Treatment of localized gingival recessions. Part I. Lateral sliding flap. J Periodontol 1978;49:351–356.
29. Zabalegui I, Sicilia A, Cambra J, Gil J, Sanz M. Treatment of multiple adjacent gingival recessions with the tunnel subepithelial connective tissue graft: A clinical report. Int J Periodontics Restorative Dent 1999;19:199–206.
30. McGuire MK, Scheyer ET, Nunn M. Evaluation of human recession defects treated with coronally advanced flaps and either enamel matrix derivative or connective tissue: Comparison of clinical parameters at 10 years. J Periodontol 2012;83:1353–1362.
31. Deshpande A, Koudale SB, Bhongade ML. A comparative evaluation of rhPDGF-BB + beta-TCP and subepithelial connective tissue graft for the treatment of multiple gingival recession defects in humans. Int J Periodontics Restorative Dent 2014;34:241–249.
32. Tatakis DN, Chambrone L, Allen EP, et al. Periodontal soft tissue root coverage procedures: A consensus report from the AAP Regeneration Workshop. J Periodontol 2015;86(2 suppl):S52–S55.
33. Kim DM, Neiva R. Periodontal soft tissue non-root coverage procedures: A systematic review from the AAP Regeneration Workshop. J Periodontol 2015;86(2 suppl):S56–S72.
34. Leong DJ, Wang HL. A decision tree for soft tissue grafting. Int J Periodontics Restorative Dent 2011;31:307–313.
35. Richardson CR, Allen EP, Chambrone D, et al. Periodontal soft tissue root coverage procedures: Practical applications from the AAP Regeneration Workshop. Clini Adv Periodontics 2015;5:2–10.
36. Chambrone L, Tatakis DN. Long-term outcomes of untreated buccal gingival recessions: A systematic review and meta-analysis. J Periodontol 2016;87:796–808.
37. Agudio G, Cortellini P, Buti J, Pini Prato G. Periodontal conditions of sites treated with gingival augmentation surgery compared with untreated contralateral homologous sites: An 18- to 35-year long-term study. J Periodontol 2016;87:1371–1378.
38. Greenwell H, Fiorellini J, Giannobile W, et al. Oral reconstructive and corrective considerations in periodontal therapy. J Periodontol 2005;76:1588–1600.
39. Chambrone L, Pini Prato GP. Clinical insights about the evolution of root coverage procedures: The flap, the graft, and the surgery. J Periodontol 2019;90:9–15.
40. Chambrone L, Tatakis DN. Periodontal soft tissue root coverage procedures: A systematic review from the AAP Regeneration Workshop. J Periodontol 2015;86(2 suppl):S8–S51.
41. Harris RJ. Creeping attachment associated with the connective tissue with partial-thickness double pedicle graft. J Periodontol 1997;68:890–899.
42. Pini Prato G, Clauser C, Cortellini P, Tinti C, Vincenzi G, Pagliaro U. Guided tissue regeneration versus mucogingival surgery in the treatment of human buccal recessions. A 4-year follow-up study. J Periodontol 1996;67:1216–1223.
43. Leknes KN, Amarante ES, Price DE, Boe OE, Skavland RJ, Lie T. Coronally positioned flap procedures with or without a biodegradable membrane in the treatment of human gingival recession. A 6-year follow-up study. J Clin Periodontol 2005;32:518–529.
44. Spahr A, Haegewald S, Tsoulfidou F, et al. Coverage of Miller class I and II recession defects using enamel matrix proteins versus coronally advanced flap technique: A 2-year report. J Periodontol 2005;76:1871–1880.
45. Nickles K, Ratka-Krüger P, Neukranz E, Raetzke P, Eickholz P. Ten-year results after connective tissue grafts and guided tissue regeneration for root coverage. J Periodontol 2010;81:827–836.
46. Moslemi N, Mousavi Jazi M, Haghighati F, Morovati SP, Jamali R. Acellular dermal matrix allograft versus subepithelial connective tissue graft in treatment of gingival recessions: A 5-year randomized clinical study. J Clin Periodontol 2011;38:1122–1129.
47. Rosetti EP, Marcantonio E Jr, Zuza EP, Marcantonio RA. Root coverage stability of the subepithelial connective tissue graft and guided tissue regeneration: A 30-month follow-up clinical trial. J Dent 2013;41:114–120.
48. Pini Prato GP, Franceschi D, Cortellini P, Chambrone L. Long-term evaluation (20 years) of the outcomes of subepithelial connective tissue graft plus coronally advanced flap in the treatment of maxillary single recession-type defects. J Periodontol 2018;89:1290–1299.
49. Yilmaz HG, Boke F, Ayali A. Cone-beam computed tomography evaluation of the soft tissue thickness and greater palatine foramen location in the palate. J Clin Periodontol 2015;42:458–461.
50. Tomaszewska IM, Tomaszewski KA, Kmiotek EK, et al. Anatomical landmarks for the localization of the greater palatine foramen: A study of 1200 head CTs, 150 dry skulls, systematic review of literature and meta-analysis. J Anat 2014;225:419–435.
51. Wara-aswapati N, Pitiphat W, Chandrapho N, Rattanayatikul C, Karimbux N. Thickness of palatal masticatory mucosa associated with age. J Periodontol 2001;72:1407–1412.
52. Studer SP, Allen EP, Rees TC, Kouba A. The thickness of masticatory mucosa in the human hard palate and tuberosity as potential donor sites for ridge augmentation procedures. J Periodontol 1997;68:145–151.
53. Soehren SE, Allen AL, Cutright DE, Seibert JS. Clinical and histologic studies of donor tissues utilized for free grafts of masticatory mucosa. J Periodontol 1973;44:727–741.
54. Zucchelli G, Mele M, Stefanini M, et al. Patient morbidity and root coverage outcome after subepithelial connective tissue and de-epithelialized grafts: A comparative randomized-controlled clinical trial. J Clin Periodontol 2010;37:728–738.
55. Bertl K, Pifl M, et al. Relative composition of fibrous connective and fatty/glandular tissue in connective tissue grafts depends on the harvesting technique but not the donor site of the hard palate. J Periodontol 2015;86:1331–1339.

56. Al-Zahrani MS, Bissada NF, Ficara AJ, Cole B. Effect of connective tissue graft orientation on root coverage and gingival augmentation. Int J Periodontics Restorative Dent 2004;24:65–69.
57. Lafzi A, Mostofi Zadeh Farahani R, Abolfazli N, Amid R, Safaiyan A. Effect of connective tissue graft orientation on the root coverage outcomes of coronally advanced flap. Clin Oral Investig 2007;11:401–408.
58. Henderson RD, Greenwell H, Drisko C, et al. Predictable multiple site root coverage using an acellular dermal matrix allograft. J Periodontol 2001;72:571–582.
59. Wang HL, Romanos GE, Geurs NC, Sullivan A, Suárez-López Del Amo F, Eber RM. Comparison of two differently processed acellular dermal matrix products for root coverage procedures: A prospective, randomized multicenter study. J Periodontol 2014;85:1693–1701.
60. McGuire MK, Scheyer ET. Randomized, controlled clinical trial to evaluate a xenogeneic collagen matrix as an alternative to free gingival grafting for oral soft tissue augmentation. J Periodontol 2014;85:1333–1341.
61. McGuire MK, Scheyer ET. Xenogeneic collagen matrix with coronally advanced flap compared to connective tissue with coronally advanced flap for the treatment of dehiscence-type recession defects. J Periodontol 2010;81:1108–1117.
62. Chambrone L, Chambrone D, Pustiglioni FE, Chambrone LA, Lima LA. The influence of tobacco smoking on the outcomes achieved by root-coverage procedures: A systematic review. J Am Dent Assoc 2009;140:294–306.
63. Kaval B, Renaud DE, Scott DA, Buduneli N. The role of smoking and gingival crevicular fluid markers on coronally advanced flap outcomes. J Periodontol 2014;85:395–405.
64. Silva CO, Ribeiro Edel P, Sallum AW, Tatakis DN. Free gingival grafts: Graft shrinkage and donor-site healing in smokers and non-smokers. J Periodontol 2010;81:692–701.
65. Baldi C, Pini Prato G, Pagliaro U, et al. Coronally advanced flap procedure for root coverage. Is flap thickness a relevant predictor to achieve root coverage? A 19-case series. J Periodontol 1999;70:1077–1084.
66. Pini Prato G, Baldi C, Pagliaro U, et al. Coronally advanced flap procedure for root coverage. Treatment of root surface: Root planning versus polishing. J Periodontol 1999;70:1064–1076.
67. Pini Prato G, Pagliaro U, Baldi C, et al. Coronally advanced flap procedure for root coverage. Flap with tension versus flap without tension: A randomized controlled clinical study. J Periodontol 2000;71:188–201.
68. Pini Prato GP, Baldi C, Nieri M, et al. Coronally advanced flap: The post-surgical position of the gingival margin is an important factor for achieving complete root coverage. J Periodontol 2005;76:713–722.
69. Saletta D, Pini Prato G, Pagliaro U, Baldi C, Mauri M, Nieri M. Coronally advanced flap procedure: Is the interdental papilla a prognostic factor for root coverage? J Periodontol 2001;72:760–766.
70. Zucchelli G, Gori G, Mele M, et al. Non-carious cervical lesions associated with gingival recessions: A decision-making process. J Periodontol 2011;82:1713–1724.
71. Bengazi F, Wennström JL, Lekholm U. Recession of the soft tissue margin at oral implants. A 2-year longitudinal prospective study. Clin Oral Implants Res 1996;7:303–310.
72. Zucchelli G, Mazzotti C, Mounssif I, Mele M, Stefanini M, Montebugnoli L. A novel surgical-prosthetic approach for soft tissue dehiscence coverage around single implant. Clin Oral Implants Res 2013;24:957–962.
73. El Askary Ael S, Ghallab NA, Tan SC, Rosen PS, Shawkat A. Implant-related gingival recession: Pilot case series presents novel technique and scoring template. Compend Contin Educ Dent 2016;37:468–480.
74. Le B, Borzabadi-Farahani A, Nielsen B. Treatment of labial soft tissue recession around dental implants in the esthetic zone using guided bone regeneration with mineralized allograft: A retrospective clinical case series. J Oral Maxillofac Surg 2016;74:1552–1561.
75. Decker AM, Suárez-López Del Amo F, Urban IA, Miller PD Jr, Wang HL. Prognostic classification system for implant recession defects. Implant Dent 2017;26:848–852.
76. Zucchelli G, Tavelli L, Stefanini M, et al. Classification of facial peri-implant soft tissue dehiscence/deficiencies at single implant sites in the esthetic zone. J Periodontol 2019;90:1116–1124.

23

PERIODONTAL AND PERI-IMPLANT MAINTENANCE

Lucía Barallat, DDS, MS, PhD
Jose Nart, DDS, PhD

DEFINITIONS AND TERMINOLOGY

Periodontal maintenance (formerly referred to as *supportive periodontal therapy*, *preventive maintenance*, *recall maintenance*): Procedures performed at selected intervals to assist the periodontal patient in maintaining oral health. As part of periodontal therapy, an interval is established for periodic ongoing care. Maintenance procedures are under the supervision of the dentist and typically include an update of the medical and dental histories, radiographic review, extraoral and intraoral soft tissue examination, dental examination, periodontal evaluation, removal of the bacterial flora from crevicular and pocket areas, scaling and root planing where indicated, polishing of the teeth, and a review of the patient's plaque control efficacy. Periodontal maintenance procedures following active therapy are not synonymous with prophylaxis.[1]

Compliance: Action in accordance with recommendation(s).[1]

Periodontal therapy includes a variety of different phases, such as the systemic phase, nonsurgical cause-related therapy, surgical or corrective phase, and maintenance phase. **Periodontal maintenance** or *supportive periodontal therapy (SPT)* is the group of procedures performed at select intervals to assist the periodontal patient in maintaining oral health after it has been achieved during the active phase of treatment.[1]

The main goals of SPT are the following:

- To prevent the relapse and progression of periodontal or peri-implant diseases in patients who previously received treatment
- To reduce the incidence of tooth and/or implant loss
- To increase the probability of detecting and treating other conditions or diseases present in the oral cavity[2]

Importance of SPT

The importance of SPT is based on the bacterial etiology of periodontal diseases. Multiple studies have shown a causal relationship between plaque accumulation and gingivitis[3] and mucositis.[4,5] Because gingivitis always precedes periodontitis[6] and mucositis precedes peri-implantitis,[7] it appears evident that good plaque control is necessary to maintain periodontal and peri-implant health. Furthermore, it has been shown that, in the absence of adequate supragingival plaque control after scaling and root planing (SRP), recolonization of the deep pockets may take place, reaching bacterial loads similar to baseline values after 4 to 8 weeks.[8] SPT will also compensate for difficulties that patients may have in maintaining good oral hygiene. It will reinforce good oral hygiene habits and motivate the patient to continue practicing them.

TABLE 23-1 Disease progression with different levels of compliance

Study	Population	Mean annual clinical attachment loss	Mean annual tooth loss
Nyman et al[9] (1977)	Noncompliant patients after periodontal surgical therapy	1 mm/year	NR
Becker et al[10] (1984)	Compliers after periodontal therapy	NR	0.11 teeth/year
	Noncompliers after periodontal therapy		0.22 teeth/year
	No periodontal therapy		0.36 teeth/year
Costa et al[11] (2014)	Regular compliers	NR	0.12 teeth/year
	Irregular compliers		0.36 teeth/year

NR, not reported.

PROGRESSION OF PERIODONTAL DISEASE IN NONCOMPLIANT PATIENTS

Several longitudinal studies have shown that patients who are susceptible to periodontitis and do not attend the recommended maintenance visits will likely present with a relapse of the disease. Also, noncompliant patients are at a higher risk of attachment loss and tooth loss when compared with complying patients (Table 23-1).[9–11] For example, if we compare clinical attachment loss between noncompliant patients after active periodontal therapy with different surgical approaches[9] and a nontreated population,[12] the mean annual clinical attachment loss was three times greater in the noncompliant patients than in individuals who did not receive treatment.

PROGRESSION OF PERIODONTAL DISEASE IN COMPLIANT PATIENTS

Strong evidence exists regarding the effectiveness of SPT in maintaining periodontal and oral health. Axelsson et al spent 30 years following a periodontally treated population who received SPT after active periodontal therapy according to their individual needs.[13] In this study, only 2% to 4% of sites lost more than 2 mm of attachment, and the interproximal and lingual surfaces showed a mean attachment gain of 0.1 to 0.5 mm. Additionally, a mean tooth loss of 0.4 to 1.8 teeth occurred during the evaluation period, with root fracture as the main reason for tooth loss. Regarding new caries lesions, a mean of 1.2 to 2.1 new lesions were diagnosed.[13]

However, while long-term longitudinal and retrospective studies have shown that SPT is effective in the majority of patients, a small proportion of highly susceptible individuals may still present with recurrence of the disease.[14] Hirschfeld and Wasserman[15] retrospectively analyzed tooth loss in 600 periodontally treated patients and observed that in 499 patients ("well-maintained" group), only 0.68 teeth per patient were lost, whereas in 25 patients ("extreme downhill" group), it reached 13.3 teeth per patient. Teeth with furcation involvement and/or initial questionable prognosis were lost more frequently over time.

MAINTENANCE INTERVALS

During the last decades, different maintenance recall intervals have been proposed, ranging from several weeks to months. Lovdal et al[16] was the first study to establish a 3- to 6-month maintenance interval depending on disease severity. Since then, a 3-month recall has been the most widely used.[17–20] The rationale for this frequency relies on the risk of recolonization of the pockets after 8 to 11 weeks.[8,21] In addition, Ramfjord et al demonstrated that with 3-month recall intervals, the outcomes of periodontal therapy can be maintained after 3 to 4 years regardless of the different levels of oral hygiene, showing minor differences between individuals with good and poor hygiene habits.[17] However, other investigations have adapted the maintenance frequency according to the patient's individual risk of relapse: 3 to 6 months,[22,23] 4 to 6 months,[15] or 3 to 12 months.[13]

EFFECTIVENESS OF SPT ON PERI-IMPLANT HEALTH

Costa et al followed a cohort of partially edentulous patients restored with implant-supported prostheses during 5 years. The incidence of peri-implantitis was 18% for the complying patients and 43.9% in those not attending the SPT program. The lack of maintenance showed an association with peri-implantitis (odds ratio = 5.92) when compared with the well-maintained group.[24] These results are in concordance with those presented by Monje et al, in which it was observed that only 4.5% of compliant patients presented with peri-implantitis, whereas 23.9% of noncompliant patients presented with peri-implantitis. Regular SPT was associated with 86% less prevalence of peri-implantitis on a patient level.[25]

Furthermore, Rocuzzo et al followed a cohort of individuals with and without history of periodontal disease over 10 years and found that the risk of implant loss and peri-implant bone loss greater than 3 mm was significantly higher in periodontally compromised patients who did not attend SPT.[26] Therefore, implants should only be placed when periodontitis has been successfully treated and the patient is ready to comply with an SPT program.[27]

In another prospective study, 31 patients who received surgical treatment of peri-implantitis at 71 implants were enrolled in a SPT program for 5 years. At the final evaluation, only 9 implants (13%) showed clinical attachment loss, and 43 implants (60%) exhibited healthy soft tissues.[28]

In summary, all these investigations are in accordance with the outcomes of a recent systematic review in which SPT seemed to have a positive impact on the incidence of peri-implant diseases and implant survival rate.[29]

SPT Visit

Each maintenance visit should include the following procedures:

1. Update of medical and dental history
2. Clinical examination:
   - Extraoral and intraoral tissues, including cancer screening
   - Dental examination:
     - Occlusion
     - Dental caries assessment
     - Evaluation of prosthesis and abutment teeth
   - Periodontal examination:
     - Probing depths (PDs)
     - Gingival recessions and other mucogingival deformities or conditions
     - Clinical attachment level (CAL)
     - Tooth mobility
     - Furcation involvement
     - Bleeding on probing (BOP)
     - Suppuration
3. Radiographic examination and new radiographs if indicated
4. Comparison of current findings with previous records
5. Oral hygiene assessment
6. Treatment:
   - Behavioral modification
     - Motivation and reinforcement of oral hygiene habits
     - Control of other environmental factors such as smoking, stress, and more
   - Removal of supra- and subgingival calculus
   - SRP of residual pockets
   - Occlusal adjustment if indicated
   - Other additional treatments that may be indicated, such as administration of local antiseptics or antibiotics
   - Polishing and administration of fluorides or desensitizing agents
7. Inform the patient about current oral health status and communicate with other health care professionals if needed
8. Establish a recall interval determined by a careful multilevel risk assessment, including patient-, tooth-, and site-specific factors[2]

SPT Risk Assessment

According to the 2017 World Workshop, *periodontal disease stability* is that state in which periodontitis has been successfully treated through control of local and systemic factors, resulting in minimal BOP, optimal improvements in PDs and CAL, and lack of progressive destruction.[30] Thus, when performing a clinical diagnosis during an SPT visit, the final outcome after active periodontal therapy should always be taken as a reference.[31] Ideally, patients under an SPT program would maintain CAL in the long term. In clinical practice, a full-mouth bleeding on probing

(FMBOP) index of less than 10% and PDs of 4 mm or less would be accepted as a healthy periodontium.[6,30]

The SPT risk assessment should be based on three main categories: patient-, tooth-, and site-specific levels.

PATIENT LEVEL

In 2003, Lang and Tonetti proposed a periodontal risk assessment (PRA) diagram based on different aspects on a patient level to guide the clinician in determining a recall interval (see Fig 23-1).[32]

Compliance with the recall system

As mentioned previously, the lack of maintenance after periodontal therapy will lead to reinfection and progressive clinical attachment loss, whereas patients who regularly attend their SPT visits in most cases will be able to maintain a healthy and stable clinical situation.

Oral hygiene

Because dental biofilm is the main etiologic factor for periodontitis, good plaque control is essential to avoid disease recurrence. Although a plaque index threshold compatible with health varies between individuals, a percentage between 20% and 40% should be suitable for most patients.[32]

Bleeding on probing

FMBOP reflects the patient's oral hygiene and response to plaque accumulation. For this reason, it is considered the first parameter of the diagram. One prospective study observed that FMBOP under 25% was associated with periodontal stability, but patients with greater percentages showed recurrent disease.[33] Also, it has been reported that FMBOP less than 10% might be compatible with periodontal stability.[6] Therefore, more than 25% FMBOP will be considered as a high-risk patient, while FMBOP less than 10% will be a low-risk patient.

Residual pockets 5 mm or greater

The number of deep residual pockets reflects the success of active periodontal therapy. Matuliene et al observed that PD 6 mm or greater was associated with increased risk of disease progression and tooth loss.[34] This factor is considered as the second risk indicator in the diagram: four residual pockets will be considered as low risk and eight or more as high risk.

Tooth loss (out of 28 teeth)

Tooth loss is the final outcome of periodontal disease. A short arch from premolar to premolar can be compatible with a stable occlusion, but having less than 20 teeth has been related to functional alterations. For this reason, low-risk patients will include those who have lost 4 teeth or less, while high-risk patients will be those with a tooth loss of 8 teeth or more.[35]

Bone loss in relation to patient's age

Bone loss in relation to the patient's age has been used as an indirect method to evaluate the rate of disease progression.[36] Radiographic bone loss (RBL) is calculated at the most affected tooth as a percentage, in which each millimeter represents a 10% bone loss of the total root length. RBL is then divided by the patient's age to obtain the index. An index of 0.5 or less will be considered as low risk, while 1 or greater will be high risk.

Systemic and genetic factors

Diabetes mellitus (DM) has been strongly associated with higher prevalence and severity of periodontal disease, specially type 2 DM.[37,38] Also, there is some evidence that patients positive to the polymorphism interleukin-1 present with more advanced periodontitis.[39] This parameter will only be taken into consideration if it is known, and if present, it will be automatically considered as high risk.

Cigarette smoking

Smoking, the sixth parameter, is the most important modifiable risk factor for periodontitis, and a strong causal association between the two entities has been established.[40,41] Tobacco consumption affects the outcomes of periodontal therapy and increases the risk of relapse[34,42] and tooth loss[42] during the maintenance phase. The association between smoking and periodontitis is dose dependent,[43] meaning that individuals who smoke more than 20 cigarettes per day will be at high risk. On the other hand, former smokers (for more than 5 years) and nonsmokers are considered at low risk.

How to determine patient's individual periodontal risk assessment

The following diagram will help determine whether the patient is at low, moderate, or high risk for each of the factors (Fig 23-1). Once that exercise is completed,

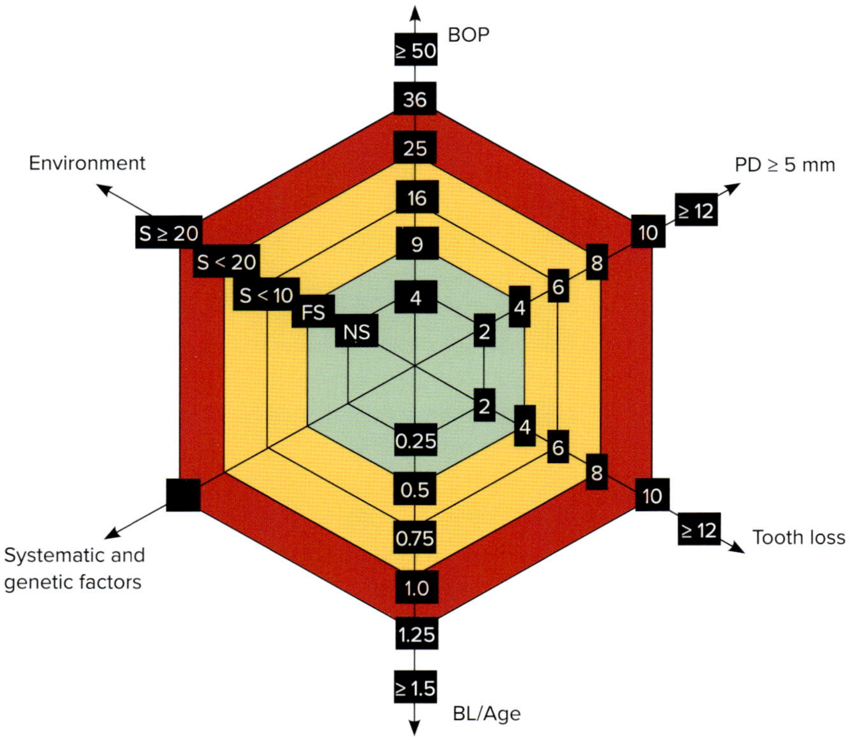

Fig 23-1 Periodontal risk assessment diagram. *Green*, low risk. *Yellow*, moderate risk. *Red*, high risk. NS, nonsmoker; FS, former smoker; S, cigarettes smoked per day.

patients will be subsequently placed in one of the following categories:

- *Low risk:* All parameters are at low risk or one parameter is at moderate risk. A 12-month recall is recommended.
- *Moderate risk:* There are two or more parameters in the moderate category and/or one in the high risk category. A 6-month recall is recommended.
- *High risk:* Two or more parameters fall under the high risk category. A 3-month recall is recommended.[32,44]

To validate PRA, Matuliene et al followed a cohort of patients under maintenance according to the patient's risk assessment during 9 years and observed that periodontitis recurred in 49.2% of the high-risk patients and 18.2% in the low-risk group.[44] High-risk patients had twice as much tooth loss as moderate- and low-risk patients.[44] Furthermore, a recent systematic review confirmed the predictive value of this tool as a predictor for tooth loss and periodontal disease progression.[45]

TOOTH LEVEL

Furcation involvement

Several longitudinal studies have observed that furcation-involved teeth are associated with increased risk of tooth loss.[15,46] Pretzl et al observed that, while 13% of multirooted teeth with furcation involvement were lost after 10 years, only 5% of uniradicular teeth were lost.[46] Similarly, Hirschfeld and Wassermann observed that most of the teeth that were lost presented with furcation involvement.[15] Another prospective study observed that the degree of furcation involvement plays an important role in periodontal stability. Molars presenting with class I furcations were more frequently maintained in the long term than class II or class III furcations.[47,48]

Iatrogenic factors

The presence of overhanging restorations may favor plaque accumulation.[49] Furthermore, subgingival margins and overcontoured crowns may produce biologic width invasions that can result in chronic inflammation, gingival recession, and/or bone loss.[50]

Tooth mobility

Tooth mobility might be present in a reduced periodontium and still be compatible with periodontal health. However, if mobility increases over time, it should be considered pathologic and should be treated.[51,52]

Residual periodontal support

As mentioned previously, after therapy, periodontally healthy teeth with a reduced clinical attachment might be maintained in the long term if occlusal forces are adequately distributed.[53,54]

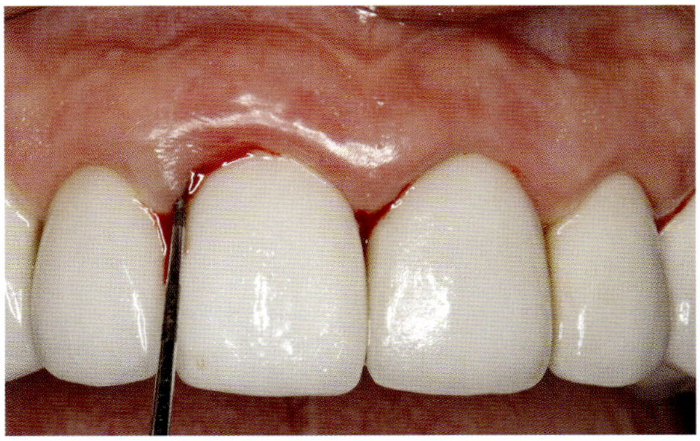

Fig 23-2 Patient presenting with BOP.

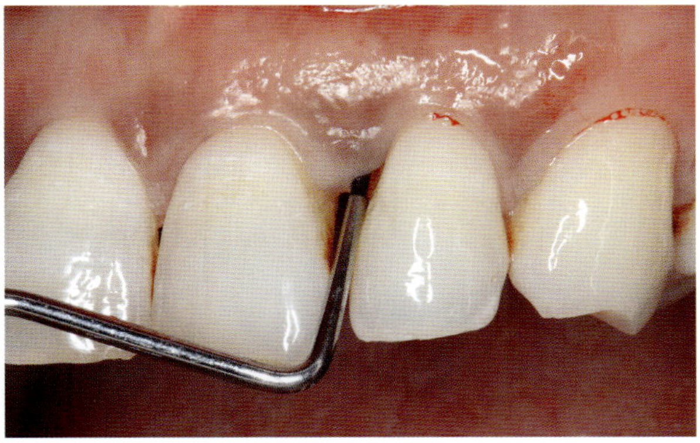

Fig 23-3 Site presenting PD of 10 mm.

Tooth position

Tooth crowding and malposition may facilitate gingival inflammation, especially in patients with poor plaque control.[55] Some studies have shown increased clinical attachment loss in misaligned anterior teeth when compared with aligned anterior dentition.[56,57]

Initial tooth prognosis

In a recent systematic review, teeth classified as questionable or hopeless at baseline were lost in a significantly higher percentage than teeth with a good prognosis at baseline.[14]

SITE LEVEL

Continuous monitoring at a site level is key during SPT because it allows for the detection of sites that are at a higher risk of future clinical attachment loss and subsequently to determine whether or not retreatment is needed.

Bleeding on probing

During maintenance, absence of BOP at a specific site has been associated with periodontal stability,[58] but its presence during subsequent maintenance appointments indicates a probability of 30% of future clinical attachment loss.[59] Thus, sites repeatedly presenting with BOP are at higher risk of disease progression than nonbleeding sites (Fig 23-2).

Probing depth

PD and clinical attachment loss reflect the changes in the periodontium that have already occurred, but they do not indicate disease activity. The only method to identify if a site is actively losing attachment is by performing different evaluations over time. However, the presence of residual deep pockets increases the probability of further attachment loss by up to 50%. Furthermore, the combination of residual pockets and BOP or suppuration was associated with a greater than 75% chance of disease progression[60] (Fig 23-3).

Suppuration

In a prospective study, suppuration on probing had a diagnostic predictability of future attachment loss of 40% to 50%.[49] Kaldahl et al observed that when suppuration was present, less PD reduction was expected after periodontal therapy.[61]

Peri-Implant Maintenance

MONITORING PERI-IMPLANT HEALTH STATUS

When implant therapy first became a common practice, it was thought that probing around implants would result in irreversible damage to the soft tissue seal. It was later demonstrated that gentle probing (ie, < 0.25 N) around implants is not harmful because the epithelial attachment is re-formed after 5 to 7 days.[62] In addition, probing is necessary to diagnose peri-implant diseases.[63,64] There is also no evidence to support the use of metallic probes rather than plastic probes.[63]

According to the 2017 World Workshop, peri-implant soft tissue health is characterized by the following[64]:

- Absence of signs of clinical inflammation (ie, BOP and/or suppuration)
- Absence of increased PD compared with previous examinations

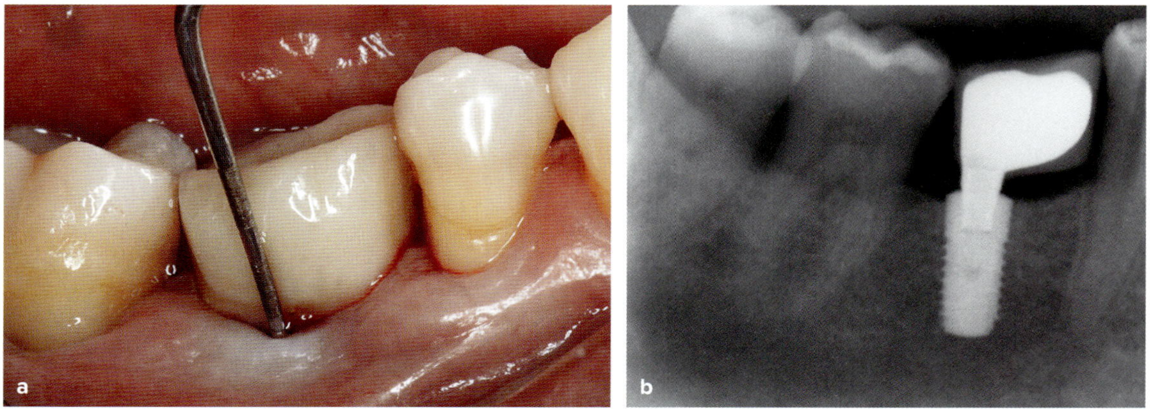

Fig 23-4 Site presenting with peri-implant mucositis. PDs are stable, and there are no crestal bone level changes. Only BOP and signs of inflammation are visible. *(a)* Clinical photograph. *(b)* Radiograph.

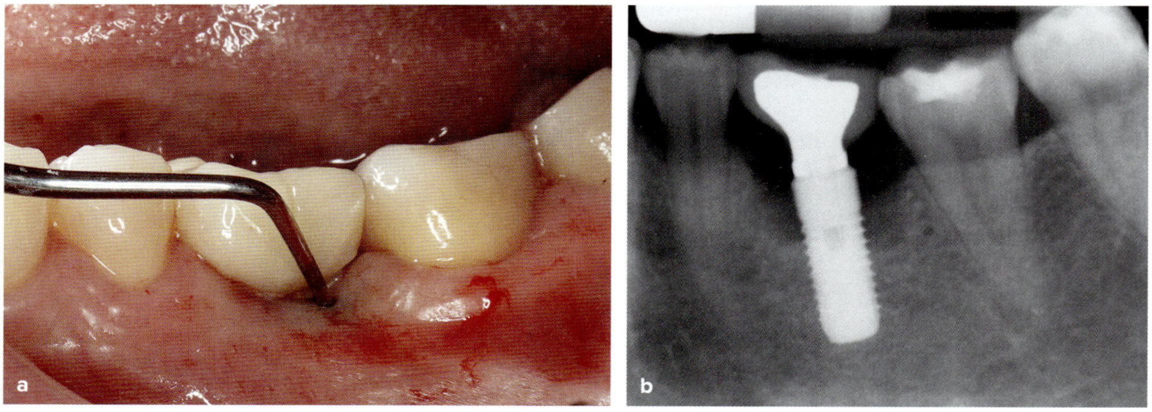

Fig 23-5 In the absence of previous records, the presence of PD greater than 6 mm and crestal bone loss greater than 3 mm apical to the intraosseous part of the implant is diagnosed as peri-implantitis. *(a)* Clinical photograph. *(b)* Radiograph.

- No bone loss beyond crestal bone level changes after initial bone remodeling

Due to the variability in the apicocoronal placement of implants, it is not possible to define a range of PDs compatible with health.[64] Therefore, to monitor peri-implant health status, implants should be probed after placement of the prosthetic rehabilitation to determine baseline levels. Additionally, baseline clinical radiographs should be taken once the remodeling phase after implant loading has occurred.[65,66]

Previous records should be obtained if possible. However, if previous clinical and radiographic information is not available, peri-implantitis will be diagnosed if the following is present[64]:

- BOP and/or suppuration
- PD of 6 mm or greater
- Bone loss of 3 mm or greater (ie, the bone level is 3 mm or more apical from the intraosseous part of the implant)

At every maintenance visit, signs of inflammation, BOP, suppuration, PDs, and apical migration of the peri-implant mucosa should be recorded. If changes with respect to the baseline records are identified, periapical radiographs can be taken to help determine if bone loss has occurred.[66] If there are signs of inflammation (mucosal redness and BOP) but PDs and bone levels have remained stable, the diagnosis is peri-implant mucositis (Fig 23-4). On the contrary, if increased PDs and/or crestal bone level changes are detected, the diagnosis is peri-implantitis[64] (Fig 23-5).

MAINTENANCE OF DENTAL IMPLANTS

The treatment approach for implants during maintenance visits will depend on the peri-implant conditions. In the presence of peri-implant health, polishing of the crown with a rubber cup and low-abrasive paste might be enough.[27] In the case of mucositis lesions, the goal will be to return peri-implant tissues to health because there is evidence that mucositis increases the risk for developing peri-implantitis.[24] Treatment options include oral hygiene instructions, modification of the implant-supported prosthesis,[67] mechanical debridement, air polishing, use of adjunctive chemotherapeutic agents, probiotics,[68] and/or laser therapy. However, there is still no consensus on the best treatment approach, and complete resolution of inflammation might not always be achieved.[69] If peri-implantitis is diagnosed, a more advanced treatment is needed to stop disease progression (see chapter 18).

Regarding the instruments to be used during mechanical debridement around implants, conventional steel curettes are not recommended because they are harder than titanium and might damage the implant surface. For this reason, plastic and titanium curettes have been proposed, although plastic curettes might not be sufficiently efficient with respect to biofilm removal.[70] Ultrasonic devices with nonmetallic or copper tips have also been developed to avoid altering the implant surface.[27]

As with SPT, the recall interval will vary for each case as well as the type of treatment performed during maintenance. Thus, in low-risk patients, a recall interval of 5 to 6 months has been suggested.[29] However, a more frequent recall regime would be advisable in patients with a previous history of periodontal disease.[26]

References

1. American Academy of Periodontology. Glossary of Periodontal Terms. American Academy of Periodontology, 2001.
2. Cohen RE, Research, Science and Therapy Committee, American Academy of Periodontology. Position paper: Periodontal maintenance. J Periodontol 2003;74:1395–1401.
3. Löe H, Theilade E, Jensen SB. Experimental gingivitis in man. J Periodontol 1965;36:177–187.
4. Pontoriero R, Tonelli MP, Carnevale G, Mombelli A, Nyman SR, Lang NP. Experimentally induced peri-implant mucositis. A clinical study in humans. Clin Oral Implants Res 1994;5:254–259.
5. Zitzman NU, Berglundh T, Marinello CP, Lindhe J. Experimental peri-implant mucositis in man. J Clin Periodontol 2001;28:517–523.
6. Chapple ILC, Mealey BL, Van Dyke TE, et al. Periodontal health and gingival diseases and conditions on an intact and a reduced periodontium: Consensus report of workgroups 1 of the 2017 World Workshop on the Classification of Periodontal and Peri-implant Diseases and Conditions. J Clin Periodontol 2018;89(1 suppl):S74–S84.
7. Berglundh T, Armitage G, Araugo MG, et al. Peri-implant diseases and conditions: Consensus report of workgroup 4 of the 2017 World Workshop on the Classification of Periodontal and Peri-implant Diseases and Conditions. J Clin Periodontol 2018;45(20 suppl):S286–S291.
8. Magnusson I, Lindhe J, Yoneyama T, Liljenberg B. Recolonization of a subgingival microbiota following scaling in deep pockets. J Clin Periodontol 1984:11;193–207.
9. Nyman S, Lindhe J, Rosling B. Periodontal surgery in plaque-infected dentitions. J Clin Periodontol 1977;4:240–249.
10. Becker W, Becker BE, Berg LE. Periodontal treatment without maintenance. A retrospective study in 44 patients. J Clin Periodontol 1984;55:505–509.
11. Costa FO, Lages EJ, Cota LO, Lorentz TC, Soares RV, Cortelli JR. Tooth loss in individuals under periodontal maintenance therapy: 5-year prospective study. J Periodontal Res 2014;49:121–128.
12. Löe H, Ånerud Å, Boysen H, Morrison EC. Natural history of periodontal disease in man. Rapid, moderate and no loss of attachment in Sri Lankan laborers 14–46 years of age. J Clin Periodontol 1986;13:431–440.
13. Axelsson P, Nyström B, Lindhe J. The long-term effect of a plaque control program on tooth mortality, caries and periodontal disease in adults. Results after 30 years of maintenance. J Clin Periodontol 2004;31:749–757.
14. Chambrone L, Chambrone D, Lima LA, Chambrone LA. Predictors of tooth loss during long-term periodontal maintenance: A systematic review of observational studies. J Clin Periodontol 2010;37:675–684.
15. Hirschfeld L, Wasserman, B. A long-term survey of tooth loss in 600 treated periodontal patients. J Periodontol 1978;49:225–237.
16. Lovdal A, Arno A, Schei O, Waerhaug J. Combined effect of subgingival scaling and controlled oral hygiene on the incidence of gingivitis. Acta Odontol Scand 1961;19:537–555.
17. Ramfjord SP, Morrison EC, Burgett FG, Nissle RR, Shick RA, Knowles JW. Oral hygiene and maintenance of periodontal support. J Periodontol 1982;53:26–30.
18. Knowles JW, Burgett FG, Nissle RR, Shick, RA, Morrison EC, Ramfjord SP. Results of periodontal treatment related to pocket depth and attachment level. Eight years. J Periodontol 1979;50:225–233.
19. Fleszar TJ, Knowles JW, Morrison EC, Burgett FG, Nissle RFR, Ramfjord SP. Tooth mobility and periodontal therapy. J Clin Periodontol 1980;7:495–505.
20. Hill RW, Ramfjord SP, Morrison EC, et al. Four types of periodontal treatment compared over two years. J Periodontol 1981;52:655–662.
21. Greenstein G. Periodontal response to mechanical non-surgical therapy: A review. J Periodontol 1992;63:118–130.
22. Lindhe J, Nyman S. The effect of plaque control and surgical pocket elimination on the establishment and maintenance of periodontal health. A longitudinal study of periodontal therapy in cases of advanced disease. J Clin Periodontol 1975;2:67–79.
23. Lindhe J, Nyman S. Long-term maintenance of patients treated for advanced periodontal disease. J Clin Periodontol 1984;11:504–514.

24. Costa FO, Takenaka-Martinez S, Cota LO, Ferreira SC, Silva GL, Costa JE. Peri-implant disease in subjects with and without preventive maintenance: A 5-year follow-up. J Clin Periodontol 2012;39:173–181.
25. Monje A, Wang HL, Nart J. Association of preventive maintenance therapy compliance and peri-implant diseases: A cross-sectional study. J Periodontol 2017;88:1030–1041.
26. Rocuzzo M, De Angelis N, Bonino L, Aglietta M. Ten-year results of a three-arm prospective cohort study on implants in periodontally compromised patients: Part I: Implant loss and radiographic bone loss. Clin Oral Implants Res 2010;21:490–496.
27. Armitage GC, Xenoudi P. Post-treatment supportive care for the natural dentition and dental implants. Periodontol 2000 2016;71:164–184.
28. Serino G, Turri A, Lang NP. Maintenance therapy in patients following surgical treatment of peri-implantitis: A 5-year follow-up study. Clin Oral Implants Res 2015;26:950–956.
29. Monje A, Aranda L, Diaz KT, et al. Impact of maintenance therapy for the prevention of peri-implant diseases: A systematic review and meta-analysis. J Dent Res 2016;95:372–379.
30. Lang NP, Bartold PM. Periodontal health. J Clin Periodontol 2018;45(20 suppl):S9–S16.
31. Claffey N. Decision making in periodontal therapy. The re-evaluation. J Clin Periodontol 1991;18:384–389.
32. Lang, NP, Tonetti MS. Periodontal risk assessment (PRA) for patients in supportive periodontal therapy (SPT). Oral Health Prev Dent 2003;1:7–16.
33. Joss A, Adler R, Lang NP. Bleeding on probing. A parameter for monitoring periodontal conditions in clinical practice. J Clin Periodontol 1994;21:402–408.
34. Matuliene G, Pjetursson BE, Salvi GE, et al. Influence of residual pockets on progression of periodontitis and tooth loss: Results after 11 years of maintenance. J Clin Periodontol 2008;35:685–695.
35. Käyser AF. Shortened dental arches and oral function. J Oral Rehabil 1981;8:457–462.
36. Papapanou PN, Wennström JL, Grondahl KA. A 10-year retrospective study of periodontal disease progression. J Clin Periodontol 1989;16:403–411.
37. Chapple IL, Genco R, working group 2 of the joint EFP/AAP workshop. Diabetes and periodontal diseases: Consensus report of the Joint EFP/AAP Workshop on Periodontitis and Systemic Diseases. J Periodontol 2013;84(4 suppl):S106–S112.
38. Chávarry NG, Vettore MV, Sansone C, Sheiham A. The relationship between diabetes mellitus and destructive periodontal disease: A meta-analysis. Oral Health Prev Dent 2009;7:107–127.
39. Kornman KS, Crane A, Wang HY, et al. The interleukin-1 genotype as a severity factor in adult periodontal disease. J Clin Periodontol 1997;24:72–77.
40. Bergström J, Eliasson S, Dock J. A 10-year prospective study of tobacco smoking and periodontal health. J Periodontol 2000;71:1338–1347.
41. Baljoon M, Natto S, Berström J. Long-term effect of smoking on vertical periodontal bone loss. J Clin Periodontol 2005;32:789–797.
42. Kaldahl WB, Johnson GK, Patil KD, Kalkwarf KL. Levels of cigarette consumption and response to periodontal therapy. J Periodontol 1996;67:675–681.
43. Martínez-Canut P, Lorca A, Magán R. Smoking and periodontal disease severity. J Clin Periodontol 1995;22:743–749.
44. Matuliene G, Studer R, Lang NP, et al. Significance of periodontal risk assessment on the recurrence of periodontitis and tooth loss. J Clin Periodontol 2010;37:191–199.
45. Lang NP, Suvan JE, Tonetti MS. Risk factor assessment tools for the prevention of periodontitis progression a systematic review. J Clin Periodontol 2015;42(16 suppl):S59–S70.
46. Pretzl B, Kaltschmitt J, Kim TS, Reitmeir P, Eickholz P. Tooth loss after active periodontal therapy. 2: Tooth-related factors. J Clin Periodontol 2008;35:175–182.
47. Salvi GE, Mischler DC, Schmidlin K, et al. Risk factors associated with the longevity of multi-rooted teeth. Long-term outcomes after active and supportive periodontal therapy. J Clin Periodontol 2014;41:701–707.
48. Graetz C, Schützhold S, Plaumann A, et al. Prognostic factors for the loss of molars: An 18-years retrospective cohort study. J Clin Periodontol 2015;42:943–950.
49. Highfield JE, Powell RN. Effects of removal of posterior overhanging metallic margins of restorations upon the periodontal tissues. J Clin Periodontol 1978;5:169–181.
50. Lang NP. Periodontal considerations in prosthetic dentistry. Periodontol 2000 1995;9:118–131.
51. Giargia M, Lindhe J. Tooth mobility and periodontal disease. J Clin Periodontol 1997;24:785–795.
52. Anderreg CR, Metler DG. Tooth mobility revisited. J Periodontol 2001;72:963–967.
53. Lulic M, Brägger U, Lang NP, Zwahlen M, Salvi GE. Ante's (1926) law revisited: A systematic review on survival rates and complications of fixed dental prostheses (FDPs) on severely reduced periodontal tissue support. Clin Oral Implants Res 2007;18(3 suppl):63–72.
54. Nyman S, Ericsson I. The capacity of reduced periodontal tissues to support fixed bridgework. J Clin Periodontol 1982;9:409–414.
55. Behfelt K, Ericsson I, Jacobson L, Liner-Aronson S. The occurrence of plaque and gingivitis and its relationship to tooth alignment within the dental arches. J Clin Periodontol 1981;8:329–337.
56. Artun J, Osterberg SK. Periodontal status of secondary crowded mandibular incisors. Long-term results after orthodontic treatment. J Clin Periodontol 1987;4:261–266.
57. Silness J, Roynstrand T. Relationship between alignment conditions of teeth in anterior segments and dental health. J Clin Periodontol 1985;12:312–320.
58. Lang NP, Joss A, Orsanic T, Gusberti FA, Siegriest BE. Bleeding on probing: A predictor for the progression of periodontal disease? J Clin Periodontol 1986;13:590–596.
59. Lang NP, Adler R, Joss A, Nyman S. Absence of bleeding on probing: An indicator of periodontal stability. J Clin Periodontol 1990;17:714–721.
60. Claffey N, Nylund K, Kiger R, Garret S, Egelberg J. Diagnostic predictability of scores of plaque, bleeding, suppuration and probing depth for probing attachment loss. 3½ years of observation following initial periodontal therapy. J Clin Periodontol 1990;17:108–114.
61. Kaldahl WB, Kalwarf KL, Patil KD, Molvar MP. Evaluation of gingival suppuration and supragingival plaque following 4 modalities of periodontal therapy. J Clin Periodontol 1990;17:642–649.
62. Etter TH, Håkanson I, Lang NP, Trejo PM, Caffesse RG. Healing after standardized clinical probing of the periimplant soft tisse seal: A histomorphometric study in dogs. Clin Oral Implants Res 2002;13:571–580.
63. Heitz-Mayfield LJA. Peri-implant diseases: Diagnosis and risk indicators. J Clin Periodontol 2008;35(8 suppl):292–304.
64. Berglundh T, Armitage G, Araujo MG, et al. Peri-implant diseases and conditions: Consensus report of workgroup 4 of the 2017 World Workshop on the Classification of Periodontal and Peri-implant Diseases and Conditions. J Clin Periodontol 2018;45(20 suppl):S286–S291.

65. Sanz M, Chapple IL, Working Group 4 of the VIII European Workshop on Periodontology. Clinical research on peri-implant diseases: Consensus report of Working Group 4. J Clin Periodontol 2012;39(12 suppl):202–206.
66. Lindhe J, Meyle J, Group D of European Workshop on Periodontology. Peri-implant diseases: Consensus report of the Sixth European Workshop on Periodontology. J Clin Periodontol 2008;35(8 suppl):282–285.
67. de Tapia B, Mozas C, Valles C, Nart J, Sanz M, Herrera D. Adjunctive effect of modifying the implant-supported prosthesis in the treatment of peri-implant mucositis. J Clin Periodontol 2019;46:1050–1060.
68. Peña M, Barallat L, Vilarrasa J, Vicario M, Violant D, Nart J. Evaluation of the effect of probiotics in the treatment of peri-implant mucositis: A triple-blind randomized clinical trial. Clin Oral Investig 2019; 23:1673–1683.
69. Schwarz F, Becker K, Sager M. Efficacy of professionally administered plaque removal with or without adjunctive measures for the treatment of peri-implant mucositis. A systematic review and meta-analysis. J Clin Periodontol 2015;42(16 suppl):S202–S213.
70. Porras R, Anderson GB, Caffesse R, Narendran S, Trejo PM. Clinical response to 2 different therapeutic regimens to treat peri-implant mucositis. J Periodontol 2002;73:1118–1125.

24

INTERDISCIPLINARY TREATMENT

Gonzalo Blasi, DDS, MS
Ignacio Blasi, DDS, MS, PhD
Alvaro Blasi, DDS, CDT

DEFINITIONS AND TERMINOLOGY

Active eruption: The process by which a tooth moves from its germinative position to its functional position in occlusion with the opposing arch.[1]

Gingival zenith: The most apical postion of the gingival margin.

Passive eruption: Tooth exposure secondary to apical migration of the gingival margin to a location at or slightly coronal to the cementoenamel junction.[1]

Recession: The migration of the marginal soft tissue to a point apical to the cementoenamel junction of a tooth or the platform of a dental implant.[1]

A treatment plan often involves the combined effort of different specialties. Therefore, it is essential for the various dentists and specialists involved to understand and closely collaborate with one another. This chapter reviews the orthodontic, endodontic, periodontal, functional, and esthetic considerations when approaching interdisciplinary treatment. In addition, it describes critical parameters for diagnosis and successful treatment planning.

Periodontic–Orthodontic Interrelationship

Orthodontics can play a key role for the periodontal patient by managing several local contributing factors that promote periodontal tissue breakdown. As such, orthodontic treatment can reduce crowding, eliminate occlusal trauma, assist with the treatment of intrabony defects, upright molars, and extrude hopeless teeth to facilitate posterior implant treatment, among many other objectives. On the other hand, in the presence of an unstable periodontium, orthodontic treatment can cause more rapid attachment loss than would otherwise occur with bacterial biofilm on its own. This section of the chapter focuses on the orthodontic–periodontal interrelationship as well as the impact of orthodontic treatment in the periodontium.

ORTHODONTIC TREATMENT AND GINGIVAL RECESSION

Gingival **recession** is defined as the migration of the gingiva to a point apical to the cementoenamel junction (CEJ).[1] Although the main etiology of gingival recession remains unclear, orthodontic treatment can be considered a predisposing factor to these mucogingival deformities. The movement of teeth outside the alveolar housing results in a thin buccal bone plate or even in the development of buccal dehiscence[2] (Fig 24-1). Moreover, tooth displacement outside the bony envelope may lead to reduced soft tissue volume.[2,3] Therefore, these sites act with low resistance to the development of gingival recession.

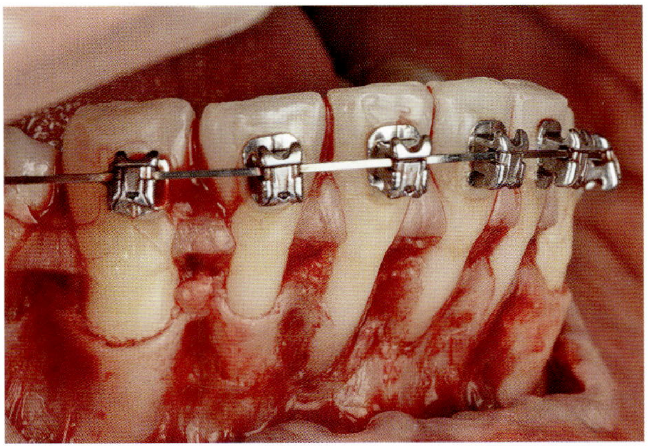

Fig 24-1 Full-thickness flap showing a bone dehiscence on orthodontic patient.

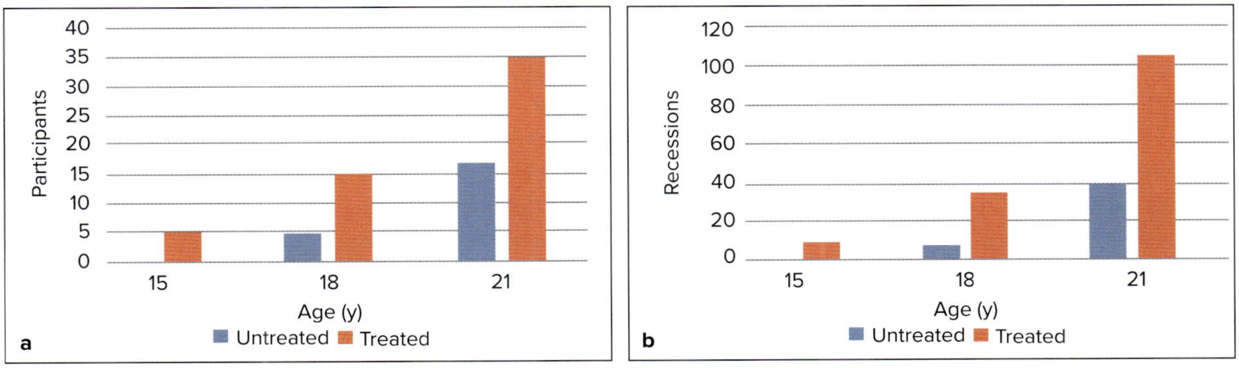

Fig 24-2 *(a)* Number of participants with at least one recession. *(b)* Total number of recessions. (Data from Renkema et al.[4])

In 2013, Renkema et al performed a case-control study and demonstrated that 35% of patients treated with orthodontics developed at least one gingival recession over a period of 9 years as compared to 16.7% of untreated patients (Fig 24-2a).[4] Furthermore, the total number of recessions were 105 in the treated group as compared to 39 in the untreated group[4] (Fig 24-2b).

RESPONSE OF THE PERIODONTIUM TO ORTHODONTIC MOVEMENT

When forces are applied to a tooth, the surrounding bone will respond as follows: On the pressure side, bone resorption will occur; while on the tension side, bone apposition will occur. When the periodontal ligament is compressed, there is an initial phase of immediate and rapid tooth movement, resulting in a hyalinized zone. Hyalinization is produced by a restriction of blood supply to the periodontal ligament and localized necrosis. When this happens, the tooth stops moving until the hyalinized zone is eliminated by macrophages and multinucleate giant cells. Once the hyalinized tissue is resorbed, the tooth movement can occur, and bone apposition takes place on the tension side.[5]

ORTHODONTIC TREATMENT AND PERIODONTAL HEALTH

Orthodontic treatment may also have a detrimental effect on periodontal health. Animal studies have demonstrated that in the presence of bacterial plaque, orthodontic movement can cause a more rapid periodontal breakdown than would occur with inflammation alone[6] (Fig 24-3). On the other hand, in a reduced but healthy periodontium, orthodontics can be performed without further periodontal destruction[7] (Fig 24-4). A clinical study performed on 20 adults (10 with reduced periodontium) and 20 adolescents showed that adult patients had no significant increase in attachment loss after orthodontic treatment.[8]

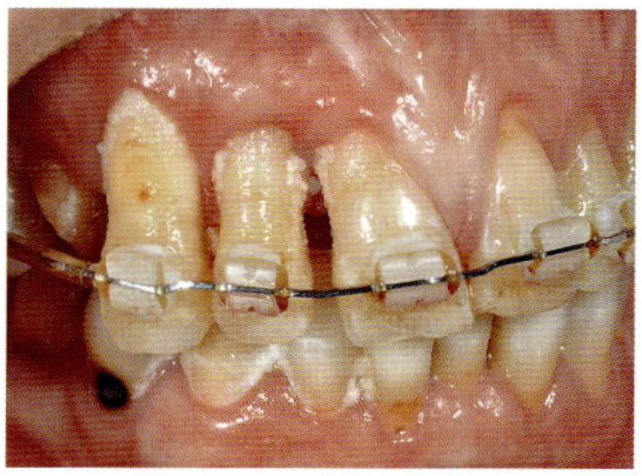

Fig 24-3 Orthodontic treatment on a periodontally noncontrolled patient.

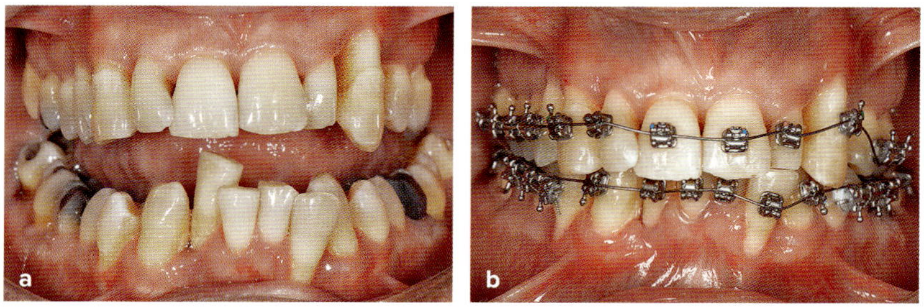

Fig 24-4 *(a and b)* Orthodontic treatment on a periodontally controlled patient.

TIMING BETWEEN ORTHODONTIC AND PERIODONTAL TREATMENT

As previously mentioned, in the presence of inflammation, orthodontics can lead to a more rapid periodontal breakdown. Therefore, it is mandatory for orthodontic treatment to be preceded by periodontal therapy. In addition, orthodontic appliances can sometimes hinder the performance of adequate oral hygiene, and a close monitoring of the periodontal health status is necessary.[5]

ORTHODONTIC MOVEMENT INTO INTRABONY DEFECTS

The movement of teeth into intrabony defects is a controversial topic. The available evidence is ambiguous when identifying the true effects on the periodontium after orthodontic movements are performed in this type of defect.

Some animal studies have shown that when inflammation has been eliminated, bodily movement into an intraosseous defect can be performed without further loss of attachment.[6,9] The results showed an epithelial lining covering the root to its initial position. Thus, it was concluded that teeth could be moved into an intrabony defect without additional damage. Moreover, this movement resulted in slight bone apposition and no changes in connective tissue attachment levels. Other investigations using a rat model have demonstrated that there could be up to a 6.5-fold increase in bone apposition when moving teeth into intrabony defects.[10]

Contrarily, in the presence of poor plaque control, bodily tooth movement on experimentally induced intrabony defects resulted in increased pocket depth and loss of connective tissue attachment in a dog model. These findings have been reproduced in similar studies using different animal models.[10,11] Hence, more studies are needed in order to clarify the periodontal response to this type of orthodontic movements.

In some cases, intrabony defects are associated with mesially tilted molars. In 1973, Brown performed a case series on five patients with mesially tipped molars that underwent an uprighting movement.[12] Photographs, models, and histologic sections were used to determine the effects of the movement. Pocket reduction from a combination of scaling and orthodontics averaged 3.5 mm (down from a mean of 8 mm). In addition, the teeth resulted in a favorable axial inclination and contributed to the restoration of a normal occlusal plane.[12]

EXTRUSION AND ITS EFFECTS ON THE PERIODONTIUM

Forced eruption is a type of orthodontic movement that has many different applications. It is an effective treatment for managing angular bony defects and unleveled gingival margins as well as implant site development.

Many case reports have illustrated the effectiveness of orthodontic extrusion on soft and hard tissues. It was first introduced by Ingber on a case report for the treatment of intraosseous defects.[13] By stretching the periodontal ligament fibers, there will be a more coronal positioning of the connective tissue attachment, and the angular defect will become shallower.[13,14] These findings were also confirmed by animal studies where bony defects were created surgically and teeth were extruded. The results showed that there was a greater cementum width, wider periodontal ligament space, and increased bone height on the tested teeth as compared with controls.[15]

On the other hand, while there could be an improvement of the periodontal parameters when performing forced eruption, it should be taken into consideration that the crown will often have to be shortened, and endodontic treatment may be needed due to supraclusion. In addition,

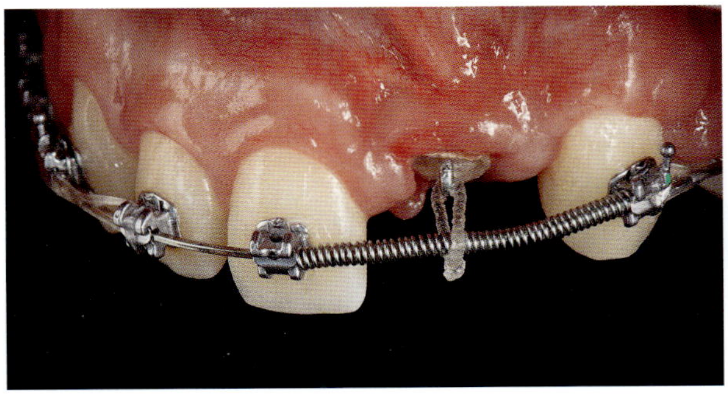

Fig 24-5 Orthodontic forced eruption of a hopeless tooth.

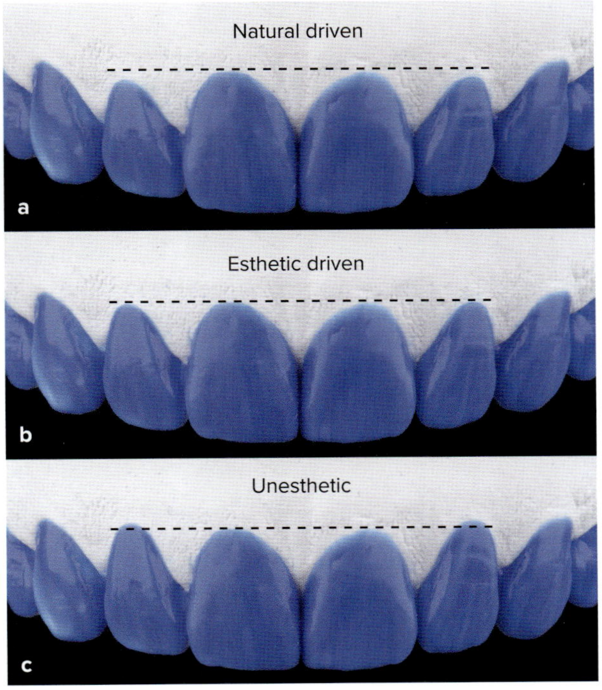

Fig 24-6 Gingival levels of maxillary anterior dentition. *(a)* Natural driven. *(b)* Esthetic driven. *(c)* Unesthetic.

the crestal bone of the healthy side of the extruded tooth will follow the movement pattern as well. Its final position will be even more occlusal than the affected side and should be surgically reduced according to the bone height of the adjacent teeth.

Forced eruption of a hopeless tooth that needs to be replaced by a dental implant is also an excellent approach to improve the bone crest and gingival margins (Fig 24-5). For example, an animal study evaluated the gingival alterations that occurred following orthodontic extrusion and showed an increase in keratinized tissue, while the position of mucogingival junction remained unchanged. Therefore, orthodontic forced eruption represents a valid alternative to improve misalignment of gingival margins and marginal bone levels.[16]

Periodontic–Prosthodontic Interrelationship

Interdisciplinary treatment involving periodontal and prosthodontic specialists is often crucial to achieve optimal functional and esthetics results. Thus, there are certain parameters that the periodontist and restorative dentists have to take into consideration together to achieve these outcomes. This section focuses on the esthetic and functional parameters to consider in order to perform a properly combined periodontal–prosthetic treatment.

ESTHETIC PARAMETERS FOR PERIODONTAL TREATMENT

Gingival esthetics is an important component in interdisciplinary treatment. The ideal gingival architecture has been defined by Chiche and Pinault[17] and describes several parameters that must be taken into account to achieve satisfactory results.

First, esthetic apicocoronal positions of the gingival margins are considered when maxillary central incisors and canines are at the same level and the lateral incisor is between 0.5 to 1 mm more coronal. However, in situations when the patient wants a more symmetric smile rather than more natural smile, the lateral incisor could be located at the same level as the central incisor and canine. An unesthetic gingival display would be if the lateral incisor gingival margin is located in a more apical position than the central incisors and canines[18,19] (Fig 24-6).

Second, the ideal length of a maxillary central incisor should be between 10 and 11.5 mm. It is established from the vertical height of the patient's face and the amount of tooth exposure with the upper lip at rest. This exposure

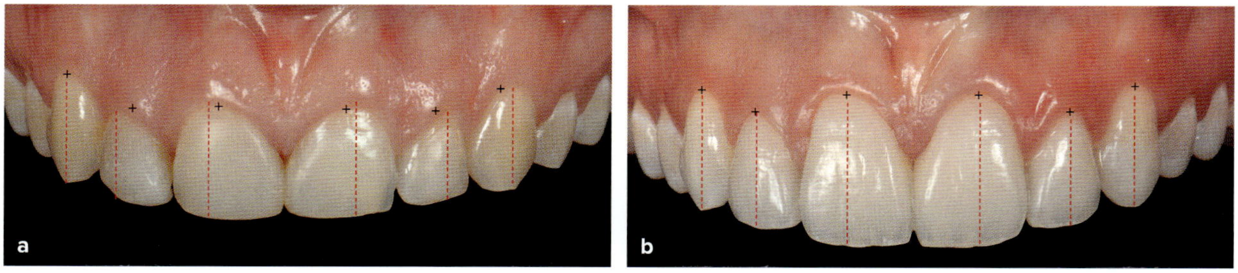

Fig 24-7 *(a)* Ideal zenith location marked with +. Actual zenith location marked with *red line*. *(b)* Same patient after zenith location corrected with periodontal and prosthetic treatment.

is based on the patient's gender and age and should be between 1 and 4.5 mm.[20] Moreover, the incisor width should be 75% to 80% of its length. Following these parameters and defining "X" as the width of the central incisor, the ideal width of the lateral incisor should be X – 2 mm and the canine X – 1 mm.

Third, the proximal contact areas, papilla levels, and zenith positions are also important parameters. The ideal mesial proximal contact area for the maxillary central incisor should be 40% of its length, for the lateral incisor should be 30%, and for canine and first premolar should be 20% of their lengths. Mesial papillae for the maxillary central and lateral incisors should be 41% of their length, and for the canine should be 43% of their length.[21,22]

Last, the **gingival zenith** is defined as the most apical position of the gingival margin. On a central incisor, the zenith should be located 1 mm distal from the vertical midline axis of the crown. On lateral incisors and canines, the gingival zenith should be located concurrent to the vertical midline axis of the crown[23] (Fig 24-7).

All of these parameters have to be taken into consideration when performing periodontal esthetic procedures such as crown lengthening, root coverage, and implant placement.

ESTHETIC CROWN LENGTHENING

Esthetic crown lengthening is often performed to treat the so-called gummy smile. A *gummy smile* is a colloquial term frequently used to refer to excessive gingival display when smiling, approximately 3 mm or more. This can be to the result of multiple factors:

- Vertical maxillary excess
- Upper lip incompetence or hypermobility
- Altered passive eruption (APE)
- Compensatory eruption
- Gingival overgrowth

This section focuses on the etiology, diagnosis, and treatment of APE.

During the dental eruption process, two marked phases can be differentiated:

Active eruption: This is the period during which the tooth emerges through the gingiva until it is in its final position. During this time, the gingival margin is covering part of the anatomical crown, so the clinical crown is shorter than the anatomical crown.

Passive eruption: This is the process by which the gingival margin migrates apically until the anatomical crown is completely exposed. This process allows the gingival margin to be located 1 to 3 mm coronal to the CEJ, with the coronal end of the junctional epithelium coinciding with the CEJ. At the end of the passive eruption, clinical and anatomical crown height should coincide. The process of passive eruption may continue throughout adolescence and may extend up to the early to mid 20s of adulthood. On the other hand, APE occurs when the gingival margin does not migrate apically once the process of tooth eruption has been completed. Coslet et al described a classification for APE in which each site has both a type and a subgroup[24]:

- Type 1: There is a wide band of keratinized tissue, and the mucogingival junction is apical to the bone crest.
- Type 2: There is a normal or minimal band of keratinized tissue, which is on the anatomical crown, so the mucogingival junction is situated at or near the CEJ.
- Subgroup A: The distance from the bone crest to the CEJ is 1.5 to 2 mm.
- Subgroup B: The bone crest is located close to or at the level of the CEJ.

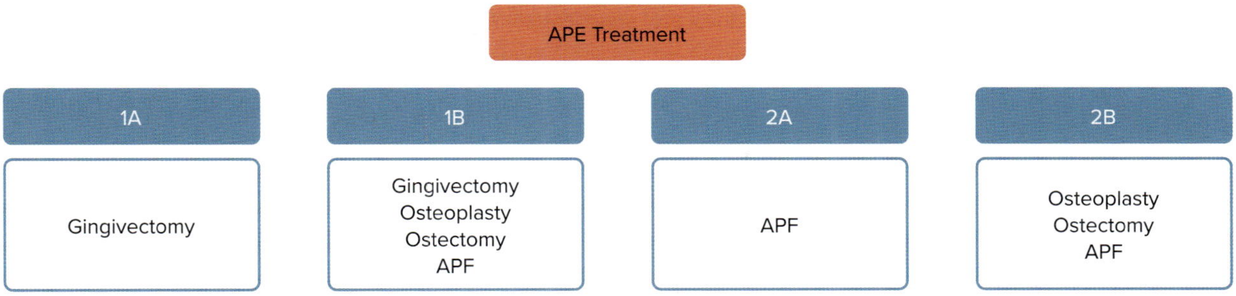

Fig 24-8 Treatment approaches for APE. APF, apically positioned flap.

Fig 24-9 Assessment of the location of the CEJ. *(a)* Using an explorer/periodontal probe to feel the CEJ. *(b)* CBCT image with retracted lips, showing the gingival margin coronal to the CEJ.

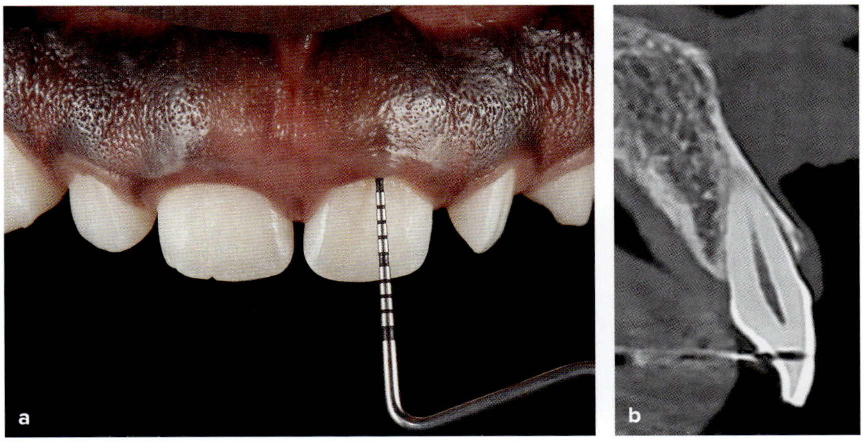

This classification is crucial to understand the treatment of crown lengthening. Depending on the type of APE that a patient presents with, the surgical approach will vary (Fig 24-8).

When the treatment of APE is considered in the anterior maxilla, two approaches have to be differentiated: *(1)* surgical and *(2)* combination of surgical and prosthetic.

When only surgical crown lengthening is needed, the CEJ will be used as reference. The distance from the gingival margin to the CEJ has to be evaluated to determine how much reduction in soft and hard tissues is necessary. On the other hand, when the treatment requires surgical and prosthetic treatment, the references of how much soft and hard tissue reduction is needed are going to be based on an esthetic evaluation on a wax-up model.

The position of the CEJ in regard to the gingival margin can be assessed by different methods:

- Clinical: Using an explorer or periodontal probe to feel the CEJ (Fig 24-9a).
- Periapical radiographs: Placing a radiopaque material on the gingival margin.
- CBCT: Placing plastic retractors or cotton rolls to separate the lips and cheeks, allowing the gingival margin to be assessed[25] (Fig 24-9b).

OSSEOUS SURGERY FOR NONRESTORABLE TEETH

The presence of at least 2 mm of tooth structure coronal to the gingival margin is known as the *ferrule effect*, and it has been reported to be one of the most important factors that increase the resistance to fracture of the restoration.[26,27] Whenever the tooth to be restored has less than 1.5 mm of height from the gingival margin with a sufficient root length, a crown lengthening procedure can be performed.

While performing a surgical crown lengthening, two main parameters should to be taken into consideration from a restorative point of view. First, the distance from the bone crest to the future margin of the restoration has to be at least 3 mm for the formation of the biologic width and sulcus. Secondly, the remaining tooth structure has to be at least 1.5 mm in height to have enough ferrule effect (Fig 24-10).

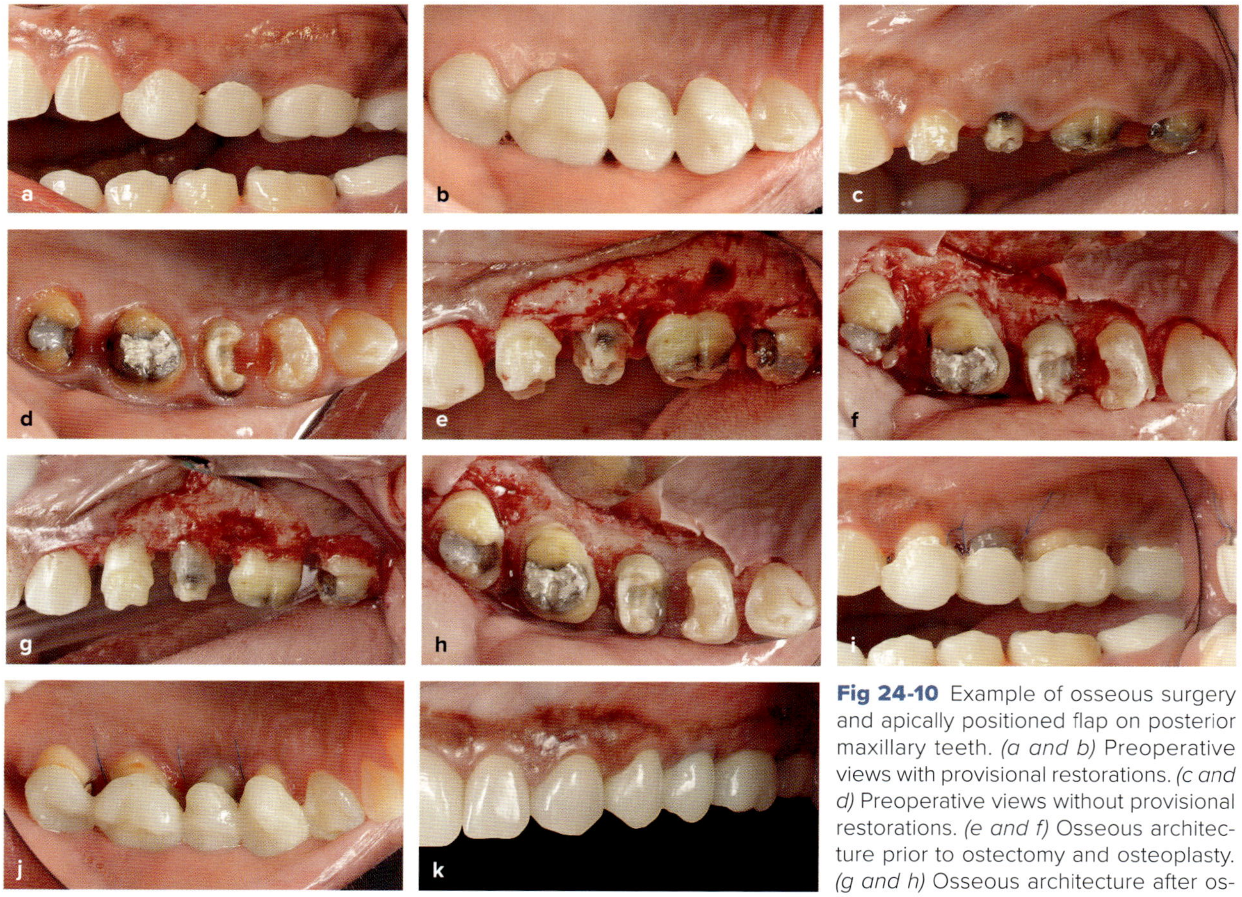

Fig 24-10 Example of osseous surgery and apically positioned flap on posterior maxillary teeth. *(a and b)* Preoperative views with provisional restorations. *(c and d)* Preoperative views without provisional restorations. *(e and f)* Osseous architecture prior to ostectomy and osteoplasty. *(g and h)* Osseous architecture after ostectomy and osteoplasty. *(i and j)* Postoperative view with provisional restorations. *(k)* Definitive restorations.

As demonstrated by Herrero et al, it is sometimes challenging to achieve these measurements.[28] In this clinical study on 21 teeth requiring surgical crown lengthening, the results showed that the objective of 3 mm between planned restoration margin and alveolar crest was routinely not achieved. It was also shown that the least amount of ostectomy was achieved on the distolingual sites.[28]

Pontoriero and Carnevale carried out a clinical study performing surgical crown lengthening on 30 patients with a 12-month follow-up assessing the position of the gingival margin (Table 24-1).[29] The patients were divided in three groups: thin, normal, and thick phenotype. The results demonstrated a coronal migration of the gingival margin during the healing phase, which was more significant in patients with a thick phenotype. It was concluded that when resective surgery is performed to achieve crown elongation, a greater removal of supporting bone should be considered in thick phenotypes. It was also concluded that in esthetic areas, close monitoring of tissue regrowth is recommended to assess the ideal time to restore.[29]

In contrast, in a similar study performed by Brägger et al with 25 patients, it was shown that the position of the gingival margin immediately after surgery remained almost identical after 6 months. Moreover, in most cases, no change was observed between 6 weeks and 6 months postoperatively. Only 12% of the sites showed changes with 2 to 4 mm of recession from 6 weeks to 6 months.[30]

PROSTHETIC CONSIDERATIONS FOR RESTORING TEETH WITH A REDUCED PERIODONTIUM

Crown-to-root ratio

When restoring teeth with indirect restorations, one of the most critical aspects is the crown-to-root ratio. A comprehensive analysis should include length as well as shape of the crown and root. The main characteristics that

TABLE 24-1 Postsurgical gingival margin regrowth at 1-, 3-, 6- and 12-month examinations*

Examination	Interproximal (mm)	Buccolingual (mm)
1 month	2.1 ± 0.8†	1.6 ± 0.6‡
3 months	2.5 ± 0.7	2.1 ± 0.5
6 months	2.9 ± 0.6	2.5 ± 0.4
12 months	3.2 ± 0.8†	2.9 ± 0.6‡

*Data from Pontoriero and Carnevale.[29]
†$P < .001$
‡$P < .002$

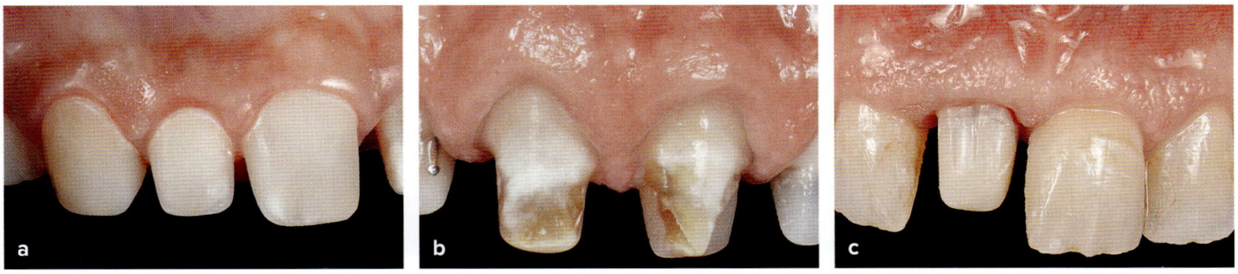

Fig 24-11 Different preparation designs. *(a)* Chamfer. *(b)* Shoulder. *(c)* Feather-edge.

make a root properly absorb occlusal forces are width and length. Consequently, the weakest root would be short and narrow.

On a reduced periodontium, it is more important to analyze the clinical rather than anatomical crown and root. It is a common finding to have a clinical crown longer than the anatomical crown and a clinical root shorter than the anatomical root.

The ideal crown-to-root ratio is 1:2, the root being two times the length of the crown. A tooth with a good prognosis is up to 1:1. When the clinical root becomes shorter than the clinical crown, the prognosis of the tooth begins to be significantly compromised. When this occurs and the patient develops secondary occlusal trauma, splinting teeth should be considered.[31–33]

Splinting teeth

Splinting is a viable option for teeth with a clinical crown-to-root ratio less than 1:1 and secondary occlusal trauma. There are many options available for splinting teeth with fixed and removable prostheses, and the splinting may be unilateral or bilateral. Splinting teeth has been demonstrated to improve long-term prognosis if performed properly.

When considering splinting teeth as a treatment of choice, unilateral splinting should be the first option. Bilateral splinting should be considered only when all of the abutments are mobile and to prevent movement of the entire complex. As bilateral splinting may present biomechanical complications, it should be performed carefully with proper adjustment of centric and eccentric occlusion. Overall, fixed definitive restorations splinting teeth unilaterally have better prognoses than bilateral splints.[31,34]

Preparation design

Indirect restorations are influenced by material selection and tooth abutment geometry. There are three main preparation designs for an indirect full-coverage crown based on the margin: shoulder, chamfer, and feather-edge. On one hand, when restoring teeth with anatomical crowns similar to clinical crowns, shoulder and chamfer are more conservative preparations. On the other hand, when restoring teeth with elongated clinical crowns, vertical feather-edge will be the most recommended preparation design to optimize preservation of the tooth structure. Shoulder and chamfer margin would require more aggressive preparation for long teeth[35,36] (Fig 24-11).

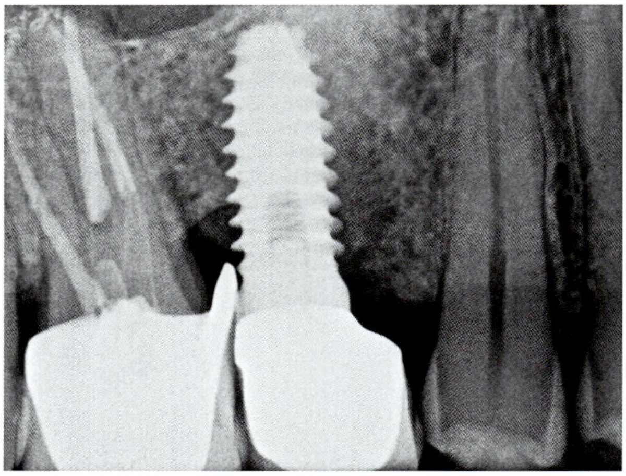

Fig 24-12 Overhanging crown affecting a dental implant.

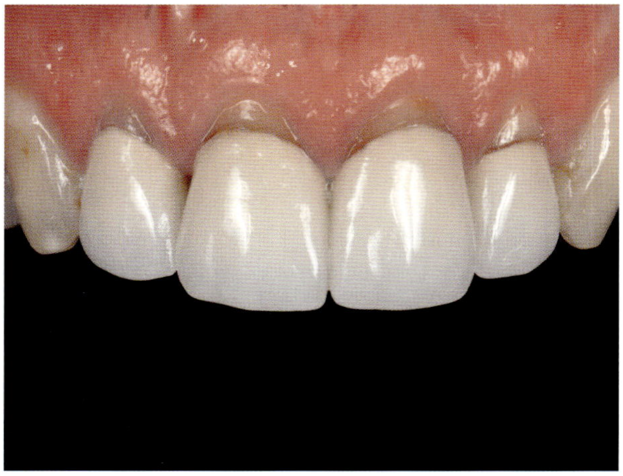

Fig 24-13 Gingival recession due to biologic width violation.

INFLUENCE OF RESTORATIONS ON THE PERIODONTIUM

Overhanging restorations and periodontal health

Overhanging restorations result in plaque retention, and there are numerous studies showing an association between plaque-retentive restorations and increased risk of periodontal disease progression (Fig 24-12). A clinical study performed on nine patients testing the subgingival microflora on ill-fitting onlays was performed by Lang et al.[37] Following the placement of overhanging onlays, there was a shift in the subgingival flora, which closely resembled that of chronic periodontitis, and there were also increases in gingival and plaque indices. In contrast, following the placement of restorations with properly fitting margins, there was a shift on the microflora that was characteristic of gingival health. After 20 to 27 weeks, all the percentages for plaque, gingival, and bleeding indices reached preexperimental levels.[37]

A cross-sectional study by Jeffcoat and Howell was also performed to evaluate the effect of defective amalgams on the periodontium. This study was achieved by pairing 100 defective amalgams with the contralateral tooth without restoration. It was concluded that overhanging restorations cause statistically significant greater bone loss than control teeth.[38]

Pack et al evaluated 1,319 teeth in which 2,117 restored surfaces were evaluated. Periodontal disease was more advanced when overhangs were present. However, when proximal overhanging margins were adjacent to an edentulous space, the periodontal effects were lessened. When adjacent to neighboring teeth, overhanging margins also significantly affected the periodontal status of those teeth.[39]

Violation of the biologic width

Biologic width was defined by Gargiulo et al as 0.97 mm of junctional epithelium and 1.07 mm of connective tissue attachment.[40] When this is invaded by a subgingival restoration, it may lead to inflammation and periodontal breakdown (Fig 24-13).

In an animal study with beagle dogs, after performing a full-thickness flap, Class 5 amalgam restorations were placed, and the apical border of each restoration was located at the alveolar bone crest. The flaps were repositioned and sutured, leaving the restorations in subgingival locations. The authors found that the continuous abuse of the biologic width resulted in attachment loss. Also, it was observed that remodeling will occur until the biologic width reestablishes itself apical to the restoration.[41]

In a human study with histologic analysis, Tarnow et al had similar findings. Provisional crowns were placed below the base of the crevice on 13 teeth, and block extractions were performed after 1 to 8 weeks. Histologic data revealed reformation of the dentogingival junction on a more apical and lateral position, resulting in marginal recession.[42]

Interdental contacts

It has been suggested that food impaction within interproximal spaces favors bacterial plaque accumulation. Some of the anatomical factors that influence food impaction are open and deficient contacts, crowded teeth, plunger cusps, and abnormal or defective marginal ridge relationships. Larato evaluated the presence of these factors on 121 dry human skulls on intrabony defects.[43] Of the 206 lesions encountered, 39 (18%) were associated with factors that were able to cause food impaction.

While there seems to be a correlation between open contacts and increased attachment loss, Hancock et al could not find a significant relationship between contact type and gingival index or pocket depth. Nevertheless, the significant relationship observed between food impaction and open or improper contacts, and between food impaction and probing depth, reinforced the observations that food impaction contributes to periodontal breakdown.[44]

Periodontic–Endodontic Interrelationship

Endo-perio lesions often represent a challenging scenario for determining a diagnosis and treatment plan. Adequate diagnosis is a key factor to determine the treatment sequence.[45] This section focuses on diagnosis, prognosis, and treatment plan selection for these types of lesions. It is important to bear in mind that the periodontal ligament and the dental pulp can be connected through three different pathways: dentinal tubules, accessory canals, and the apex. Endo-perio lesions can be classified into six categories: primary endodontic; primary periodontal; primary endodontic, secondary periodontal; primary periodontal, secondary endodontic; true combined; and concomitant.

PRIMARY ENDODONTIC LESION

This is an apical lesion that drains coronally through the periodontal ligament and mimics a periodontal abscess. The pocket is normally deep and narrow, and the pulp is necrotic. No signs of plaque or calculus are found in the pocket. This may also occur in the furcation area due to the presence of accessory canals. This type of lesion heals after endodontic treatment.

PRIMARY PERIODONTAL LESION

Periodontitis progresses far apically. In these cases, the pulp is vital and the pocket is wide. Plaque and calculus are present. The treatment depends on the periodontal prognosis of the tooth, and no endodontic treatment is necessary.

PRIMARY ENDODONTIC, SECONDARY PERIODONTAL LESION

When a primary endodontic lesion remains untreated, it may develop a combined lesion as bacterial plaque accumulates in the gingival sulcus, communicating with the sinus tract and resulting in further periodontal tissue breakdown. The treatment sequence should start with endodontic therapy first, and periodontal therapy would follow once it has been ensured that the endodontic therapy was successful.

PRIMARY PERIODONTAL, SECONDARY ENDODONTIC LESION

These lesions are the result of periodontal disease progressing up to the apex of a tooth involving the apical tissues. The therapy should be similar to primary endodontic, secondary periodontal lesions.

TRUE COMBINED LESION

These lesions occur when an endodontic lesion progresses coronally and meets a periodontal pocket migrating apically. The prognosis of these teeth is usually guarded. Both therapies will be necessary. In these cases, it is recommended to perform endodontic therapy first.

CONCOMITANT LESION

Concomitant endodontic-periodontal lesions occur when an endodontically induced periapical lesion exists at a tooth that is also affected by periodontitis. The two lesions exist separately and do not merge. Both treatments can commence at the same time, although it is typically suggested to perform endodontic therapy first.

References

1. American Academy of Periodontology. Glossary of Periodontal Terms. American Academy of Periodontology, 2001.
2. Wennström JL, Lindhe J, Sinclair F, Thilander B. Some periodontal tissue reactions to orthodontic tooth movement in monkeys. J Clin Periodontol 1987;14:121–129.

3. Danz JC, Bibby BM, Katsaros C, Stavropoulos A. Effects of facial tooth movement on the periodontium in rats: A comparison between conventional and low force. J Clin Periodontol 2016;43:229–237.
4. Renkema AM, Fudalej PS, Renkema AAP, Abbas F, Bronkhorst E, Katsaros C. Gingival labial recessions in orthodontically treated and untreated individuals: A case-control study. J Clin Periodontol 2013;40:631–637.
5. Blasi I Jr, Pavlin D. Minimally and noninvasive approaches to accelerate tooth movement. In: Graber LW, Vanarsdall RL Jr, Vig KWL, Huang GJ (eds). Orthodontics: Current Principles and Technique, ed 6. St Louis: Elsevier, 2017:913–925.
6. Ericsson I, Thilander B, Lindhe J, Okamoto H. The effect of orthodontic tilting movements on the periodontal tissues of infected and non-infected dentitions in dogs. J Clin Periodontol 1977;4:278–293.
7. Vanarsdall RL, Jr, Blasi I, Jr, Secchi AG. Periodontal-orthodontic interrelationships. In: Graber LW, Vanarsdall RL, Vig KWL, Huang GJ (eds). Orthodontics: Current Principles and Techniques, ed 6. St Louis: Mosby, 2016:621–668.
8. Boyd RL, Leggott PJ, Quinn RS, Eakle WS, Chambers D. Periodontal implications of orthodontic treatment in adults with reduced or normal periodontal tissues versus those of adolescents. Am J Orthod Dentofacial Orthop 1989;96:191–198.
9. Polson A, Caton J, Polson AP, Nyman S, Novak J, Reed B. Periodontal response after tooth movement into intrabony defects. J Periodontol 1984;55:197–202.
10. Vardimon AD, Nemcovsky CE, Dre E. Orthodontic tooth movement enhances bone healing of surgical bony defects in rats. J Periodontol 2001;72:858–864.
11. Nevins M, Wise RJ. Use of orthodontic therapy to alter infrabony pockets. 2. Int J Periodontics Restorative Dent 1990;10:198–207.
12. Brown IS. The effect of orthodontic therapy on certain types of periodontal defects. I. Clinical findings. J Periodontol 1973;44:742–756.
13. Ingber JS. Forced eruption. I. A method of treating isolated one and two wall infrabony osseous defects: Rationale and case report. J Periodontol 1974;45:199–206.
14. Ingber JS. Forced eruption: Part II. A method of treating nonrestorable teeth—Periodontal and restorative considerations. J Periodontol 1976:47:203–216.
15. Van Venrooy JR, Yukna RA. Orthodontic extrusion of single-rooted teeth affected with advanced periodontal disease. Am J Orthod 1985;87:67–74.
16. Kajiyama K, Murakami T, Yokota S. Gingival reactions after experimentally induced extrusion of the upper incisors in monkeys. Am J Orthod Dentofacial Orthop 1993;104:6–47.
17. Chiche GJ, Pinault A. Esthetics of Anterior Fixed Prosthodontics. Chicago: Quintessence, 1994.
18. Vig RG, Brundo GC. The kinetics of anterior tooth display. J Prosthet Dent 1978;39:502–504.
19. Mangne P, Belser U. Bonded Porcelain Restorations in the Anterior Dentition: A Biomimetic Approach. Chicago: Quintessence, 2003.
20. Chiche GJ. Proportion, display, and length for successful esthetic planning. In: Cohen M (ed). Interdisciplinary Treatment Planning. Vol 1: Principles, Design, Implantation. Chicago: Quintessence, 2008:1–48.
21. Chu SJ, Tarnow DP, Tan JHP, Stappert CFJ. Papilla proportions in the maxillary anterior dentition. Int J Periodontics Restorative Dent 2009;29:385–93.
22. Stappert CFJ, Tarnow DP, Tan JHP, Chu SJ. Proximal contact areas of the maxillary anterior dentition. Int J Periodontics Restorative Dent 2010;30:471–477.
23. Chu SJ, Tan JHP, Stappert CFJ, Tarnow DP. Gingival zenith positions and levels of the maxillary anterior dentition. J Esthet Restor Dent 2009;21:113–120.
24. Coslet JG, Vanarsdall R, Weisgold A. Diagnosis and classification of delayed passive eruption of the dentogingival junction in the adult. Alpha Omegan 1977;70:24–28.
25. Ferrari M, Vichi A, Fadda GM, et al. A randomized controlled trial of endodontically treated and restored premolars. J Dent Res 2012;91:72S–78S.
26. Mancebo JC, Jiménez-Castellanos E, Cañadas D. Effect of tooth type and ferrule on the survival of pulpless teeth restored with fiber posts: A 3-year clinical study. Am J Dent 2010;23:351–356.
27. Schertel Cassiano L, Barriviera M, Suzuki S, et al. Soft tissue cone beam computed tomography (ST-CBCT) for the planning of esthetic crown lengthening procedures. Int J Esthet Dent. 2016;11:482–493.
28. Herrero F, Scott JB, Maropis PS, Yukna RA. Clinical comparison of desired versus actual amount of surgical crown lengthening. J Periodontol 1995;66:568–571.
29. Pontoriero R, Carnevale G. Surgical crown lengthening: A 12-month clinical wound healing study. J Periodontol 2001;72:841–848.
30. Brägger U, Lauchenauer D, Lang NP. Surgical lengthening of the clinical crown. J Clin Periodontol 1992;19:58–63.
31. Abduo J, Lyons KM. Interdisciplinary interface between fixed prosthodontics and periodontics. Periodontol 2000 2017;74:40–62.
32. Bennani V, Ibrahim H, Al-Harthi L, Lyons KM. The periodontal restorative interface: Esthetic considerations. Periodontol 2000 2017;74:74–101.
33. Amsterdam M. Periodontal prosthesis. Twenty-five years in retrospect. Alpha Omegan 1974;67:8–52.
34. Blasi A, Chiche G, Torosian A, Aimplee S, Londono J, Arias SR. Key factors in treatment planning for complex cases: Orthodontics as a tool to manage severely worn dentitions. J Cosmet Dent 2016;32:88–105.
35. Goto Y, Nicholls JI, Phillips KM, Junge T. Fatigue resistance of endodontically treated teeth restored with three dowel-and-core systems. J Prosthet Dent 2005;93:45–50.
36. Morgano SM. Restoration of pulpless teeth: Application of traditional principles in present and future contexts. J Prosthet Dent 1996;75:375–380.
37. Lang NP, Kiel RA, Anderhalden K. Clinical and microbiological effects of subgingival restorations with overhanging or clinically perfect margins. J Clin Periodontol 1983:10;563–578.
38. Jeffcoat MK, Howell TH. Alveolar bone destruction due to overhanging amalgam in periodontal disease. J Periodontol 1980;51:599–602.
39. Pack AR, Coxhead LJ, McDonald BW. The prevalence of overhanging margins in posterior amalgam restorations and periodontal consequences. J Clin Periodontol 1990;17:145–152.
40. Gargiulo AW, Wentz FM, Orban B. Dimensions and relations of the dentogingival junction in humans. J Periodontol 1961:32;261–267.
41. Tal H, Soldinger M, Dreiangel A, Pitaru S. Periodontal response to long-term abuse of the gingival attachment by supracrestal amalgam restorations. J Clin Periodontol 1989:16;654–659.

42. Tarnow D, Stahl SS, Magner A, Zamzok J. Human gingival attachment responses to subgingival crown placement. Marginal remodelling. J Clin Periodontol 1986;13:563–569.
43. Larato DC. Relationship of food impaction to interproximal intrabony lesions. J Periodontol 1971;42:237–238.
44. Hancock EB, Mayo CV, Schwab RR, Wirthlin MR. Influence of interdental contacts on periodontal status. J Periodontol 1980;51:445–449.
45. Rotstein I. Interaction between endodontics and periodontics. Periodontol 2000 2017;74:11–39.

25

EVIDENCE-BASED DENTISTRY

Guo-Hao Lin, DDS, MS

DEFINITIONS AND TERMINOLOGY

False negatives: Incorrect negative diagnoses.[2]

Meta-analysis: A statistical method to quantitatively pool data from several independent but similar studies, collected through a systematic review, to allow testing for significance from a larger, and more diverse, data set.[2]

Specificity: The ability of a diagnostic test to detect the absence of a disease in a healthy population. Specificity = true negatives divided by the sum of true negatives plus false positives, or TN / (FN + TN).[2]

Statistical sensitivity: The ability of a diagnostic test to detect a disease, when present, in a diseased population. Sensitivity = true positives divided by the sum of true positives plus false negatives, or TP / (FN + TP).[2]

Systematic review: A topic-focused literature review designed to answer specific research questions and performed using specific criteria to identify, collect, and critically evaluate published studies. A systematic review may include a meta-analysis of the available data, and as such, typically constitutes the highest level of hierarchical evidence.[2]

True positives: Correct positive diagnoses.[2]

Evidence-based practice is defined as "the integration of best research evidence with clinical expertise and patient values."[1] In dentistry, this concept has been enforced for decades. Consequently, practicing evidence-based dentistry is the standard of patient care that should be applied in every scenario. Clinicians should keep themselves up-to-date on the best current evidence so that patients can benefit from the state-of-the-art diagnosis, treatment planning, surgical techniques, and more.

Study Protocol

PICOS QUESTION

To facilitate an effective search, a clinical question should be defined based on the participants, interventions, comparisons, outcomes, and study design (PICOS). A clearly defined PICOS question will aid with the location of the most currently available evidence in a database.

NULL HYPOTHESIS

After facilitating a PICOS question, a hypothesis should be established regarding the current view or explanation that the researcher wants to challenge.

POWER ANALYSIS/CALCULATION

Before conducting a clinical study, researchers should perform a statistical analysis to determine the ideal sample size that is suitable to detect the effect of a given test at the designated level of significance.

Frequency Distribution

CONTINGENCY TABLE

A contingency table[3] is often used to display the frequency distribution of the variables (Table 25-1).

- True positive: A, the people with disease who tested positive.
- True negative: D, the people without disease who tested negative.
- False positive: B, also called *type I error*; the people without disease who tested positive.
- False negative: C, also called *type II error*; the people with disease who tested negative.
- Sensitivity: A / (A + C), measures the proportion of actual people with the disease who tested positive.
- Specificity: D / (B + D), measures the proportion of actual people without the disease who tested negative.
- Positive predictive value (PPV): A / (A + B), measures the proportions of those who tested positive who actually have the disease.
- Negative predictive value (NPV): D / (C + D), measures the proportions of those who tested negative and who actually do not have disease.
- Odds ratio (OR): (A × D) / (B × C), measures the association between an exposure and an outcome. This ratio represents the odds that an outcome will occur with a particular exposure compared to the odds of the outcome occurring without exposure. It can be calculated based on the probability that an event happened divided by the probability that an event did not happen.
- Prevalence: (A + C) / (A + B + C + D), measures the percentage of people found to have disease with the total number of people studied.
- Incidence: Not shown in the contingency table. *Incidence* is the rate of newly diagnosed cases of a disease within a period of time, eg, 1 year.

TABLE 25-1 Contingency table

		Disease	
		+ (with)	– (without)
Test	+ (positive)	A	B
	– (negative)	C	D

Types of Studies

LEVELS OF EVIDENCE

Several types of studies are conducted and applied in dentistry. Table 25-2 lists the various types of studies in order from highest to lowest level of evidence.

EXPERIMENTAL STUDIES

These types of studies could potentially provide cause-and-effect because they demonstrate what outcome occurs when a particular variable is manipulated. The researchers can change an independent variable and observe the dependent variables based on the study design. This type of study (ie, randomized controlled trials) offers a higher level of evidence due to its experimental nature.

OBSERVATIONAL STUDIES

These types of studies could possibly provide association but not causation. The independent variable is not under the control of the researchers but simply an outcome being observed.

Systematic Reviews and Meta-Analyses

PRISMA

Preferred reporting items for systematic reviews and meta-analyses (PRISMA) is an evidence-based guideline describing the required items for reporting in systematic reviews and meta-analyses (Table 25-3).[4] When conducting a systematic review or meta-analysis, researchers are recommended to follow this protocol to ensure the comprehensiveness of the study.

TABLE 25-2 Levels of evidence

Level of evidence	Study type	Description
Highest	Systematic reviews/ meta-analyses	Systematically collect secondary data with clearly defined inclusion and exclusion criteria, critically evaluate studies and their heterogeneity, and statistically synthesize studies.
	Randomized clinical trials	Participants are allocated at random to receive one of the interventions. One of these interventions serves as control or standard of care. It is an experimental design.
	Nonrandomized clinical trials	Participants are allocated without randomization to receive one of the interventions. It is an experimental design.
	Cohort studies	Studies analyze data in a prospective or retrospective longitudinal manner without active manipulation of variables. It is usually an observational design.
	Case-control studies	Studies analyze data in a retrospective manner without longitudinal follow-up. This type of study compares those with the disease or condition (cases) and a group of participants who do not have the disease or condition (controls). It can provide evidence of association but not causation. It is an observational design.
	Cross-sectional studies	Observe a population and collect data at a given time. It is an observational design.
Lowest	Case reports/expert opinions	Provide description of a case or cases or personal opinions regarding an outcome.

TABLE 25-3 Required items for systematic reviews and meta-analyses*

	Section/topic	Checklist item
	Title	
1	Title	Identify the report as a systematic review, meta-analysis, or both.
	Abstract	
2	Structured summary	Provide a structured summary including, as applicable: background; objectives; data sources; study eligibility criteria, participants, and interventions; study appraisal and synthesis methods; results; limitations; conclusions and implications of key findings; systematic review registration number.
	Introduction	
3	Rationale	Describe the rationale for the review in the context of what is already known.
4	Objectives	Provide an explicit statement of questions being addressed with reference to participants, interventions, comparisons, outcomes, and study design (PICOS).
	Methods	
5	Protocol and registration	Indicate if a review protocol exists, if and where it can be accessed (eg, web address), and, if available, provide registration information including registration number.
6	Eligibility criteria	Specify study characteristics (eg, PICOS, length of follow-up) and report characteristics (eg, years considered, language, publication status) used as criteria for eligibility, giving rationale.
7	Information sources	Describe all information sources (eg, databases with dates of coverage, contact with study authors to identify additional studies) in the search and date last searched.

→

TABLE 25-3 Required items for systematic reviews and meta-analyses* *(cont)*

	Section/topic	Checklist item
	Methods	
8	Search	Present full electronic search strategy for at least one database, including any limits used, such that it could be repeated.
9	Study selection	State the process for selecting studies (ie, screening, eligibility) included in systematic review and, if applicable, included in the meta-analysis.
10	Data collection process	Describe methods of data extraction from reports (eg, piloted forms, independently, in duplicate) and any processes for obtaining and confirming data from investigators.
11	Data items	List and define all variables for which data were sought (eg, PICOS, funding sources) and any assumptions and simplifications made.
12	Risk of bias in individual studies	Describe methods used for assessing risk of bias of individual studies (including specification of whether this was done at the study or outcome level) and how this information is to be used in any data synthesis.
13	Summary measures	State the principal summary measures (eg, risk ratio, difference in means).
14	Synthesis of results	Describe the methods of handling data and combining results of studies, if done, including measures of consistency (eg, I^2) for each meta-analysis.
15	Risk of bias across studies	Specify any assessment of risk of bias that may affect the cumulative evidence (eg, publication bias, selective reporting within studies).
16	Additional analyses	Describe methods of additional analyses (eg, sensitivity or subgroup analyses, meta-regression), if done, indicating which were prespecified.
	Results	
17	Study selection	Give numbers of studies screened, assessed for eligibility, and included in the review, with reasons for exclusions at each stage, ideally with a flow diagram.
18	Study characteristics	For each study, present characteristics for which data were extracted (eg, study size, PICOS, follow-up period), and provide the citations.
19	Risk of bias within studies	Present data on risk of bias of each study and, if available, any outcome-level assessment (see item 12).
20	Results of individual studies	For all outcomes considered (benefits or harms), present, for each study: *(1)* simple summary data for each intervention group and *(2)* effect estimates and confidence intervals, ideally with a forest plot.
21	Synthesis of results	Present results of each meta-analysis done, including confidence intervals and measures of consistency.
22	Risk of bias across studies	Present results of any assessment of risk of bias across studies (see item 15).
23	Additional analysis	Give results of additional analyses, if done (eg, sensitivity or subgroup analyses, meta-regression [see item 16]).
	Discussion	
24	Summary of evidence	Summarize the main findings, including the strength of evidence for each main outcome; consider their relevance to key groups (eg, health care providers, users, and policymakers).
25	Limitations	Discuss limitations at study and outcome level (eg, risk of bias), and at review level (eg, incomplete retrieval of identified research, reporting bias).
26	Conclusions	Provide a general interpretation of the results in the context of other evidence, and implications for future research.
	Funding	
27	Funding	Describe sources of funding for the systematic review and other support (eg, supply of data); role of funders for the systematic review.

*Reproduced with permission from Moher et al.[4]

TABLE 25-4 Forest plot to represent the outcome of a meta-analysis*

	Wide			Narrow				Mean difference	Mean difference
Study	Mean	SD	Total	Mean	SD	Total	Weight	IV, Random, 95% CI	IV, Random, 95% CI
Adibrad et al[6] (2009)	1.2	0.71	36	1.87	0.59	30	8.3%	−0.67 [−0.98, −0.36]	
Bouri et al[7] (2008)	1.25	0.53	110	1.78	0.78	90	10.4%	−0.53 [−0.72, −0.34]	
Boynuegri et al[8] (2012)	0.25	0.486	15	0.583	0.532	15	7.5%	−0.33 [−0.70, 0.03]	
Chung et al[9] (2006)	1.26	0.8	255	1.51	0.82	84	10.2%	−0.25 [−0.45, −0.05]	
Crespi et al[10] (2010)	1.18	0.09	125	1.71	0.12	39	12.0%	−0.53 [−0.57, −0.49]	
Esper et al[11] (2012)	0.6	0.62	133	0.67	0.71	69	10.2%	−0.07 [−0.27, 0.13]	
Kim et al[12] (2009)	0.74	0.83	186	0.74	0.91	90	9.8%	0.00 [−0.22, 0.22]	
Mericske-Stern[13] (1990)	0.71	0.72	142	0.83	0.79	132	10.5%	−0.12 [−0.30, 0.06]	
Mericske-Stern et al[14] (1994)	0.54	0.66	79	0.49	0.6	49	9.8%	0.05 [−0.17, 0.27]	
Schrott et al[15] (2009)	0.31	0.62	595	0.57	0.81	177	11.2%	−0.26 [−0.39, −0.13]	
Total (95% CI)			1,676			775	100.0%	−0.27 [−0.43, −0.11]	

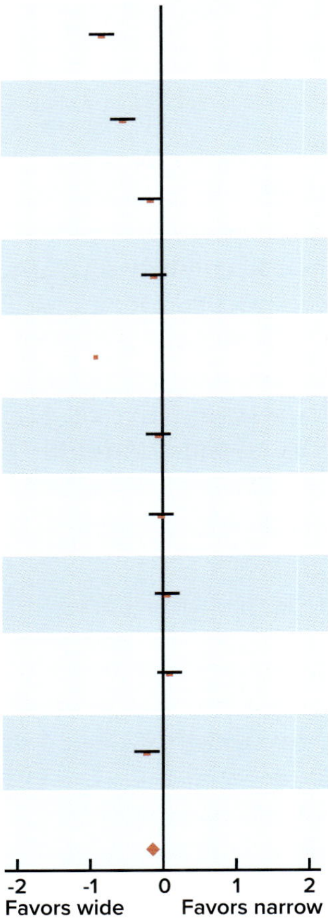

Heterogeneity: $Tau^2 = 0.06$; $Chi^2 = 92.04$; df = 9 ($P < .00001$); $I^2 = 90\%$
Test for overall effect: Z = 3.25 ($P = .001$)
*Adapted with permission from Lin et al.[5]

SYSTEMATIC REVIEW

A systematic review uses scientific studies to accumulate information, grade existing literature, and then combine literature findings into a synthesized analysis of new research. A systematic review generally analyzes data in a descriptive or statistical way if the articles reflect literature that comes from a high level of evidence and if the material is generally homogenous in nature. A systematic review should be conducted with a structured search strategy based on a clear PICOS question and inclusion and exclusion criteria. If there is more than one person conducting the literature search process, an analysis of interexaminer agreement should be reported to demonstrate the quality of the search.

META-ANALYSIS

A meta-analysis is a statistical analysis for combining data from multiple studies. Each included study is considered to have an unbiased estimate of the true effect when meta-analyzed. An advantage of meta-analyses is to increase statistical power. A forest plot is often generated to demonstrate the outcome of an analysis.

Table 25-4 includes an example of a forest plot.[5–15] This forest plot represents an analysis of 10 included studies with a similar focused question. The final test outcome is shown with a diamond-shaped mark at the bottom of the plot. If the diamond crosses the middle line, representing "no difference" between the test and control groups, this outcome is considered to have no statistically significant difference between the two groups. On the contrary, if the diamond does not cross the middle line, then this analysis is considered as statistically significant. In the example shown in Table 25-4, since the diamond does not cross the "no difference" line, the outcome is statistically significant, with an overall test effect *P*-value of .001.

HETEROGENEITY ANALYSIS

Because data from multiple studies are synthesized together in meta-analyses, an evaluation to identify heterogeneity among studies is required to assess the variation in study outcomes. Heterogeneity analysis is often done by reporting I-square (I^2) value, which ranges between 0% and 100% with the lower values representing less heterogeneity. Another commonly used analysis is chi-square test; if a *P*-value for chi-square test is less than .05, a high heterogeneity among the selected studies is identified.

RISK-OF-BIAS ASSESSMENT

A bias of an individual study is a deviation from the truth due to potential confounding factors. Therefore, assessing the quality of each included study is crucial to identify any potential biased data. Biased data can underestimate or overestimate the true effect and are often excluded from a meta-analysis due to high risk of jeopardizing the study outcomes.

Several risk-of-bias assessment guidelines[16–18] have been proposed to evaluate the potential risk of bias. For randomized controlled trials, the checklist of the Cochrane Center[15] is widely used. This checklist consists of several items, such as random sequence generation, allocation concealment method, blinding of participants and personnel, blinding of outcome assessment, incomplete outcome data addressed, and selective reporting. A high-quality study should be graded with low risk of bias in most of the checklist items. If a study is considered to have a high risk of bias, the extracted data from the study must be interpreted cautiously or even excluded from statistical analysis because other confounding factors may influence the results.

References

1. Sackett DL, Straus SE, Richardson WS, Rosenberg W, Haynes RB. Evidence-Based Medicine: How to Practice and Teach EBM, ed 2. Edinburgh: Churchill Livingstone, 2000:1–2.
2. American Academy of Periodontology. Glossary of Periodontal Terms. American Academy of Periodontology, 2001.
3. Pearson K. Mathematical Contributions to the Theory of Evolution. XIII. On the Theory of Contingency and its Relation to Association and Normal Correlation. London: Dulau and Co, 1904:1–37.
4. Moher D, Liberati A, Tetzlaff J, Altman DG, PRISMA Group. Preferred reporting items for systematic reviews and meta-analyses: The PRISMA statement. PLoS Med 2009;6:e1000097.3.
5. Lin GH, Chan HL, Wang HL. The significance of keratinized mucosa on implant health: A systematic review. J Periodontol 2013;84:1755–1767.
6. Adibrad M, Shahabuei M, Sahabi M. Significance of the width of keratinized mucosa on the health status of the supporting tissue around implants supporting overdentures. J Oral Implantol 2009;35:232–237.
7. Bouri A Jr, Bissada N, Al-Zahrani MS, Faddoul F, Nouneh I. Width of keratinized gingiva and the health status of the supporting tissues around dental implants. Int J Oral Maxillofac Implants 2008;23:323–326.
8. Boynuegri D, Nemli SK, Kasko YA. Significance of keratinized mucosa around dental implants: A prospective comparative study. Clin Oral Implants Res 2013;24:928–933.
9. Chung DM, Oh TJ, Shotwell JL, Misch CE, Wang HL. Significance of keratinized mucosa in maintenance of dental implants with different surfaces. J Periodontol 2006;77:1410–1420.
10. Crespi R, Capparè P, Gherlone E. A 4-year evaluation of the peri-implant parameters of immediately loaded implants placed in fresh extraction sockets. J Periodontol 2010;81:1629–1634.
11. Esper LA, Ferreira SB Jr, de Oliveira Fortes Kaizer R, de Almeida AL. The role of keratinized mucosa in periimplant health. Cleft Palate Craniofac J 2012;49:167–170.
12. Kim BS, Kim YK, Yun PY, et al. Evaluation of periimplant tissue response according to the presence of keratinized mucosa. Oral Surg Oral Med Oral Pathol Oral Radiol Endod 2009;107:e24–e28.
13. Mericske-Stern R. Clinical evaluation of overdenture restorations supported by osseointegrated titanium implants: A retrospective study. Int J Oral Maxillofac Implants 1990;5:375–383.
14. Mericske-Stern R, Steinlin Schaffner T, Marti P, Geering AH. Peri-implant mucosal aspects of ITI implants supporting overdentures. A five-year longitudinal study. Clin Oral Implants Res 1994;5:9–18.
15. Schrott AR, Jimenez M, Hwang JW, Fiorellini J, Weber HP. Five-year evaluation of the influence of keratinized mucosa on peri-implant soft-tissue health and stability around implants supporting full-arch mandibular fixed prostheses. Clin Oral Implants Res 2009;20:1170–1177.
16. Higgins JP, Green S. Cochrane Handbook for Systematic Reviews of Interventions. Version 5.1.0 (updated March 2011). The Cochrane Collaboration, 2011. Available at http://handbook-5-1.cochrane.org/
17. Wells GA, Shea B, O'Connell D, et al. The Newcastle-Ottawa Scale (NOS) for assessing the quality of nonrandomized studies in meta-analyses. Available at http://www.ohri.ca/programs/clinical_epidemiology/oxford.htm
18. Slim K, Nini E, Forestier D, Kwiatkowski F, Panis Y, Chipponi J. Methodological index for non-randomized studies (MINORS): Development and validation of a new instrument. ANZ J Surg 2003;73:712–716.

26

ORAL MEDICINE AND PATHOLOGY

Vivian Petersen Wagner, DDS, PhD
Manoela Domingues Martins, DDS, PhD

DEFINITIONS AND TERMINOLOGY

Cyst: A pathologic cavity lined by epithelium and usually containing fluid or semisolid material.[1]

Desquamative gingivitis: A nonspecific term describing erythema and ulceration of the free and attached gingiva. It reflects diffuse inflammation of the gingiva with sloughing of the surface epithelium. It can be a manifestation of one or more of vesiculoerosive mucosal conditions.[1]

Granuloma: A reactive nodule consisting of modified macrophages resembling epithelial cells surrounded by a rim of mononuclear cells, usually lymphocytes, and often containing giant cells.[1]

Keratosis: Any keratinous growth, such as a wart or callus.[1]

Nikolsky sign: Occurs when the apparently normal, superficial layer of skin or oral mucosa may be rubbed off with slight trauma. Originally associated with pemphigus vulgaris, but can be seen in several bullous conditions.[1]

Ulcer, ulceration: A lesion on the surface of the skin or mucosa characterized by discontinuation of the epithelium deeper than erosion, exhibits gradual tissue disintegration and necrosis.[1]

This chapter aims to review the main diseases affecting the periodontal tissues from the perspective of oral medicine and pathology. Due to the great variety of disorders that can occur in the periodontium and jawbones, only the most clinically relevant or prevalent conditions are included.

Developmental Disorders

EXOSTOSES

Exostoses are characterized by limited protuberances arising from cortical bone. The most common types of exostoses in the jaws are the torus palatinus and the torus mandibularis (Fig 26-1), which occur in the midline of hard palate and along the lingual aspect of the mandible, respectively. Other types of exostoses include bilateral hard swellings along the facial aspect of the alveolar process or in the lingual aspect of maxillary tuberosities. Most exostoses are asymptomatic and can be diagnosed by clinical and radiographic assessment. In edentulous patients, surgical intervention might be necessary to accommodate dentures.[2]

Local Soft Tissue Lesions

TRAUMATIC ULCERS

Traumatic **ulcers** can occur in any site of the oral mucosa. The etiologic factor can be usually detected during anamnesis (eg, trauma during brushing) or physical examination (eg, denture hooks). Their clinical features and location can vary, and both characteristics are directly correlated with the cause of the injury (Fig 26-2). Traumatic ulcers regularly present as an exposure of the connective tissue recovered by a yellowish-white necrotic pseudomembrane with slightly erythematous borders. Biopsies are not indicated to achieve a final diagnosis once the microscopic aspect consists of exposed connective tissue without any particular feature that allows for a specific diagnosis. Other ulcerative conditions might have a similar microscopic appearance. The etiologic factor must be identified and removed (eg, polishing a cutting edge of a broken tooth or prosthesis adjustment). The gradual or complete regression of the lesion confirms the diagnosis of a traumatic ulcer. Ulcers that do not regress or do not heal completely within 10 days should be reevaluated. A new hypothesis should be considered, and a biopsy may be indicated.

Other ulcerative lesions caused by thermal and chemical agents can also occur. Hot foods, hot dental instruments, electrical burns, or cryosurgery can cause thermal lesions. Chemical etiologic factors include acids used during dental procedures, mouthwashes, and medications or recreational drugs (eg, analgesic tablets or cocaine deliberately rubbed into the gingiva). The diagnosis also needs to be established based on clinical history and physical examination, supplemented by the regression of the lesion.

FRICTIONAL KERATOSIS

This reactive condition is caused by a constant trauma with low intensity (ie, chronic), leading to more keratin production by the epithelium. Frictional **keratosis** frequently occurs in the ridge of edentulous areas or in the retromolar area due to constant trauma from mastication (Fig 26-3). To confirm the diagnosis, the dentist should remove the traumatic agent and observe the regression of the lesion. If the clinical differential diagnosis includes leukoplakia, a potentially malignant disorder, a biopsy can be performed.

RECURRENT APHTHOUS STOMATITIS

The involvement of gingiva and other keratinized mucosa (hard palate and dorsal surface of the tongue) by recurrent aphthous stomatitis (RAS) is rare and usually represents the extension of a large wound that originates in nonkeratinized areas. However, this condition is among the most prevalent oral mucosa diseases, so it is important to understand. It is considered an immunologic reaction that can be triggered by different events, such as hormonal changes, stress, and spicy foods or foods with citric acid. RAS is more common in younger patients

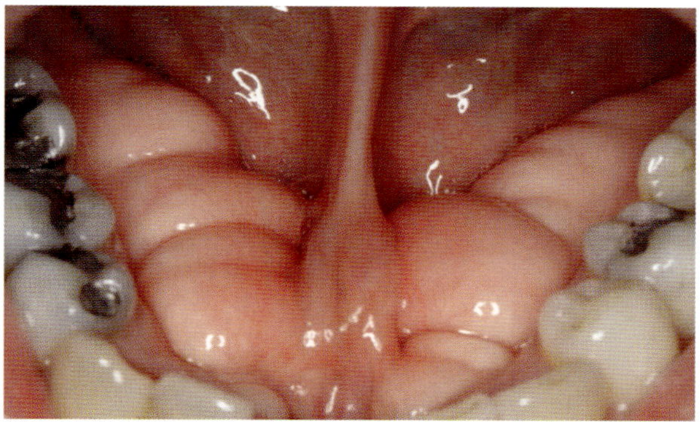

Fig 26-1 Bilateral tori mandibularis.

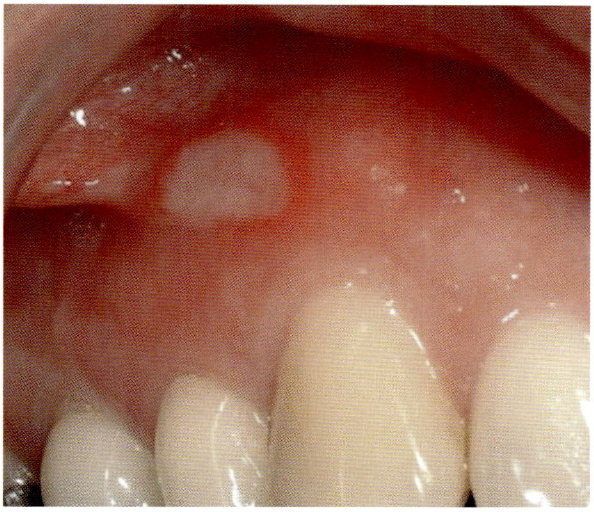

Fig 26-2 Traumatic ulcer located in the gingiva caused by trauma during tooth brushing.

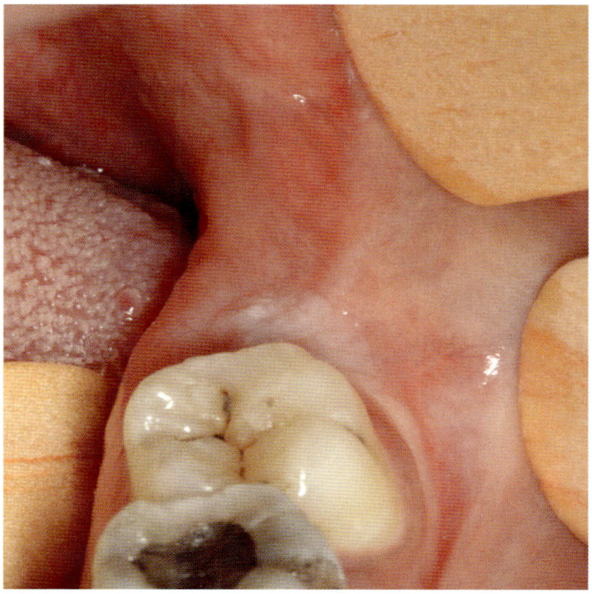

Fig 26-3 Frictional keratosis in the retromolar area due to trauma during mastication.

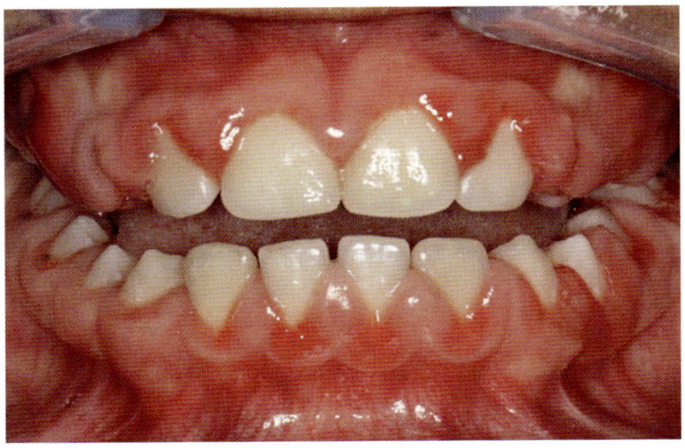

Fig 26-4 Drug-related gingival lesions in a patient taking cyclosporine.

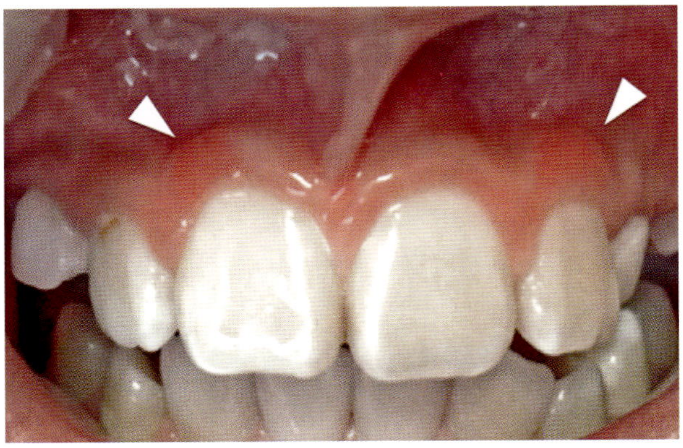

Fig 26-5 The patient presented with two reddish macules in the attached gingiva above the maxillary right central incisor and left lateral incisor *(arrowheads)*. The biopsy revealed an inflammatory infiltrate composed mostly of plasma cells. Modifications to the patient's diet resulted in regression of the lesions.

BOX 26-1 Drugs associated with gingival hyperplasia[5]

Anticonvulsants
- Ethosuximide
- Ethotoin
- Mephenytoin
- Methsuximide*
- Phenobarbital
- Phenytoin
- Primidone
- Sodium valproate
- Vigabatrin

Immunosuppressants
- Cyclosporine
- Sirolimus
- Tacrolimus

Calcium channel blockers
- Amlodipine
- Diltiazem
- Felodipine
- Manidipine
- Nicardipine
- Nifedipine
- Nimodipine
- Nisoldipine
- Nitrendipine
- Verapamil

*Alternately spelled *mesuximide*, *methosuximide*, or *methosuxinimide*.

such as adolescents. There are three clinical variants: minor, major, and herpetiform. The minor form is the most common, in which lesions are usually small and heal in a shorter time than other variants. Major lesions take more time to heal and are usually associated with scar formation. The herpetiform variant demonstrates the greatest number of lesions per episode, and patients experience frequent recurrences. The diagnosis is based on clinical features associated with a history of recurrences after excluding systemic conditions that may also trigger aphthous-like ulcerations. The treatment usually involves the use of topical agents such as corticosteroids and aims to relieve pain and accelerate repair. It is important to differentiate RAS from other autoimmune diseases such as oral lichen planus, pemphigus vulgaris, and bullous pemphigoid, in which lesions usually persist for a longer time and occur mostly in individuals older than 40 years.[3]

DRUG-INDUCED GINGIVAL LESIONS

Drug-related gingival enlargement is characterized by firm, pale to reddish, and enlarged gingival papillae secondary to the use of a systemic medication[4] (Fig 26-4). Box 26-1 provides a list of medications that have been demonstrated to produce gingival overgrowth.[5] The prevalence of gingival hyperplasia among drugs varies, and the patient's susceptibility appears to play an important role. Additionally, poor oral hygiene exacerbates the symptoms. The treatment should be planned in collaboration with the professional who prescribed the drug. Discontinuation and drug substitution are the main treatment modalities, usually resulting in cessation of gingival overgrowth. In some circumstances, regression can also be observed. Systemic and topical agents can be used to increase plaque control when attempting to ameliorate the gingival hyperplasia. In a significant number of cases, surgical removal of excess gingiva is necessary.

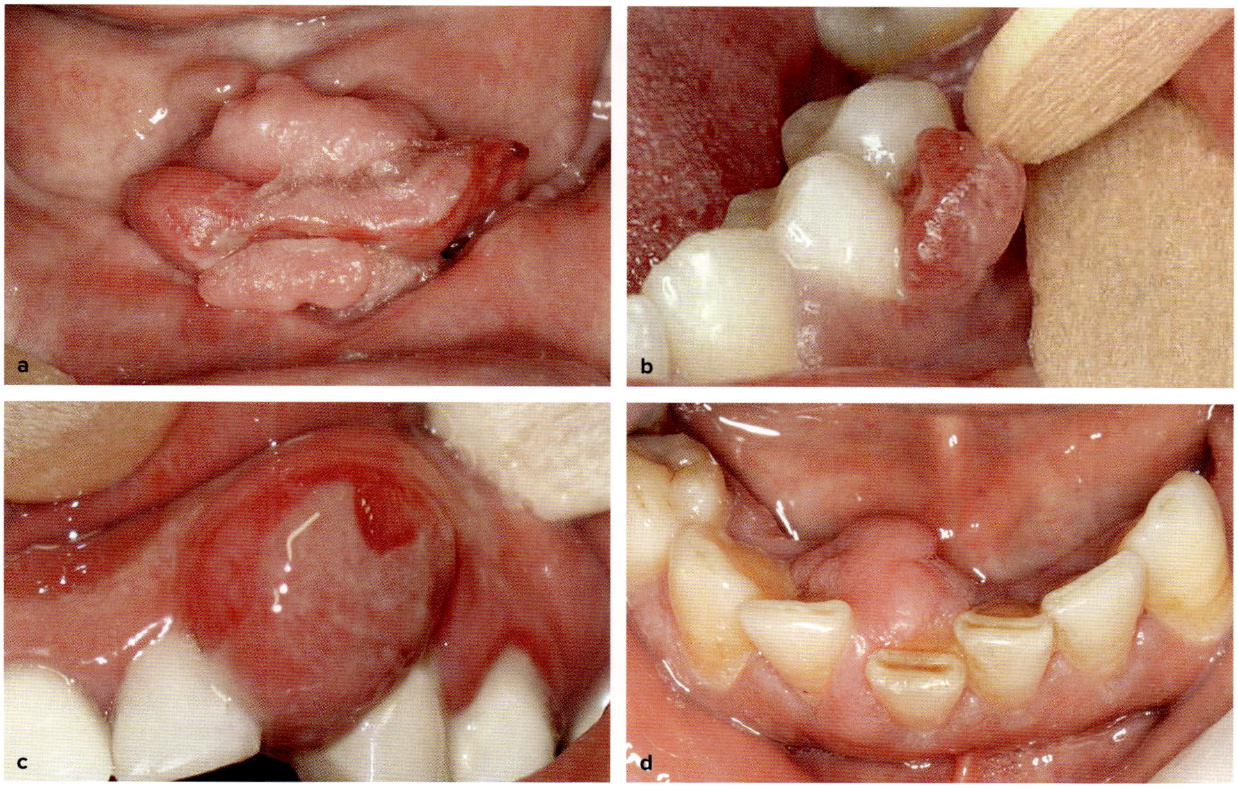

Fig 26-6 *(a)* Focal fibrous hyperplasia. *(b)* Pyogenic granuloma. *(c)* Peripheral giant cell granuloma. *(d)* Peripheral ossifying fibroma.

PLASMA CELL GINGIVITIS

Plasma cell gingivitis is a rare and distinct type of gingival alteration characterized by a sharply demarcated bright erythematous area in the free and attached gingiva (Fig 26-5). Plasma cell gingivitis is considered a hypersensitive allergic reaction, and several substances have been associated with this condition, such as cinnamon oil, mint, peppers, and herbal toothpastes, among others. The inflammatory infiltrate is composed mainly of plasma cells, and investigation of the clonality of these cells might be necessary to rule out a plasma cell neoplasm in atypical cases. Possible allergens should be identified and eliminated.

NONNEOPLASTIC PROLIFERATIVE LESIONS

Nonneoplastic proliferative lesions are especially relevant because they affect the gingiva more frequently or exclusively. Several inflammatory stimuli can be present in the periodontal region, such as local irritation from calculus, trauma, food impaction, and restorations with irregular margins, among others. Four forms of localized reactive hyperplastic lesions of the gingiva are currently recognized: fibrous hyperplasia, pyogenic **granuloma**, peripheral giant cell granuloma, and peripheral ossifying fibroma.[6] All four types are mainly characterized by slow-growing nodular masses arising from the dental papilla (Fig 26-6). Edentulous areas may also be affected. Some clinical features, such as surface and color, may vary between lesions; however, these characteristics may also overlap. The final diagnosis can only be established through histopathologic investigation. The main differences among these lesions are presented in Table 26-1.

The main clinical diagnosis hypothesis can be constructed based on clinical aspects and patients' history. Nevertheless, the final diagnosis will be established according to the microscopic features (Fig 26-7). All lesions need to be completely excised. Strategies such as root surface instrumentation and curettage can be performed to prevent recurrence of the lesions by eliminating possible sources of irritation.

GIANT CELL FIBROMA

Giant cell fibroma also occurs with greater frequency in the gingiva. However, this condition is not as common

TABLE 26-1 Clinical and histopathologic features of the most frequent nonneoplastic proliferative lesions

	Focal fibrous hyperplasia	Pyogenic granuloma	Peripheral giant cell granuloma	Peripheral ossifying fibroma
Surface	Smooth	Smooth or lobulated	Smooth or lobulated	Smooth
Color	Same as mucosa	Pink to fiery red	Red to reddish-blue	Same as mucosa to red
Ulceration	Usually absent, unless secondary trauma	Usually present, bleeds easily	Usually present, bleeds easily	Usually absent, unless secondary trauma
Exclusive in the gingiva	No	No	Yes	Yes
Peculiarities	Frequently associated with ill-fitting complete or partial denture	Frequently develops in pregnant women, may exhibit rapid growth	Can cause "cupping" resorption of the adjacent alveolar bone	Hard mass at physical examination, might have radiopaque image
Histopathology	Mass of dense collagenous connective tissue in a scar-like pattern	Marked proliferation of endothelial cells that line capillary channels and mixed inflammatory cells	Proliferation of mesenchymal cells and multinucleated giant cells	Cellular fibroblastic tissue and formation of mineralized products

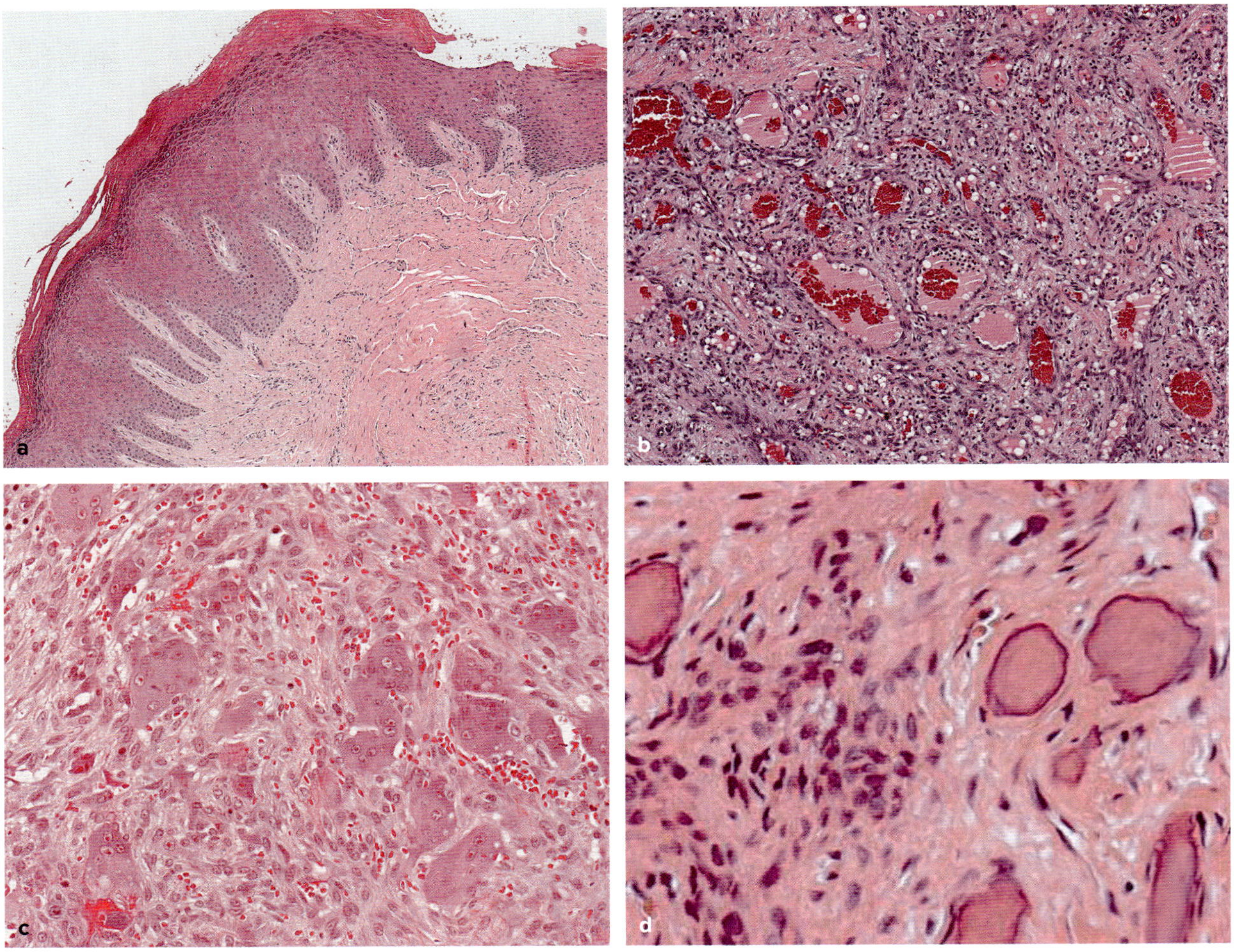

Fig 26-7 *(a)* Focal fibrous hyperplasia. *(b)* Pyogenic granuloma. *(c)* Peripheral giant cell granuloma. *(d)* Peripheral ossifying fibroma.

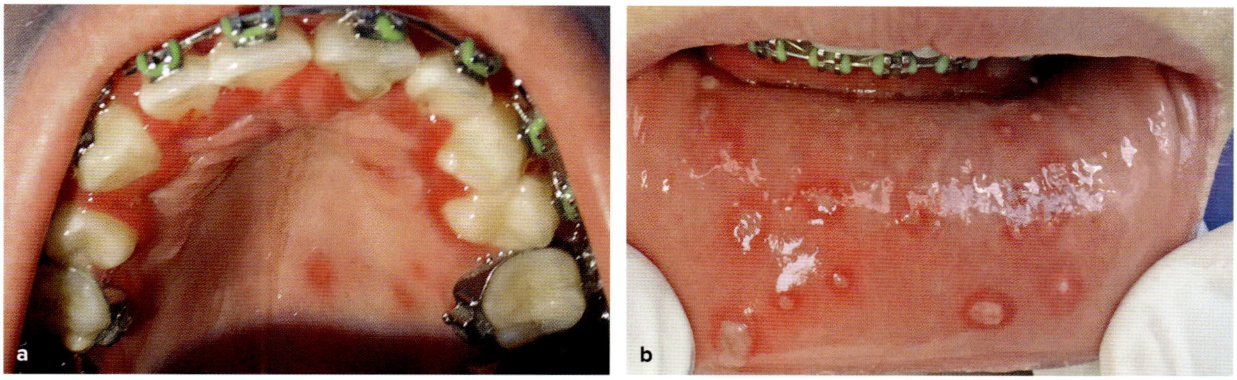

Fig 26-8 Primary herpetic gingivostomatitis in a teenaged patient. The area demonstrated gingival erythema and multiple erosive areas or ulcers in the palate *(a)* and labial mucosa *(b)*.

as localized reactive hyperplastic lesions. Moreover, giant cell fibroma does not seem to be associated with chronic irritation. The diagnosis of giant cell fibroma also relies on the histopathologic examination, which reveals numerous large, stellate fibroblasts that may contain multiple nuclei.

Infectious Diseases

VIRAL INFECTIONS

Herpetic

The oral infection by herpes simplex virus (HSV) can be divided into *primary infection* and *secondary* or *recurrent infection*. The infection is usually caused by type 1 HSV (HSV-1) that is transmitted in saliva. The primary infection is asymptomatic in the majority of patients or causes insignificant signs and symptoms. However, in a subset of patients, an acute manifestation known as *herpetic gingivostomatitis* can occur. Most cases arise between the ages of 6 months to 5 years, directly related to the first contact with the virus. The onset is abrupt and accompanied by general malaise, high fever, and regional lymphadenopathy. Different mucosa sites, such as tongue, buccal mucosa, palate, and lips, can be affected and demonstrate numerous vesicles that collapse rapidly, resulting in erosive areas or ulcers. The gingival involvement is extremely common in primary infection and is characterized by erythema, edema, and pain (Fig 26-8).

After the primary infection, either asymptomatic or symptomatic, the virus is transported retrograde by neurons to the trigeminal ganglion, where latency is established. Different stimuli such as acute sun exposure, stress, and low immunity can trigger virus reactivation. The virus uses the sensory neurons axons to "travel back," and the manifestation usually occurs at the site of primary inoculation. The most common affected site is the outer edge of the vermilion border. Nevertheless, oral mucosal involvement can also occur, mostly in the attached gingiva and hard palate. As in primary infection, the manifestation initiates with fluid-filled vesicles that rapidly collapse, leaving erythematous or ulcerated lesions. Patients usually report prodromal signs and symptoms such as burning, itching, or pain.

The diagnosis of both primary and recurrent forms is generally based on clinical history and features but can also be supplemented by laboratory confirmation. Patients should be advised to avoid contact with active lesions (vesicles) in order to prevent spread to other sites (autoinoculation) or infection of other individuals. In a primary infection, the treatment is usually symptomatic, involving the prescription of analgesics and antipyretics (in cases of fever). In addition, local hygiene measures with gauze soaked in serum, hydration, liquid diet, and rest should be recommended. In recurrent lesions, antiviral medications are more effective if initiated in the prodromal period.

Human papillomavirus

Human papillomaviruses (HPVs) include a large group of DNA viruses that are capable of infecting the skin and mucosa of animal species. Based on their oncogenic potential, HPV types are categorized as low risk or high risk. Among the high-risk HPV types, HPV-16 is the most frequently associated with cervical cancer and oropharyngeal cancer. The incidence of HPV-positive oropharyngeal cancer has been increasing significantly in the past 30 years. The tonsils and base of the tongue represent the

BOX 26-2 Predisposing factors to oral candidiasis

Systemic factors	Local factors
Physiologic factors • Extreme ages (children and elderly)	**Dentures (acidic and anaerobic conditions)** • Reduced vertical dimension (saliva accumulation and a moist environment)
Endocrine disorders • Diabetes, hypothyroidism	**Xerostomia** • Sjögren syndrome, radiotherapy, or drug-induced xerostomia
Nutritional factors • Deficiency of vitamin B_{12}, iron, or folate	**Medications (changes in normal microbiota)** • Broad-spectrum antibiotics, corticosteroids (systemic or inhaled)
Immunosuppression • AIDS, drug-induced immunosuppression (transplanted patients)	

sites most commonly affected by HPV-positive carcinomas. Compared with conventional oral squamous cell carcinoma (SCC; associated with tobacco and alcohol), these tumors are frequently diagnosed with a smaller size. Yet, nodal metastasis (cystic type in most cases) is commonly present at diagnosis. The 3-year survival rates of HPV-positive oropharyngeal carcinoma are significantly higher than HPV-negative oropharyngeal carcinoma.[7]

Oral papilloma is the most common HPV-associated benign lesion of the oral cavity, and it occurs especially in the palate, tongue, and lips. Verruca vulgaris, another benign HPV-associated lesion, is more common in the skin; however, due to autoinoculation, lesions in the oral mucosa can also occur. Both lesions are characterized as small nodules with a papillary or verrucous surface. Oral papilloma is usually solitary, while patients with verruca vulgaris usually present with multiple lesions.

HPV vaccine

Three HPV vaccines have been licensed for use in the United States. Currently, routine vaccination is recommended for *(1)* girls at age 11 or 12 years (series can be started at age 9 years) and through age 26 years if not vaccinated previously; and *(2)* boys at age 11 or 12 years (series can be started at age 9 years), through age 21 years if not vaccinated previously and through age 26 years for men who have sex with men. Two doses of the vaccine are recommended for immunocompetent individuals starting series at age 9 to 14 years, and three doses for individuals starting series at older ages and for individuals with immunocompromised conditions.[8]

Other viral infections

Infection by varicella zoster virus (varicella or chickenpox) and enteroviruses (hand-foot-and-mouth disease and herpangina) can also cause oral lesions. These situations are more common in children. Varicella is well known by its skin lesions; however, oral mucosa involvement may occur and even precede the skin manifestation. Oral lesions are very common in hand-foot-and-mouth disease and herpangina, which are considered two distinct manifestations of the same disease. In all these conditions, the gingiva does not represent the most common oral site affected.

FUNGAL INFECTIONS

Oral candidiasis

Candida species are commensal yeast present at the oral mucosa that can cause infection in specific circumstances, such as a weakening of the host's immune defenses or changes in the local environment (Box 26-2). *Candida albicans* is the most commonly observed species in health and disease situations. The clinical manifestation of oral candidiasis is very broad and depends mainly in the type of predisposing factors present.[9] Table 26-2 summarizes the clinical aspects and etiology associated with the most common types of primary oral candidiasis and *Candida*-associated lesions.

The diagnosis of oral candidiasis is usually based on clinical signs and symptoms associated with a comprehensive investigation of medical and dental history. It is important to identify and correct the underlying predisposing factors. Treatment with antifungal agents without removal of the predisposing factor might result in only temporary relief, and relapses will probably occur. Topical antifungals are generally the drug of choice for localized

TABLE 26-2 Most common types of oral candidiasis and *Candida*-associated lesions

	Etiology	Clinical manifestation
Pseudomembranous candidiasis (oral thrush)	Infants, elderly, corticosteroid or prolonged broad-spectrum antibiotic therapy, diabetes mellitus, AIDS	Creamy white plaques on the tongue, palate, and buccal mucosa that can be removed by wiping gently, leaving behind an underlying erythematous tissue that may bleed slightly.
Denture-related stomatitis (erythematous candidiasis)	Dentures associated with poor oral hygiene, nocturnal denture wear, ill-fitting prostheses, or low salivary flow	Varies from pinpoint hyperemia, diffuse erythematous, or papillary type. Lesions are asymptomatic and present only in the area supporting the denture.
Angular cheilitis	Reduced vertical dimension (elderly denture patients), vitamin B_{12} or iron deficiency	Erythematous or ulcerated fissures affecting the commissures of the lip.
Median rhomboid glossitis	Etiology is poorly understood (smoking and inhalation steroids have been implicated)	Well-demarcated depapillated area (atrophy) located in the midline of the dorsum of the tongue anterior to the circumvallate papillae.

lesions in patients with normal immune function, while systemic drugs will be indicated for disseminated disease and/or patients with a compromised immune system.

Systemic mycoses

Histoplasmosis. Histoplasmosis is the most common systemic fungal infection in the United States and is caused by the environmental dimorphic fungus *Histoplasma capsulatum*. Human infection occurs once the microorganism is inhaled from the environment, and there is no person-to-person transmission. Usually, infected individuals are asymptomatic; however, the disease will manifest in 1% of the infected population, which might have different clinical presentations, including acute pulmonary disease, disseminated disease, or chronic pulmonary histoplasmosis. Histoplasmosis oral lesions are rare but can occur in the disseminated form of the disease. The clinical manifestation is usually indistinguishable from a malignancy, appearing as a solitary chronic ulceration. The most classic microscopic aspect is epithelioid granulomas. Special stains, such as the periodic acid–Schiff (PAS) and Grocott-Gomori methenamine silver (GMS) methods, evidence the small yeasts of *Histoplasma capsulatum*. The treatment is based on systemic antifungals, mainly itraconazole.

Other systemic mycoses. Examples include the following, though there are others as well:

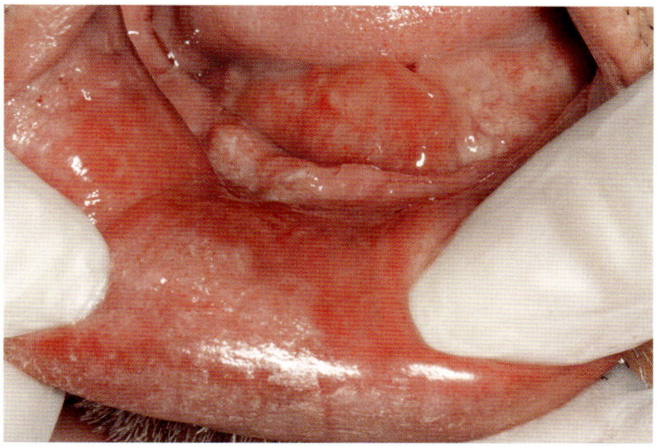

Fig 26-9 Multiple paracoccidioidomycosis lesions in the labial mucosa and alveolar ridge.

- Blastomycosis, caused by the fungus *Blastomyces dermatitidis*
- Paracoccidioidomycosis, caused by *Paracoccidioides brasiliensis*
- Coccidioidomycosis (valley fever), caused by *Coccidioides immitis*
- Cryptococcosis, caused by *Cryptococcus neoformans*

The contamination usually occurs due to fungus inhalation. In paracoccidioidomycosis, gingival involvement is very common and presents as mulberry-like ulcerations (Fig 26-9). This condition is endemic in several areas of Brazil, including the Southeast, Midwest, and South.

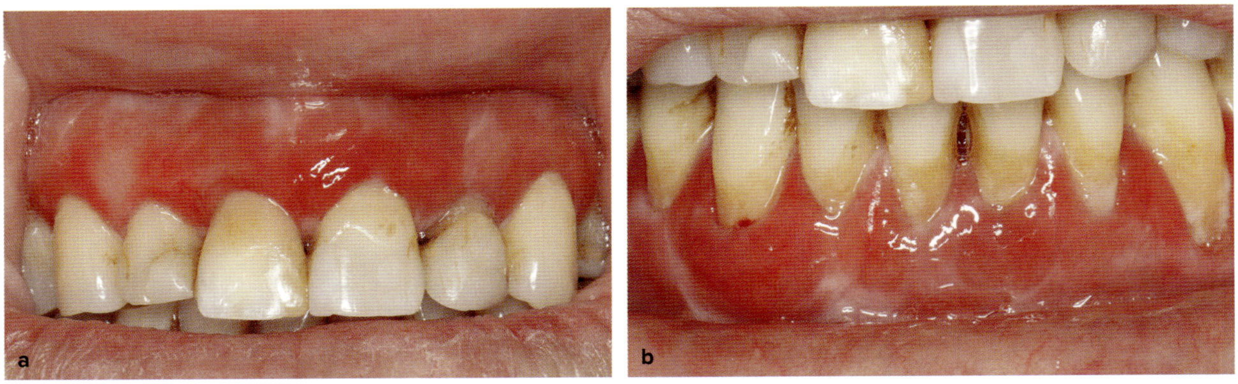

Fig 26-10 Desquamative gingivitis diagnosed as LP through a clinical and histopathologic examination. *(a)* Clinical appearance of maxilla. *(b)* Clinical appearance of mandible.

Autoimmune Diseases

An autoimmune disease is characterized by the recognition and attack of autoantigens by the immune system (cellular and/or humoral). This response can persist for an indeterminate time; therefore, most of these conditions are chronic, with periods of remission and exacerbation. Currently, autoimmune diseases are manageable but incurable. The therapy consists of modulating the immune response to reduce or control the clinical repercussion. Oral lesions of autoimmune diseases are usually symptomatic. The gingival involvement, termed **desquamative gingivitis**, is frequent and can be very similar between the different diseases: presence of erythema, desquamation, erosion, and blistering of attached and marginal gingiva. The main differential diagnosis is between mucocutaneous autoimmune disorders; however, chemical and electric burns and allergic reactions can produce similar clinical features. A biopsy should be performed to establish the final diagnosis. This procedure is very important because the different mucocutaneous autoimmune disorders can have very distinct outcomes.

LICHEN PLANUS

Lichen planus (LP) is an immune-mediated mucocutaneous condition that can affect the skin, nails, hair, and mucous membranes. Oral lesions are common and might represent the first or only manifestation of the disease. Oral LP lesions may persist for years with periods of remission and exacerbation. It is common for periods of exacerbation to be associated with episodes of emotional stress or low immunity. Based on the clinical characteristics and symptomatology, oral LP is classified as reticular or erosive. The same patient can also present with both forms of the disease. Reticular is the more prevalent type and is characterized by asymptomatic white lacy streaks called *Wickham striae*, surrounded by erythematous borders. The lesions are typically symmetric, bilateral, and predominantly found in the buccal mucosa and border of the tongue. In the erosive form, patients report symptomatology that can range from slight discomfort to severe pain. In this type of LP, areas of erosion or ulceration are present, showing radiating white striae. Some patients present with lesions restricted to the gingiva, termed *desquamative gingivitis* (Fig 26-10), which can be either symptomatic or asymptomatic.

The diagnosis should be confirmed through histopathologic study. The typical microscopic features include epithelial rete ridges with a pointed or "saw-toothed" shape, "liquefaction degeneration" of the epithelial basal cell layer, presence of degenerating keratinocytes (civatte bodies), and presence of a band-like zone of inflammatory infiltrate, mainly lymphocytes, confined to the superficial part of the connective tissue. The absence of epithelial dysplasia is also considered an important feature to confirm the microscopic diagnosis of LP (Fig 26-11).

Reticular LP usually does not require drug-based treatment once patients have no symptoms. In these situations, orientation and monitoring is sufficient. For erosive cases, corticosteroids are frequently recommended to control symptoms such as pain. The choice of drug and route of administration will depend on the intensity of symptoms and periodicity of the episodes. The potential for malignant transformation of LP is still controversial.

PEMPHIGUS VULGARIS

Pemphigus vulgaris (PV) is an autoimmune mucocutaneous disease characterized by the formation of intraepithelial blisters. Exclusive mucosal involvement is frequent, but the skin can also be affected concomitantly or exclusively. Mucosal lesions are characterized by flaccid blisters that break easily, resulting in erosions or painful ulcers distributed along the oral cavity. The **Nikolsky sign** is positive, which is stimulated by an oblique pressure to the mucosa and/or skin, resulting in new blisters or the easy desquamation of a superficial layer of the epithelium. PV oral lesions are often the first sign of the disease and are considered the most difficult to resolve with treatment. Exclusive gingival involvement (desquamative gingivitis) appears to be less frequent in PV compared to LP and mucous membrane pemphigoid (MMP). Direct immunofluorescence of perilesional tissue represents the most reliable and sensitive way to diagnose PV. The presence of immunoglobulin G (IgG) antibodies and occasionally components of the complement system (eg, component complement 3 or C3) are evident in the intercellular spaces between the epithelial cells, resulting in a "honeycomb" or "chicken wire" pattern. Prolonged treatment associated with immunosuppression is usually necessary and should be performed by an experienced immunosuppressive therapist.[10]

MUCOUS MEMBRANE PEMPHIGOID (CICATRICIAL PEMPHIGOID)

MMP is characterized by a subepithelial blistering formation that predominantly involves the oral and ocular mucosae and infrequently the skin. Mucosal lesions start as vesicles or blisters that rupture, leaving an area of superficial ulceration. Ulcerated lesions are usually painful and can persist for weeks or months if left untreated. In general, this process is diffusely observed in the mouth, but it may be limited to certain locations, especially the gingiva (desquamative gingivitis). The most significant complication of MMP, however, is ocular involvement. More severe cases can progress to eyelid and corneal damage and sometimes blindness. The diagnosis should be established through the association of clinical manifestations and direct immunofluorescence, revealing linear deposition of IgG, IgA, or C3 along the epithelial basement membrane zone. Follow-up by an ophthalmologist is imperative to prevent or treat ocular complications.

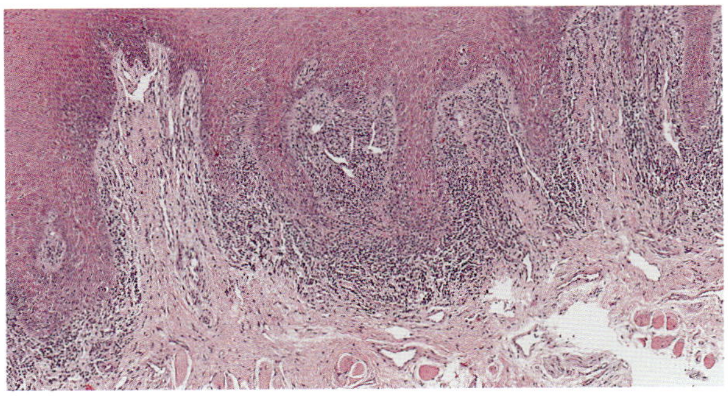

Fig 26-11 Microscopic features of oral LP. Note the inflammatory infiltrate composed mainly of lymphocytes in a band-like pattern and liquefaction degeneration of the epithelial basal cell layer.

Oral lesions can be managed with topical corticosteroids. If there is no adequate response, systemic corticosteroids or immunosuppressive agents may be used.[11]

SJÖGREN SYNDROME

Sjögren syndrome is a chronic systemic autoimmune condition involving the salivary and lacrimal glands, and it is frequently associated with a diffuse connective tissue disease (collagenosis). The lymphocytic infiltrate destroys the glandular parenchyma, causing ocular dryness (xerophthalmia or keratoconjunctivitis sicca) and buccal dryness (xerostomia). The syndrome mainly affects women (male:female ratio of 1:9) between 40 and 60 years of age. Clinicians should be alert to clinical signs such as dry and shiny mucosa and foaming residual saliva, which might result in the mucosa becoming adhered to the mirror or presence of sedimented remains of food. Other signs include depapillated tongue and swelling of salivary glands. The low salivary flow might also result in dental caries, worsening periodontal disease, candidiasis, bacterial sialadenitis, or sialolithiasis. Regular monitoring is important to prevent these complications. Treatment should focus on the relief of symptoms through constant hydration, stimulation of saliva with sugar-free chewing gum or drugs, and artificial saliva. Patients should avoid drugs that can worsen xerostomia and should avoid smoking and drinking alcoholic beverages. Also, patients should follow up with a rheumatologist once other autoimmune connective tissue diseases present or develop.

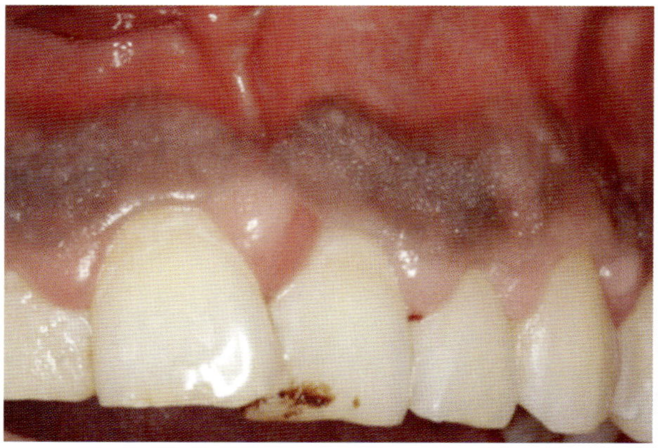

Fig 26-12 Physiologic pigmentation of the attached gingiva.

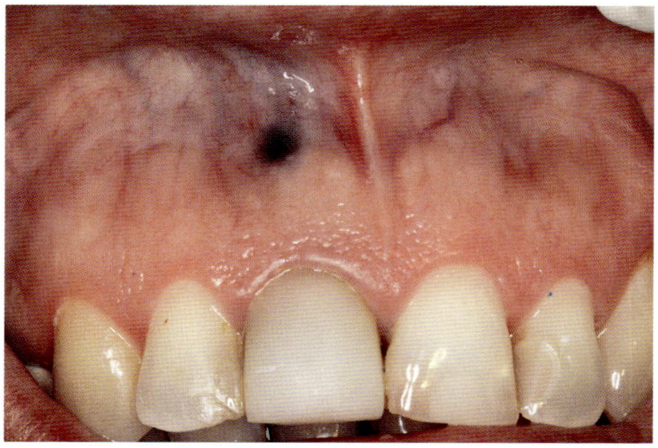

Fig 26-13 Clinical features of amalgam tattoo. The patient had a history of endodontic retrofill procedures at the maxillary right central incisor.

Pigmented Disorders

PHYSIOLOGIC PIGMENTATION

Physiologic pigmentation does not represent a true pathology; instead, it is a variation of normality related to race. This condition is very common in patients with dark skin (ie, populations of African, Asian, or Mediterranean origin). The marginal gingiva is the most affected intraoral site, characterized by bilateral well-demarcated brown pigmentation with a band appearance that generally spares the attached gingiva (Fig 26-12). No treatment is necessary.

SMOKER'S MELANOSIS

Smoking causes pigmentation in light-skinned patients and accentuates brown pigmentation in dark-skinned patients. Smoker's melanosis is observed in approximately 20% of smokers. The intensity of pigmentation is related to the duration and number of cigarettes consumed. The lesions usually involve the anterior facial gingiva. The diagnosis is based on clinical features and history. No treatment is necessary, and the pigmentation usually disappears within 3 years of smoking cessation.

AMALGAM TATTOO

Implantation of dental amalgam in the oral mucosa represents the main cause of exogenous pigmentation and is known as *amalgam tattoo*. The gingiva is the most affected site (Fig 26-13). The presence of amalgam restorations or endodontic retrofill procedures near the pigmented area should be investigated if an amalgam tattoo is suspected. In some cases, especially when the amalgam particles are sufficiently large, radiopaque granules can be observed on intraoral radiography. In these cases, the final diagnosis can be established based on clinical and radiographic findings. If in doubt, a biopsy may be performed, and microscopic evaluation will permit the identification of amalgam particles in the connective tissue.

MELANOTIC MACULE AND NEVUS

Melanotic macule and nevus represent two forms of localized pigmentation. From a clinical perspective, both lesions are very similar, characterized by a brown macule, usually small and well demarcated. The main differences between theses lesions are summarized in Table 26-3. For both conditions, the clinician may choose between monitoring or surgical removal. If changes in size, color, texture, surface, and/or borders are identified, a biopsy should be performed and the tissue examined microscopically to exclude oral melanoma (Fig 26-14).

MELANOMA

Oral mucosa melanoma is extremely rare, accounting for less than 1% of all oral malignancies. The most common location is the palate followed by the gingiva. Clinically, early lesions are usually characterized as a brown to

TABLE 26-3 Main features of melanotic macule and nevus

	Melanotic macule	Nevus
Nature	Reactive	Neoplastic (benign)
Most affected site	Lower lip	Palate or gingiva
Distinct clinical features	Usually flat surface	Surface can be elevated
Microscopic features	Increased melanin deposition in the basal and parabasal layers. Melanin also seen free or within melanophages in the connective tissue.	Unencapsulated yet well-demarcated proliferation of nevus cells that demonstrate variable capacity to produce melanin. Cells tend to be organized in small aggregates known as *theques*. Lesions are classified as junctional, compound, and intramucosal.
Peculiarities	Systemic and genetic conditions can cause lesions clinically and microscopically similar to the melanotic macule.	Melanocytic nevus has other clinical-pathologic variants such as congenital nevus, halo nevus, spitz nevus, and blue nevus.

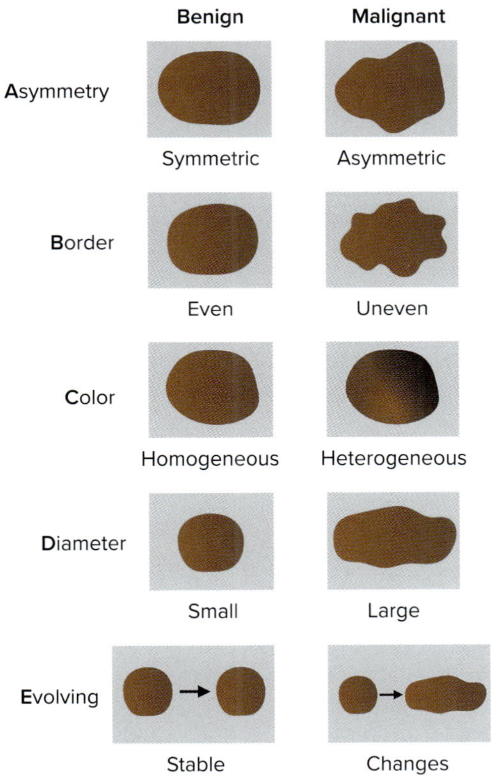

Fig 26-14 ABCDE system used to differentiate benign and malignant pigmented lesions.

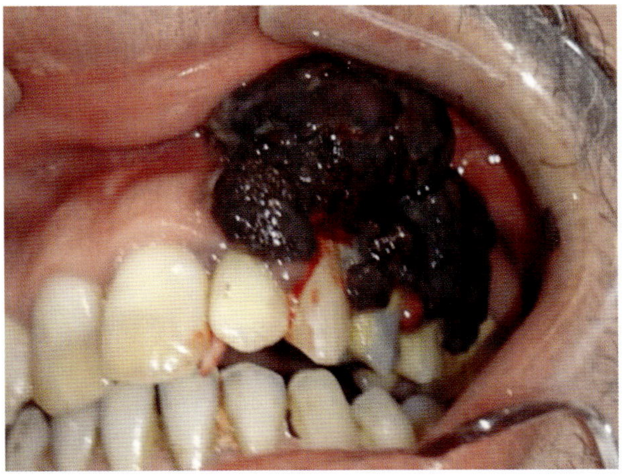

Fig 26-15 Advanced mucosal melanoma.

black macula with irregular borders. Melanomas tend to exhibit an initial radial growth phase followed by a vertical growth phase. Thus, advanced lesions usually evolve to exophytic nodular masses that may or may not be ulcerated (Fig 26-15). When there is bone involvement, the radiographic pattern is described as "moth-eaten" destruction. A useful method to identify if the lesion has malignant characteristics is to follow the ABCDE system initially developed for skin cancer (see Fig 26-14). All oral macules that demonstrate at least some aggressive features should be submitted for microscopic examination. If the diagnosis of melanoma is confirmed, the patient should be referred to a head and neck surgeon or oncologist for treatment.

TABLE 26-4 Examples of oral lesions characterized by white plaque or macule to be excluded for a diagnosis of leukoplakia

Lesion	Etiology	Clinical features
Frictional keratosis	Reactive, caused by a chronic irritative agent	White asymptomatic homogeneous macule or plaque. Commonly seen in the alveolar ridges.
Morsicatio	Reactive, caused by chronic habit of biting the mucosa	White plaques of irregular surface, possibly but not necessarily associated with areas of erythema. Usually occurs in the occlusion line (buccal mucosa).
Burn	Reactive, caused by thermal or chemical injury	White plaques or macules removable by scraping.
Leukoedema	Unknown cause (more common in dark-skinned individuals)	Milky-white alteration affecting the buccal mucosa bilaterally that disappears when stretched.
Nicotine stomatitis	Reactive, caused by tobacco smoking (no potentially malignant nature)	White to grayish palatal mucosa with slightly elevated reddish papules.
Pseudomembranous candidiasis	Infectious, caused by the fungus *C albicans*	"Milk curd" or "cottage cheese" appearance; can be scraped off, leaving a red base.
White sponge nevus	Genetically determined skin disorder	Bilateral and symmetric thick plaques, with corrugated or velvety surface in the buccal mucosa (present since birth, childhood, or adolescence).
Hairy leukoplakia	Infectious, caused by Epstein-Barr virus (EBV) in immunosuppressed patients (usually HIV)	Plaques with rough surface and vertical fissures in the lateral border of tongue.
Lichen planus	Autoimmune condition	Bilateral presentation and Wickham striae are usually present.

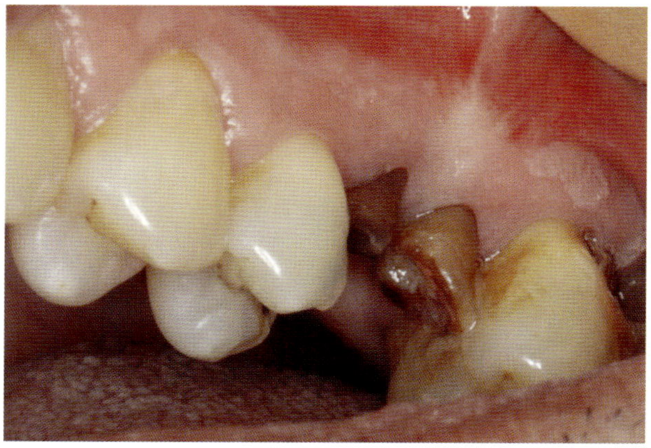

Fig 26-16 Leukoplakia in the attached gingiva.

Potentially Malignant Disorders

LEUKOPLAKIA

Leukoplakia is a clinical term used to designate a predominantly white plaque or macule that cannot be characterized clinically or pathologically as any other disease. The World Health Organization (WHO) currently defines leukoplakia as "a white plaque of questionable risk having excluded (other) known diseases or disorders that carry no increased risk for cancer."[12]

Leukoplakia is the most common potentially malignant disorder. The main risk factors are tobacco and alcohol use. Clinically, lesions can be classified into homogeneous and nonhomogeneous based on color and texture. Nonhomogeneous lesions tend to present more aggressive microscopic characteristics and clinical behavior. These lesions are also more common in the lateral border of the tongue and floor of the mouth, and less frequently at the gingiva. The diagnosis of leukoplakia depends on the exclusion of other entities that appear as white oral plaques (Table 26-4). If all other possibilities are excluded, the provisional clinical diagnosis of leukoplakia is established (Fig 26-16).

TABLE 26-5 Main clinical and microscopic features of benign and malignant neoplasms

	Benign neoplasms	Malignant neoplasms
Clinical features		
Growth rate	Low	High
Type of growth	Expansive	Infiltrative
Lesion borders	Well defined	Poorly defined
Local and systemic effects	Inexpressive	Usually severe
Recurrences	Usually absent	Might occur
Metastasis	Absent	Might occur
Capsule	Usually present	Usually absent
Microscopic features		
Degree of cell differentiation	Well differentiated	Poorly differentiated
Cellular and architectural atypia	Rare	Frequent
Mitotic figures	Rare	Frequent
Necrosis and degeneration	Absent	Present

In these cases, an incisional biopsy is mandatory. The diagnosis of leukoplakia is confirmed when there are no microscopic characteristics of another known lesion. The histopathologic diagnosis can vary from hyperkeratosis to epithelial dysplasia (characterized by cellular and architectural atypia). The presence of dysplasia represents the most important risk factor for malignant transformation.

Patients should be informed regarding the potentially malignant nature of the disease and the importance of cessation of tobacco and alcohol use. Periodic follow-ups must also be completed. The treatment of the lesion can be surgical or nonsurgical and can only be performed after a previous biopsy has established the final diagnosis. Surgical treatment is more common and includes the use of laser, cryotherapy, and conventional surgery. Nonsurgical treatment comprises the use of pharmacologic agents (topical or systemic), also known as *chemoprevention*. Recurrence of the lesion is more commonly observed after nonsurgical approaches.

The annual malignant transformation rate is approximately 2%.[13] In addition to the presence of dysplasia, other known risk factors for malignant transformation include the following:

- Presence of multiple lesions
- Lesions located in the tongue or floor of the mouth
- Lesions larger than 2 cm at the largest diameter
- Nonhomogeneous lesions

LICHEN PLANUS

The malignant transformation potential of oral LP remains highly controversial in the literature. Currently, the WHO recognizes LP as a potentially malignant disorder.[12] A systematic review published in 2017 evaluated the rate of malignant transformation in 57 studies accounting for a total of nearly 20,000 LP patients. The average malignant transformation rate was 1.1%. There was a greater risk of malignant transformation in smokers, alcoholics, and patients with hepatitis C, demonstrating that cofactors may contribute to the risk of malignant transformation.[14]

Neoplasms

Neoplasms can be classified as benign or malignant (Table 26-5). The final diagnosis of neoplasms can only be achieved after microscopic analysis. Thus, a biopsy is mandatory in these situations. This complementary

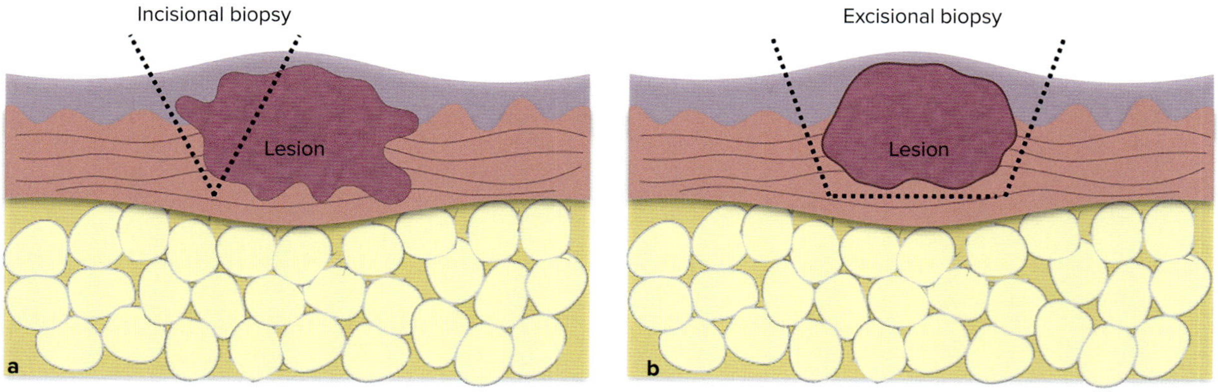

Fig 26-17 Schematic illustration of incisional *(a)* and excisional *(b)* biopsies.

TABLE 26-6 Indications for incisional and excisional biopsies

	Incisional biopsy (removal of part of the lesion)	Excisional biopsy (removal of the entire lesion*)
Type of lesion	Multiple or poorly circumscribed lesions	Solitary and well circumscribed lesions
Size	Extensive lesions	Small lesions
Nature of lesion	Hypothesis of a malignant nature	Hypothesis of a reactive† or benign nature

*This examination aims to obtain a final diagnosis, but in many situations, the lesion is treated concomitantly by surgical removal.
†For reactive lesions, it is essential to eliminate the irritative factor.

examination is always indicated when the clinical features are not sufficient to achieve a final diagnosis. In addition, cases in which the clinical course is not consistent with the initial diagnosis should also be biopsied. This examination can be classified as incisional or excisional based on the amount of lesional tissue removed (Fig 26-17 and Table 26-6). For incisional biopsies, the selection of the area is also important and should involve healthy tissue at the lesion margin, allowing the analyses of lesional tissues and its relation to adjacent normal tissues. Central areas of necrosis (in ulcerated cases) must be avoided.

BENIGN NEOPLASMS

Benign neoplasms are very frequent in the oral mucosa. Oral papilloma represents one of the main benign neoplasms in this region. Oral fibroma is another frequent type of benign neoplasm; however, some lesions appear to have a reactive etiology rather than a true neoplastic origin. Oral fibroma and other common types of oral benign neoplasms are described in Table 26-7.

MALIGNANT NEOPLASMS

Squamous cell carcinoma

Nearly 95% of all oral malignant tumors are SCCs. The main risk factors for oral SCC are smoking and alcohol. Tobacco is a complete carcinogen and acts as a cancer initiator and promoter. The synergistic effect of both habits, however, represents the most alarming risk factor. Genetic predisposition plays an important role, especially in patients not exposed to the usual risk factors. The most frequent locations are tongue (border) and floor of the mouth. The most commonly observed clinical presentation is an ulcer with elevated and hard edges. The lesion exhibits rapid growth (Fig 26-18) and in more advanced stages can cause pain, tooth mobility, difficulty swallowing (dysphagia), and speech problems. Nodal metastasis can be present at diagnosis and usually occurs in ipsilateral lymph nodes in the chin that drain the region of the primary tumor (Table 26-8).

Microscopically, oral SCC is characterized by the invasion of the epithelial lining into the underlying connective tissue

TABLE 26-7 Examples of benign neoplasms that can occur in the oral cavity

Neoplasm	Cell of origin	Most common oral site	Other notes
Fibroma	Fibroblasts	Buccal and labial mucosa	Might represent a reactive hyperplasic lesion in some cases.
Lipoma	Adipocytes	Buccal mucosa and vestibule	The most common benign neoplasm in the body. The lesion floats in liquids due to its fat content.
Neurilemoma (schwannoma)	Schwann cells	Tongue	In rare occasions, the tumor can arise centrally within bone (intraosseous).
Neurofibroma	Schwann cells and perineural fibroblasts	Tongue and buccal mucosa	Can arise as solitary tumors or be a component of neurofibromatosis.
Hemangioma	Vascular endothelial cells	–	Lesion of infancy characterized by a rapid growth phase followed by gradual involution.
Lymphangioma	Lymphatic endothelial cells	Tongue	Most likely represents a developmental malformation rather than neoplastic.

–, not applicable.

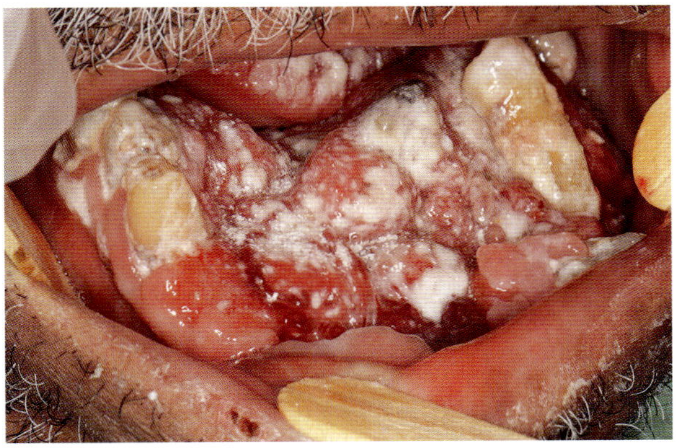

Fig 26-18 Advanced case of oral squamous cell carcinoma at the floor of the mouth and gingiva, leading to mandibular bone destruction.

TABLE 26-8 Differences between reactive and metastatic lymph nodes

	Reactive lymph nodes	Neoplastic/metastatic lymph nodes
Pain	Yes	No
Mobility	Yes	No
Texture	Smooth and fibroelastic texture	Firm and rough texture

(Fig 26-19). Neoplastic cells demonstrate atypia and loss of differentiation. Histologic subtypes of oral SCC recognized by the WHO include basaloid, spindle cell, adenosquamous, cuniculatum, verrucous, lymphoepithelial, papillary, and acantholytic. Carcinoma cuniculatum represents a well-differentiated type that usually occurs on the mucoperiosteum. This variant is locally destructive and recurs with high frequency, but it rarely if ever metastasizes.[12]

After diagnosis, patients should be referred to a head and neck surgeon for treatment. Surgical resection with safety margins remains the main treatment line for oral SCC. In a large number of patients, neck dissection and/or adjuvant radiotherapy are indicated. When chemotherapy is used, platinum-based regimens are the most commonly applied. Currently, according to the National Cancer Institute, there are seven drugs approved by the

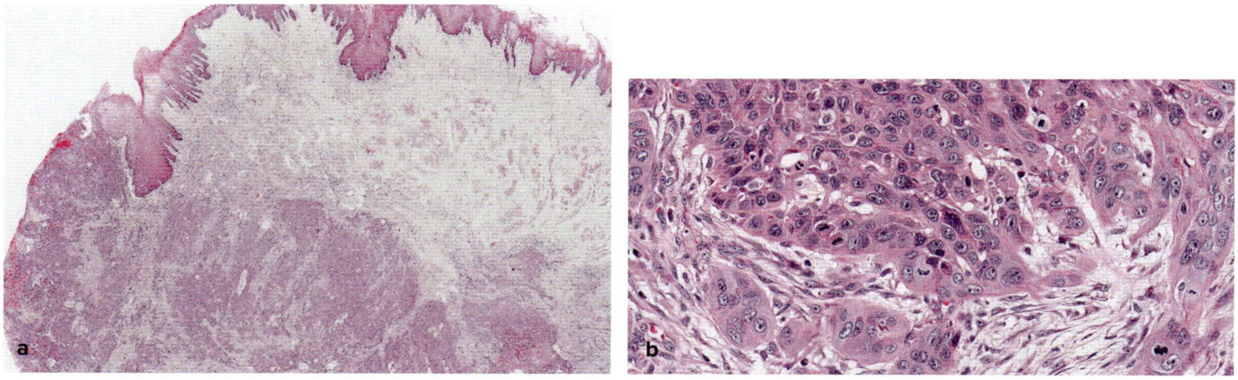

Fig 26-19 Microscopic features of oral SCC. *(a)* Malignant epithelial cells invading the connective tissue. *(b)* Epithelial pleomorphic malignant cells. Mitotic figures can also be observed.

U.S. Food and Drug Administration (FDA) to treat head and neck cancer:

1. Bleomycin
2. Cetuximab
3. Docetaxel
4. Hydroxyurea
5. Methotrexate
6. Nivolumab
7. Pembrolizumab

The prognosis of oral SCC is considered poor, especially for patients diagnosed at late stages. The 5-year overall survival is around 50%, and this rate has not been increasing significantly over the years.

TNM staging

The American Joint Committee on Cancer (AJCC) cancer staging is based on the evaluation of three categories at the time of diagnosis:

1. Tumor (T): Analyzes the size and extent of the primary tumor
2. Lymph node (N): Analyzes the degree regional lymph nodes spread
3. Metastasis (M): Analyzes the presence of metastasis

In 2016, the AJCC released the 8th edition of the Cancer Staging Manual, introducing substantial modifications from the previous edition. The most significant update was a separate staging system for high-risk HPV-associated cancer of the oropharynx (HR-OC), discriminating it from oropharyngeal cancer with other causes. The AJCC along with the American College of Pathology states that high-risk HPV testing is recommended for all new oropharyngeal SCC patients through p16 immunohistochemistry (IHC). For oral cavity cancer, the most important modifications were in the tumor (T) and lymph node (N) categories. The T category now incorporates the depth of invasion (DOI), thereby discerning tumors that are small but invasive. To determine the N pathologic category, it is now necessary to evaluate if there is extranodal extension (ENE) in metastatic lymph nodes. These changes were made to significantly increase the power of the TNM staging in predicting patients' prognoses and therefore have a major clinical relevance.[15]

Osteosarcoma

An *osteosarcoma* is a malignant bone tumor characterized by the production of bone or osteoid by neoplastic cells. Genetic predisposition, Paget disease, and previous irradiation at the site have been pointed out as risk factors. In 90% of cases, the osteosarcoma is located in the metaphysis of the long bones. Osteosarcomas of the jawbones are very rare. Radiographic aspects of osteosarcomas may vary from a fully radiolucent image with irregular ill-defined borders (Fig 26-20) to predominantly radiopaque areas, due to the to greater deposition of osteoid matrix within the lesion. Some peculiar but nonpathognomonic

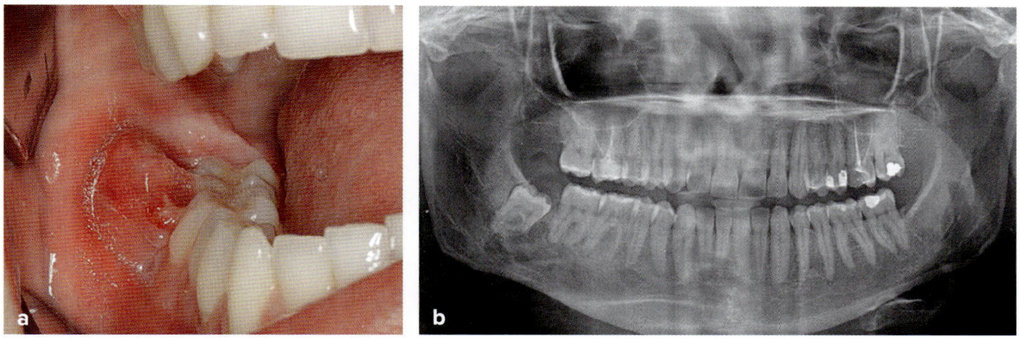

Fig 26-20 Clinical *(a)* and radiographic *(b)* features of a mandibular osteosarcoma with gingival involvement.

radiographic findings include a symmetric thickening of the periodontal space due to neoplastic infiltration and the presence of a periosteal reaction characterized by osteophytic bone production on the surface of the lesion, a pattern classically described as "sunburst" or "sunray," which is more evident in occlusal radiographs. The clinical manifestation varies from a slight swelling to destruction of the cortical bones, dental mobility, mucosal ulceration, pain, and paresthesia. Osteosarcomas of the gnathic bones are usually treated through radical surgery followed by radiotherapy.

Lymphomas

Oral cavity lymphomas are quite rare. Approximately 2% of extranodal lymphomas arise in the oral cavity. These lesions most often involve the palate or gingiva and can invade subjacent bone. Diffuse large B-cell lymphoma is the most common type. Plasmablastic lymphoma represents a rare non-Hodgkin lymphoma with plasma cell immunophenotype; however, this tumor has a predilection for extranodal sites, with the oral cavity as the most affected site (Fig 26-21). Epstein-Barr virus (EBV) infection appears to play an important role in the pathogenesis of this tumor, and most patients are HIV positive.

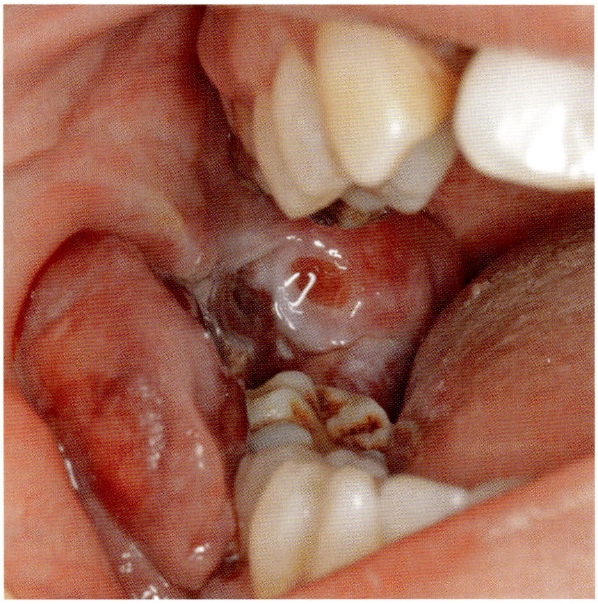

Fig 26-21 Plasmablastic lymphoma arising in the gingiva.

Leukemic gingival infiltration

Leukemias are malignant tumors of the body's blood-forming tissues and are classified according to their clinical behavior (acute/chronic) and histogenesis (lymphocytic/lymphoblastic). Systemic signs and symptoms include fatigue, easy tiring, dyspnea, fever, and easy bruising or bleeding. These symptoms occur due to a striking decrease in normal white and red blood cells counts as well as thrombocytopenia. Due to the compromised ability of patients to combat the normal microbial flora, gingival ulcerations with a grayish-white necrotic base can also occur. Frequently, in the myelomonocytic types of leukemia, malignant cells infiltrate the oral mucosa tissues, resulting in diffuse gingival enlargement. In the gingiva, this event produces firm and reddish generalized gingival overgrowth that bleeds easily. Association with other systemic symptoms might lead the differential diagnosis to a leukemic gingival infiltration.

Oral metastasis

The oral cavity is an uncommon site for spread of metastatic tumors. When it occurs, the most common malignant tumor primary sites are the lung and prostate for men and breast and genital organs for women. Clinicians

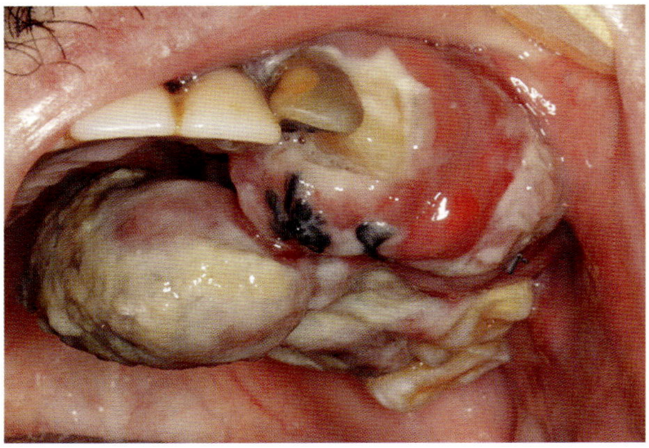

Fig 26-22 Oral metastasis of kidney cancer. The primary tumor was discovered after the oral lesion was biopsied.

should be alert that, though it is rare, when this event occurs, the gingiva and jawbones are the most affected sites, particularly the mandible. The clinical presentation varies but is usually highly suggestive of an aggressive and destructive lesion. In the jawbones, the most common symptoms are rapidly progressing swelling, pain, and paresthesia. In the gingival region, early lesions can mimic hyperplastic or reactive lesions and in more advanced cases present extensive tumor growths and/or ulcers (Fig 26-22). The overall survival rate of patients after diagnosis of an oral metastasis is extremely poor; life expectancy is around 7 months.

Odontogenic Cysts and Tumors

Odontogenic lesions are thought to originate from remnants of odontogenesis, including the following:

- Epithelial cell rests of Malassez: Remnants of the disintegration of the Hertwig epithelial root sheath
- Reduced enamel organ epithelium: Remnants of the enamel organ collapse after complete formation of the crown of the tooth
- Rests of Serres: Remnants of the dental lamina after disintegration
- Ectomesenchymal remnants of dental papilla or dental follicle

Odontogenic tumors may also originate from the epithelial lining of odontogenic **cysts**, which have origins in the same epithelial remnants previously mentioned.[16] The 2017 WHO classification of odontogenic lesions is presented in Box 26-3.[12]

ODONTOGENIC TUMORS

Ameloblastic carcinoma

This is the malignant counterpart of ameloblastoma and, though it is rare, is the most common type of malignant odontogenic tumor. The tumor can arise de novo or in preexisting ameloblastomas. The posterior part of the jaw is the most affected site, and lesions are characterized by poorly defined or irregularly marginated radiolucencies that might cause cortical expansion or perforation and infiltration into adjacent structures. The final diagnosis relies on the identification of a histologic pattern of ameloblastoma associated with cytologic features of malignancy. Radical surgical excision is the primary treatment, and the prognosis is reserved.

Ameloblastoma

Ameloblastomas are common and potentially aggressive odontogenic tumors. Recurrent gene mutations associated with the mitogen-activated protein kinase (MAPK) signaling pathway have been identified in nearly 90% of ameloblastomas, suggesting an important role of this pathway in the pathogenesis of the tumor. Mutations in the *BRAF* gene have been found in approximately 60% of cases, and *RAS* mutations have also been detected less frequently. Besides the MAPK pathway, mutations in the *SMO* gene from the hedgehog pathway have also been identified.[12]

The tumor occurs in a wide age range with a peak of incidence in younger patients and does not show a predilection for sex or skin color. The posterior region of the mandible is usually affected. Included teeth may or may not be associated with injury. Radiographically, a corticated multilocular so-called soap-bubble or honeycomb radiolucency represents the most common presentation (Fig 26-23). An incisional biopsy should be taken to establish the diagnosis prior to treatment. The microscopic evaluation reveals sheets and islands of epithelial cells in a fibrous mature stroma. The peripheral cells resemble preameloblasts, while the cells at the central core resemble the stellate reticulum (Fig 26-24). According to the microscopic appearance, tumors can be classified as follicular, plexiform, acanthomatous, granular, and basaloid. This classification has no impact on the patient's prognosis.

The treatment consists of wide surgical excision, including an area of apparently normal bone beyond

BOX 26-3 WHO classification of odontogenic and maxillofacial bone tumors[12]

Odontogenic carcinomas
- Ameloblastic carcinoma
- Primary intraosseous carcinoma
- Sclerosing odontogenic carcinoma
- Clear cell odontogenic carcinoma
- Ghost cell odontogenic carcinoma

Odontogenic carcinosarcoma

Odontogenic sarcoma

Benign epithelial odontogenic tumors
- Ameloblastomas
  - Ameloblastoma, unicystic type
  - Ameloblastoma, extraosseous/peripheral type
  - Metastasizing (malignant) ameloblastoma
- Squamous odontogenic tumor
- Calcifying epithelial odontogenic tumor
- Adenomatoid odontogenic tumor

Benign mixed epithelial and mesenchymal odontogenic tumors
- Ameloblastic fibroma
- Primordial odontogenic tumor
- Odontomas
  - Odontoma, compound type
  - Odontoma, complex type
- Dentinogenic ghost cell tumor

Benign mesenchymal odontogenic tumors
- Odontogenic fibroma
- Odontogenic myxoma/myxofibroma
- Cementoblastoma
- Cementoossifying fibroma

Odontogenic cysts of inflammatory origin
- Radicular cyst
- Inflammatory collateral cyst

Odontogenic and nonodontogenic developmental cysts
- Dentigerous cyst
- Odontogenic keratocyst
- Lateral periodontal and botryoid odontogenic cyst
- Gingival cyst
- Glandular odontogenic cyst
- Calcifying odontogenic cyst
- Orthokeratinized odontogenic cyst
- Nasopalatine cyst

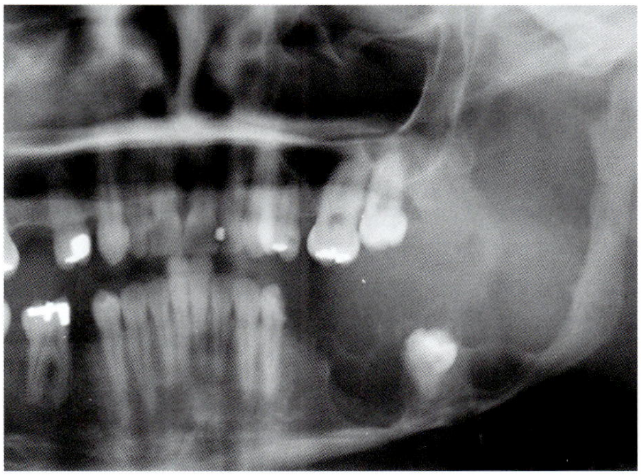

Fig 26-23 Radiographic aspect of ameloblastoma.

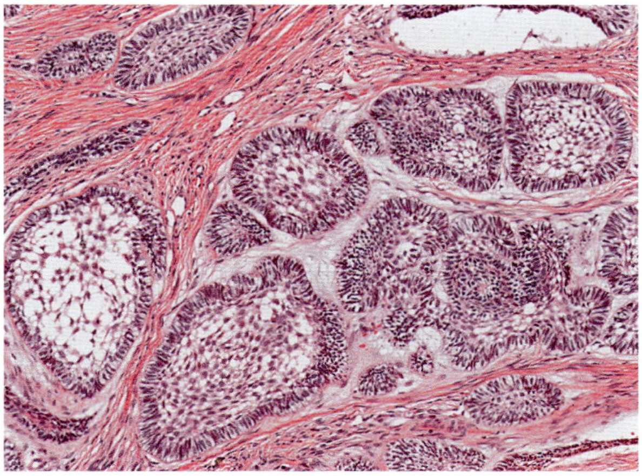

Fig 26-24 Microscopic features of ameloblastoma. Observe odontogenic epithelial islands with peripheral columnar to cuboidal cells with hyperchromatic nuclei arranged in a palisading pattern with reverse polarity. The central cells are angular and loosely arranged. The stroma is composed of mature connective tissue. This example represents a follicular microscopic variant.

radiographic margins. Recurrence rates increase significantly when conservative approaches are attempted. Lifelong follow-up should be considered because late recurrences might occur.

Unicystic ameloblastoma

Unicystic ameloblastoma (UAM) represents a variant of ameloblastoma that occurs as a single cystic cavity. Therefore, the radiographic image consists of a well-defined

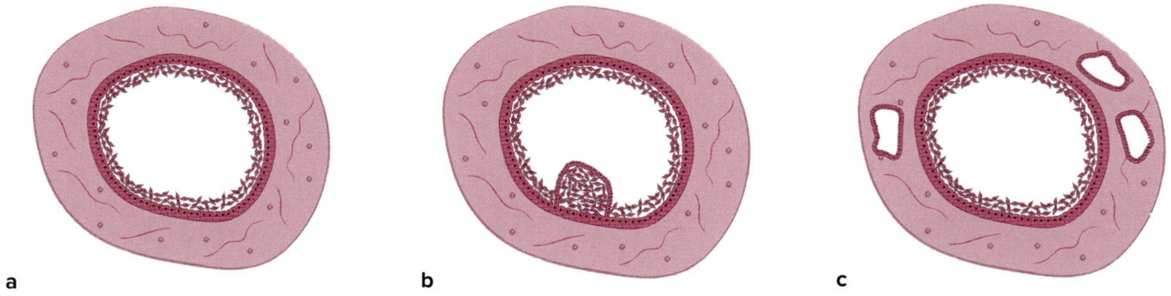

Fig 26-25 Histopathologic variants of unicystic ameloblastoma: *(a)* luminal, *(b)* intraluminal, and *(c)* mural.

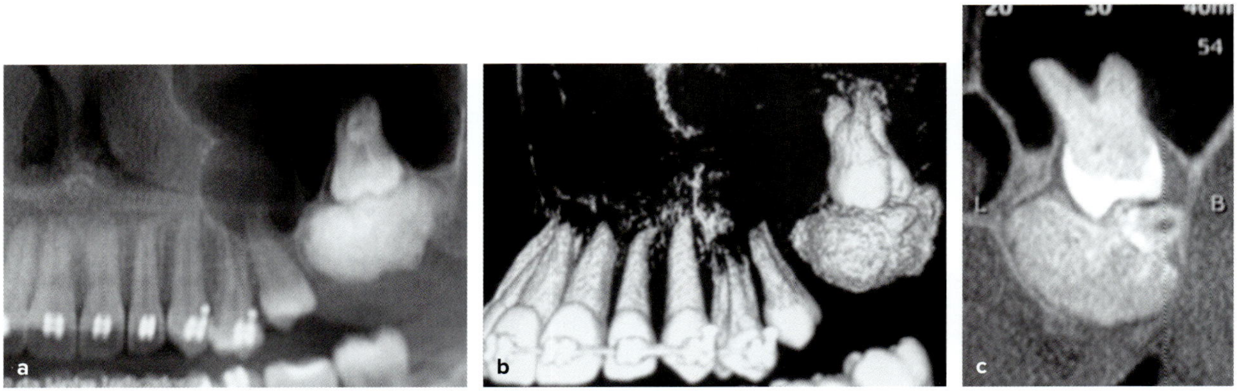

Fig 26-26 A complex odontoma occurring adjacent to the crown of the maxillary left first molar. *(a)* Radiograph. *(b)* CBCT scan. *(c)* CT scan.

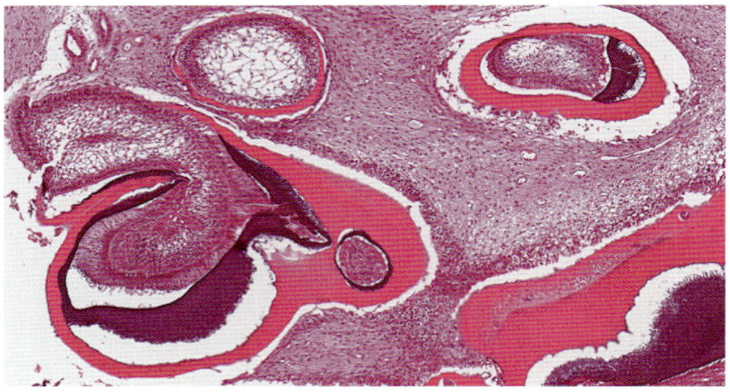

Fig 26-27 Microscopic features of a complex odontoma showing disorganized dental soft and hard tissues.

unilocular radiolucency, mimicking a cyst. A conclusive diagnosis of UAM can be made only after careful examination of the entire specimen. Unlike conventional ameloblastoma, the microscopic subtype of UAM has an impact on prognosis. Lesions are classified as luminal, intraluminal, and mural (Fig 26-25). Mural involvement denotes a more aggressive behavior (similar to conventional ameloblastoma). This variant requires either additional surgery or a closer follow-up.

Odontoma

Odontomas are the most common odontogenic tumors. It is believed that they represent tumor-like malformations (hamartomas) rather than a true neoplasia. They are classified into compound and complex. Both are mainly diagnosed in young patients. Compound odontomas occur mainly in the anterior maxilla, while complex odontomas are found more often in the posterior mandible. Radiographically, compound odontomas appear as numerous tooth-like structures, and complex odontomas are characterized by a disorganized mass of radiopaque calcified tissue (Fig 26-26). Early-stage odontomas might demonstrate a well-defined radiolucent lesion with radiopaque foci. The treatment consists of conservative surgery, and the prognosis is excellent. The histopathologic examination reveals dental soft and hard tissues (pulp, dentin, cementum, and enamel matrix) that can be disorganized (complex odontoma; Fig 26-27) or form rudimentary teeth (compound odontoma). Early-stage odontomas show variable amounts of odontogenic epithelium and mesenchyme with little mineralized product.

TABLE 26-9 Main features of other benign odontogenic tumors

Tumor	Radiographic image	Most common site	Other notes
Adenomatoid odontogenic tumor	Well-defined unilocular radiolucent lesion. About two-thirds present small foci of radiopacity.	Anterior maxilla	Commonly associated with impacted canines
Calcifying epithelial odontogenic tumor	Well-defined uni- or multilocular radiolucent lesion. Two-thirds are mixed radiolucent and radiopaque.	Posterior mandible	Also known as *Pindborg tumor*
Ameloblastic fibroma	Well-defined uni- or multilocular radiolucent lesion.	Posterior mandible	Occurs in young patients
Odontogenic fibroma	Well-defined uni- or multilocular radiolucent lesion with cortical margins.	Maxilla and mandible	Peripheral odontogenic fibroma is more common than the central

Other benign odontogenic tumors

Table 26-9 summarizes the main features of other benign odontogenic tumors.

ODONTOGENIC AND NONODONTOGENIC CYSTS

Periapical cyst and other apical inflammatory lesions

Apical inflammatory lesions occur as a consequence of bacteria or their toxic products in the root canal of a nonvital tooth. Acute lesions, such as acute apical periodontitis and dentoalveolar abscess, are usually symptomatic and associated with sensitivity to percussion, extrusion of the tooth, and tissue swelling. Radiographically, a thickening of the apical periodontal ligament or an ill-defined radiolucency might be observed.

Chronic lesions such as apical granuloma and radicular cyst represent the most prevalent lesions associated with pulp necrosis. Both lesions are usually asymptomatic, and the majority are discovered on routine radiographic examinations, which demonstrates a radiolucency of variable size at the apex. An overlap of clinical and radiographic features can occur between these lesions; however, a radicular cyst can reach large dimensions and cause cortical expansion or even rupture (Fig 26-28). Tooth mobility and root resorption can also occur. The treatment of both conditions consists of eliminating the etiologic factor, which can be attempted by conventional endodontic treatment. The apex region needs to be reevaluated after a few months to ensure that bone repair is occurring. If the treatment is unsuccessful, endodontic retreatment can be performed. Periapical surgery is usually indicated when the two attempts failed or for larger lesions. The tissue removed from the periapical site must be submitted for histopathologic examination. Other cysts and neoplasms can simulate an apical lesion, which could also justify the failure of previous treatments. Histologically, apical granuloma is characterized by chronic inflammatory infiltrate surrounded by a fibrous connective tissue. Radicular cysts are lined by nonkeratinized stratified squamous epithelium with a variable degree of inflammation in the capsule.

Oral fistula

An oral fistula is a suppurative channel that allows for draining of accumulated suppuration to the exterior. The presence of oral fistula indicates an active inflammatory process; however, pain is usually absent (as long as the fistula is open). It is important to establish the origin of the fistula, which can be performed by introducing a radiopaque and malleable instrument (eg, gutta-percha) in the fistula channel through its orifice followed by a radiographic examination.

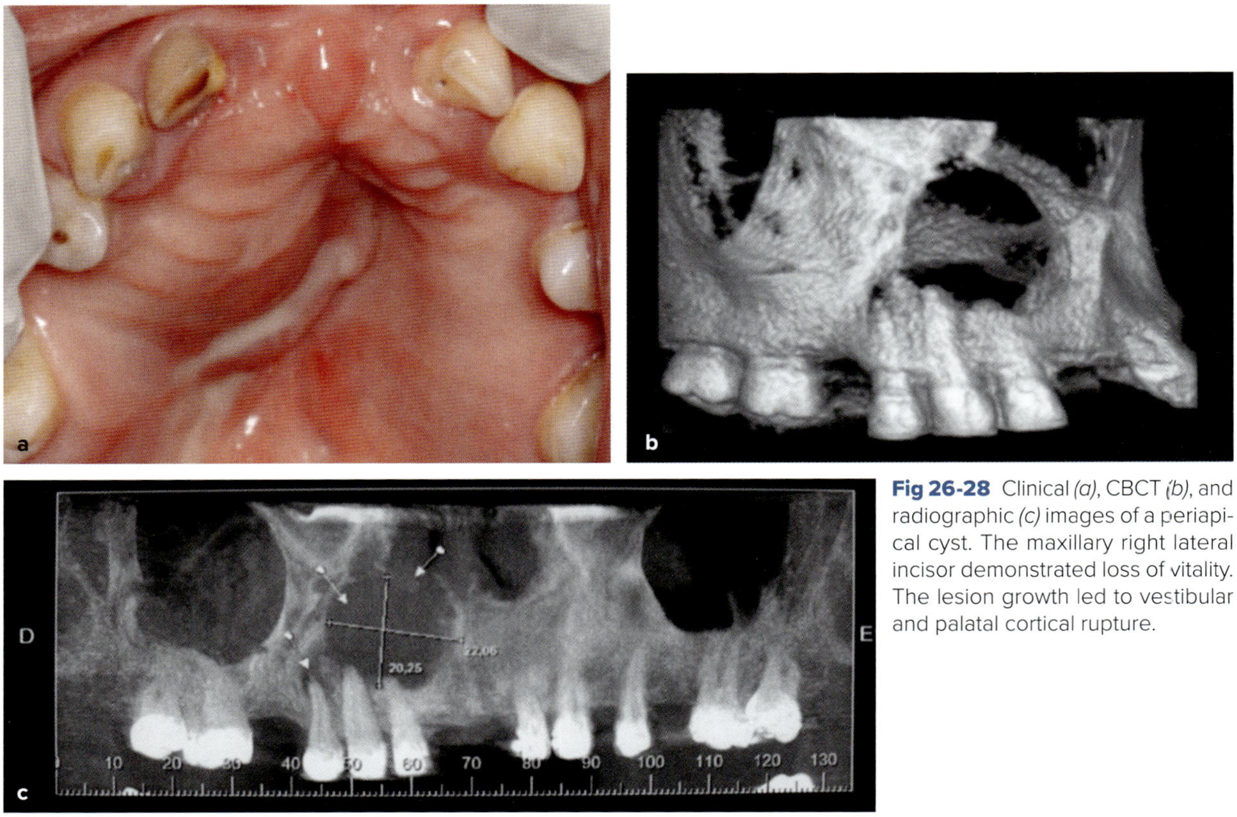

Fig 26-28 Clinical *(a)*, CBCT *(b)*, and radiographic *(c)* images of a periapical cyst. The maxillary right lateral incisor demonstrated loss of vitality. The lesion growth led to vestibular and palatal cortical rupture.

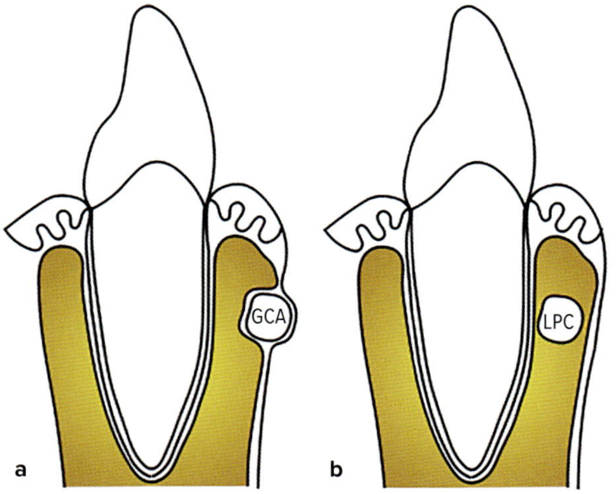

Fig 26-29 Differences in location between *(a)* GCA, which occurs in the soft tissue, and *(b)* LPC, which is an intraosseous lesion.

Gingival cyst of adult and periodontal lateral cyst

Gingival cyst of the adult (GCA) and lateral periodontal cyst (LPC) are very rare developmental cysts thought to arise from rests of the dental lamina. The microscopic appearance of both cysts is similar, with the location as the most important piece of information to distinguish these lesions. The GCA arises in soft tissues, while an LPC is an intraosseous lesion (Fig 26-29). This difference results in important clinical and radiographic divergences described in Table 26-10. Enucleation is curative for both lesions, with a low recurrence rate. The botryoid variant of LPC has a greater risk of recurrence.

Dentigerous and eruption cysts

Dentigerous cyst is associated with the crown of an impacted or partially erupted tooth. The radiographic aspect is a unicystic well-demarcated radiolucency connected at the cervical portion of the tooth in the cementoenamel junction; however, the 3D relationship with the tooth can vary, leading to different aspects (Figs 26-30 and 26-31). It is important to note that radiographic appearance is not unique; ameloblastoma, odontogenic

TABLE 26-10 Differences and similarities between GCA and LPC

	GCA	LPC
Location	Soft tissue	Intraosseous
Clinical features	Well-defined nodule at the attached gingiva with a smooth surface and bluish color	No clinical features
Radiographic appearance	No radiographic image	Well-demarcated unilocular radiolucency seen between the roots of vital teeth
Description	Cystic space covered by thin nonkeratinized squamous or cuboidal luminal epithelium. Areas with focal plaque-like/nodular thickenings and epithelial cells with clear cytoplasm (glycogen rich) might be seen.	

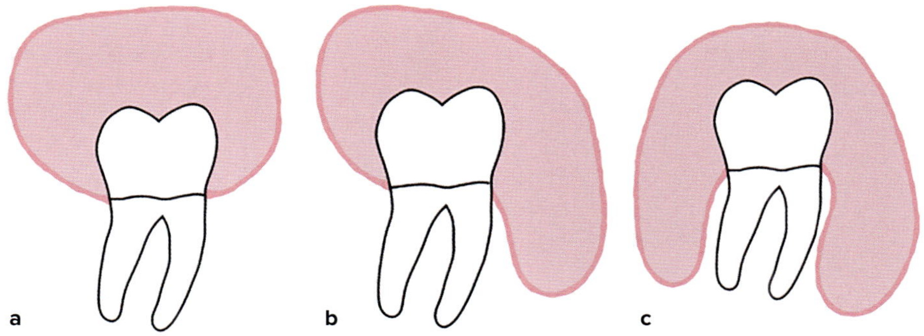

Fig 26-30 Different positions of dentigerous cysts: *(a)* central, *(b)* lateral, and *(c)* circumferential. Note that despite the position, the cyst always begins in the cementoenamel junction.

keratocyst, and other lesions can mimic dentigerous cysts. Treatment consists of the extraction of the involved tooth with curettage and enucleation of the cyst. The recurrence rate is very low. The specimen should be evaluated microscopically to confirm the diagnosis. The final diagnosis is established based on the correlation of clinical, radiographic, and microscopic features.

An eruption cyst is an extraosseous variant of a dentigerous cyst. It is found in the soft tissues overlying an erupting tooth and therefore has no radiographic image and causes gingival swelling. Permanent molars and maxillary incisors are the most affected teeth. If the cyst does not rupture spontaneously, a simple excision of the roof of the cyst allows the affected tooth to erupt normally.

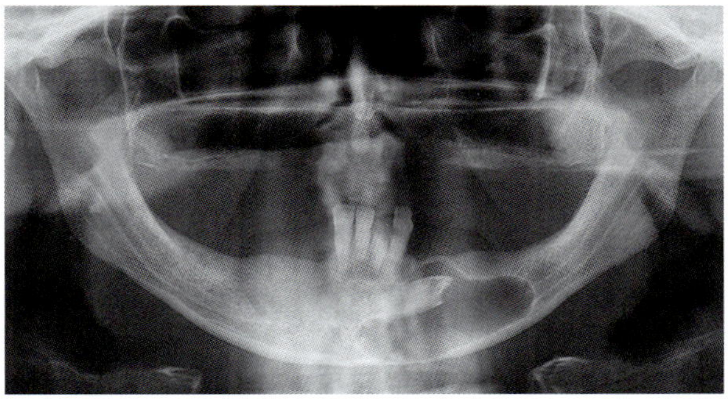

Fig 26-31 Dentigerous cyst in a circumferential configuration arising from an impacted canine in an adult patient.

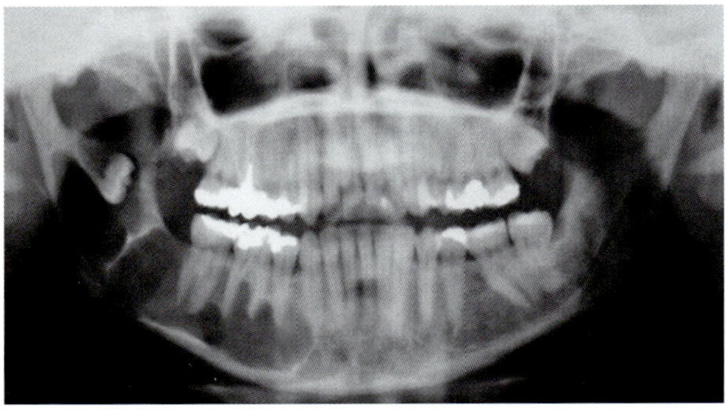

Fig 26-32 Radiographic view of odontogenic keratocyst.

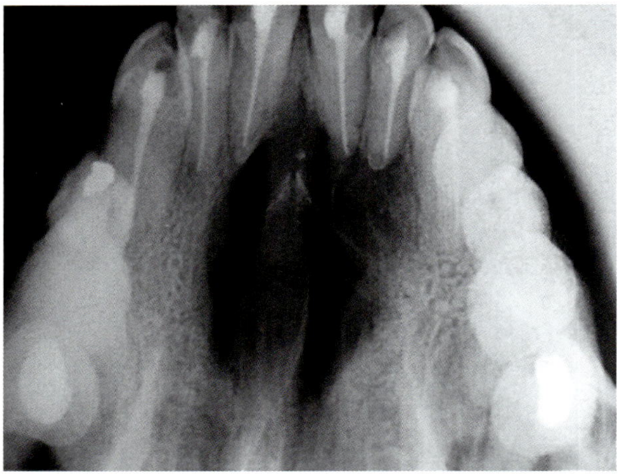

Fig 26-34 Well-defined radiolucent area with a rounded shape located in the midline region of the anterior maxilla. Note that the maxillary incisors had received endodontic treatment, probably due to a misdiagnosis of inflammatory cyst. The vitality test is important to determine the differential diagnosis.

Odontogenic keratocyst

The odontogenic keratocyst deserves a special consideration among all developmental odontogenic cyst due to unique features, such as the following:

- Great growth potential compared with most odontogenic cysts
- High recurrence rate
- Possible association with nevoid basal cell carcinoma syndrome

This cyst is believed to originate from cell rests of the dental lamina. The mandible is affected in 60% to 80% of cases, with a pronounced tendency to involve the posterior region of the mandibular body and the ascending ramus. The cyst has a tendency toward an anteroposterior growth pattern without causing cortical expansion. Radiographically, a uni- or multilocular radiolucent area with well-defined borders is observed (Fig 26-32).

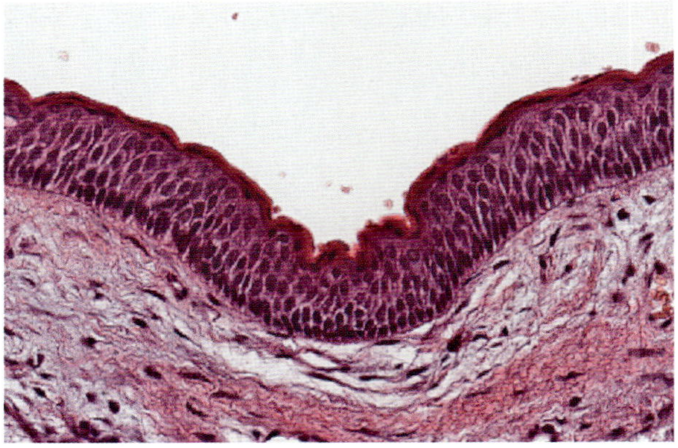

Fig 26-33 Microscopic features of odontogenic keratocyst. Observe a cystic cavity lined with parakeratinized epithelium with fewer layers and columnar basal cells with palisade arrangement. Note the corrugated surface and the flat interface between the epithelial and the connective tissues.

Histologic analysis reveals a rather irregular cystic cavity lined by a parakeratinized epithelium with fewer layers and columnar or cubic hyperchromatic basal cells with palisade arrangement. The parakeratinized surface is corrugated, and the interface between the epithelial tissue and the connective tissue is flat (Fig 26-33). The epithelial lining is quite friable, so areas of detachment from the fibrous capsule might occur.

With regard to the treatment, simple enucleation may increase the chances of relapse, so a peripheral ostectomy or the use of cryotherapy in the surgical bed is recommended. The likely causes of the high rates of recurrence are the friable capsule that breaks easily during surgery and the presence of satellite cysts in the capsule.

Nasopalatine duct cyst

This is a nonodontogenic cystic lesion of developmental origin that originates in the epithelial remains of the nasopalatine duct located within the incisive canal. Cysts might be detected in routine radiographic examinations or by clinical examination, in cases where a swelling of the anterior palatal region is observed. Radiographically, a well-defined radiolucent area with sclerotic borders located in the midline region of the anterior maxilla is observed. In most cases, the lesion is oval, rounded, inverted, or heart-shaped (Fig 26-34). Radicular cysts

TABLE 26-11 Main features of fibroosseous lesions

	Fibrous dysplasia	Cementoosseous dysplasia	Ossifying fibroma (OF)
Etiology	Developmental disorder caused by *GNAS1* mutation	Reactive	Neoplastic
Types	• Monostotic • Polyostotic • McCune–Albright syndrome (associated with café au lait spots and endocrine disorders)	• Periapical (apical areas of mandibular anterior teeth) • Focal • Florid (multiquadrant involvement)	• Juvenile trabecular OF • Juvenile psammomatoid OF • Cemento-OF
Clinical features	Slow-growing painful mass that starts growing at a young age and stops during adult life. More common in the maxilla.	Predilection for middle-aged women. Periapical type occurs mostly in Black women. Lesions are usually asymptomatic and nonexpansive (florid cases are the exception).	Lesions can grow slowly and progressively or fast and aggressively. Most common in young patients. Psammomatoid type occurs more frequently in frontal bone. Cemento-OF occurs predominantly in the mandible.
Radiographic features	Initial stage is more radiolucent. Later stage is a radiopaque area with a frosted glass aspect. There may be narrowing of the periodontal ligament. Usually presents ill-defined borders. The radiopaque density increases as the lesion matures.		Well-demarcated lesion that might be radiolucent or may show various degrees of opacification.
Microscopic features	Immature bone irregular trabeculae with curvilinear forms assuming the aspect of "Chinese characters" in a fibrous stroma. The normal (cortical) bone fuses directly with the lesional bone.	The mineralized tissues consist of osteoid, bone, and cementum-like material. Osteoblastic rimming is generally absent.	Well encapsulated. The mineralized tissues consist of variable amounts of osteoid, bone, and lobulated basophilic masses (cementum-like tissue). Osteoblastic rimming is usually evident.
Management and treatment	Investigation to determine the extent of the condition. If facial deformities exist, cosmetic surgery is recommended.	Patients should be monitored for dental complications (specifically osteomyelitis for florid type).	Treatment consists of conservative surgical excision. Recurrences are rare.

must be excluded from the differential diagnosis. In nasopalatine duct cysts, the teeth involved are vital.

Other Bone Lesions

FIBROOSSEOUS LESIONS

Fibroosseous lesions of the gnathic bones represent distinctive processes characterized by the replacement of normal bone by fibrous tissue containing neoformed mineralized material.[17] The microscopic aspects of these lesions are quite similar; however, lesions have different etiologies, behaviors, and prognoses. The diagnosis should be established through clinical, radiographic, and histopathologic correlations. Table 26-11 describes the main differences between fibroosseous lesions.

OSTEOMYELITIS

Osteomyelitis is a generic term given to acute or chronic inflammatory processes affecting the bone. In the jawbones, this event can occur as a complication following tooth extraction at the dental alveolus and therefore is called alveolar osteitis or *dry socket*. Clinical manifestations include severe pain that lasts several days after exodontia, redness, edema, and heat in the area. Systemic manifestations such as fever and lymphadenopathy may also be present. There may be drainage of suppuration through the alveolus, common in acute alveolar osteitis, or

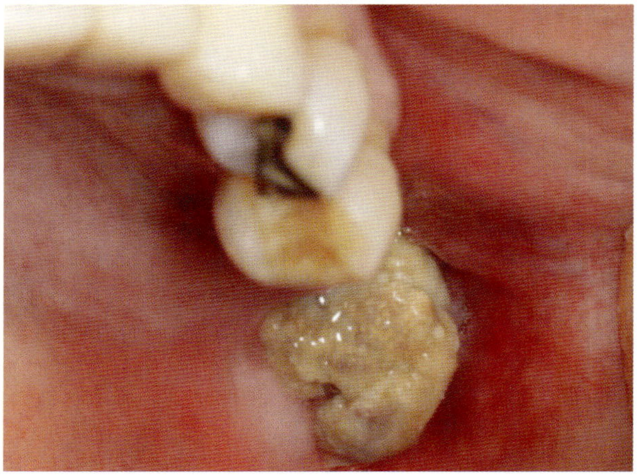

Fig 26-35 Patient under treatment with zoledronate for prostate cancer bone metastasis presented with MRONJ at the retromolar area.

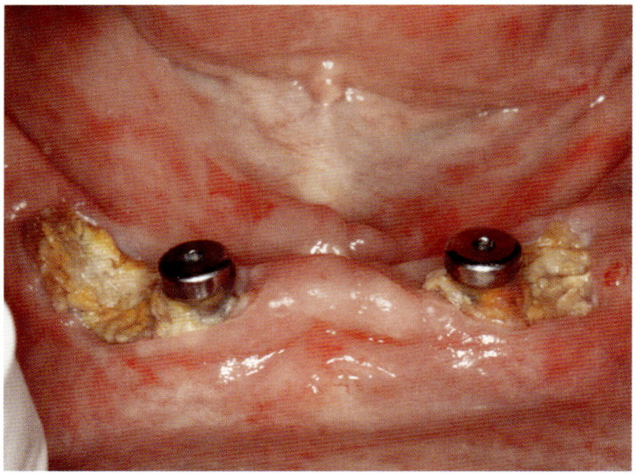

Fig 26-36 Patient with history of radiotherapy in the head and neck region with two mandibular implants. ORN followed this procedure.

extraoral fistulas in cases of chronification. Bone sequestration might occur and represents a fragment of the necrotic bone that has become separate from normal adjacent bone by granulation tissue. This necrotic tissue must be removed to allow the healing of the alveolus. Antibiotic therapy is also necessary.

MEDICATION-RELATED OSTEONECROSIS OF THE JAW

The diagnosis of medication-related osteonecrosis of the jaw (MRONJ) is established when three criteria are present[18]:

1. Patient is currently receiving or has previously received treatment with antiresorptive or antiangiogenic agents.
2. Presence of exposed bone or bone that can be probed through an extraoral or intraoral fistula in the maxillofacial region that has persisted more than 8 weeks.
3. No history of radiation therapy to the jaws or evident metastatic disease.

Bisphosphonates and denosumab are among the antiresorptive drugs related to MRONJ. These drugs are used to manage bone metastases (intravenous administration) and osteoporosis (oral administration). Most cases of MRONJ have an associated triggering factor, especially exodontia. However, cases of spontaneous onset have been reported in the literature. Different aspects are implicated in an increased risk of MRONJ, including therapeutic indications, type of medications, dose and duration of drug use, periodontal disease, and diabetes, among others. MRONJ lesions occur more frequently in the mandible than in the maxilla. Clinically, the most common feature is bone exposure (Fig 26-35), which is usually accompanied by pain, erythema or ulceration, drainage of secretion in the mouth, osteomyelitis, and, in advanced cases, pathologic fracture. Prevention is the best approach. All cancer patients who are planned to receive antiresorptive drugs should receive a comprehensive oral evaluation prior to initiating therapy, and all possible foci of infection should be eliminated. Different therapeutic modalities are proposed for MRONJ, including conservative treatment (prolonged antibiotic therapy and wound care), surgery, hyperbaric oxygenation, platelet-rich plasma, laser therapy, ultrasound, and often the combined use of several approaches.

OSTEORADIONECROSIS OF THE JAWS

Osteoradionecrosis (ORN) of the jaws is considered one of the worst and most severe long-term complications of head and neck radiotherapy. ORN is defined as a slow-healing radiation-induced ischemic necrosis of the bone associated with a variable degree of soft tissue necrosis occurring in the absence of local primary tumor necrosis, recurrence, or metastatic disease.[19] Most cases of ORN present with an etiologic triggering factor such as local trauma, dental extractions, infection, immune defects, and malnutrition (Fig 26-36). In some patients, however, ORN occurs spontaneously. Patients suffering from ORN can experience severe clinical symptoms

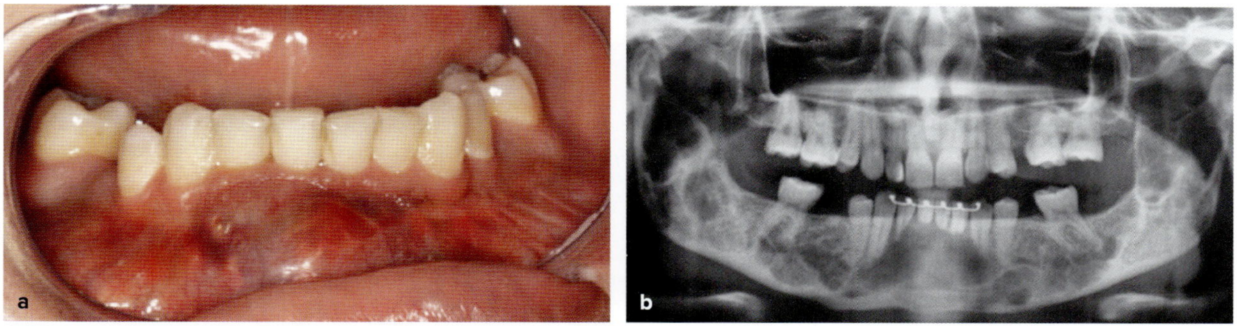

Fig 26-37 Patient with a CGCG located in the midline that caused cortical bone rupture. *(a)* Clinical view. *(b)* Radiograph.

such as chronic spontaneous pain and facial deformation, which has a direct impact in their quality of life. As in MRONJ, prevention is the best approach. A dental evaluation should be performed in all patients planned to receive radiotherapy in the head and neck region. Once the ORN is established, the treatment is challenging and, as in MRONJ, the association of different therapeutic modalities is usually necessary.

CENTRAL GIANT CELL GRANULOMA

Central giant cell granuloma (CGCG) is a nonneoplastic localized, benign but sometimes aggressive lesion of the jaws. The lesions are more frequent in the anterior jaws (frequently crossing the midline), particularly the mandible. CGCGs are usually characterized as slow growing, asymptomatic, expansile, well-defined radiolucencies (Fig 26-37). Lesions can be classified as aggressive CGCG by the presence of one or more of these features: pain, paresthesia, root resorption, rapid growth, cortical perforation, and high recurrence rate after treatment. Histopathologic features include an unencapsulated proliferation of mononuclear spindle-shaped and polygonal cells with a diverse quantity of osteoclast-type multinucleated giant cells. Surgical treatment is usually required. Most lesions respond favorably to curettage; however, some aggressive lesions require more radical surgery. Intralesional or systemic drugs can be used in an attempt to limit the extent of resection. Different agents such as steroids, calcitonin, interferon, and denosumab (RANKL inhibitor) have been proposed.

Oral Manifestations of Genetic Disorders

Some genetic disorders have important oral manifestations. Table 26-12 describes some of the disorders of special interest to periodontists.[20]

Oral Complications of Chemotherapy and Head/Neck Radiation

The multidisciplinary team responsible for the care of oncologic patients is composed by many specialists (eg, medical doctors, dietitians, psychologists), including dentists. Prior to the beginning of oncologic treatment, it is extremely important to appropriately treat any foci of oral infections, such as caries, residual roots, abscesses, periapical lesions, and periodontal disease. The presence of these foci may lead to local or systemic complications during the treatment. Periodic monitoring during and after cancer treatment is critical because patients may develop several complications from head and neck radiation and/or chemotherapy. Some complications are acute and last only during treatment. However, several side effects are chronic and can persist for months, years, or throughout the patient's life. Table 26-13 describes the acute and chronic side effects of chemotherapy and head and neck irradiation in the oral cavity.

TABLE 26-12 Main genetic disorders with gingival or periodontal manifestations

Genetic disorder	Main features	Oral manifestations
Papillon-Lefèvre syndrome	Autosomal recessive disorder caused by a mutation of the *CTSC* gene (affects the immune response). Skin manifestations include palmoplantar keratosis, follicular hyperkeratosis, and keratosis on the elbows and knees.	Generalized hyperplastic and hemorrhagic gingivitis and rapidly progressing periodontitis seen in primary and permanent dentitions.
Hereditary gingival fibromatosis (HGF)	Familial or idiopathic condition. Familial variant may be an isolated finding or associated with hereditary syndromes (eg, Zimmermann-Laband, Murray-Puretic-Drescher, Rutherfurd). Manifestations that can accompany HGF include hypertrichosis, epilepsy, intellectual disability, hypothyroidism, chondrodystrophia, growth hormone deficiency, and sensorineural deafness.	Gingival overgrowth may be generalized or localized to one or more quadrants. It usually begins with tooth eruption and can cause failure or delay in eruption of following teeth. The overgrowth is highly fibrotic, firm, and has a normal mucosa color.
Cowden syndrome	Autosomal dominant disorder caused by a mutation in the *PTEN* gene. Skin manifestations include multiple small papules (hamartomas) located mainly in the face (mouth, nose, and ears). Patients also have increased risk to develop cancers (thyroid, breast, and uterine).	Multiple papules (hamartomas) located mainly in the gingiva, dorsal tongue, and buccal mucosa. Other manifestations such as high arched palate, periodontitis, and extensive dental caries have been reported.
Down syndrome	Caused by the trisomy of chromosome 21, which alters the course of development. Common physical traits include low muscle tone, small stature, and an upward slant to the eyes. Patients have increased risk of congenital heart defects, respiratory and hearing problems, among others.	Relative macroglossia (small oral cavity), fissured and protruded tongue. Poor oral seal and suck. Class III malocclusion and presence of dental anomalies are frequent. Patients have greater risk for periodontitis.
Ehlers-Danlos syndromes	Group of inherited connective tissue disorders currently classified in 13 subtypes. Typical features include overly flexible joints and stretchy, fragile skin, dystrophic scars, and a tendency for excessive bleeding. Approximately 50% of patients can touch the end of their nose with their tongue (Gorlin sign).	Patients demonstrate early onset of periodontitis, fibrinoid deposits, and excessive gingival bleeding. The mucosa tears easily when touched by instruments. Numerous dental anomalies and temporomandibular joint disorders can be present.

TABLE 26-13 Acute and chronic oral side effects of chemotherapy and head and neck radiotherapy

	Chemotherapy		Head and neck radiotherapy	
	Acute	Chronic	Acute	Chronic
Caries		X		X
Dysgeusia	X		X	X
Bleeding	X			
Infections (candidiasis, herpes)	X		X	
Mucositis	X		X	
Osteoradionecrosis				X
Trismus			X	
Xerostomia	X		X	X

ACKNOWLEDGMENTS

The authors would like to thank the Department of Oral Pathology and Medicine from the Federal University of Rio Grande do Sul, Porto Alegre, Brazil.

References

1. American Academy of Periodontology. Glossary of Periodontal Terms. American Academy of Periodontology, 2001.
2. Neville BW, Damm DD, Allen C, Chi A (eds). Oral and Maxillofacial Pathology, ed 4. St Louis: Saunders, 2015.
3. Regezi J, Sciubba J, Jorda R (eds). Oral Pathology Clinical Pathologic Correlations, ed 7. St Louis: Saunders, 2016.
4. Brown RS, Arany PR. Mechanism of drug-induced gingival overgrowth revisited: A unifying hypothesis. Oral Dis 2015;21:e51–e61.
5. Bharti V, Bansal C. Drug-induced gingival overgrowth: The nemesis of gingiva unravelled. J Indian Soc Periodontol 2013;17:182–187.
6. Buchner A, Shnaiderman-Shapiro A, Vered M. Relative frequency of localized reactive hyperplastic lesions of the gingiva: A retrospective study of 1675 cases from Israel. J Oral Pathol Med 2010;39:631–638.
7. Pytynia KB, Dahlstrom KR, Sturgis EM. Epidemiology of HPV-associated oropharyngeal cancer. Oral Oncol 2014;50:380–386.
8. Harper DM, DeMars LR. HPV vaccines: A review of the first decade. Gynecol Oncol 2017;146:196–204.
9. Patil S, Rao RS, Majumdar B, Anil S. Clinical appearance of oral candida infection and therapeutic strategies. Front Microbiol 2015;6:1391.
10. Kasperkiewicz M, Ellebrecht CT, Takahashi H, et al. Pemphigus. Nat Rev Dis Primers 2017;3:17026.
11. Xu HH, Werth VP, Parisi E, Sollecito TP. Mucous membrane pemphigoid. Dent Clin North Am 2013;57:611–630.
12. El-Naggar AK, Chan JKC, Grandis JR, Takata T, Slootweg PJ (eds). WHO/IARC Classification of Tumours, ed 4. Lyon: International Agency for Research on Cancer, 2017.
13. Brouns E, Baart J, Karagozoglu Kh, Aartman I, Bloemena E, van der Waal I. Malignant transformation of oral leukoplakia in a well-defined cohort of 144 patients. Oral Dis 2014;20:e19–24.
14. Aghbari SMH, Abushouk AI, Attia A, et al. Malignant transformation of oral lichen planus and oral lichenoid lesions: A meta-analysis of 20095 patient data. Oral Oncol 2017;68:92–102.
15. Lydiatt WM, Patel SG, O'Sullivan B, et al. Head and neck cancers-Major changes in the American Joint Committee on Cancer Eighth Edition Cancer Staging Manual. CA Cancer J Clin 2017;67:122–137.
16. Bilodeau EA, Collins BM. Odontogenic cysts and neoplasms. Surg Pathol Clin 2017;10:177–222.
17. MacDonald DS. Maxillofacial fibro-osseous lesions. Clin Radiol 2015;70:25–36.
18. Ruggiero SL, Dodson TB, Fantasia J, et al. American Association of Oral and Maxillofacial Surgeons position paper on medication-related osteonecrosis of the jaw: 2014 update. J Oral Maxillofac Surg 2014;72:1938–1956.
19. Chrcanovic BR, Reher P, Sousa AA, Harris M. Osteoradionecrosis of the jaws—A current overview—Part 1: Physiopathology and risk and predisposing factors. Oral Maxillofac Surg 2010;14:3–16.
20. Nualart Grollmus ZC, Morales Chávez MC, Silvestre Donat FJ. Periodontal disease associated to systemic genetic disorders. Med Oral Patol Oral Cir Bucal 2007;12:E211–E215.

27

PHARMACOLOGY

Alexandra Plonka Hosking, DDS, MS
Rachel Sheridan Sinacola, DDS, MS

DEFINITIONS AND TERMINOLOGY

Anesthesia: Loss of feeling or sensation caused by an anesthetic agent to permit diagnostic and treatment procedures.[1]

Antibiotic: Molecules or agents produced by microorganisms that have the capacity to kill or inhibit the growth of other microorganisms.[1]

Bactericide: An agent capable of destroying bacteria. Also termed *bacteriocide*.[1]

Bacteriostatic: Inhibiting or retarding the growth of bacteria.[1]

Drug: Any chemical that alters the physiologic processes of living systems. Used in the diagnosis, cure, mitigation, treatment, or prevention of disease.[1]

Half-life (drug): The amount of time for plasma concentration of a drug to be reduced by 50%.[1]

Pharmacology: The study of the interaction of chemicals with biologic systems.[1]

Placebo: An inactive substance resembling one having therapeutic value; used in controlled studies to determine the effect of drugs without the influence of bias.[1]

Medications are used in periodontal therapy for a variety of purposes. This chapter outlines the most commonly prescribed medications in periodontics and implant dentistry. In addition, sample prescriptions are provided with some of the most common dosages.

Disclaimer: The examples provided in this chapter are not intended to be a guide nor recommendations for the prescription of the mentioned medications. The practitioner must always evaluate the individual patient's medical and dental histories, and when appropriate, consult with the patient's physician prior to administering any medications.

ASA Classification

The American Society of Anesthesiologists (ASA) Physical Status (PS) Classification System assesses patients to determine their fitness for general anesthesia.[2] The ASA PS classification can also assist in evaluating the medical status of a patient, and it may alert the periodontal provider to consult with the patient's physician. The most recent ASA PS classification was approved by the ASA House of Delegates in 2019. The classification and examples are detailed in Table 27-1.[2]

Antibiotics

Antibiotics function by selectively inhibiting bacterial cell growth (bacteriostatic) or killing bacteria (bactericidal) while leaving the human cells intact. The mechanism of action is important when considering prescribing multiple antibiotics: avoid combining **bacteriostatic** and **bactericidal** drugs, which could antagonize each other.[3] Bactericidal antibiotics are usually preferred for periodontal applications.[4] Antibiotics that are commonly prescribed in periodontal patient care are shown in Table 27-2.[4] Examples of common dosing regimens in periodontics are provided in Table 27-3.[4–6]

TABLE 27-1 ASA PS classification system*

Classification	Definition	Examples
ASA I	Normal, healthy patient	Healthy, nonsmoker, no or minimal alcohol use
ASA II	Patient with mild systemic disease	Mild diseases only without substantive functional limitations (eg, current smoker, social alcohol drinker, pregnancy, obesity [BMI between 30 and 40], well-controlled DM or HTN, mild lung disease)
ASA III	Patient with severe systemic disease	Substantive functional limitations or one or more moderate to severe diseases (eg, poorly controlled DM or HTN; COPD; morbid obesity [BMI ≥ 40]; active hepatitis; alcohol dependence or abuse; implanted pacemaker; moderate reduction of ejection fraction; ESRD undergoing regularly scheduled dialysis; premature infant PCA < 60 weeks; history [> 3 months] of MI, CVA, TIA, or CAD/stents)
ASA IV	Patient with severe systemic disease that is a constant threat to life	Recent (< 3 months) MI, CVA, TIA, or CAD/stents; ongoing cardiac ischemia or severe valve dysfunction; severe reduction of ejection fraction; sepsis; DIC; ARD; or ESRD not undergoing regularly scheduled dialysis
ASA V	Moribund patient who is not expected to survive without the operation	Ruptured abdominal/thoracic aneurysm, massive trauma, intracranial bleed with mass effect, ischemic bowel in the face of significant cardiac pathology, or multiple organ/system dysfunction
ASA VI	Declared brain-dead patient whose organs are being removed for donor purposes	NA

DM, diabetes mellitus; HTN, hypertension; BMI, body mass index; COPD, chronic obstructive pulmonary disease; ESRD, end-stage renal disease; PCA, postconceptual age; MI, myocardial infarction; CVA, cerebrovascular accident; TIA, transient ischemic attack; CAD, coronary artery disease; DIC, diffuse intravascular coagulation; ARD, ascites reinfusion dialysis; NA, not applicable.

Note: The addition of "E" denotes emergency surgery. An *emergency* is defined as existing when delay in treatment of the patient would lead to a significant increase in the threat to life or body part.

*Reprinted with permission from the ASA.[2]

INDICATIONS FOR ANTIBIOTICS IN PERIODONTAL THERAPY

Antibiotics are prescribed in the dental and periodontal fields for a variety of purposes.[4] These purposes include but are not limited to treatment of abscess or infection[7] and as an adjunct to periodontal therapy, as a preventive method, or for premedication.

Treatment of abscess or infection

Examples include but are not limited to gingival abscess, pericoronitis, periodontal abscess, endodontic abscess, and postsurgical infection. Signs of infection include but are not limited to edema, erythema, pain, fever, increase in temperature, and/or exudate after 72 hours. It may be possible, however, to overestimate the incidence of infections because symptoms may be similar to normal postoperative sequalae such as lymphadenopathy, pain, necrosis, and swelling.[8] Nevertheless, the incidence of postsurgical infections is low, ranging from 1% to 2%.[8,9]

Adjunct to periodontal therapy

An antibiotic may be prescribed at the completion of mechanical periodontal therapy for certain patient groups, such as immunocompromised patients, and those with refractory or aggressive forms of periodontitis.

Preventive

As part of dental implant or bone grafting procedures, for example.

Premedication

Similar to preventive antibiotics, which are based on procedure type, some patients are prescribed antibiotic prophylaxis based on their medical history (see the following section).

ANTIBIOTIC PROPHYLAXIS

Without specific medical indications, prophylactic antibiotics are generally not indicated. Several studies found

TABLE 27-2 Common antibiotics in periodontal therapy

	Penicillin	Tetracyclines	Macrolides (clindamycin, azithromycin)	Fluoroquinolones (levofloxacin, ciprofloxacin)	Metronidazole
Inhibits	Cell wall synthesis	Protein synthesis: Translation (30S ribosomal subunit)	Protein synthesis: Translation (50S ribosomal subunit)	Nucleic acid synthesis	Anaerobes
Mechanism	β-lactam ring inhibits peptidoglycan synthesis	30S ribosomal subunit: blocks tRNA attachment to ribosome	50S subunit: prevents continuation of protein synthesis	Inhibits DNA metabolism	Target key chemical reaction unique to anaerobes
Effect on cell	Bactericidal	Bacteriostatic	Bacteriostatic	Bactericidal	Bactericidal
Targets	Gram +	Broad-spectrum (Gram +/–)	Broad-spectrum (Gram +/–)	Broad-spectrum (Gram +/–)	Anaerobes
Potential side effects[4]	Hypersensitivity (rash) Diarrhea	Photosensitivity; tooth discoloration in children	Diarrhea (clindamycin, azithromycin); clindamycin has risk of pseudomembranous colitis	Nausea/vomiting, photosensitivity, risk of tendon damage on exercise	Nausea/vomiting "Disulfiram-like" reaction to alcohol
Notes	Amoxicillin is often used for antibiotic prophylaxis; can be prescribed with clavulanic acid due to susceptibility to β lactamases	Alternative use with subantimicrobial doses (20 mg) of doxycycline as an adjunct therapy for periodontitis	Clindamycin: alternative to amoxicillin for prophylaxis in patients allergic to penicillin	Sinusitis; ciprofloxacin suitable for alternative to amoxicillin for combination therapy with metronidazole	Combination with amoxicillin commonly used for treatment of aggressive periodontitis
Usual dose for adults in periodontics[4]	Amoxicillin: 250–500 mg tid	200 mg qd	Clindamycin: 300 mg tid or qid	500 mg bid	500 mg bid or tid

tid, three times per day; qd, once per day; qid, four times per day; bid, twice per day.

TABLE 27-3 Common dosages of adjunctive antibiotics in periodontics[4–6]

Antibiotic	Microbes targeted	Common adult dosage
Doxycycline	Nonspecific	Disp: 100–200 mg Sig: qd for 21 days
Minocycline	Nonspecific	Disp: 50 mg Sig: qd for 2 weeks
Metronidazole	*Porphyromonas gingivalis*, *Tannerella forsythia*, *Treponema* species	Disp: 500 mg Sig: tid for 8 days
Azithromycin	Periodontal pathogens, with some resistance	Disp: 500 mg Sig: qd for 4–7 days
Clindamycin	Gram-negative anaerobes	Disp: 300 mg Sig: tid for 8 days
Metronidazole + amoxicillin	*Aggregatibacter actinomycetemcomitans* or *P gingivalis* with high numbers of Gram-positive pathogens	Disp: 250 mg metronidazole and 375 mg amoxicillin Sig: tid for 8 days (each)
Metronidazole + ciprofloxacin	*A actinomycetemcomitans* or presence of susceptible enteric microorganisms	Disp: 500 mg (each) Sig: bid for 8 days (each)

qd, once per day; tid, three times per day; bid, twice per day.

TABLE 27-4 Common antibiotic premedication regimens

Drug	Adult dose	Child dose
Amoxicillin	2 g	50 mg/kg
Clindamycin*	600 mg	20 mg/kg
Azithromycin or clarithromycin*	500 mg	15 mg/kg
Cephalexin*	2 g	50 mg/kg

*Potential alternative for patients with an allergy to penicillin.

that prescribing penicillin or tetracycline at the time of periodontal surgery did not significantly reduce infection compared with **placebo**. This finding held regardless of the technique or surgery type, use of membranes or dressings, or postsurgical use of chlorhexidine rinse.[8–12] Interestingly, setting and practitioner experience may play a role: Incidence of infection has been reported as 1.2% for board-certified periodontists versus 2.5% for residents and general dentists. The study suggested that there is no clear benefit of perisurgical antibiotics for prevention of infection in healthy patients.[9] For dental implant therapy, a systematic review and meta-analysis found that for healthy patients, antibiotic prophylaxis may not be indicated for prevention of postoperative infections.[13]

Candidates for antibiotic prophylaxis

Antibiotic prophylaxis is most often prescribed for patients with *(1)* a history of joint replacement, *(2)* history of infective endocarditis, or *(3)* specific cardiac considerations (eg, certain congenital conditions, certain repaired heart defects and/or valves, and presence of artificial heart valves). If prophylaxis is indicated, antibiotics are administered prior to nearly all dental procedures that involve manipulation of gingival tissue or the periapical region of teeth or perforation of the oral mucosa. Exceptions include the following:

- Routine anesthetic injections through noninfected tissue
- Radiographs
- Placement of removable prosthodontic or orthodontic appliances
- Adjustment of orthodontic appliances
- Shedding of primary teeth and bleeding from trauma to the lips or mucosa

Antibiotic selection

Oral regimens are most commonly administered 30 to 60 minutes prior to treatment (Table 27-4). If a candidate for antibiotic prophylaxis fails to take the prescribed medication prior to the appointment for treatment, it may safely protect the patient if administered up to 2 hours after the procedure. If the patient is already taking an antibiotic for another purpose, it is recommended to select an alternative class of **drug** rather than increasing the dosage of the antibiotic to the premedication dose.[14] An alternative is to wait until 10 days after completion of the antibiotic. If the antibiotic is penicillin, avoid cephalosporin.[14]

Nonnarcotic Pain and Anti-Inflammatory Medications

POSTSURGICAL PAIN OVERVIEW

For the majority of periodontal procedures, postsurgical pain is usually not significant. Comparing periodontal procedures with conventional dental treatment, 97% of patients found no difference in discomfort between the two types.[15] Moreover, periodontal surgery has minimal impact on quality of life. Curtis et al found that 94.8% of patients did not miss work or school after surgery, and 81.3% did not change their eating habits.[16]

NONSTEROIDAL ANTI-INFLAMMATORY DRUGS (NSAIDs)[17]

- **Properties**
  - Anti-inflammatory
  - Antipyretic
  - Analgesic
- **Mechanism of action**

- Reversible inhibition of cyclooxygenase (COX) enzymes and limiting formation of prostaglandin precursors. Possible additional anti-inflammatory effects (effect on immune cells).
- COX-1 and COX-2 (ibuprofen, naproxen).
- COX-2 selective (celecoxib [Celebrex, Pfizer]).

- **Contraindications and precautions**
  - Contraindications: Hypersensitivity (allergy), gastrointestinal (GI) bleed (increased risk of bleeding), kidney disease, severe hepatic impairment, and pregnancy.
  - Potential contraindication: Concomitant use of an anticoagulant medication, such as warfarin. Recommend consultation with the patient's physician.
  - Some patients who report an allergy have a leukotriene intolerance. NSAID blockage of the COX pathway may increase the lipooxygenase pathway. A subsequent accumulation of leukotrienes may cause some patients to experience redness.
  - Use caution in asthmatic patients and those with decreased hepatic function.
- **Association with blood loss during surgery**
  - NSAIDs and other medication-induced inhibition of thromboxanes can reduce platelet function and increase bleeding. Preoperative ibuprofen was shown to significantly increase bleeding with almost twice the blood loss at the halfway point of the surgery, but blood loss still fell within normal limits.[18]
  - May prolong bleeding time and inhibit platelet aggregation. Less effect on platelet function than aspirin.
- **Dosages**
  - Ibuprofen
    - Ceiling for analgesia: 400 mg
    - No ceiling dose for anti-inflammatory properties
    - Maximum dosage: 3,200 mg in 24 hours
- **Sample Rx**
  - Ibuprofen
    - 600 mg q6h. Do not exceed 4 tablets in 24 hours.
    - 800 mg q8h. Do not exceed 3 tablets in 24 hours.
- **Naproxen**
  - 220 mg q12h. Do not exceed 2 tablets in 24 hours.

ASPIRIN[17]

- **Properties**
  - Antipyretic
  - Analgesic
  - Anti-inflammatory
- **Mechanism of action**
  - Irreversible inhibition of COX-1 and COX-2 enzymes, resulting in decreased prostaglandin precursors. Irreversible inhibition of thromboxane A2, which inhibits platelet aggregation.
- **Contraindications and precautions**
  - Children (< 16 years of age) with viral infections due to risk of Reye syndrome. Use caution for patients with asthma, tinnitus/hearing impairment, and nasal polyps.
- **Association with blood loss during surgery**
  - Risk of increased bleeding due to irreversible inhibition of platelet function. This effect on bleeding persists for the life of the platelet, 7 to 10 days. Despite bleeding risk, there is limited evidence to support discontinuing aspirin ahead of dental surgery. It was found that discontinuing daily low-dose aspirin is not necessary prior to surgery because local measures effectively controlled increased bleeding.[19] It is important to consult with the patient's physician prior to discontinuing or modifying an aspirin regimen.
- **Adult dosages**
  - Extra-strength: 500 mg
  - Regular strength: 325 mg
  - Cardiovascular dose (baby aspirin): 81 mg
- **Sample Rx**
  - 325–650 mg q4–6h. Maximum 4,000 mg in 24 hours.

ACETAMINOPHEN[17]

- **Properties**
  - Antipyretic
  - Analgesic (not anti-inflammatory)
- **Mechanism of action**
  - Mechanism not fully understood. Antipyretic properties stem from inhibition of hypothalamic heat-regulation center. Possible action in central nervous system (CNS) to inhibit prostaglandins. Possible action in peripheral nervous system to inhibit pain sensations.
- **Contraindications and precautions**
  - Hypersensitivity, severe hepatic impairment, or hepatic disease. Consuming alcohol with

acetaminophen increases risk of acetaminophen-induced liver failure.

- **Maximum dose**
  - 3,000 mg in 24 hours.
  - When using alcohol, maximum dose is 2,000 mg in 24 hours. Consider avoiding alcohol use with acetaminophen.[17]
- **Sample Rx**[20]
  - Regular-strength Tylenol (Janssen Pharmaceutical): 325-mg tablets
    - 2 tablets q4–6h while symptoms last
    - Do not exceed 10 tablets in 24 hours
  - Extra-strength Tylenol: 500-mg tablets
    - 2 tablets q6h while symptoms last
    - Do not exceed 6 tablets in 24 hours

SYSTEMIC CORTICOSTEROIDS[17]

- **Properties**
  - Anti-inflammatory (mainly anti-edema)
  - Minimally analgesic[21]
- **Mechanism of action**
  - Bind to intracellular receptors and enter the cell nucleus, thus exerting a wide range of actions. Anti-inflammatory properties result from suppressing polymorphonuclear neutrophil (PMN) migration, decreasing formation of inflammatory mediators, and reducing capillary permeability, thus reducing edema.[17]
- **Contraindications and precautions**
  - Contraindications
    - Hypersensitivity
    - Recent fungal infection
    - Herpes
    - HIV
    - Tuberculosis infections
    - Recent vaccines
  - Caution[12]
    - Diabetes
    - Heart, liver, kidney, and mental/mood diseases
    - Hypertension
    - Thyroid disease
    - GI disorders
    - Osteoporosis
    - Myasthenia gravis
    - Seizures or risk of seizures
    - Allergies
    - Pregnancy/breastfeeding
    - Glaucoma
    - Cataracts
    - Osteoporosis
- **Adult dosage considerations**
  - Physiologic secretion is 30 to 45 mg in 24 hours but peaks at 300 mg.
  - Prescribed steroid dosage should exceed 300 mg cortisol, the maximum physiologic daily output.[22]
  - In order to avoid rebound edema, maintain steroid levels for at least 3 days.[23]
  - It is recommended that steroids be administered 2 to 4 hours prior to significant surgery, at doses exceeding the maximum equivalent daily output, and for at least 2 days to avoid rebounds.[4]
  - Generally, dosing regimens taper down dosages over a period of days.
- **Example oral forms**
  - Methylprednisolone
    - Dosages available: 2, 4, 8, 16, 24, 32 mg
    - Example brand name: Medrol (Pfizer)
  - Dexamethasone
    - Dosages available: 0.25, 0.5, 0.75, 1, 1.5, 2, 4, 6 mg
    - Example brand name: Decadron (Merck)
- **Sample Rx**
  - Rx: Medrol Dosepak.
  - Disp: 1 pack.
  - Sig: Follow instructions on package insert until gone. Start morning of procedure.

TOPICAL CORTICOSTEROIDS[17]

- **Properties**
  - Anti-inflammatory
  - Antipruritic
- **Mechanism of action**
  - Mechanism not fully understood. Likely anti-inflammatory, anti-proliferative, and immunosuppressant.[22] Used to treat intraoral autoimmune conditions with symptomatic mucosal manifestations such as lichen planus.
- **Contraindications and precautions**
  - Contraindications
    - Hypersensitivity
    - Skin lesions (viral, fungal, tubercular)
    - Herpes simplex virus infection
- **Caution**
  - If topical forms are absorbed systemically, systemic absorption could cause suppression of

TABLE 27-5 Continuum of depth of sedation[24]

	Minimal sedation (anxiolysis)	Moderate sedation (conscious sedation)	Deep sedation	General anesthesia
Responsiveness	Normal response	Purposeful response	Purposeful response to repeated or painful stimulation	Unarousable
Airway	Unaffected	No intervention required	Intervention may be required	Intervention often required
Spontaneous ventilation	Unaffected	Adequate	May be inadequate	Frequently inadequate
Cardiovascular function	Unaffected	Usually maintained	Usually maintained	May be impaired

hypothalamic-pituitary-adrenal axis. Topical steroid may be applied to affected area several times per day, depending on severity. Use should be discontinued when symptoms resolve. Plan to reevaluate the patient 2 weeks after starting therapy. It is not recommended to prescribe topical corticosteroids in the dental setting for patients younger than 12 years.[17]

- **Sample Rx**
  - 0.05% fluocinonide gel.
  - Disp: 45-g tube.
  - Sig: Apply thin layer to affected area 4 times per day.
  - Do not use higher strength (0.1%) for greater than 2 weeks.
  - Also available in cream (0.05%) and ointment (0.05%) forms.

Oral and Intravenous Sedation Medications, Reversal Agents, and Opioid Analgesics

Author's note: This section does not intend to provide instructions on how to practice sedation. This is solely intended to be an informational overview of concepts and drugs that may be used during sedation.

OVERVIEW

Continuum of depth of sedation

There are degrees of intensity of sedation, with various levels of increasing depth (Table 27-5).[24] The level of sedation is not related to route of administration of the drug(s). The goal of intravenous (IV) and oral in-office sedation is usually minimal or moderate sedation.[24] The common combination of nitrous oxide and oxygen along with sedative agent(s) may provide minimal, moderate, or deep sedation or general **anesthesia**.[25]

According to the American Dental Association:

> Because sedation and general anesthesia are a continuum, it is not always possible to predict how an individual patient will respond. Hence, practitioners intending to produce a given level of sedation should be able to diagnose and manage the physiologic consequences (rescue) for patients whose level of sedation becomes deeper than initially intended. For all levels of sedation, the qualified dentist must have the training, skills, drugs, and equipment to identify and manage such an occurrence until either assistance arrives (emergency medical service) or the patient returns to the intended level of sedation without airway or cardiovascular complications.[25]

In dosing, apply a margin of safety so that unintended loss of consciousness is unlikely. Prior to administering IV sedation, patients are required to fast for 2 to 8 hours (Table 27-6).[24] The purpose of fasting is to minimize risk of aspiration in case of vomiting.

BENZODIAZEPINES

- **Properties**
  - Antiseizure (all benzodiazepines), skeletal muscle relaxation, anxiolysis, sedation, hypnosis, amnesia.
  - Onset: Related to lipid solubility. High lipid solubility enhances the drug's ability to cross the blood–brain barrier, allowing the drug to take effect faster.
  - Duration of action: Related to **half-life**. IV drugs are eliminated from the plasma by two mechanisms. The time in which a drug is eliminated by each mechanism is identified as the α and β half-life phase.
    - α half-life: Related to distribution of the drug from the plasma into other body tissues. This occurs most rapidly and ends when an equilibrium is formed between plasma and tissues.
    - β half-life: More gradual. This decrease in plasma concentration is a result of metabolism and excretion of the drug from the body.
  - Metabolism: Liver (cytochrome p450 enzymes).
  - Excretion: Kidney.
- **Mechanism of action**
  - Promote the binding of neurotransmitter gamma-aminobutyric acid (GABA) to chlorine ion channel in cell membrane. Binding of GABA to an ion channel causes cell hyperpolarization, making it harder for the cell to depolarize and create an action potential. Thus, GABA acts as a neuroinhibitor where it is found physiologically in the CNS.[17]
- **Contraindications and precautions**[26]
  - Relative contraindications: Antidepressants (ie, selective serotonin reuptake inhibitors [SSRIs]) due to their inhibition of cytochrome p450 enzymes that may increase the effect of benzodiazepines.
  - Absolute contraindications: Narrow angle glaucoma.[26]
- **Complications**
  - Paradoxical reaction: Due to removal of inhibitions. May cause aggressiveness, agitation, and/or crying, which occur more commonly in women or older patients.[27]
  - Possible respiratory depression. Benzodiazepines generally do not cause respiratory depression, except for midazolam. There is a synergistic effect on respiratory depression when combining midazolam and other sedative agents, such as fentanyl.[28]
- **Example IV sedatives**
  - Midazolam
    - Example IV sedation administration rate: 1 mg/minute in 15- to 30-minute period.
    - Example total dose for moderate conscious sedation: 2 to 5 mg.
    - Metabolism: Liver cytochrome p450 (CYP) 3A4 enzyme.
    - Excretion: 1 to 12 hours.
    - Note: No active metabolites.
  - Diazepam (Valium, Roche)
    - Example IV sedation administration rate: 5 mg/minute in 30 to 45 minutes.
    - Example dose: 5 to 10 mg. Ceiling dose is 20 mg. Most patients need 0.6 to 1 mg.
    - Half-life: 24 to 72 hours.
    - Not water-soluble; allow IV to be run for a period of time before administering.
- **Example oral sedatives**[26]
  - Triazolam (Halcion, Pfizer): 0.25-mg tablet
    - Properties: Hypoxic, amnesic, anxiolytic, sedative, anticonvulsant, and muscle relaxant.
    - Onset: 15 to 30 minutes.
    - Half-life: 1.5 to 5 hours, appropriate for 2- to 4-hour appointment.
    - Side effects: Somnolence, dizziness, altered coordination.
    - Sample Rx:
      - Triazolam 0.25-mg tabs.
      - Disp: 1 tab.
      - Sig: Take 1 tab 1 hour prior to dental appointment.
  - Lorazepam (Ativan, Pfizer): 0.5-mg tablet (dose: 0.25 to 4 mg)
    - Properties: Sedation, anxiolytic, potent amnesia.
    - Onset: 30 to 60 min.
    - Half-life: ≤ 8 hours, appropriate for ≤ 3-hour appointment.
    - Adverse effects: Hypotension, severe sedation.

TABLE 27-6 Fasting guidelines from the ASA[24]

Ingested material	Minimum fasting period
Clear liquids	2 hours
Breast milk	4 hours
Infant formula	6 hours
Nonhuman milk	6 hours
Light meal	6 hours
Fatty meal	8 hours

BOX 27-1 Action of opioids on receptors

Agonist	Agonist/antagonist	Antagonist
• Morphine • Meperidine • Fentanyl • Codeine	• Butorphanol • Nalbuphine • Pentazocine • Buprenorphine	• Naloxone • Nalmefene

    - Note: Does not convert to an active metabolite.
    - Sample Rx:
      - Lorazepam 1 mg.
      - Disp: 2 tabs.
      - Sig: Take 1 to 2 tabs 2 hours prior to appointment.
  - Diazepam (Valium, Roche): 2-mg tab (dosage: 2, 5, 10)
    - Properties: Treat anxiety and insomnia.
    - Onset: 20 to 40 minutes.
    - Note: Has an active metabolite.
    - Half-life: 24 hours. May be prescribed the night before the procedure so the patient can sleep well.
    - Adverse effects: anterograde amnesia, confusion, excess sedation.
  - Alprazolam (Xanax, Pfizer)
    - Properties: Treat anxiety and panic disorders.
    - Half-life: 11 hours.
    - Adverse effects: Change in libido, ataxia, slurred speech.
    - Sample Rx: 0.25 to 0.5 mg 1 hour prior.
- **Reversal agent: Flumazenil**
  - Mechanism of action: Benzodiazepine antagonist; competitive inhibitor. Inhibits GABA action.
    - Onset: Rapid.
    - Duration of action: Shorter than benzodiazepines. Repeat dosing may be needed.
    - Reverses: Respiratory depression, sedation, anxiolysis, amnesia, psychomotor impairment, laryngospasm, paradoxical reactions.
  - Availability: Packaged 0.1 mg/mL in 5- or 10-mL vial.
  - Administration
    - IV: 0.2 mg over 15 seconds. Wait 45 seconds, repeat up to 1 mg (five times).
    - Intramuscular (IM): 0.25-mg dose every 60 to 120 seconds. Maximum 1 mg. Insert into middle deltoid muscle.

OPIOIDS FOR SEDATION AND ANALGESIA

- **Properties**
  - Desired: Analgesia, sedation, euphoria.
  - Undesired: Respiratory depression, dysphoria, nausea/vomiting, constipation, dependence, withdrawal.
- **Mechanism of action**
  - Act on naturally occurring receptors (mu, kappa, sigma, delta).
  - Agonist: Bind to receptor and activate a response.
  - Antagonist: Block action of agonist.
  - Mixed agonist/antagonist: Drug possesses properties of both agonist and antagonist, depending on the conditions (Box 27-1).
  - An opioid may act as an agonist at one type of receptor and an antagonist at another. Example: Kappa agonist but mu antagonist.
  - Agonist/antagonist may act as an agonist, but when mixed with another opioid, they can act as antagonist and cause withdrawal.
  - Warning: Mixed agonist/antagonist can induce withdrawal symptoms in patients who regularly take opioids.
- **Adverse effects**
  - Respiratory depression
  - Chest wall rigidity
  - Nausea/vomiting
  - Histamine release (morphine)
  - Pruritus
- **Contraindications and precautions**
  - Hypersensitivity.
  - Administration of meperidine.
  - Recent or current use of monoamine oxidase inhibitors (risk of serotonin syndrome).
  - Renal failure or impairment.

- Use caution with other sedative medications such as benzodiazepines due to synergistic effect on respiratory depression.
- Use caution with other drugs that cause CNS depression, because sedatives can potentiate CNS depression.[29]

- **Example IV dosages (sedation)**
  - Meperidine (Demerol, Pfizer): Pure opioid agonist
    - Example administration rate: 25 mg/minute (maximum).
    - Example dose: 25 to 75 mg. Ceiling dose is typically 50 to 100 mg.
    - Duration: 30 to 60 minutes, short 2- to 4-hour half-life.
    - Metabolism: CYP3A4, active metabolites.
  - Fentanyl: 100 times more potent than morphine
    - Example dose: 25 to 50 mcg.
    - Half-life: 4 hours.
- **Example oral formulations (analgesia)**
  - Vicodin (AbbVie): Hydrocodone Bitartrate (5 mg, 7.5 mg, or 10 mg) + acetaminophen 500 mg
  - Norco (Allergan): Hydrocodone Bitartrate (5 mg, 7.5 mg, or 10 mg) + acetaminophen 325 mg
  - Percocet (Endo International): Oxycodone (5 mg, 7.5 mg, 10 mg) + acetaminophen 325 mg
  - Tylenol with codeine #3: Acetaminophen 300 mg + 30 mg codeine phosphate
  - Tylenol with codeine #4: Acetaminophen 300 mg + 60 mg codeine phosphate
- **Reversal agent: Naloxone**
  - Mechanism of action: Pure opioid antagonist.
  - Half-life: Shorter than opioid drugs. Additional doses of naloxone may be needed.
  - Side effects: Catecholamine release due to activation of sympathetic nervous system response. Epinephrine release could theoretically lead to cardiac arrest or stroke.
  - Dosage: 0.4 to 2 mg/minute IV or IM until patient is responsive. Packaged in 0.4 mg per 1-mL vial.
  - Example administration: 0.1 to 0.2 mg every 2 to 3 minutes, maximum dose is 10 mg.

NITROUS OXIDE[30]

- **Properties**
  - Odorless
  - Colorless
  - Non-irritating
  - Nonflammable but supports combustion
  - Low potency
  - Safe
  - Effective
  - Reliable
  - Effects
    - Anxiolysis
    - Minimal analgesia
    - Minimal cardiovascular and respiratory depression
    - No motor or sensory impairment
  - Onset
    - Almost immediate
    - Possible to titrate
    - Rapid recovery on exhalation
- **Mechanism of action**
  - Unknown. Likely stimulates release of enkephalins, an endogenous compound that binds to and activates opioid receptors.
- **Contraindications/precautions**
  - Inability to use nasal mask (physical or psychologic reasons)
  - Recent ear surgery
  - Use caution in patients with a history of obstructed bowel, pneumothorax, middle ear inflammation (risk of rupturing tympanic membrane), or recent retinal surgery. Nitrous oxide will fill gas spaces faster than naturally occurring nitrogen (present in room air).
  - Absolute contraindication for patients with chronic obstructive pulmonary disease (COPD) who rely on hypoxemic drive to breathe oxide. Nitrous oxide may reduce hypoxemic drive.
  - A medical consultation and caution are recommended for:
    - Patients with psychiatric disorders
    - Pregnant patients
  - Do not administer nitrous oxide when using a dental laser, unless the nitrous oxide is delivered with a closed system and the use of a scavenger. Relative contraindication is due to risk of combustion, especially with 100% oxygen flush.
- **Adverse effects**
  - Nausea/vomiting.
  - Diffusion hypoxia: After terminating nitrous oxide administration, the high partial pressure in the blood transfers N_2O to alveoli rapidly, which can lead to hypoxemia. Avoid diffusion hypoxia by administering 100% O_2 flush when finished administering nitrous.

- **Sample dose**
  - 30% to 50% combined with oxygen, flow rate 4 L/minute.
  - Start low and titrate to desired effect.
  - Minimum 5-minute 100% O_2 flush at completion of nitrous administration.

Local Anesthesia

Local anesthetics (LAs) bind to sodium (Na+) channels in nerves and inactivate them. This inhibits Na+ ions from entering the neuron, so neurons cannot depolarize. Thus, there is no reaction to the LAs. LAs works better on rapid, firing, and small fibers (autonomic, sensory, motor fibers in order). Trigeminal nerve branches are rapid and small, facilitating the effect of LAs in dentistry. Pain fibers are more sensitive than fibers that detect pressure or sense proprioception.

- **Structure**
  - Lipophilic ring
  - Ester or amide link
  - Tertiary amine
- **Time of onset**
  - Dependent on diffusion into the nerve.[31,32]
  - The drug exists as a mix of two states, ionized and nonionized, depending on the local pH. The pKa of the drug determines how much of each form is present at a given pH. The nonionized form penetrates tissue better than the ionized form. The nonionized form can diffuse through the neural membrane (lipid bilayer; cannot be polarized). Once inside the nerve, the ionized form of the drug binds to the Na+ channel and inactivates it, allowing the LA to take effect. Thus, since onset is dependent on speed of drug diffusing into the cell, the onset is related to the pKa of each specific anesthetic.
  - ↑ pKa = more ionized forms at physiologic pH = slower onset.
  - ↓ pKa = less ionized forms at physiologic pH = faster onset.
- **Metabolism**
  - Amides: Liver
    - The primary site of biotransformation of amide is the liver.
    - Virtually the entire metabolic process occurs in the liver for lidocaine, mepivacaine, and bupivacaine.
  - Esters: In blood plasma
    - Metabolized by pseudocholinesterase. This is rapid and results in water-soluble metabolites excreted in urine.
    - Historically, the chemical structure of LAs was an ester. However, some patients had allergic reactions to para-aminobenzoic acid (PABA), a product of metabolism with by plasma esterases. LAs are now amide in structure, which are metabolized by the liver.
    - Esters may still be used for topical purposes (eg, benzocaine).
- **Excretion:** Kidneys.
- **Contraindications/precautions**
  - Significant liver dysfunction or heart failure (ASA IV, V).
  - Significant renal disease (IV, V).
  - Avoid use in those with allergy to local anesthetic or any of the formulated drug's contents (eg, preservatives).
  - Use epinephrine with caution in patients with cardiac history. As an alternative, mepivacaine has naturally occurring vasoconstrictor properties and is packaged without epinephrine.
- **Adverse reactions**
  - Prilocaine can cause methemoglobinemia.
  - Local anesthetic allergy: Very rare, usually due to the preservative (methylparaben or sulfites). Treatment: Benadryl (Johnson & Johnson); epinephrine if anaphylaxis.
  - Signs of overdose
    - Local anesthetic: Metallic taste, convulsions possible. Activate emergency response system.
    - Epinephrine: Tachycardia. Treat by monitoring the patient, reassuring them of transient nature, administer oxygen if needed. Should normalize in 15 to 30 minutes.

Anticoagulants

TESTS FOR BLEEDING RISK

- **Prothrombin time (PT)**
  - Normal range is 8.8 to 11.5 seconds
- **International normalized ratio (INR)**
  - INR = (Patient's PT) / (A standardized normal PT)

- Physicians usually aim for patients taking warfarin (Coumadin, Bristol-Myers Squibb) to be between 2.5 to 3.5.
- The therapeutic range for periodontal treatment is usually 2 to 3.

- **Partial thromboplastin time (PTT)**
  - Normal range is < 35 seconds.
- **Bleeding time**
  - Normal range is 3 to 8 minutes.

COMMON MEDICATIONS FOR PATIENTS WITH COAGULATION DISORDERS

- **Warfarin/Coumadin**
  - Mechanism of action: Vitamin K antagonist
- **Heparin**
  - Mechanism of action: Inactivates thrombin and Factor X, inhibiting thrombin-induced activation of platelets, Factor 4, Factor 8, and fibrin formation.
  - Lovenox (Sanofi) is a low-molecular-weight heparin.
- **Direct-acting medications**
  - Dabigatran (Pradaxa, Boehringer Ingelheim): A thrombin inhibitor
  - Rivaroxaban (Xarelto, Janssen Pharmaceutical): A Factor X inhibitor
  - Apixaban (Eliquis, Bristol-Myers Squibb): A Factor X inhibitor
- **Anti-platelet medications**
  - Aspirin
    - Mechanism of action: Irreversible inhibition of COX-1 and COX-2
  - Clopidogrel (Plavix, Bristol-Myers Squibb)
    - Mechanism of action: Inhibits adenosine diphosphate (ADP)-induced platelet aggregation

Antiviral Agents

Antiviral agents are most effective when given at the prodrome or first signs of herpes simplex virus (HSV). The prodrome may present as tingling or numbness in the area. Antiviral agents may also be considered for early-stage lesions in which vesicles are present but have not ruptured. When lesions are present, the patient is at risk of spreading the herpetic virus; therefore, dental procedures are not recommended at this time.

- **Sample dose**
  - Topical acyclovir: 5% 15-g tube 6 times per day for 1 week.
  - Systemic acyclovir: 200 mg, 70 tabs, take 1 q4h for 2 weeks.

Antifungal Agents

- **Oral candidiasis**
  - Clotrimazole (Mycelex, Bayer): 10-mg troches, prescribed qid for 10 days.
  - Nystatin: 300-mL oral suspension, prescribed 1-tsp rinse qid for 2 minutes for 14 days.
- **Denture stomatitis**
  - Treatment for oral candidiasis listed above with dentures removed.
  - Treatment of the denture is also required.
- **Actinic cheilitis**
  - Clotrimazole 1% cream or ointment applied to the corners of the mouth qid.

References

1. American Academy of Periodontology. Glossary of Periodontal Terms. American Academy of Periodontology, 2001.
2. American Society of Anesthesiologists. ASA Physical Status Classification System. https://www.asahq.org/standards-and-guidelines/asa-physical-status-classification-system. Accessed 10 February 2020.
3. Ocampo PS, Lázár V, Papp B, et al. Antagonism between bacteriostatic and bactericidal antibiotics is prevalent. Antimicrob Agents Chemother 2014;58:4573–4582.
4. Slots J, Research and Therapy Committee. Systemic antibiotics in periodontics. J Periodontol 2004;75:1553–1565.
5. Lindhe J, Karring T, Lang NP. Clinical Periodontology and Implant Dentistry. Malden: Blackwell Munksgaard, 2003.
6. van Winkelhoff AJ, Winkel EG. Microbiological diagnostics in periodontics: Biological significance and clinical validity. Periodontol 2000 2005;39:40–52.
7. Herrera D, Retamal-Valdes B, Alonso B, Feres M. Acute periodontal lesions (periodontal abscesses and necrotizing periodontal diseases) and endo-periodontal lesions. J Periodontol 2018;89(1 suppl):85S–102S.
8. Pack PD, Haber J. The incidence of clinical infection after periodontal surgery. A retrospective study. J Periodontol 1983;54:441–443.
9. Powell CA, Mealey BL, Deas DE, McDonnell HT, Moritz AJ. Post-surgical infections: Prevalence associated with various periodontal surgical procedures. J Periodontol 2005;76:329–333.
10. Pendrill K, Reddy J. The use of prophylactic penicillin in periodontal surgery. J Periodontol 1980;51:44–48.
11. Checchi L, Trombelli L, Nonato M. Postoperative infections and tetracycline prophylaxis in periodontal surgery: A retrospective study. Quintessence Int 1992;23:191–195.

12. Greenstein G, Greenstein B, Cavallaro J, Elian N, Tarnow D. Flap advancement: Practical techniques to attain tension-free primary closure. J Periodontol 2009;80:4–15.
13. Khouly I, Braun RS, Chambrone L. Antibiotic prophylaxis may not be indicated for prevention of dental implant infections in healthy patients. A systematic review and meta-analysis. Clin Oral Investig 2019;23:1525–1553.
14. Wilson W, Taubert KA, Gewitz M, et al. Prevention of infective endocarditis: Guidelines from the American Heart Association: A guideline from the American Heart Association Rheumatic Fever, Endocarditis and Kawasaki Disease Committee, Council on Cardiovascular Disease in the Young, and the Council on Clinical Cardiology, Council on Cardiovascular Surgery and Anesthesia, and the Quality of Care and Outcomes Research Interdisciplinary Working Group. J Am Dent Assoc 2008;139(3 suppl):3S–24S.
15. Fardal O, Johannessen AC, Linden GJ. Patient perceptions of periodontal therapy completed in a periodontal practice. J Periodontol 2002;73:1060–1066.
16. Curtis JW Jr, McLain JB, Hutchinson RA. The incidence and severity of complications and pain following periodontal surgery. J Periodontol 1985;56:597–601.
17. Wynn RL, Meiller TF, Crossley HL. Drug Information Handbook for Dentistry, ed 25. Hudson: Lexi-Comp, 2020.
18. Braganza A, Bissada N, Hatch C, Ficara A. The effect of non-steroidal anti-inflammatory drugs on bleeding during periodontal surgery. J Periodontol 2005;76:1154–1160.
19. Ardekian L, Gaspar R, Peled M, Brener B, Laufer D. Does low-dose aspirin therapy complicate oral surgical procedures? J Am Dent Assoc 2000;131:331–335.
20. Johnson & Johnson. Tylenol dosage for adults. http://www.tylenol.ca/safety-dosing/adult/dosage-for-adults. Accessed 10 February 2020.
21. Sisk AL, Bonnington GJ. Evaluation of methylprednisolone and flurbiprofen for inhibition of the postoperative inflammatory response. Oral Surg Oral Med Oral Pathol 1985;60:137–145.
22. Gersema L, Baker K. Use of corticosteroids in oral surgery. J Oral Maxillofac Surg 1992;50:270–277.
23. Alexander RE, Throndson RR. A review of perioperative corticosteroid use in dentoalveolar surgery. Oral Surg Oral Med Oral Pathol Oral Radiol Endod 2000;90:406–415.
24. American Society of Anesthesiologists Task Force on Sedation and Analgesia by Non-Anesthesiologists. Practice guidelines for sedation and analgesia by non-anesthesiologists. Anesthesiology 2002;96:1004–1017.
25. American Dental Association. Guidelines for the Use of Sedation and General Anesthesia by Dentists. October 2016. http://www.ada.org/~/media/ADA/Education%20and%20Careers/Files/anesthesia_use_guidelines.pdf. Accessed 10 February 2020.
26. Calixto N, André de Costa Maia J. Influence of lorazepam on ocular pressure in patients with glaucoma. Curr Ther Res Clin Exp 1975;17:156–160.
27. Weinbroum AA, Szold O, Ogorek D, Flaishon R. The midazolam-induced paradox phenomenon is reversible by flumazenil. Epidemiology, patient characteristics and review of the literature. Eur J Anaesthesiol 2001;18:789–797.
28. Bailey PL, Pace NL, Ashburn MA, Moll JW, East KA, Stanley TH. Frequent hypoxemia and apnea after sedation with midazolam and fentanyl. Anesthesiology 1990;73:826–830.
29. Becker DE. Adverse drug interactions. Anesth Prog 2011;58:31–41.
30. Becker DE, Rosenberg M. Nitrous oxide and the inhalation anesthetics. Anesth Prog 2008;55:124–130.
31. Becker DE, Reed KL. Essentials of local anesthetic pharmacology. Anesth Prog 2006;53:98–108.
32. Haas DA. An update on local anesthetics in dentistry. J Can Dent Assoc 2002;68:546–551.

28

MEDICAL EMERGENCIES

Farah Asa'ad, BDS, MSc, PhD

Medical emergencies may arise in dental practices at any time before, during, or after treatment. If dental care providers are not prepared on how to manage these conditions on site, they might find themselves in a critical situation. In this chapter, the most common medical emergencies that may be encountered are presented with a focus on their causes, signs and symptoms, and successful management (Box 28-1).

Disclaimer: The examples provided in this chapter are not intended to be a guide for the management of medical emergencies. The practitioner must always evaluate the individual patient's medical and dental histories, and when appropriate, consult with the patient's physician prior to administering any medications and/or performing any procedure.

BOX 28-1 Summary of medical emergencies

- Loss of consciousness
  - Vasovagal syncope (faint)
  - Postural hypotension
  - Hypoglycemic coma
  - Adrenal insufficiency
- Respiratory distress
  - Asthma
  - Hyperventilation (panic attack)
- Allergic reactions
  - Anaphylaxis
  - Angioedema
- Epileptic seizures
  - Tonic-clonic seizures (grand mal seizures)
- Bleeding disorders
- Chest pain
  - Angina pectoris
  - Myocardial infarction (heart attack)
- Cardiac arrest
- Foreign body aspiration and choking

DEFINITIONS AND TERMINOLOGY

Allergy: The altered reactivity of a sensitized individual on exposure to an allergen.[1]

Anaphylactic shock: A severe, sometimes fatal, immediate allergic reaction, usually occurring seconds to minutes after exposure to an antigen and mediated via histamine.[1]

Angina pectoris: Paroxysmal thoracic pain with feeling of suffocation and impending death; usually due to anoxia of the myocardium and precipitated by effort or excitement.[1]

Astringent: An agent that causes contraction of the tissues, arrests secretion, or controls bleeding.[1]

Cardiopulmonary resuscitation (CPR): An emergency procedure involving manual compression of the chest overlying the heart and forcing air into the lungs, maintaining circulation when circumstances render the heart unable to pump blood. Follow current standards as advised by the American Heart Association.[1]

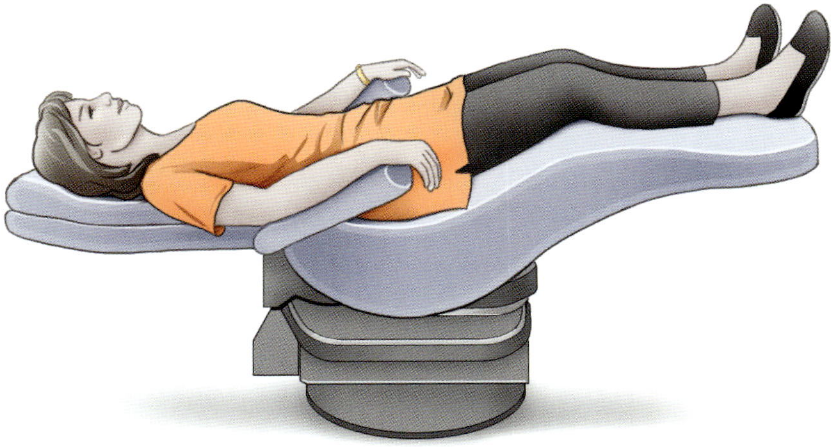

Fig 28-1 Trendelenburg position.

Loss of Consciousness

VASOVAGAL SYNCOPE (FAINT)

In general, *syncope* is defined as a transient loss of consciousness. *Vasovagal syncope*, also referred to as the "simple faint," is the most commonly encountered medical emergency in the dental practice. It is a reflex mediated by autonomic nerves in which there is vasodilatation in the splanchnic and skeletal vessels, bradycardia, and loss of consciousness due to diminished cerebral perfusion.

Causes at the dental chair

- Emotional stress
- Pain
- Fear at the sight of blood or injection needle
- Changes in posture
- Hypoxia
- Carotid sinus syndrome: Due to mild pressure on the neck in elderly patients, resulting in a vagal effect and eventually producing syncope

Signs and symptoms

- Patient feels dizzy, light-headed, or faint
- Pallor
- Sweating
- Slow pulse rate
- Low blood pressure
- Nausea and/or vomiting
- Loss of consciousness

Treatment and management

- Reassure the patient.
- Lay patient flat and raise the legs (Trendelenburg position; Fig 28-1).
- Maintain a patent airway.
- Administer oxygen to the patient in case recovery is delayed, and take into consideration other causes for loss of consciousness.

POSTURAL HYPOTENSION

Postural hypotension usually occurs when the position of the patient is changed rapidly on the dental chair from treatment position to resting position.

Causes at the dental chair

- Prompt elevation of dental chair from treatment position

Signs and symptoms

- Dizziness in an upright position

Treatment and management

- Reassure the patient.
- Lay the patient in the Trendelenburg position.
- Consider administration of oxygen.

Prevention

- This condition can be prevented by gradual elevation of the dental chair.

HYPOGLYCEMIC COMA

Diabetic patients can experience hypoglycemia or hypoglycemic coma due to an imbalance in their blood glucose.

Causes at the dental chair

- Abnormally low levels of blood glucose usually described as less than 70 mg/dL. It can occur in both type 1 and type 2 diabetes patients.

Signs and symptoms

- Rapid onset, resembling fainting
- Sweaty skin
- Shakiness
- Confusion
- Fast pulse
- Headache
- Hunger and nausea
- Lack of coordination
- Patient may convulse
- Adrenaline release, often with anxiety, irritability, and disorientation before consciousness is lost

Treatment and management

- The cause should be established as soon as possible because hypoglycemia needs urgent treatment.
- Check breathing and circulation.
- If there is uncertainty about the cause, **never administer insulin** but immediately give glucose as a diagnostic test, as this will cause little harm in hyperglycemic coma but will improve hypoglycemic coma. (Note: Insulin can cause brain damage or kill a hypoglycemic patient.)
- Administer oxygen and record vitals.
- If the patient is conscious, provide 15 to 20 g of glucose or simple carbohydrates. Glucose solution by mouth can also be administered.
- If the patient is unconscious, give 1 mg of glucagon intramuscularly (IM) and call 911.

Prevention

- Schedule morning appointments and ensure that patients have followed their medication regimen and have eaten prior to their visit to the dentist.
- Patients with well-controlled diabetes are less likely to suffer from hypoglycemic episodes.

ADRENAL INSUFFICIENCY

Adrenal insufficiency, also known as *adrenal crisis*, is a serious condition caused by suppression of the adrenocortical response (adrenocortical hypofunction) that results in hypotension, shock, and death.

Causes at the dental chair

- In patients on systemic corticosteroids: Stress induced by trauma, surgery, anesthesia, and infection.
- Adrenal disorders (causes of stress as above): Addison disease, postadrenalectomy, Waterhouse-Friderichsen syndrome, and congenital adrenal hyperplasia.
- Hypopituitarism.

Signs and symptoms

- Loss of consciousness
- Rapid fall in blood pressure
- Weak or impalpable pulse

Treatment and management

- Lay patient flat and raise the legs (Trendelenburg position).
- Maintain a patent airway and administer oxygen.
- Administer 200 mg hydrocortisone intravenously (IV).
- Administer normal saline or glucose-saline intravenously.
- Call 911.

Prevention

A thorough medical history is essential to confirm if the patient has recently used or is currently on corticosteroid therapy. Adrenal insufficiency can be prevented by the administration of a boost of corticosteroid prior to oral surgical procedures (ie, steroid cover). For patients suffering from adrenal disorders, such as Addison disease, the steroid doese should be doubled before significant dental treatment (eg, surgical procedures) under local anesthesia and continue this for 24 hours.

Respiratory Distress

ASTHMA

Bronchial asthma is a state of bronchial hyperreactivity characterized by paroxysmal expiratory wheezing and dyspnea. This condition can be life-threatening, and it should be managed immediately. Therefore, a thorough health history is necessary to understand the frequency and severity of asthmatic attacks.

Causes at the dental chair

- Anxiety
- Infection
- Physical exertion
- Exposure to allergens
- Irritating fumes

Signs and symptoms

- Breathlessness
- Expiratory wheezing
- Rapid pulse

Treatment and management

- Reassure the patient.
- Do not lay the patient flat.
- Patient should use his or her own β_2-agonist inhaler (eg, salbutamol).
- Administer oxygen to the patient.
- Administer adrenaline (epinephrine) IM if the symptoms persist or if the asthma is part of a more generalized **anaphylactic reaction** (see "Anaphylaxis").
- If there is no rapid response or the patient shows any signs of severe or life-threatening asthma, emergency protocol should be activated and 911 should be contacted.

HYPERVENTILATION (PANIC ATTACK)

Hyperventilation is commonly encountered in the dental practice. In case of persistence, this condition can become very distressing to the patient.

Causes at the dental chair

- Anxiety

Signs and symptoms

- Anxiety
- Weakness
- Lightheadedness
- Dizziness
- Disturbed consciousness
- Tetany
- Muscle pain or stiffness
- Paresthesia
- Chest pain and/or palpitations
- Breathlessness
- Dry mouth

Treatment and management

- Reassure the patient.
- Let the patient breathe CO_2-enriched air by providing them with a paper bag and instructing them to breathe into it. If a paper bag is not available, the patient should be instructed to breathe into their cupped hands.
- Administer benzodiazepines IM or IV if reassurance was ineffective.

Allergic Reactions

ANAPHYLAXIS

Anaphylaxis is a type I hypersensitivity reaction that involves Immunoglobulin E (IgE) and the release of histamine and vasoactive peptides. It is the most dangerous form of **allergic** reactions as it could lead to death if not promptly managed.

Causes at the dental chair

- β-lactams (penicillins and cephalosporins)
- Latex
- Local anesthetics (rarely)

Signs and symptoms

- Itchy rashes/erythema
- Facial flushing or pallor
- Laryngeal edema and bronchospasm
- Respiratory arrest that might result in cardiac arrest
- Acute hypotension and collapse due to vasodilatation that might result in cardiac arrest

Treatment and management

- Apply the ABCDE approach (airway, breathing, circulation, disability, exposure).
- Administer oxygen.

- Administer adrenaline (epinephrine) IM in the anterolateral mid-third of the thigh (0.5 mL of 1:1,000).
- IM adrenaline should be followed by an antihistamine such as Benadryl (Johnson & Johnson) and IV 200 mg hydrocortisone (to be performed as needed by emergency team personnel).
- Perform **cardiopulmonary resuscitation** (CPR) in case of cardiac arrest.
- Medical assistance is required, and the patient should be transferred as soon as possible for monitoring or further treatment because relapse may occur within 24 hours.

ANGIOEDEMA

Acute allergic edema can develop alone or may be associated with anaphylaxis. This condition occurs when histamine is released into the blood by mast cells, resulting in rapid swelling that might be fatal if the airway is involved. Angioedema can be either hereditary or acquired.

Causes at the dental chair

- β-lactams (penicillins and cephalosporins)
- Latex
- Minute amount of allergen can trigger the reaction

Signs and symptoms

- Rapid swelling of the head and neck region (eyes, lips, throat) and extremities
- Laryngeal edema and bronchospasm

Treatment and management

- Mild angioedema may respond to antihistamines or to sympathomimetic agents such as ephedrine, which can be taken orally.
- In severe cases that also involve airway obstruction, case management should be the same as anaphylactic reaction.
- Corticosteroids may be required in intractable chronic cases.

Prevention

Since there is deficiency of C1 esterase inhibitor in angioedema, administration of C1 esterase inhibitor concentrates prior to dental treatment could be considered for selected cases. Administration should be done at a hospital setting.

Epileptic Seizures

TONIC-CLONIC SEIZURES (GRAND MAL SEIZURES)

Epilepsy is a group of disorders of brain function that lead to episodic disturbances of consciousness, usually of motor or sensory function. Although most of the cases are idiopathic, that is, without any identifiable cause, few cases are secondary to generalized brain disease, drug addiction, or metabolic disorders. The most common type of epilepsy is *tonic-clonic epilepsy*, also known as *grand mal seizure*.

Causes at the dental chair

- Withdrawal of anticonvulsant drug
- Alcohol
- Fatigue
- Starvation
- Stress
- Flashing lights

Signs and symptoms

A typical seizure is characterized by an aura, which consists of mood change, irritability, brief hallucination or headache, followed by loss of consciousness, tonic and clonic convulsions, and ending with recovery. However, it must be noted that this sequence might not be fully completed.

Treatment and management

- Airway maintenance.
- Administer oxygen if possible.
- Remove any objects in the mouth, then rotate face down if vomiting occurs.
- Patient must be positioned away from any equipment, tools, or furniture to prevent injuries.
- Continue monitoring the patient; if the seizure is uncomplicated and short in duration, then discharge the patient to an adult companion.
- If the seizure persists, administer benzodiazepines as needed.

Bleeding Disorders

Patients with bleeding disorders are usually recognized when their medical history is obtained. However, the practitioner could still face situations in which prolonged bleeding might occur during surgical procedures or postoperatively. Prolonged bleeding related to oral surgery procedures usually has a local cause, but it is also one of the most common signs of hemorrhagic diseases. In some occasions, bleeding might be the first symptom in which the disease is recognized.

Causes at the dental chair

- Local causes:
  - Primary hemorrhage (at the time of procedure) due to excessive trauma, damage to vital structures, etc.
  - Reactionary hemorrhage (few hours after procedure) due to wearing off of the vasoconstrictor element of adrenaline in the anesthetic solution.
  - Secondary hemorrhage (a few days after procedure).
- Systemic causes (congenital and acquired):
  - Bleeding disorders: Hemophilia A, hemophilia B (Christmas disease or factor IX deficiency), von Willebrand disease, and thrombocytopenia
  - Liver impairment and/or alcoholism
  - Chronic kidney disease
  - Medications: Anticoagulants (eg, aspirin, warfarin, heparin)
  - Patients undergoing radiotherapy or receiving cytotoxic medication

Signs and symptoms

- Prolonged bleeding during or after surgical procedures such as tooth extraction, implant placement, periodontal surgical procedures, and so forth.

Treatment and management

- Patients with congenital bleeding disorders are best treated in specialized centers.
- Patients with hemophilia A, hemophilia B, or von Willebrand disease may require replacement therapy before surgery and an antifibrinolytic agent (eg, tranexamic acid) postoperatively.
- Consider the postextraction use of local hemostatic agents such as oxidized cellulose (ie, Surgicel, Johnson & Johnson) with suturing.
- Intraoperatively, a variety of techniques can be used to minimize or stop bleeding. These include but are not limited to pressure, suturing, blood vessel ligation, administration of more local anesthetic with vasoconstriction, electrosurgery and cauterization, hemostatic agents, etc. If bleeding cannot be stopped or managed intraoperatively and it represents a life-threating condition, call 911 immediately.
- Warfarin should not be discontinued unless specified by the physician, as it might increase the risk of thromboembolism even further. Patients on warfarin should have their international normalized ratio (INR) measured before any surgical procedure. If needed, the physician should be consulted for temporarily warfarin discontinuation. In this case, warfarin is stopped 2 days before surgery and then resumed on the evening of the day of the procedure. Local hemostatic agents can be employed as needed. For other medications altering bleeding, the appropriate test should be performed, and physicians should be consulted if/when indicated.
- Several antifibrinolytic agents can reduce postoperative bleeding in anticoagulated patients.
- The practitioner must be aware of drug interactions with certain medications. For example, erythromycin enhances the anticoagulant effect of warfarin. Metronidazole inhibits the metabolism of warfarin, and tetracycline may enhance the effect of warfarin.
- In patients with hepatic impairment, lower doses should be used for drugs metabolized by the liver. In cases of significant liver impairment, certain drugs should be avoided, such as acetaminophen.

Prevention

- A thorough medical history must be obtained.
- Certain patients should not be treated without consulting their physicians, including those with liver impairment and/or alcoholism, chronic kidney disease, or bleeding disorders, as well as patients undergoing cytotoxic medication or radiotherapy.
- Patients taking anticoagulants should be evaluated prior to the procedure for potential risk of bleeding, and consultations should be performed if indicated.

Chest Pain

ANGINA PECTORIS

Angina pectoris represents paroxysms of severe ischemic chest pain. It is reversible damage to the myocardium caused by insufficient oxygen and emboli.

Causes at the dental chair

- Anxiety
- Anger
- Physical exertion, especially in cold weather

Signs and symptoms

- Crushing tightness, heaviness, and compression of the chest, which might radiate to the left arm or mandible.
- The pain is usually described as a sense of strangling or choking and thus is often unmistakable.

Treatment and management

- Keep the patient in an upright position.
- Administer a nitroglycerin (glyceryl trinitrate) tablet (0.3 to 0.5 mg) sublingually.
- Administer oxygen.
- If chest pain is not relieved after 2 to 3 minutes or increases in severity or intensity, then myocardial infarction is probably the cause (see the following section).

MYOCARDIAL INFARCTION (HEART ATTACK)

Myocardial infarction (often referred to as *coronary thrombosis* or *heart attack*) is irreversible damage to the myocardium and is the most severe and lethal form of coronary heart disease.

Signs and symptoms

- Severe crushing chest pain, which usually radiates to the left arm, shoulders, and mandible (more severe than the pain in angina pectoris)
- Shortness of breath
- Pale skin
- Sweating
- Weak pulse and possible hypotension
- Nausea and vomiting (common)

Treatment and management

- Call 911.
- Patients should be managed in the sitting position, unless they are feeling faint, in which case the patient should be laid flat.
- Administer oxygen.
- Administer nitroglycerin (glyceryl trinitrate) sublingually.
- Administer aspirin orally (300 mg).
- Start CPR if the patient is unresponsive.

Cardiac Arrest

Cardiac arrest is a sudden loss of heart function in which the heart stops beating. It is a serious condition that can lead to immediate collapse followed by death within a few minutes if left untreated. It must be kept in mind that patients with heart diseases, mainly ischemic heart disease, have the greatest risk to develop this condition.

Causes at the dental chair

- Myocardial infarction
- Hypoxia
- Anesthetic overdose
- Anaphylaxis
- Bleeding
- Choking

Signs and symptoms

- Loss of consciousness
- Breathlessness
- Cyanosis
- Absence of pulse
- Severe hypotension

Treatment and management

CPR is considered one of the cornerstones in the management of cardiac arrest. Not only do the practitioners need to recognize the causes of a cardiac arrest, but they should also know how to perform CPR (Table 28-1).

TABLE 28-1 CPR in patients of different age groups

	Compression-to-breath ratio (one rescuer)	Compression-to-breath ratio (two rescuers)	Compressions	Compression technique
Adult CPR (≥ 14 years old)	30:2	30:2	100–120/minute, 2 inches deep	Two hands, with one on top of the other
Child CPR (1 to 13 years old)	30:2	15:2	100–120/minute, 2 inches deep	One or two hands
Infant CPR (≤ 11 months)	30:2	15:2	100–120/minute, 1.5 inches deep	Two-finger compression technique

Rescue breaths

If there is a pulse (> 60 beats per minute), then rescue breathing should be provided as follows:

- Adult (≥ 14 years old): For 1 second every 5 seconds
- Child (1 to 13 years old): For 1 second every 3 to 5 seconds
- Infant (≤ 11 months): For 1 second every 3 to 5 seconds

Foreign Body Aspiration and Choking

Foreign body aspiration means the lodgment of an object in the larynx or trachea. It could result in a life-threatening condition.

Causes at the dental chair

- Accidental aspiration of a foreign body such as endodontic files, dental restoration materials, implant components, etc.

Signs and symptoms

- Mild airway obstruction: Patient is choking and is able to speak, cough, and breathe.
- Severe airway obstruction: Patient is choking and is unable to speak. Patient may respond by nodding.
- Wheezing.
- Loss of consciousness.

Treatment and management

- Mild airway obstruction: Coughing is usually effective in these cases. Monitoring of the cough is recommended to determine relief of obstruction or deterioration.
- Severe airway obstruction (conscious patient): Perform five back blows. If the blows are ineffective, perform abdominal thrusts.
- Severe airway obstruction (unconscious patient): Perform CPR.

Prevention

- Use of rubber dam, instrument chains, and mouth sponges when performing dental procedures.
- Risk of choking and aspiration can be minimized by efficient suction around the oral cavity and careful observation when performing dental procedures.
- The dentist should be attentive when handling small instruments, especially when the patient is placed in a supine or semisupine position.

Emergency Kit

The drugs mentioned for the previously listed conditions should be present in an emergency kit available at the dental office. These drugs are summarized in Table 28-2.

TABLE 28-2 Emergency kit drugs

Drug	Condition	Comments
Oxygen	Loss of consciousness, chest pain, asthma, anaphylaxis	Usually high-flow oxygen is needed
Nitrous oxide	Myocardial infarction	Administered as a mixture with oxygen to relieve pain
Adrenaline (epinephrine)	Asthma, anaphylaxis	Administered IM
Nitroglycerine (glyceryl trinitrate)	Angina pectoris, myocardial infarction	Administered sublingually
β_2 agonist	Asthma	Usually brought by the patient
Aspirin	Angina pectoris, myocardial infarction	Administered orally
Glucose	Hypoglycemia	Any form of glucose or simple carbohydrates given orally
Glucagon	Hypoglycemia	Administered IM
Benzodiazepines	Hyperventilation, epileptic seizures	Administered IV or IM
Hydrocortisone	Adrenal crisis, anaphylaxis, angioedema	Administered IV
Antihistamine	Anaphylaxis	May be used as supplementary treatment or for minor allergic reactions

IM, intramuscularly; IV, intravenously.

Conclusions

Medical emergencies might be encountered in everyday dental practice, and thus, dentists must be aware of these conditions and be able to recognize their signs and symptoms. Moreover, dental practitioners must remain calm if an emergency situation should occur, as they must have sufficient knowledge on how to manage such conditions and—most importantly—how to prevent them from occurring. Thorough evaluation and complete health history are the key elements for prevention. Lastly, the dental clinic must be properly equipped to efficiently handle these critical situations on site.

Reference

1. American Academy of Periodontology. Glossary of Periodontal Terms. American Academy of Periodontology, 2001.

Further Reading

- American Academy of CPR and First Aid. Online BLS CPR (Adult/Infant/Child) Certification & CPR AED Training Recertification. https://www.onlinecprcertification.net/blscprcourse.php. Accessed 11 February 2020.
- Greenwood M, Corbett I (eds). Dental Emergencies. Ames: Wiley-Blackwell, 2012.
- Scully C. Scully's Medical Problems in Dentistry, ed 7. London: Elsevier, 2014.
- American Diabetes Association. Hypoglycemia (low blood sugar). http://www.diabetes.org/living-with-diabetes/treatment-and-care/blood-glucose-control/hypoglycemia-low-blood.html. Accessed 11 February 2020.

INDEX

Page numbers followed by "t" denote tables; those followed by "f" denote figures; and those followed by "b" denote boxes.

B

D

E

F

N

O

T